A SHORT TEXTBOOK
OF
MEDICINE

Sixth edition

J. C. HOUSTON
M.D., F.R.C.P.
Physician and Dean of the Medical and Dental Schools, Guy's Hospital, London

C. L. JOINER
M.D., F.R.C.P.
Physician, Guy's Hospital, London
Honorary Consultant Physician to the British Army

J. R. TROUNCE
M.D., F.R.C.P.
Professor of Clinical Pharmacology, Guy's Hospital, London

HODDER AND STOUGHTON
LONDON SYDNEY AUCKLAND TORONTO

British Library Cataloguing in Publication Data

Houston, James Caldwell
  A short textbook of medicine.—6th ed—
  (University medical texts).
  1. Pathology   2. Medicine
  I. Title   II. Joiner, Charles Louis
  III. Trounce, John Reginald   IV. Series
  616   RB111

ISBN 0–340–24288–4
ISBN 0–340–24289–2 Pbk

ISBN 0 340 24288 4 boards edition
ISBN 0 340 24289 2 paper edition

First Edition 1962. Reprinted 1964
Second Edition 1966. Reprinted 1967
Third Edition 1968. Reprinted 1970, 1971 (with revisions)
Fourth Edition 1972. Reprinted with revisions 1973
Fifth Edition 1975. Reprinted with revisions 1977
Sixth Edition 1979

Printed and bound in Great Britain
for Hodder and Stoughton Educational, a division of
Hodder and Stoughton Ltd, Mill Road, Dunton Green, Sevenoaks, Kent
by Hazell Watson & Viney Ltd, Aylesbury, Bucks

A SHORT TEXTBOOK OF MEDICINE

$\dfrac{11}{79}$

UNIVERSITY MEDICAL TEXTS

General Editor
SELWYN TAYLOR
D.M., M.Ch. (Oxon.), F.R.C.S.

A Short Textbook of Surgery
(Fourth Edition)
SELWYN TAYLOR
D.M., M.Ch. (Oxon.), F.R.C.S.
Surgeon, Royal Postgraduate Medical School, Hammersmith Hospital

L. T. COTTON
M.Ch. (Oxon.), F.R.C.S.
Consultant Surgeon, King's College Hospital, London

A Short Textbook of Paediatrics
P. CATZEL
M.B.Bch., F.R.C.P., D.C.H.
Transvaal Memorial Hospital for Children, Johannesburg, South Africa

A Short Textbook of Chemical Pathology
(Third Edition)
D. N. BARON
M.D., D.Sc., M.R.C.P., F.R.C.Path.
Professor of Chemical Pathology, Royal Free Hospital School of Medicine, London

A Short Textbook of Medical Microbiology
(Fourth Edition)
D. C. TURK
D.M., M.R.C.P., M.R.C.Path.
Consultant Microbiologist, Regional Public Health Laboratory, Sheffield

and

I. A. PORTER
M.D., M.R.C.Path.
Consultant Bacteriologist, City Hospital, Aberdeen;
Hon. Clinical Senior Lecturer in Bacteriology, University of Aberdeen

A Short Textbook of Orthopaedics and Traumatology
(Second Edition)
J. N. ASTON
F.R.C.S.
Orthopaedic Surgeon, St. Bartholomew's Hospital, London

and

S. HUGHES
F.R.C.S.
Orthopaedic Surgeon, Royal Postgraduate Medical School, Hammersmith

A Short Textbook of Psychiatry
(Second Edition)
W. L. LINFORD REES
B.Sc., M.D., F.R.C.P., D.P.M.
Professor of Psychiatry, St. Bartholomew's Hospital Medical School

A complete list of titles in the Series is available from the Publisher

EDITOR'S FOREWORD

'Books must follow sciences, and not sciences books'
FRANCIS BACON

Textbooks of medicine are all too often so vast that the student could not possibly read them through but only use them as works of reference. Alternatively they are so brief and synoptic as merely to provide aides-mémoires in those crowded revision weeks before the final examination. This text is intended for the medical student during his clinical apprenticeship. It is a concise account of the subject with more than enough material to satisfy the examiners for the final medical degree. It is intended to be read and reread until, with tattered covers, it is discarded, having served its purpose well.

Medicine is developing so rapidly at the present time that any textbook is out of date almost before it is published, therefore the days of great and comprehensive textbooks, like those of William Osler and Clifford Allbutt, are departed. The authors of this book have wisely called upon colleagues to help with some of the more specialised branches of medicine. There are thus eight additional authors, three of them new to this edition.

Seventeen years and six editions have seen extraordinary strides in medicine and the extensive revision which has once again been necessary is apparent throughout the text. Skilful editing and pruning still justifies its title of a Short Textbook, although it might equally well be called a modern textbook; certainly it is a very readable textbook.

It is a great compliment that it is used in so many European countries both in English and in Italian and Spanish translations, while for hotter climates there is a tropical edition. I am confident it will not be long before another edition becomes necessary.

SELWYN TAYLOR

PREFACE TO SIXTH EDITION

It has again been necessary to carry out extensive revisions throughout this new edition, particularly in the sections on cardiovascular disease and on endocrine disorders. The section on the lymphomas has been rewritten and a certain amount of additional material has been incorporated. In line with established practice SI units have been used throughout.

We should like to thank those who have given us advice, help and criticism.

J. C. HOUSTON
C. L. JOINER
J. R. TROUNCE

Guy's Hospital
London
1979

PREFACE TO FIFTH EDITION

This edition has been very extensively revised, in particular the sections on endocrinology, skin diseases, and psychiatry have been entirely rewritten and we welcome Dr. Hicks, Dr. Wells and Dr. Willis to our list of authors.

We are very sorry to lose Dr. Stafford-Clark, who has been responsible for the psychiatric section since the first edition.

We would like to thank Professor Stuart Cameron for considerable help in the chapter on diseases of the kidney and Dr. D. C. Deuchar for permission to reproduce figures from his book *Clinical Phonocardiography*. Finally we would like to thank all those who have given advice or criticism.

PREFACE TO FIRST EDITION

The need for an inexpensive short textbook of medicine has been long felt and frequently expressed. Both the theory and practice of medicine are changing so quickly at the present time that any textbook is out of date within a very few years; what the clinical student requires, therefore, is a convenient and expendable manual of current medical practice rather than a large and comprehensive work 'which he can use all his life'. For wider reading he should be encouraged into the habit of consulting original sources in his medical school library, and to this end we have appended a few key references to the principal chapters. The practitioner anxious to keep abreast of the times may also welcome a book of this size, for we have deliberately given rather fuller treatment to the more rapidly developing branches of medicine.

Apart from four special chapters, the whole book has been written jointly by the three authors, the original draft of each section, written by one of us, being subjected to very free criticism and discussion by the other two before its final form was agreed. Our aim has been to write of medicine as we have seen it and practised it and to avoid wherever possible second-hand information and traditional statements. The book has not been produced with any examination in mind, but in spite of its small size we believe it provides a sound basis of reading for the Membership and more than enough to satisfy the Finals' examiners. There is no section on diseases of children, but all the other specialities which come from time to time within the province of the general physician have been included.

We are particularly grateful to Dr. A. G. Bearn for the chapter on human genetics; to Professor W. J. H. Butterfield for the chapter on medical aspects of radiation; to Dr. I. C. K. Mackenzie for the chapter on the nervous system; and to Dr. D. Stafford-Clark for the chapter on psychiatry.

Our thanks are due also to Mrs. C. Dawbarn and Mrs. K. Hasler of the Department of Medical Illustrations, Guy's Hospital; to Mr. W. H. G. Hill, who prepared the index; to Mr. J. Fennel, who reviewed the names of the drugs and the doses quoted throughout the book; and to the publishers, for their help and forbearance during the book's long gestational period.

CONTRIBUTORS

A. G. BEARN, M.D.

*Professor and Chairman, Dept. of Medicine,
Cornell University Medical College,
Physician-in-Chief, The New York Hospital, New York.*

SIR JOHN BUTTERFIELD, O.B.E., M.D., F.R.C.P.

*Regius Professor of Physic, University of Cambridge
formerly Professor of Medicine, Guy's Hospital Medical School, London.*

S. COHEN, C.B.E., PH.D., F.R.C.PATH., M.D., F.R.S.

Professor of Chemical Pathology, Guy's Hospital Medical School, London.

B. HICKS, M.D., M.R.C.P.

Senior Lecturer, Dept. of Medicine, Guy's Hospital, London.

I. C. K. MACKENZIE, M.D., F.R.C.P.

Physician for Nervous Diseases, Guy's Hospital, London.

G. W. SCOTT, M.D., F.R.C.P.

*Physician, Guy's Hospital, London.
Physician to the Chest Clinic, Guy's Hospital, London.*

R. S. WELLS, M.D., F.R.C.P.

*Consultant Dermatologist, Guy's Hospital, London.
Senior Lecturer in Clinical Dermatology, Institute of Dermatology,
St. John's Hospital, London.*

J. WILLIS, M.B., F.R.C.P.(E.), M.R.C.PSYCH., D.P.M.

*Consultant Psychiatrist in Drug Dependence, Guy's, King's College and
Bexley Hospitals.*

To the Reader

A special Tropical Edition of this book is now available for students in the tropical and subtropical regions of the world. It contains a new chapter on *Tropical Diseases and Worms* giving far more detailed information than is required by readers in temperate areas, who will find sufficient coverage of these topics in the existing Chapters 17 and 18.

CONTENTS

CHAPTER ONE

HUMAN GENETICS

Most diseases which affect man are occasioned by the interaction of genetic and environmental influences. In some diseases, such as those caused by infectious agents, the hereditary component is relatively trivial whereas in diseases such as haemophilia and muscular dystrophy, the genetical influence is crucial and environmental factors unimportant. The subsequent discussion will focus on genetic principles and their application to human disease, with particular reference to those diseases in which hereditary influences predominate.

It should be emphasised at the outset that not all familial diseases are genetically determined. The clustering of disease among family members may simply reflect the presence of a common environmental influence. Pulmonary tuberculosis and certain vitamin deficiencies were at one time erroneously considered to be genetically determined because of their concentration in certain families. Congenital diseases are diseases recognisable at birth and are not necessarily genetically determined. In some instances the aetiology of the malformation is due to the exposure of the developing foetus to irradiation or certain viral infections, while in other congenital defects, such as X-linked hydrocephalus, genetic influences are causal. It is apparent that in most congenital malformations both environmental and genetic influences play an important role.

Chromosomes, the bearers of the hereditary material, are present in the cell nucleus of all tissues. In man, all somatic (diploid) cells have 46 chromosomes; 44 of these chromosomes are the same in both males and females and are called the autosomes. In addition to the 44 autosomes, females have two X chromosomes while males have one X and one Y chromosome. It has been estimated that there are approximately 100,000 genes in man of which about 1,000 have been identified. Thus, despite the rapid advances in human genetics during the past 25 years, about 99 per cent of the human genome remains to be discovered.

Mitosis, Meiosis and the Structure and Function of Genes

During *mitosis* each chromosome duplicates, and when cell division takes place one of the identical daughter chromosomes passes to each daughter cell. In this way, each daughter cell preserves the identical chromosomal constitution that occurred in the parental cell.

During the development of ovum and sperm the number of chromosomes halve. This process of halving is called *meiosis* and results in a gamete with a haploid number of chromosomes (23). Fertilisation of the ovum restores the chromosome complement to 46, the number characteristic of all somatic cells.

Genes are arranged in linear fashion along the chromosome and are composed of double-stranded deoxyribonucleic acid (DNA). DNA directs the synthesis of single-stranded messenger RNA which migrates from the nucleus to the cytoplasm and becomes attached to ribosomal RNA, where it serves as a template on which the amino acids are assembled to form proteins. Within the cytoplasm, there is another RNA species, called transfer RNA. There are twenty different species forms of transfer RNA each one of which serves to bring the twenty amino acids to the messenger RNA, for incorporation into the polypeptide. As the messenger RNA moves along the ribosome the amino acids are brought into position by the transfer RNA which, in addition to recognising the specific amino acid, also recognises a specific site on the messenger RNA. Thus, the amino acids are lined up on the template in an order specified by the sequence of triplets in the messenger RNA, which in turn have been specified by the triplets in the DNA. Thus, DNA specifies RNA, and the RNA specifies the amino acid sequence of the protein synthesised.

CHROMOSOMAL ABNORMALITIES

Disturbances in the normal mechanism of meiosis or mitosis may result in the formation of cells with an abnormal number of chromosomes. Abnormal segregation of the chromosomes during meiosis or mitosis leaves cells with an unequal number of chromosomes. The most frequent abnormality of cell division is non-disjunction in which two chromosomes, members of the same pair, are incorporated into one daughter nucleus. Meiotic non-disjunction occurs more frequently with increasing maternal age. Mitotic (post-zygotic) non-disjunction is also not uncommon and leads to individuals in whom there are cells of differing chromosome number. Such individuals are called *chromosomal mosaics*.

Transfer of a chromosomal segment of one chromosome to a non-homologous chromosome is called a *translocation*. In this way structural chromosomal aberrations may occur despite the presence of a normal chromosomal complement. If the translocation results in a genetic imbalance (unbalanced translocation), a specific error of a development such as mongolism will occur. Although the frequency of chromosome abnormality is only about 0·5 per cent in the newborn, about 50 per cent of spontaneous abortions, in the first trimester, are chromosomally abnormal. Thus, the majority of chromosomal aberrations lead to death during early fetal life. Chromosomal abnormalities also occur in about 5–20 per cent of multiple congenital malformations, 1–10 per cent of patients with sterility and up to 3 per cent of patients with mental retardation.

Mongolism (Down's Syndrome) (1 in 650 live births)

This disease, which accounts for 5 per cent of institutionalised patients with mental deficiency, is usually associated with trisomy of chromosome 21. In about 9 per cent of children born to mothers under the age of thirty, and in 1·5 per cent of mothers over the age of thirty, the additional chromosomal material is rearranged so that although 46 chromosomes are present, one chromosome is longer than its normal partner (unbalanced translocation). The translocation usually occurs between one of the chromosomes of the D group (13–15) and a 21. One of the normal parents (usually the mother) of such mongols carries the translocation chromosome and has a total chromosome complement of 45 (balanced translocation carrier). The mean age of the mother at the birth of a mongol child is approximately thirty-seven, compared with a mean of twenty-nine for all births. The risk rises steeply with increasing maternal age; at the age of twenty-five the risk of a mongol child is approximately 1 in 2,000, while at the age of forty-five the risk is 1 in 50. The recurrence risk of having a second affected child is only slightly increased in patients with trisomy 21, whereas in clinically normal mothers in whom a balanced translocation is present the recurrence risk may be as high as 20 per cent. The recurrence risk for a mongol child when the father carries the translocation is only 5 per cent.

Mitotic non-disjunction leads to chromosomal mosaicism in which some of the patient's cells are trisomic 21 and some are normal. Although some of these mosaic mongols are only mildly affected, they have a significant risk of having mongol offspring, as cells in the gonadal tissue may be trisomic 21.

Klinefelter's Syndrome (1 in 450 males) and Turner's Syndrome (1 in 1500, females)

These conditions are examples of non-disjunction of the X chromosome. Individuals with Klinefelter's syndrome have 47 chromosomes with an XXY constitution, whereas in Turner's syndrome the chromosomal constitution is XO and the total complement only 45 chromosomes. Mosaicism due to mitotic non-disjunction is particularly common in Turner's syndrome. Approximately one-half of the patients have a 45 XO chromosomal constitution, about one-third have 45 XO/46 XY, and a small proportion have a structural defect in one of the X chromosomes. Klinefelter's syndrome should be suspected in males with infertility, gynecomastia, or eunuchoidism. Behavioural disorders (particularly incessant insubstantial talkativeness) and mental deficiency are not uncommon. Turner's syndrome is frequently associated with dwarfism, webbing of the neck, and congenital bone abnormalities. Coarctation of the aorta, before the age of puberty, may be an early symptom.

XYY Syndrome

This recently described syndrome occurs in 1/1000 male births and is characterised by a chromosomal complement of 47 with an extra Y chromosome. Individuals with this syndrome are often unusually tall and may be mentally retarded; they are particularly liable to exhibit aggressive, psychopathic or criminal behaviour. In many instances, however, such individuals are physically and mentally normal.

GENETIC VARIATION

The position of the chromosome occupied by a gene is called a *locus* and at each locus there may be one or more alternative forms of the gene (*alleles*).When both chromosomes carry the same gene at a particular locus, individuals are said to be homozygous at that locus; if the genes are different they are said to be heterozygous. Five main types of inheritance can be recognised from the examination of human pedigrees, *autosomal dominant, autosomal recessive, autosomal co-dominant, sex-linked (X-linked) dominant,* and *sex-linked (X-linked) recessive.* It is becoming increasingly evident that certain diseases that are clinically almost indistinguishable may be inherited in more than one way. For example, the mucopolysaccharidoses may be caused by genes on autosomes, of which the classical *Hurler's syndrome* is the most common, or by a gene on the X-chromosome (*Hunter's syndrome*). Considerable genetic heterogeneity is also evident in the severe inherited forms of muscular dystrophy.

Autosomal Dominant Traits

Dominant traits are those which are determined by a gene in the heterozygous state. Except for mutation, each affected individual will have one parent affected. On the average, affected individuals will have normal and abnormal offspring in equal proportions; the usual 1 : 1 ratio of a dominant gene. Normal offspring have all normal children, whereas abnormal children have normal and abnormal offspring in equal proportions. Sometimes the gene may be incompletely manifest, so that the descendants of the apparently unaffected person may be affected. This phenomenon is known as 'skipping a generation'. Dominant disorders are usually mild, and are characterised by extreme variability in the expression of the gene. The disease may be manifest only late in life, as is common in congenital polycystic disease of the kidneys, and Huntington's chorea. Many dominant disorders are due to new mutational events and should be suspected, in those instances when an affected individual does not have an affected parent, provided extra-marital paternity can be excluded. About 80 per cent of patients with achondroplasia, and 40 per cent of patients with Marfan's syndrome are due to new mutations. Common dominant disorders include familial hypercholesterolemia, hereditary haemorrhagic telangiectasia, acute intermittent porphyria, and hereditary spherocytosis. The primary genetic defect in dominant disorders, in contrast to recessive diseases, is usually poorly understood. In many instances the gene appears to affect rate-limiting enzymes under feed-back control, as in hypercholesterolemia or to affect a structural protein with a non-enzymatic function such as collagen or haemoglobin.

Autosomal Recessive Traits

A disease or trait which is only recognisable when a gene is present in the homozygous state is called recessive. Both parents of an affected individual are usually heterozygous for the gene in question, but are clinically normal. Although parents and all immediate ancestors are normal, siblings are likely to be affected. On the average, one quarter of the offspring of parents heterozygous for the same gene will be affected, one quarter will be normal and one half will be unaffected heterozygous carriers, like their parents. All children of affected individuals will be heterozygous for the abnormal gene. Due to the bias in locating families through an affected individual, the proportion of affected members in small groups of siblings will usually exceed one quarter.

The incidence of consanguinity in the parents of individuals suffering from a rare recessive disease will be much greater than in the normal population. In some instances, the incidence of first-cousin marriage may be as high as 35 per cent. An increased consanguinity rate is not found however if the disease is very common, and is not observed in *cystic fibrosis*, the most frequently occurring recessively inherited disease of man. Most of the classical inborn errors of metabolism are inherited in an autosomal recessive fashion. Such conditions include *phenylketonuria, albinism, alkaptonuria, Wilson's disease* and *galactosaemia*. In contrast to dominant disorders, recessively inherited diseases are commonly severe, uniform in expression and manifest early in life. The primary genetic defect usually affects an enzyme that participates in normal catabolism. As a consequence of the defective enzyme, the metabolic substrate, anterior to the metabolic block, accumulates in the blood and tissues. In phenylketonuria, for instance, there is an abnormality in the enzyme which metabolises phenylalanine to tyrosine; in galactosaemia there is a defect in the normal metabolism of galactose. In certain recessive diseases the enzyme affected is located in the lysozome. As a result, unmetabolised substrate accumulates within the lysozome. The mucopolysaccharidoses (e.g. Hurler's syndrome, Hunter's syndrome) and lipoidoses (e.g. Gaucher's disease) are examples of lysozomal disorders. Detection of heterozygous carriers of recessively determined disease is becoming increasingly important for genetic counselling.

Autosomal Co-dominant Traits

In this form of inheritance, illustrated by the genetics of the abnormal haemoglobins, the products of both alleles are recognisable. If an individual is homozygous (AA) for the gene which directs the synthesis of normal haemoglobin, only normal haemoglobin is synthesised. If he is homozygous for sickle haemoglobin (SS), only sickle haemoglobin is formed. The heterozygote (AS), in whom there is one gene for normal haemoglobin and one gene for sickle haemoglobin, will produce approximately equal amounts of normal and sickle haemoglobin.

Dominant X-linked Traits

Females are affected twice as often as males. Affected males will transmit the trait to their daughters but not to their sons. Heterozygous affected females will transmit the trait to half their sons and half their daughters. *Vitamin D resistant rickets* and *pseudohyper-parathyroidism* are transmitted as a dominant X-linked trait.

Recessive X-linked Traits

Haemophilia is the classical example of an X-linked recessive disease. About 20 per cent of patients with haemophilia are the result of new mutations. If an X-linked recessive disease is so severe that none of those affected can reproduce, one-third of the cases will be due to new mutations. This situation is seen in the severe form of *Duchenne muscular dystrophy*. The pedigree is highly characteristic. The disease is restricted to males but transmitted by females. Affected individuals frequently have affected maternal uncles. An affected man who marries a normal woman will have normal sons and normal daughters. All his daughters, however, will be carriers. When such a carrier marries a normal man, half of the sons on average will be affected and half of the daughters will be carriers. Additional examples of X-linked recessive disease include *glucose-6-phosphate dehydrogenase deficiency, testicular feminisation, and diabetes insipidus* (*nephrogenic type*). Colour blindness is an example of an X-linked recessive trait which confers only minimal disability. Indeed, it is so frequent that, in contrast to most X-linked recessive diseases, the condition is seen in an appreciable number of females (1 per cent).

BIOCHEMICAL GENETICS

Understanding the classical Mendelian genetics is a necessary prerequisite to the interpretation of pedigrees of diseases, but human genetics extends beyond these narrow bounds. Biochemical genetics, as a result of the early work of Archibald Garrod, has progressed so far that it is possible to identify the specific enzymatic defect in several hundred inborn errors of metabolism. In some inherited diseases, particularly those conditions that are inherited in a dominant or co-dominant fashion, the defective protein serves a structural or regulatory function rather than an enzymatic one. The large number of abnormal haemoglobins that have now been recognised are examples of genetic variations affecting a non-enzymatic protein. The only detectable difference between normal and sickle haemoglobin is that in the molecule of sickle haemoglobin valine has been substituted for glutamic acid in one peptide; a remarkable example of how the substitution of a single amino acid in a protein molecule can determine the difference between health and disease.

GENETIC ENVIRONMENTAL INTERACTION

The interaction between genes and specific environmental factors is nowhere more evident than in the area of drug metabolism. It has, for instance, been estimated that there are approximately one hundred million people in the world with X-linked *glucose-6-phosphate deficiency*. Severe haemolytic anaemia in patients with this inherited deficiency can be brought on by the administration of sulphonamides, anti-malarials, and certain analgesics, including aspirin. This trait is particularly frequent in patients of African, Asiatic or Mediterranean origin. *Acute intermittent porphyria*, a dominantly inherited disease is exacerbated by barbiturates and acute haemolytic anaemia in individuals with an unstable haemoglobin, such as haemoglobin Zürich and haemoglobin M, may be precipitated by sulphonamides. Smoking has a particularly deleterious effect on patients predisposed, by an inherited deficiency of *alpha-1 antitrypsin*, to *pulmonary emphysema*. Most of the common congenital defects are also a consequence of genetic environmental interaction although in these instances neither the genetic susceptibility nor the environmental insult can be well identified.

Histocompatibility Locus and Disease

The genetic control of tissue graft rejection is determined by a series of histocompatibility antigens that are expressed on the surface of cells. These antigens, more than thirty, can be detected on lymphocytes and are called the histocompatibility antigens. They are determined by multiple alleles (numbered for convenience) at two distinct separable loci, termed A and B. An association between HLA types and certain diseases has become increasingly evident in recent years. Thus, 90 per cent of patients with ankylosing spondylitis possess the B-27 antigen on their lymphocytes (compared to only 7 per cent in control subjects), and approximately 15 per cent of all individuals with the allele will eventually develop the disease. Eighty per cent of patients with *coeliac disease* have the B8 antigen, compared to 30 per cent in controls. *Reiter's syndrome* occurs approximately 40 times as frequently in patients possessing the B27 antigen. There is also an association between *multiple sclerosis* and *psoriasis* and certain HLA antigens but in these conditions the association is not strong. Although the biological reasons for these associations are not understood they are probably due to the proximity of the HLA locus to an 'immune response locus' that, in turn, controls the ability of the body to respond effectively to various immune stimuli.

GENETIC COUNSELLING AND AMNIOCENTESIS

The need for genetic counselling in families with an inherited disease is increasing rapidly. The first prerequisite is to make an accurate diagnosis of the disease in question and then to provide the patient with information about the natural history of the disease, the risk of transmitting the disease to the next generation and the available alternatives to bearing affected children, such as adoption and artificial insemination. The possibility of amniocentesis and abortion should be discussed in those instances where prenatal diagnosis is reliable and the patient is willing to have an abortion if a defective fetus is diagnosed. The risk to the fetus of an amniocentesis is less than 1 per cent.

In clear cut inherited disease the risk of affected offspring follows Mendelian laws as outlined above. It is unfortunate that many of the common congenital deformities do not conform to simple Mendelian inheritance; the genetic and environmental interaction is complex and the recurrence depends on 'empiric risk' figures. For most congenital malformations the risk of recurrence following the birth of an affected child is small; it is seldom greater than 10 per cent and is usually, as with cleft lip, with or without cleft palate, and congenital dislocation of the hip, closer to 5 per cent. Although it is hard to quantitate the importance of genetic factors in diseases such as hypertension, the collagen vascular diseases and schizophrenia, their existence is beyond dispute. Emphysema is usually caused by environmental influences. However, in those patients with a specific deficiency of alpha-l antitrypsin, genetic counselling is indicated.

The development of prenatal diagnosis by amniocentesis has added a new dimension to genetic counselling. Examination of amniotic fluid obtained by transabdominal puncture is usually performed between the fourteenth and sixteenth week of pregnancy. Indications for an amniocentesis include:

(1) Couples having a previous child with a chromosomal aberration, particularly Down's syndrome.

(2) Couples known to have a balanced chromosomal translocation for Down's syndrome.

(3) Couples who have a high risk for giving birth to an individual with an inborn error of metabolism detectable in cultivated fibroblasts, e.g. Tay Sachs disease.

(4) Women known to be carriers of a serious X-linked disorder, such as the Duchenne form of muscular dystrophy; only 50 per cent of the male fetuses from such a union would be affected but since affected males cannot be identified in cultured cells, all males would have to be aborted; all females would be clinically normal, though 50 per cent would be carriers.

(5) Previous birth of a child with anencephaly and spina bifida.

An elevation of alpha fetoprotein in the amniotic fluid indicates with extremely high probability that the fetus is anencephalic. (The recurrent risk for anencephaly is about 5 per cent.)

(6) All women over the age of 35, since they have an approximately 2 per cent chance of having a child with Down's syndrome.

FURTHER READING

Fraser, F. C. and Nora, J. J. *Genetics of Man.* Lea and Febiger, Philadelphia, 1975.

Fraser Roberts, J. A. and Pembrey, M. C. *An Introduction to Medical Genetics,* 7th edition, Oxford University Press, Oxford, 1978.

Stanbury, J. B., Wyngaarden, J. B. and Frederickson, D. S., *The Metabolic Basis of Inherited Disease,* 5th edition, McGraw-Hill, New York, 1978.

CHAPTER TWO

PSYCHIATRY

INTRODUCTION

Many students are mystified by psychiatry, a branch of medicine that started when primitive medicine men tried to explain odd or eccentric behaviour as punishment inflicted by the Gods for misdeeds. In the ancient cultures of Greece and Rome 'madness' was recognised as a form of illness but this influence was lost in the Middle Ages when eccentric and psychotic behaviour—even distress—were regarded as manifestations of demonic possession. With scientific and humane progress there emerged a sensible type of medical practice in which deluded and disturbed people were regarded as ill and in need of care, and in the past one hundred years clinical psychiatry has developed in various ways. First there was great interest in the naming and classifying of syndromes, and later there came the dynamic theories of psychiatric disorder put forward by Freud and his followers. In more recent times there has been more interest in the effects of psychotropic drugs, the whole area of psychopharmacology, which has opened up not only therapeutic possibilities but has also given clues to better understanding of brain biochemistry and its relationship to psychiatric disorder.

At the same time there has developed a better awareness that epidemiology can clarify many dimly lit areas in psychiatry, first by finding out accurate incidence and prevalence rates and secondly by identifying social aspects of aetiology. But psychiatry remains a clinical subject in which diagnosis is made after history taking and examination; yet students are somehow put off by the suspicion that psychiatric examination is unformulated and vague. This is not so. It is merely that psychiatric symptoms encompass unfamiliar territory, e.g. changes in

> General behaviour.
> Personality.
> Mood.
> Thought.
> Perception.
> Intellectual function.

Changes in any or all of these human characteristics, if intense or persistent, can cause symptoms which cluster into recognisable syndromes. Clear understanding of aetiology is scanty, but not to the extent that the 'medical model' of psychiatry needs to be discarded, since to date it is the best we have. However the 'medical model' should not be extended beyond credible limits; not everyone who consults a psychiatrist is ill, and it is wrong to suppose that psychiatry comprises a set of esoteric assertions that would include every human abnormality under the rubric of illness. To do this would be as illogical as to regard them all as forms of demonic possession. The medical model of psychiatry was reinforced when general paresis was discovered to be caused by neurosyphilis, and even more so when it was shown that this common 'mental illness' could be halted by malarial therapy. This established psychiatry as a medical specialty, although before then psychiatrists such as Kraepelin had started to classify mental disorders. At the same time aetiology *is* badly understood except in syndromes caused by organic brain disease. A broad and comprehensive approach to aetiology includes consideration of the following influences:

Heredity.
Childhood experience and upbringing.
Family relationships.
Social and cultural factors.
Physical factors, e.g. birth injury, brain damage and epilepsy.
Biochemical disturbance.

In this way there emerges a rational model of aetiology which assumes that aetiology is multifactorial.

NORMALITY AND ABNORMALITY

These are not idealistic terms; normality is not a state of absolute freedom from symptoms any more than abnormality is as recognisable as a wart on the nose. In psychiatry these terms are used in a statistical sense and refer to varieties of behaviour, experience and perception which lie outside commonly accepted norms and which cause a person to complain and ask for help. In addition to this such abnormalities may cause distress and trouble to the family and handicap in the patient's total experience. This is the frame of reference of clinical psychiatry.

Human beings are not merely complex systems governed by biochemical control. They are unique individuals who possess a wide range of comparable psychological functions and characteristics. We know that disordered brain function does produce recognised syndromes, e.g. inherited biochemical defects such as porphyria may present a wide range of symptoms masquerading as 'neurosis', 'personality disorder' or organic mental states, whilst an acquired biochemical upset such as pellagra can present an equally wide spectrum of psychiatric disorder. These examples are rare biochemical disorders which lend weight to a medical model of psychiatric illness, since they exemplify the way in which illnesses with an aetiology that is now understood have been extracted from a previously seemingly amorphous mass of 'mental illness'.

THE PSYCHIATRIC HISTORY AND EXAMINATION

A psychiatric history is a careful account of the changes and symptoms that the patient has experienced; it is as simple as that. Nevertheless students often find psychiatric history taking rather daunting since the symptoms seem indefinite and not as well defined or measurable as physical signs and symptoms. In addition to this the patient may conceal or minimise symptoms or even be genuinely unaware of them. For this reason a psychiatric history is never complete if based on self report and should always be reinforced by another informant—family member, spouse, friend, colleague, etc. (N.B. These sources are not necessarily unbiased!) Psychiatric symptoms involve highly personal aspects of life and often touch on problems, feelings and experience which cause the patient embarrassment, shame and guilt. The interview should be conducted in a tactful, sympathetic and understanding way that allows the patient to tell his story spontaneously whilst preventing him from straying from the point and avoiding putting words in his mouth. This means that time is needed.

The history should be recorded in a formal way, but this does not mean that history taking should be a rigid procedure. The history should be set out as follows:

1. *Reason for Referral:* i.e. What is the problem?
  What are the symptoms that trouble the patient?
  What has caused the patient to regard himself as ill or be regarded as such?

This should be summarised in a succinct way, e.g. 'Patient c/o persistent sadness, insomnia and weight loss for three months and was admitted to hospital after an overdose of sleeping tablets.'

2. *Family History:* This should include
  Parents' ages, state of health and occupation and any relevant information about psychiatric disorder in parents or collaterals.
  Also a general comment on parental marital situation particularly if there is frank discord, divorce or separation.
  Siblings should be enumerated and enquired about in a similar way.

In all cases there should be specific enquiry about familial incidence of
  Known inherited disorder.
  Formal psychiatric disorder, and when possible, details of treatment.
  Suicide or attempted suicide.
  Epilepsy (fits, faints and blackouts).
  Delinquency.
  Alcohol and drug abuse.
  Mental handicap.

3. *Personal History*. (a) Start with the date and place of birth and set out information about infant development both physical and emotional, noting not only milestones but also topics such as fits, blackouts, temper tantrums, school refusal, enuresis and unexplained childhood illnesses.

(b) School history and attainments are important; in particular any history of persistent truancy or delinquency.

(c) Work record. Higher education, job training and general job-holding ability are important because they may give clues about personality development and stability.

(d) Physical health record ⎱ covering diagnoses, treatment,
(e) Psychiatric health record ⎰ admission, etc.

(f) Menstrual history/obstetric history.

(g) Psychosexual and marital history, e.g. sexual development, practice and problems.

Premorbid Personality. This is neither a label nor a series of epithets but rather a picture of the person before the illness. It should be comprehensive and cover general and specific topics, e.g. personal and social behaviour, ability to relate to other people, sociability, interests, gregariousness, etc., and also emotional responsiveness, stability, volition, drive, energy and ambitions, and moral standards. The object is to describe as many attributes as possible. It is usually the least reliable and most difficult part of the history since self description is highly subjective whilst other informants may be biased.

History of the Present Illness. Should cover as fully as possible the onset of symptoms, mode of onset and relationship to any possible precipitants. Prominent symptoms and associated symptoms should be listed. Also changes in interpersonal relationships, work efficiency, etc., in short a detailed account of the changes that have occurred. One of the most useful tactics here is to ask the patient to describe in detail a typical day in his life. This often gives far more information about changes in behaviour, feeling and general performance than a set series of questions about suspected symptoms.

Psychiatric Symptoms—Examination of the Mental State

The manifestations of psychiatric disorder are not as measurable as physical signs. This means that the examination of and description of the mental state relies heavily on self report, since objective phenomena are not likely to be present in the way that is familiar in physical examination. Also the student's observations and interpretations of how the patient behaves and talks may be coloured by his own feelings and attitudes. But if these possible sources of error are recognised, then it is possible to make a clinical assessment of the mental state and set it out in a systematic way. The usefulness of the interview will depend too on how much sensible understanding and empathy the student can give to the patient without putting words into his mouth or prejudging the diagnosis.

The format of the mental state examination is usually and conveniently set out as follows:

1. General behaviour.
2. Talk.
3. Emotion.
4. Thought content.
5. Perception.
6. Cognitive function.
7. Insight.

General Behaviour. When this is extravagantly abnormal it is not hard to see that something is amiss! Often the family will describe a change in behaviour which may not be obvious at interview, since the patient may be concealing his feelings, etc., so that the student should try to assess the patient's behaviour as carefully as possible, noting such points as the facial expression, gesture, dress, and the patient's general activity, which may be exaggerated as in states of excitement, or sluggish and slow (retardation), as in severe depression. Schizophrenic patients may make poor contact and seem remote and aloof or they may display odd mannerisms (habitual expressive movements), grimace in an inappropriate way or adopt odd postures.

Talk. Here the form of the patient's talk should be noted. Is it fast or slow? Is the patient evasive or reluctant to talk? Does he drift off into irrelevant topics or does he stick to the point? Is he over-talkative or does his talk contain oddities such as puns, rhymes, etc. (often a feature of hypomania).

Gross abnormalities of speech such as incoherence are found in severe organic cerebral syndromes and in severe schizophrenia, where talk may be fragmentary and disconnected and contain words invented by the patient (*neologisms*).

Emotion. Feelings are notoriously hard to describe; the range of available words to encompass feeling is immense so that it is rarely possible to sum up a patient's feelings in a single sentence. The most useful tactic is to gauge the *prevailing emotional state of the patient*. Many psychiatric syndromes are associated with extensive change of mood. Sadness, misery, dejection, pessimism and an overall feeling of unhappy wretchedness are commonplace in psychiatric disorders, particularly *depression*, but they are also found in other syndromes, e.g. in *organic mental states* and *early schizophrenia*.

It is important to assess whether the patient's emotional state is appropriate to the rest of his mental condition and whether it is constant or variable. Shallow emotional responses and lability of mood are other features to look out for—they can occur in *organic mental* states and in *schizophrenia*. Many patients are apathetic and say that they have lost all feeling. Others may be unnaturally elated, breezy or euphoric, whilst others may describe states of bliss or ecstasy. These latter exalted feelings are found in mania and in schizophrenia whilst *episodic ecstatic states* must raise the suspicion of *temporal lobe epilepsy.*

Thought. Normally we take it for granted that a person is able to control his thoughts, but schizophrenic patients often feel that they neither possess nor control their own thoughts, or they may feel that thoughts are inserted into their minds or are removed from them, or even that their thoughts are being broadcast. Sudden gaps in thinking, often referred to as *thought blocking*, may be pathological as in *schizophrenia*, but can occur in normal people under stress and in anxiety states.

Excited patients may experience *pressure of thought*, when thoughts seem to crowd through the mind. Difficulty in thinking clearly is a relatively non-specific symptom which may occur in fatigue, in depression, in states of intoxication with drugs or alcohol, in organic mental states and in the early stages of schizophrenia.

Delusions and Other Abnormal Thought Contents. A delusion is a demonstrably false belief, held with absolute conviction which is inappropriate to the person's socio-cultural background. True delusions are usually the main abnormalities in schizophrenia where they arise spontaneously and cannot be understood, as opposed to *delusional ideas*, which are false beliefs that are an *understandable consequence of severe mood disturbance.* Persecutory and grandiose delusions of exalted status, etc. are usually referred to as *paranoid.*

Obsessions. These include recurrent ideas, phrases or acts which intrude on a person's mental life in an unpleasant way. The content is often obscene, blasphemous or ridiculous.

Perception. The collection of sense data from all modalities—perception —is the basis of interaction with the environment. Perceptions may be heightened or dulled as in certain toxic and delirious states or under the influence of hallucinogenic drugs. Hallucinations are perceptions which occur in the absence of an outside stimulus. Dreams are good examples of normal hallucinosis.

Hallucinations may occur in organic mental states and in psychoses such as schizophrenia, where they are usually auditory. False perceptions or *illusions* can occur in states of fatigue, drug intoxication and in organic mental states and in schizophrenia.

Cognitive Function. Cognition is the means by which information is stored and retrieved. To test it involves giving simple formal tests of memory, general information, concentration and orientation for time and place. Cognitive function is always impaired in organic mental states.

Orientation. Ask the patient to give the day, date and time of day. Also make sure that he knows where he is.

Memory. Give the patient a name and address. Ask him to repeat it and then ask him to reproduce it in five minutes. This is a simple but useful test of the ability to register, retain and reproduce recently learnt material. Ask about the activities of the day before.

Concentration. Ask the patient to subtract 7 from 100 and to go on subtracting—again a simple but useful test.

General Information. Usually this can be assessed in interview, but if there is any doubt a good simple test is to ask the patient to name the capitals of six countries, the names of six large cities, the names of prominent public figures, etc.

Insight. Ask the patient if he feels that he is ill in any way. The object is to find out not only whether the patient is aware of his illness but also to find out whether he has a reasonable idea of its extent and implications.

General Comments. Not every patient needs full testing of cognitive function, it is most useful when there is the slightest suspicion of organic impairment.

PSYCHIATRIC SYNDROMES

First of all it has to be said that there is considerable disagreement about psychiatric diagnostic classifications. Extreme views about this range from those who discount totally the value of diagnosis to those who rely on highly detailed diagnostic schemata. The International Classification of Disease Nomenclature has as yet had little effect on diagnostic habits. In the U.K. psychiatrists use relatively simple diagnostic labels which are based on the main diagnostic groups described by Kraepelin. This has the merit of being simple and it covers groups of recognisable disorders. It comprises:

1. Affective disorders.
2. Schizophrenia.
3. The neuroses.
4. Organic syndromes.
5. Personality disorders.
6. Mental subnormality (mental handicap).

AFFECTIVE DISORDERS

Definition. Affective disorders are all characterised by a primary disturbance of mood with associated symptoms of altered behaviour and alterations in energy, sleep, appetite and weight. The polar extremes of affective disorder range from intense excitement and elation (*mania and hypomania*) to severe *depressive states*. The original name given to these disorders was *manic depressive psychosis*, but over the past 80 years it has become increasingly recognised that this is too narrow a term, since the majority of depressives are in no sense psychotic, i.e. so disturbed that they are out of contact with reality, but that pathological states of depression are relatively common.

Depression

In depression a person becomes persistently sad and unhappy but the disturbance exceeds in extent and duration the everyday shades of feeling and emotional response that colour human life. Abnormally depressed mood is disproportionate to any cause, real or fancied and extends in time to such an extent that family and friends soon recognise that something is wrong, often before the patient does. Depression may come on suddenly or may develop in an insidious way and become chronic. There has been a fair amount of controversy about *endogenous* and *reactive* depressions, which have been thought to be different and mutually exclusive types of depression that may have different causes and require different treatment. The differences may be summarised as follows:

Endogenous	Reactive
Severe mood change	Less severe
Diurnal mood variation	No diurnal mood variation
Insomnia—early waking	No early waking
Onset spontaneous	Reaction to outside events
Responds to E.C.T. and drugs	Treated with psychotherapy—drugs less useful
Genetic factor	No genetic factor

However, many believe that the distinction is neither valid nor useful, and that the apparent dichotomy is mainly a matter of severity of symptoms in a syndrome of depression that is really a continuum of mood disturbance unrelated to endogenous and reactive aetiologies. This view is shared by the author. The most important clinical fact is that depression is common, treatable, still missed by doctors and still causes people to kill themselves.

Aetiology. A *genetic* factor operates in unipolar affective psychosis (depressive or mania) and in bipolar affective psychoses (i.e. manic depressive). These psychoses breed true, show a definite family incidence and a high concordance rate in monozygotic twins. Certain races, e.g. the Irish and Jewish people, are more prone to affective disorders than others. Also *physical build* is important: the endomorph with small hands and feet and large visceral cavities is more liable to affective illness. *Brain biochemistry* is important. Current theory stresses the importance of C.N.S. transmitters—the catecholamines, dopamine and noradrenaline and the indoleamine, 5 hydroxytryptamine (5 HT or serotonin)—as being involved in depression when their concentration in the hypothalamus and brainstem is decreased. Medication produces higher concentration and relief of depression, but the mechanism is not fully understood (see psychopharmacology).

Life events such as bereavement, moving house or losing a job, etc., can all contribute to depression. Also certain physical illnesses such as jaundice and virus infections can set off depression. The same is true of various drugs including reserpine, methyldopa, the sulphonamides, phenobarbitone and 'the pill'.

Social and family influences are hard to pinpoint, but there is at least more than a suggestion that loss of a parent in early childhood can lead to depression much later. An unduly strict and repressive family climate can mould children into depression-prone adults whose aggressive feelings cannot be expressed but can only be turned inwards.

Clinical Features

Mood. Mood disturbance is usually prominent and may be described in terms of despair, pessimism, sadness, gloom, solemnity, apathy, hopeless self scrutiny and tearfulness—in short a range of feeling that cannot easily be summarised. Mood change may be constant or show diurnal variation and may be responsive or unresponsive to outside events.

Behaviour. Is usually slow, faltering and weary; this is called retardation. Smiles are rare, fleeting and rueful. There may be restless half-organised worried over-activity, i.e. agitation, in which state the patient walks about weeping and wringing his hands.

Thought. Is slow and laboured, concentration is poor because the patient is too careworn and preoccupied. The memory may also seem affected but this is because the patient feels too wretched to pay attention to what is going on.

Delusional Ideas. Severely depressed patients may sometimes develop delusional ideas. When this happens it is understandable in the sense that the false belief arises from exaggerated ideas of guilt and self blame. Much more commonly the depressed patient feels a sense of failure and guilt which pervades his mental life to the extent of causing him to feel unworthy and suicidal. Often the depressed patient is querulous and hypochondriacal —this may easily obscure the real diagnosis.

Perception. In depression a person sees the whole world in a dull light. Pleasant experience is no longer so, everything looks grey and lacklustre. In severe psychotic depression the patient can experience auditory hallucinations, usually voices that condemn him—the voice of the devil, etc. These symptoms are rare, since nowadays treatment starts early, but they occasionally occur in elderly people.

Insight. Is always impaired in depression. No depressed person is able to judge himself sensibly. He may appear to agree that he is ill, but inside he knows how bad it all is and that the doctor is wrong. This should not be overlooked because it is just this type of insightlessness that leads to suicide.

History. The onset may be sudden or slow, related to life events or it may come on out of the blue. Besides the symptoms as outlined it is always important to look for other symptoms which may include:

1. Sleep disturbance—particularly early waking and lying awake.
2. Loss of energy.
3. Loss of interest.
4. Loss of appetite.
5. Hypochondriasis—especially concern about bowels, abdominal churning and headache.

6. Impotence, frigidity and loss of libido.
7. Irritability.
8. Anxiety and tension.
9. Indecision and self doubt.
10. A falling off in personal relationships and in application at work.
11. Apathy and inertia.
12. A general feeling of malaise.
13. Thinking and talking about suicide.
14. Self neglect.
15. Recent abuse of alcohol or drugs.

It is justifiable to list the symptoms in this way since they are easily overlooked. Admittedly many are non-specific in that they are found in physical illness, but when viewed as a whole they add up to the picture of depression. It is still the case that a patient can be extensively investigated while the diagnosis of depression is missed, because the one symptom is followed up and the patient is ignored.

Diagnosis. Apart from mood disturbance, the key symptoms to look for include general symptoms of lost function as outlined above. Depressive states are inevitably coloured by the individual's premorbid personality, the irritable person gets more irritable, the histrionic person becomes more demonstrative and unstable. The history should point out any precipitating events. Bereavement is a typical and important example. Mourning can merge into depression. Normal mourning is a healthy reaction to loss but is generally self-limiting in that people come to accept loss and adjust to normal living. However, if mourning extends for months it is more than likely to be abnormal. Space does not permit a full examination of normal and abnormal grief, but a good rule is that someone who is still grief-stricken after six months is depressed. In chronic and painful physical illness, true depression is hard to diagnose, since anyone in pain feels unhappy and lacks zest—a state of unhappy malaise that is sometimes called *dysphoria*.

Schizophrenia. Early mood change always is overtaken by basic schizophrenic symptoms; thought disorder, delusions, etc.

Organic Cerebral Disease. May cause diagnostic difficulty especially in middle-aged depressives who do not respond to treatment. Organic brain disease may then be suspected. Inevitably if organic brain disease is present it will cause memory and intellectual defect. It is wrong to diagnose organic brain disease without evidence.

Personality Disorders. Unstable people frequently are unhappy after personal crises, but their mood disturbance, though colourful, is labile.

Physical Illness. May mimic depression and vice versa. Important illnesses to look out for include myxoedema, Parkinson's disease, and pernicious anaemia.

Treatment

Admission to hospital is most likely to be used for suicidal, elderly and physically neglected patients, but in general depression is treated at home and mostly by general practitioners. Nowadays the majority of depressives who are seen by psychiatrists are either suicidal or have not responded to treatment from their doctors.

Simple support is very important and is based on sympathetic encouragement and not on breezy admonition to 'pull yourself together' a tactic which depressives interpret as lack of interest.

Physical Treatment. The basic physical treatments of depression used nowadays are antidepressant drugs and of these the tricyclic series are the most widely used. Electroconvulsive therapy (E.C.T.) is valuable if there is suicidal risk, and there is a definite but restricted place for monoamine oxidase inhibitors (MAOI's).

Prognosis. In general the prognosis is good. Acute onset favours speedy recovery and insidious onset suggests chronicity. Relapse is common and for this reason depressed patients often need long-term supervision.

General Comments. Depression is common, it is a disagreeable and wretched state to endure. There is no justification for waiting for spontaneous remission or letting the patient 'work through' depression. Once a patient begins to feel better with treatment he sees his problem in a more sensible light. Neurotic depression—i.e. chronic mild depression—tied into personality difficulties can also be improved with medication. The most important thing is to recognise depression and do something about it.

Mania and Hypomania

Both of these are much rarer than depression.

Mania is a state of high elation and uncontrollable excitement. Psychomotor over-activity is excessive. The patient is noisy, bounds with energy and ebullient high spirits. Grandiose delusional ideas are common and the patient's clothing may be covered in fantastic decoration. Often there is a paranoid colouring and the breezy elation turns to rage. Talk is so fast and overloaded with content as to be disorganised, though connected by rhymes, puns and jokes, etc.

Hypomania is less severe than mania and more common. The onset is usually gradual and may be hard to date, since often the symptoms are an exaggeration of the patient's hypomanic personality, i.e. always more cheery and energetic than his fellows, gregarious, hardworking and the 'life and soul of the party'. In hypomania, however, an acceptable degree of energy and self-confidence becomes restless energy, mild elation and wakefulness that passes unnoticed at first until the person is seen to be a restless interfering nuisance who is doing too much, overspending and is boastful and rude. The patient is over-confident, his mood is buoyant and he is scornful of advice.

Diagnosis. In any state of excitement the basic differential is between schizophrenia and affective psychosis. In theory the schizophrenic symptoms should be easy to pick out, but the patient may be so excited as to make this virtually impossible. Time and medication usually clarify the picture.

Organic Mental States. Acute excitement, e.g. delirium, is distinguished by the clouded consciousness which is an invariable symptom in organic syndromes. General paresis may start off with a manic episode.

Drugs. Amphetamines and hallucinogens such as LSD.

Treatment. Manic patients need admission because of their wild exhausted state. Compulsory admission may be needed (see Mental Health Act). The hypomanic patient usually needs admission but is always unwilling to accept it. Compulsory admission may have to await the patient's involvement in a crisis.

Physical Treatment. E.C.T. usually shortens manic or hypomanic attacks, though nowadays the neuroleptic drugs are the first line of treatment—particularly the phenothiazines and haloperidol (see Psychopharmacology). Lithium has a definite place in recurrent manic and hypomanic attacks, but should be used only by hospital doctors, because of its toxic potential.

Prognosis. Mania and hypomania are usually short lived, episodic and recurrent. Lithium is especially valuable in controlling recurrence.

SCHIZOPHRENIA

Schizophrenia is a syndrome of personality change and other symptoms, which tends to start in early adult life and which can lead to a severe disintegration of personality. Some symptoms are relatively specific, e.g. primary delusions, thought disorder, hallucinosis and social withdrawal. The illness always occurs in clear consciousness. The personality change is global and recovery, though often apparently complete, is rarely so. This makes diagnosis crucial since diagnosis implies a prognosis.

Aetiology. The notion of there being one cause for schizophrenia is now discarded in favour of a multifactorial aetiology which encompasses biological, psychological, family interaction and sociocultural factors as playing complementary roles in determining the probability of the illness occurring.

Biological Factors. The incidence in the general population is 0·85 per cent. In Britain the admission rate for schizophrenia over the last 25 years has been around 15–20 first admissions per 100,000 psychiatric admissions per year. *Genetic inheritance* is important in that certain families do breed true, but 60 per cent of schizophrenics have no family history. In the family of a schizophrenic the expected incidence may be as high as

Parents   5–10 per cent
Children   8–16 per cent
Full siblings 10 per cent

It was formerly said that concordance rates in monozygotic twins was as high as 90 per cent but this has been refuted—the figure is probably 60 per cent. *Age* is important—most cases start early.

Biochemical and Metabolic Factors. Despite intensive searching for toxic, metabolic, serological and endocrine factors, there are really little hard data. Much contemporary research involves brain biochemistry. One hypothesis is that in schizophrenia the brain produces an abnormal central transmitter in response to stress stimuli and that the build up of the substance causes the symptoms in the same way that hallucinogenic drugs and amphetamines trigger off 'model' psychoses. *Temporal lobe epilepsy* is frequently associated with schizophrenic psychoses; this suggests a link between the TLE and the psychosis that is stronger than mere chance association.

Personality and Constitution. Many have commented on the asthenic body build of chronic schizophrenics and have described a premorbid personality—a schizoid personality characterised by aloofness, seclusiveness, shyness, emotional coolness and detachment. This is true but leaves unexplained the 50 per cent of schizophrenics who have a perfectly normal premorbid personality.

Psychological Factors. The original description of schizophrenia by Bleuler stressed the importance of 'loosening of thought processes', emotional incongruity and personality disintegration, but these were descriptions of the mental state rather than explanations of causality. Some psychological theories have postulated a basic perceptual disorder, and others have suggested a malfunction of learning processes.

Psychodynamic theories relate the development of schizophrenia to defects in the parent–child relationship in early life, causing faulty psychological maturation and hence psychosis in a specially vulnerable personality.

Life events have been shown to bear a significant relationship to onset and relapse (e.g. moving house, death of spouse, promotion, etc.).

Family Interaction and Social Factors. Sociologists and anthropologists have examined schizophrenic families and presented a number of theories. For example,

(a) Schizophrenic families use odd eccentric modes of communication which set up impossible conflicts in weaker family members who are victims of an ambiguous communication net.

(b) Schizophrenic parents use incomprehensible ways of relating to their children, e.g. the 'double-bind' situation where a child is ordered to obey a negative injunction and threatened with punishment whatever happens. This leads him to adopt immobile withdrawal as a form of self-preservation, which is then called 'psychosis'.

(c) The family may be a malign influence which edges the person into psychosis as an escape from a family which has selected one member for a psychotic role.

(d) Schizophrenia probably occurs more commonly in lower socioeconomic groups than in higher, but in addition it is easier for a person in the lower end of the social scale to be diagnosed as schizophrenic.

(e) In certain countries schizophrenia is diagnosed casually, and the 'diagnosis' is used to 'treat' 'social deviants' and 'political extremists'.

Comment. Schizophrenia is likely to be a heterogenous mixture of syndromes with no unitary cause. The aetiologies so far mentioned are not mutually exclusive.

Schizophrenia: Clinical Features. Schizophrenia seems to be a useful label for syndromes with fairly definite symptoms and a poor prognosis. Schizophrenic symptoms can never be *understood* in the same way as depressive symptoms and they are never a logical reaction to a life experience. The symptoms include

>Delusions
>Thought disorder
>Behaviour disorders
>Emotional disorders
>Perceptual disorder,

all of which add up to a real change in personality.

Delusion has already been defined. The true delusion arises out of the blue and is held with extraordinary conviction—it is a basic inexplicable error in judgement. Schizophrenic delusions are often paranoid, i.e. they involve ideas of grandiose or exalted status, of being persecuted or of being singled out in a special way. The delusion may be preceded by a premonitory feeling of unusual awareness or impending revelation.

Thought disorder is a special type of abnormal thinking often found in schizophrenia. It consists of a basic flaw of conceptual thought which impairs reasoning. The patient cannot think clearly, he may interchange cause and effect and cannot make abstractions from general or concrete statements. He may seem dull and slow, though his I.Q. is average or above. In severe cases he feels that his thoughts are not his own, they are shared by others or broadcast around. Thought block and pressure of thought can occur, also slowness and poverty of thought.

Behaviour Disorders. Many patients develop stiff awkward movements and strange symbolic movements which they repeat (stereotyped movement). They may become mute and stuporose—rare since physical treatment has been possible. Excitement and uncontrolled aggression can also occur—again rare nowadays. Rarely, too, a schizophrenic can get fixed in a weird posture with sluggish stiff limbs (waxy flexibility). Again some schizophrenics may behave impulsively and act in an inexplicable way without warning, e.g. shouting, violence or suicide. A common symptom is the feeling that the body is under outside influence or control—passivity feelings.

Emotional Disorder. Often in the early stages a patient feels unaccountably anxious and vaguely depressed. Others feel strangely blissful or ecstatic or feel that something is about to happen or be revealed. The most typical emotional abnormality is an incongruity between feeling and experience (e.g. laughing at bad news), but generally the incongruity is less extreme. Emotional responses are lowered, he becomes detached, cool, aloof, uninvolved and totally absorbed in his inner life. This comes across as a lack of empathy—like a pane of glass between him and others.

Perceptual Disorders. These are diverse, ranging from feelings of unreality (depersonalisation) to feelings of unbearably intense reality. The most common disorders are auditory hallucinations, though they can occur in any modality except vision. Auditory hallucinations include whistles, whispers and murmurs but voices (phonemes) are the most common. They repeat his words or thoughts, instruct him, abuse him or comment on his acts.

Schizophrenic Symptoms: General. The most important thing is that the personality changes in a way that often leads to total fragmentation. Drive and impetus are lost, emotions are blunted and behaviour is odd. Delusions occupy thinking and disrupt personal and social life into seclusive apathetic inertia. Diagnosis is made by recognising a total picture rather than by one or two symptoms; a hallucination and a paranoid delusion do not add up to schizophrenia.

Clinical Types. Four types are described:

1. Simple.
2. Hebephrenic.
3. Paranoid.
4. Catatonic.

Simple. This type starts early and insidiously. Florid symptoms are few; the usual picture is of a fall-off in activity, thought and feeling. The patient is unaware of symptoms; it is the family who complain that he has slipped into inert self-neglect. Talk is sparse, answers are scanty or abrupt and there is a general impression of poverty of thought and emotion. Later on hallucinations and vaguely expressed delusions can be elicited. The prognosis is bad: many end up as long-term patients, or at best rather dull, empty people doing simple jobs under careful supervision.

Hebephrenia. Onset is usually insidious in late adolescence. The clinical picture is dominated by severe thought disorder, emotional incongruity and auditory hallucinations. Personality disintegration is extensive. A typical end point is one where the patient is fatuous, euphoric, buffoonish and thought disordered. The prognosis is bad.

Paranoid Schizophrenia. Onset is usually late (30–45) with paranoid delusions often very complicated (systematised) in the forefront. The delusions are usually persecutory, though grandiose and exalted ideas are equally common. The personality is well preserved, so the patient is better able to survive in the community. Drive and energy may be high and encourage the patient to act on his delusions in a forceful way. Thought disorder is hard to detect and paranoid schizophrenics are skilful in concealing paranoid content. Survival in the community is less easy if the delusions become too forcefully expressed, leading to acute crises caused by psychotic outbursts. The prognosis is generally better than in other schizophrenias since the personality is relatively well preserved. Emotionally the paranoid schizophrenic is remote, even callous, but inevitably absorbed in his delusions to the exclusion of everyone and everything else.

Catatonic. This type is comparatively rare nowadays. Onset is usually acute with either excitement or a quickly developing state of stupor. Early symptoms include odd gestures, stiff movements and weird postures. Catatonic excitement is severe to the extent of disorganised restlessness which may be aggressive or self-destructive. Bizarre acts and postures, and also echo reactions (mechanical repetition of the words or actions of the examiner) can occur as well as fixed rigid postures leading to stupor. This state requires total nursing care—feeding, washing, etc.—though E.C.T. and neuroleptic drugs have made stupor and violent excitement short-lived and rare events.

Summary. In practice, the four clinical types are not often diagnosed unless the picture is typical. Generally psychiatrists diagnose 'undifferentiated' schizophrenia without special concern for subgroups.

Diagnosis. The diagnosis is always hampered by lack of agreement about the concept of schizophrenia; nevertheless agreement is better, or as good as, in the diagnosis of neurosis. It has also been made difficult by the over-emphasis of clinical features described by early clinicians who spoke with an authority that has only recently been questioned. Some have listed 'classical' symptoms, e.g. voices commenting on actions, thought broadcasting and thought insertion or withdrawal, etc. Diagnosis is neither simple nor unacceptably difficult, but is important, since modern treatment may alter the natural history of a disorder which reduces people to empty shells.

Affective disorder is recognised by the primary mood disorder. Delusional ideas are loose, explicable and transitory. Thought disorder is absent.

Organic Cerebral Disease. Personality change is important, but there is always cognitive impairment and the basic syndromes either of clouded states, dementia and memory loss. *Hysteria* and *personality disorder* may cause difficulty by presenting a picture of pseudopsychosis. In *old age*, people may become acutely disturbed or paranoid. Once organic damage and affective disorder are excluded, there remains the possibility of *late paraphrenia* or of an acute *paranoid reaction* in an elderly paranoid personality.

Treatment. The aims of treatment include relief of distressing symptoms and the preservation of contact with reality, so as to return the patient as speedily as possible to normal social function. Aetiology is unclear, so causes cannot be treated, on the other hand aggravating factors can be modified, e.g. in family relationships, at work, etc.

Physical treatment. This consists mainly of the use of neuroleptic drugs which calm agitation, block hallucinosis and help the person to think more clearly and feel more at ease (see psychopharmacology). E.C.T. is used mainly to shorten periods of excitement or if there is associated depression. Otherwise E.C.T. has no real lasting value and may make matters worse.

Psychotherapy. Individual therapy should be supportive rather than analytic, since the latter is usually too disruptive an experience for the patient.

Social and Community Therapy. A long stay in hospital can be bad and make the person become an institutionalised zombie. Physical treatments make it easier for quick return to the community, but it should not end there. The world and the family may seem strange and unfamiliar, the patient may be odd and quirkish, too ready to talk about his delusions and voices, and the pace of life may be overstimulating and lead to relapse. Therefore the family needs support and advice. The chronic patient who goes home after many years can set off problems at home and will need re-training and supervision. These aims can only be achieved by well-coordinated community services and good links with hospital services. Above all, there should be a high level of multi-disciplinary team care of the patient and his family.

Outcome. Hebephrenic and simple schizophrenia have the worst prognosis. Acute onset and onset following some obvious precipitant are good points. Insidious onset and low I.Q. are bad points. Approximately 50 per cent of first admissions have no relapse; of the remainder, half do relatively well and the rest do badly. But all of the 'relapsers' show permanent personality change.

THE NEUROSES

Neuroses are the commonest psychiatric disorders in general practice. In a practice with 3,000 patients, a doctor can expect about 30 new cases of depression in a year, and will probably have about 6 schizophrenics in the practice population. Depending on the age range of the practice, the doctor sees a variable number of people with organic dementia, but in any case he may expect a consultation rate of 12–20 per cent of all attendances to be about neurotic disorders which may present as either psychological or physical symptoms. Neurosis has never been easy to define, as its origins are based on the older idea that mental disorder comprised 'weak nerves' (neurosis) and psychosis 'madness' or severe mental disorder. Thus neurosis is used as an unsatisfactory catch-all which can be described more easily than defined.

Neuroses can be summed up as psychiatric disorders in which the personality remains intact, contact with reality is preserved and symptoms are subjective, persistent and troublesome. The neurotic is preoccupied with his symptoms, often morose and invariably frustrated and querulous. This is mainly because he feels that he is not improving and also because he senses an unsympathetic attitude to a disorder that appears to be self-indulgent. General neurotic symptoms include low energy, a feeling of malaise, inability to cope, insomnia, and above all feelings of anxiety and tension. There is probably a constitutional element involved, but this does not account for all cases. There are two basic theories of neurosis. The first explains neurotic behaviour as a maladaptive reaction to faulty upbringing and arrested emotional development based on early childhood experience. This would broadly summarise the psychodynamic theory. The other theoretical model is that neurosis is a learned maladaptive response—a symptom of faulty learning that has no unconscious dynamic significance. Others have suggested an existentialist basis for neurosis—the fear of 'non-being'. No theory is entirely satisfactory; the clinician must rely on recognition of these disorders and their degree of handicap. Treatment is eclectic and the outlook is in general good. Certain special syndromes are recognised. They include:

> (a) Anxiety.
> (b) Phobic anxiety.
> (c) Neurotic depression.
> (d) Obsessional neurosis.
> (e) Hysteria.
> (f) Hypochondriasis.
> (g) Depersonalisation syndrome.

Anxiety

Anxiety is a common feature in affective disorder, but also exists as a syndrome on its own. Contemporary theory makes a useful distinction between *trait* anxiety, i.e. a personality trait ('I tend to get anxious') and *state* anxiety ('I am anxious'). In state anxiety, symptoms are episodic or persistent, and are usually severe. Descriptions of anxiety stress its subjectivity and its observed biological features, which can be summarised thus:

(a) It is an unpleasant emotional disturbance like fear or dread related to fear of something that may happen.

(b) It is disproportionate in its relation to stress.

(c) It has definite autonomic accompaniments caused by sympathetic overactivity; for example:

> 1. Dry mouth, nausea and vomiting. Diarrhoea.
> 2. Tremor, muscular tension, numbness, dizziness.
> 3. Tachycardia, palpitations and chest discomfort.
> 4. Lump in the throat. Butterflies in the stomach.
> 5. Anorexia, insomnia, frequency of micturition. Impotence.

Any of these symptoms if prominent may lead the patient to see a number of doctors. Anxiety can occur at any age, though adolescence is probably the time when acute anxiety in pure culture is most commonly seen. The importance of anxiety lies in its nearness to the normal. Almost everyone experiences anxiety when faced with ordeals such as examinations or interviews, when it is a normal adaptive reaction.

Morbid anxiety is maladaptive, unpredictable, frightening and unrelated to any obvious stress. It soon becomes a burden to the patient.

Treatment of anxiety includes the relief of symptoms with tranquillisers, and psychotherapy, which may be either supportive or analytic and directed at the resolution of unconscious conflict. In many cases, behaviour therapy is used to remove symptoms rather than unravel possible dynamics (see page 60).

Phobic Anxiety. This is an anxiety syndrome in which symptoms, e.g. dread, panic, fear of collapse, palpitations, etc. are evoked by specific things or situations, e.g. cats, snakes, open spaces, closed spaces, etc. Phobic states have a compulsive and recurrent quality and are unrelenting and inexplicable. The patient is often ashamed of his 'silly fears'. Once the phobia is fixed, the patient avoids the stimulus as best he can. If this is easy, as with cats, wasps, snakes, etc., he may endure, but if the phobia involves going out then the patient may end up by becoming 'housebound'.

Treatment. Tranquillisers are used to suppress symptoms such as panic. Many regard monoamine oxidase inhibitors as the best medication (see Treatment).

Psychotherapy has been extensively used, but many feel that the results are not as good as those achieved by behaviour therapy, particularly for single phobias (see page 60).

Neurotic Depression

The problems of the classification of depression have already been mentioned. Neurotic depression is usually mild and responds well to a change of environment. Symptoms are chronic and seem to be bound up with long-standing personality difficulties. The patient finds it all worrisome and unpleasant. Mood disturbance is rarely severe and there is little in the way of sleep disorder.

Treatment consists of support and psychotherapy aimed at obvious problems. The patient may have to learn to accept something less than perfection. Medication is useful in the short term (tricyclic antidepressants) but is not as successful as in more severe depressive states.

Obsessional Neurosis

Obsessions are mental concepts including words, ideas, phrases and actions which a person feels compelled to repeat against a feeling of inner resistance. Obsesssions are always unpleasant for the sufferer and may cause anxiety and severe depression. Obsessions have a quality that is very like the common childhood experience of 'having to' avoid cracks between paving stones or like some everyday superstitions that people observe in an embarrassed way. Obsessional neurosis starts early in life and persists with remissions well into middle and later years. Recent studies suggest that the long-term prognosis is not as bad as had been suspected. Long periods of relative remission *do* occur and the end point is likely to be a compromise with symptoms. Depression is a common complication, as is a relentless state of shame and tension perpetuated by the obsessions and rituals.

Treatment. The condition is relatively rare, so there is no generally agreed treatment. Anxiety, tension and depression are treated with medication. When depression is severe, E.C.T. and antidepressants relieve it and reduce the force of the obsessions.

Psychotherapy aimed at analysing the symbolism of the obsessions is of little use and most psychotherapists rely on support. Certain patients become so crippled by their obsessions and so tense that drugs and E.C.T. are useless. In these cases psychosurgery is used in carefully selected cases, often with considerable relief of tension, though the obsessions remain untouched.

Hysteria

Hysteria is a difficult word because it is used inconsistently and can mislead. Laymen use it to describe uncontrolled behaviour, in which context it is not medically useful. It is also applied to a personality type, the hysterical personality, which many feel is better described as the histrionic personality. Its chief psychiatric use is to describe disorders in which there is *loss of function* in the central nervous system but no structural damage. These disorders are said to be caused by a dissociation of consciousness—a splitting off from consciousness of a function ordinarily under conscious awareness. Thus hysterical disorders include sensory and motor dysfunction as well as amnesia, trance-like states and fugues.

The general theory of hysteria is that these states of *conversion hysteria* are the result of unacceptable conflict which causes intolerable stress which can only be dealt with by unconsciously simulating illness. The most extreme examples of this follow severe ordeals, as in wartime and disaster, but the theory hardly accounts for long-term follow-up of people diagnosed as suffering from 'hysteria', many of whom show a disturbingly high incidence of unrecognised organic disease, suicide and mental illness. Hysterical disorders are rarer than they used to be; this is possibly because a patient no longer has to complain of physical symptoms in order to receive help. On the other hand many physically ill people develop hysterical exaggeration of symptoms, and also organic brain disease can trigger off a hysterical reaction when higher control is impaired.

Diagnosis. Bizarre mental states that mimic psychosis can be hysteria, and usually occur in highly stressed situations. The same is true of amnesia and fugues. Paresis is much harder to evaluate, particularly when it is chronic. The diagnosis should not be made because no physical signs can be found. There should be some definite conflict situation which can be shown to present the patient with a gainful solution of an impossible problem.

Treatment. The acute hysterical reaction can usually be treated by heavy sedation followed by powerful suggestion and reassurance. Chronic hysteria tends to be propagated by diagnostic uncertainty. In general, vigorous and positive support and rehabilitation with the careful use of medication are the mainstays of treatment. The chronic hysteric will need careful and skilled psychotherapy to deal with conflict and encourage the return of lost function.

Hypochondriasis

Persistent concern about fancied illness occurs in depression; it may be delusional as in schizophrenia and it often complicates the lives of people with obsessional personalities. But it is common to see patients who have a neurotic state of concern about fancied ill health. Usually that patient comes from a family in which minor childhood illnesses were regarded as grave events needing prolonged rest and fussing about trivial bodily symptoms. In adult life this hardens into a pervasive worrisome attitude to health, often related to bowel action where the slightest deviation from punctual defaecation is regarded as a sign of impending serious illness. Hypochondriacal people are often too aware of bodily sensations and minor aches and pains; they tend to react badly to simple illnesses. Often they expend much time in self-scrutiny and a good deal of money on health foods, faddy diets, baths, etc. Treatment is entirely supportive. Severe hypochondriacs resent this simple approach to their problem and find a new doctor.

Depersonalisation Syndrome

A feeling of altered reality of the self is a frightening and unpleasant experience which can be an early symptom of schizophrenia or colour a depressive illness or be set off by drugs, e.g. LSD, mescaline and steroids. It also occurs in temporal lobe epilepsy. But there is also a group of patients who become depersonalised and develop phobic anxiety. This often comes on suddenly and the prognosis is reasonably good. Treatment includes the use of tranquillisers and monoamine oxidase inhibitor antidepressants. This type of depersonalisation syndrome may follow bereavement.

Summary. The term neurosis is clinically useful in that it covers common but unpleasant and troublesome symptoms that may be uncertain in aetiology but which can be considerably relieved by giving the patient time to talk about his symptoms and problems which can too easily be dismissed as 'neurotic' and left at that.

ORGANIC SYNDROMES

Organic cerebral syndromes are caused by dysfunction at cellular level, whether resulting from ischaemia, toxins, inflammation, tumour or trauma. The damage may be transient, permanent or progressive. Organic brain disease causes symptoms of:

1. Intellectual impairment.
2. Memory defect.
3. Personality change.
4. Focal signs and symptoms.

Of these, the first three contribute to recognisable syndromes of organic brain disease, which present as psychiatric disturbance, whilst the focal symptoms usually present as neurological defect.

There are four basic types of organic cerebral syndrome. They may present in pure culture or they may overlap. They include:

1. Delirium.
2. Subacute delirium (confusional state). } 'clouded states'
3. The dysmnesic syndrome.
4. Dementia.

Delirium

Consciousness is badly clouded, concentration and attention are fleeting and narrow. The patient cannot grasp what is happening and the environment appears strange and frightening. In a sleepy state the patient misinterprets what is going on and may develop fragmentary delusions. The emotional state is usually fearful and terrified. Hallucinations often occur as well as illusions (perceptual errors). This general state of frightened uncertainty leads to excited over-activity and attempts to leave the ward. Onset of delirium is usually acute and the clouding of consciousness is worst at night when visual cues are less clear. Quiet calm nurses and doctors will do much to allay the frightened delirious patient.

Subacute Delirium (Confusional state)

These are always marked by clouded consciousness, perplexity and incoherence of thinking, feeling and activity. The onset is usually slow and the course prolonged—sometimes passing unrecognised for days or weeks. Subacute delirium is common in medical and surgical wards, and may not be spotted until the patient slips into frank delirium. Often the patient seems to be 'difficult and uncooperative', but when examined carefully he is muddled and vague or flat and querulous—all based on his perplexity.

Dysmnesic Syndrome

Severe loss of memory for immediate past events is the main symptom. This is associated with a total failure to retain immediate impressions and inability to recall them. Also there is disorientation for time and place and, most striking of all, a tendency to invent answers to make up for the memory defect (confabulation).

The emotional state is flat and mildly euphoric. The classic dysmnesic syndrome is Korsakov's syndrome where the dysmnesic syndrome and peripheral neuropathy occur in chronic alcoholism and thiamine deficiency.

The lesion affects the dorsal thalamic nuclei. A Korsakov-like picture can be caused by injury, ischaemic disease and various toxins.

Dementia

Dementia is caused by global organic cerebral deterioration following general disease, trauma and tumour, among other causes. The general failure of brain function may be associated with focal signs. The symptoms of dementia include:

1. Intellectual defect, especially memory loss.
2. Personality change.
3. Emotional change.

Intellectual Defect. The earliest symptom is failure to retain and remember recently acquired information—a reflection of the brain's inability to store and retrieve new material—though past information remains untouched until the process is so extensive as to be terminal. At first the patient cannot remember to keep appointments, etc., but can get by with a notebook. But this worsens to the point where he gets lost while out shopping or is so forgetful that everyone but he is concerned about it. Concentration falls off and thought is slow and muddled. Talk becomes sparse and repetitive. It is hard to shift from one topic to another; answers become non-committal. Flexibility of thought goes and all the while the patient becomes less aware of what is going on till disorientation is so bad that he tries to get out of bed at night and go to work.

Personality Change. Personality change is probably related to frontal lobe damage. There is a loss of control of behaviour which at first seems merely exaggeration of the normal self but soon tends to coarsening of behaviour—tactlessness and rudeness go beyond eccentricity and lead to social disgrace, e.g. sexual acts with children, shoplifting. Jokes are lewd and uttered in an insightless way. The end-point is fragmentation of the personality and babbling shadowy incoherence.

Emotional Change. Affective symptoms may come on, especially when the patient is aware of failing mental powers. Usually, however, the emotional change is caused by lack of higher cerebral control. Mood change is labile—tears and laughter may come easily but have little depth. A shallow affective state prevails and the person remains unmoved by sad family events. Irritability, distress and rage are sparked off by trivia. The emotions are infantile and egocentric. Later 'emotional incontinence' occurs, i.e. there is no control over feelings which are displayed noisily and without substance.

Aetiology of Organic Syndromes

Since organic syndromes are often caused by the destruction of cells which cannot be replaced, any condition in which there is progressive cell death will cause dementia. The causes of dementia include degenerative disease, chronic inflammation, tumour and untreated metabolic disorders such as myxoedema. At the same time a tumour or a cerebral infarct may be surrounded by partially damaged and recoverable cells. In practice this means that subacute delirium may overly dementia. For this reason every organic syndrome needs careful evaluation so that the extent and aetiology may be fully established.

Investigation of Organic Cerebral Syndromes

1. First of all the mental state should be carefully examined. The picture may be mixed, e.g. subacute delirium/dementia.

2. Physical examination may reveal systemic causes, e.g. congestive cardiac failure causing subacute delirium, chest infection, etc.

3. Blood and serological tests. These may reveal such conditions as B12 or folate deficiency, SLE and neurosyphilis, lead poisoning, etc.

4. Urine testing: barbiturates, bromides. Porphyria.

5. Lumbar puncture, e.g. to confirm neurosyphilis. Never performed if tumour is suspected.

6. Psychological testing to establish the extent of measurable organic impairment.

7. Electroencephalogram. To confirm presence and type of epilepsy. To identify space occupying lesions.

8. Echogram. Of particular use in showing up midline shift and distortion caused by space occupying lesions.

9. Air encephalogram. Useful to display midline shift. Of dubious value in demonstrating cerebral atrophy, i.e. ventricular dilatation.

10. Ventriculogram. Usually employed to localise space occupying lesions.

11. Cerebral angiography. The most useful way of showing up vascular anomalies and vascular shifts caused by space occupying lesions.

12. Brain scan.

Age may be a useful pointer—tumours are commonest in the 40–50 age group. General physical disease, e.g. cardiovascular, renal, hepatic, etc., should be regarded as causal until proved otherwise. Industrial toxins should not be overlooked, nor should syphilis and porphyria and B12 deficiency. But at present the commonest causes are senile dementia and cerebral arteriosclerosis. Never omit to check for thyroid dysfunction. Myxoedema is still missed, and also the rare but treatable normal pressure hydrocephalus.

Specific Causes of Organic Syndromes

Drugs, especially alcohol, barbiturates, bromides and steroids, may all cause clouded states.

Alcohol in heavy doses causing chronic intoxication can produce a severe withdrawal syndrome of *delirium tremens*, i.e. fits, tremors, hallucinosis and delirium. Onset is usually acute.

Treatment includes chlormethiazole which is a safe anticonvulsant and sedative plus vitamin saturation and treatment of any associated infection.

Tranquillisers such as diazepam are useful. Food fluids and good nursing are mandatory. Recovery is total. *Barbiturates* in doses over 900 mg. per 24 hours cause chronic intoxication (dysarthria, nystagmus, ataxia) and withdrawal fits. Acute withdrawal causes fits and delirium.

Treatment consists in reintoxication with pentobarbitone to a state of slight slurred speech and reducing the pentobarbitone by 100 mg. daily.

Bromide intoxication is rare nowadays, but presents a picture of rashes and sub-acute delirium with psychotic excitement and hallucinosis.

Treatment consists of nursing, phenothiazines and the use of sodium chloride to hasten excretion.

Corticosteroids can cause a wide range of psychiatric disturbance, though clouded states, excitement and labile mood disorder are the most common.

Infection. Acute infections produce delirium in high fevers, but these disappear when the infection is controlled.

Chronic infections such as neurosyphilis may present with a clouded state, the classic picture of GPI-Argyll Robertson pupils, tremor of lips, face and tongue are late signs. Early GPI often starts with headache, insomnia, irritability, fits and odd behaviour. Serology and CSF findings clinch the diagnosis. *Treatment* with antibiotics arrests the disease.

Metabolic Disorders

Renal failure causes subacute delirium and coma—barbiturates are after all urea derivatives.

Hepatic failure causes subacute delirium and coma as part of the syndrome of portal systemic encephalopathy; 'flapping tremor' and inco-ordination are well-known signs. The subacute delirious state may mimic irritable depression. Parietal dysfunction is common and for this reason a progress chart should always include the patient's writing and simple drawings.

Endocrine disorders are invariably associated with psychiatric symptoms.

Myxoedema may cause a wide range of symptoms, particularly depression, which fails to respond to antidepressive treatment if the diagnosis is missed. Untreated myxoedema leads to subacute delirious states, delirium, coma and death. If early treatment is deferred there may be permanent brain damage.

Cushing's Syndrome. The clinical picture of obesity, osteoporosis, hypertension and wasting is well known. The syndrome can result from not only basophil adenoma but also excess steroid therapy, lung cancer and ovarian tumours. Mental changes include clouded states and dementia. Appropriate treatment arrests the disease but will not reverse brain damage.

Addison's Disease. A neurotic picture may delay diagnosis or there may be a subacute delirious state. All psychiatric symptoms respond to steroid therapy.

Electrolyte Disturbances usually cause clouded states and are most commonly seen after gastro-intestinal surgery. Fluid and electrolyte replacement always correct the disorder.

Porphyria is a rare inherited metabolic disorder (mendelian dominant). Symptoms include peripheral neuropathy and mental symptoms whose real significance is overlooked. Abdominal pain, skin changes and fits are common, but the psychiatric symptoms may mimic neurosis or depression, though clouded states are common. Attacks are set off by drugs such as the barbiturates, ergot, alcohol, sulphonamides and chloroquine. Urinary findings clinch the diagnosis. Phenothiazines are useful in the acute attack.

Deficiency Diseases

Pellagra is rare in England but is occasionally seen in alcoholics. The triad of 'diarrhoea, dermatitis and dementia' is classical but psychiatric symptoms can mask everything by presenting as neurosis, depression or 'personality disorder'. Untreated cases pass through clouded states to dementia, coma and death. Treatment consists of replacing the deficient substances, niacin and tryptophan.

Pernicious Anaemia. Anaemia and neurological signs usually present first but some patients develop an organic mental state with a normal peripheral blood picture. A marrow picture and serum B12 are essential.

Folate deficiency leading to anomalous psychiatric symptoms is another possibility always to be considered in patients who are on large doses of barbiturates or anticonvulsants.

Toxic. These are rare but should not be forgotten: e.g. *lead*, encephalopathy and dementia; *manganese*, extrapyramidal signs and dementia; *mercury*, tremor and dementia; *carbon monoxide*, extrapyramidal signs and dementia.

Common causes of organic syndromes include:

Vascular and Degenerative Disorders

Cerebral arteriosclerosis causes dementia which is differentiated from senile dementia by earlier onset—as early as 45— but usually in the sixties. Focal signs are frequent but onset is slow and fitful, suggesting arrest, though inevitably dementia takes over. Prodomal signs include headache, dizziness, fainting and transient focal signs lasting for days. Often the dementia is coloured by anxiety and querulous hypochondriasis. About 50 per cent start with a clouded state.

Senile dementia is a true dementia of unknown cause unrelated to poor cerebral blood flow. It is not a variant of normal ageing and the brain shows plaques of cell damage. The onset is insidious and survival beyond two years after diagnosis is exceptional as the deterioration far exceeds normal ageing.

Tumour. There is no simple rule that when applied to an organic cerebral syndrome will identify it as being caused by cerebral tumour. Obviously if there are focal signs, or if there are signs of raised intracranial pressure such as fits, vertigo, headache, nausea and papilloedema, then the diagnosis will be simpler, but in fact 30 per cent of brain tumours start in 'silent' areas and 60 per cent start with psychiatric symptoms. There is no special 'tumour' syndrome, a fact which has always to be considered when assessing any organic cerebral syndrome. Fits are usually early symptoms and often the earliest sign is personality change and memory defect; later more clear-cut organic changes appear. Two examples may illustrate the difficulty. A nineteen-year-old man was said to be 'work shy' and idle after gastro-enteritis. He gave a history of nausea and vomiting in the morning. He had early papilloedema but no focal signs. Investigation showed an extensive fronto-temporal glioma. A thirty-five-year-old housewife was treated for anxiety and depression for three years. All her symptoms went when a meningioma was removed.

Trauma. After open or closed head injury the immediate sequel is often delirium, and depending on the extent of brain damage the outcome may be permanent organic impairment. Progressive encephalopathy is found in boxers who have had repeated knock-outs (punch drunk). Subdural haematoma should not be overlooked as a cause of dementia, especially in elderly patients, alcoholics and anyone with a history of repeated head injury.

Presenile Dementia. These are rare dementias which start before age sixty, usually around forty-five to fifty-five. They include *Pick's* and *Alzheimer's* disease. These are clinically similar though the pathology is different. In Pick's disease frontal lobe signs are predominant, and the illness is probably inherited. In Alzheimer's disease the process affects the whole brain and there is a higher incidence of fits and extrapyramidal signs.

Huntington's chorea is a rare hereditary dementia (dominant). The onset is usually in the forties or fifties. Early symptoms include involuntary and choreiform movements. Neurotic or depressive symptoms are inevitably followed by dementia. Survival is rarely for longer than 10–15 years after diagnosis and the end is total helplessness and global mental deterioration.

Normal pressure hydrocephalus is a rare but increasingly recognised type of dementia. It can start spontaneously or follow injury, tumour or sub-arachnoid haemorrhage. The ventricles are dilated but there is no obstruction of CSF flow. Surgical shunt procedures may arrest the dementia.

Psychiatric Aspects of Epilepsy. Most epileptic patients need guidance, particularly when the condition is first diagnosed. This is not a matter for psychiatric intervention but is usually provided by the family doctor, the neurologist and a body such as the British Epilepsy Association.

Epileptic psychoses are typically schizophrenic in form and are associated with temporal lobe epilepsy. Psychiatric admission may be necessary. *Fugue states* may follow a series of temporal lobe fits. *Behaviour disturbance* such as episodic aggression, ecstasy or excitement may be related to temporal lobe epilepsy; a number of temporal lobe epileptics show odd or difficult behaviour which is unrelated to fits but which may be due to associated personality disorder.

Diagnosis of Organic Syndromes

The diagnosis of organic syndromes is made by eliciting the symptoms as described and by careful investigation. Depression may resemble dementia especially in old people, where slowness, forgetfulness and apathy can look like dementia. Since depression is treatable, a confident diagnosis of dementia should always have excluded depression. *Schizophrenia*, particularly late onset and paranoid states, may appear to be organic states, but apparent clouding in schizophrenia is fleeting and there are no memory or intellectual defects.

Hysteria and Personality Disorders. Here apparent organic features fade away under careful scrutiny which reveals only a superficial resemblance to organic mental states.

Treatment of Organic Mental States. If there is an underlying treatable cause, then it should be treated appropriately. Otherwise treatment is supportive and symptomatic. Tranquillisers and neuroleptics are used to calm agitated behaviour, but for the dementing patient it is mainly a question of finding the right environment for him. Family and social pressures often dictate admission.

PERSONALITY DISORDER—ABNORMAL PERSONALITY—PSYCHOPATHY

Personality has never been easy to define. In general it is used to summarise the various characteristics of an individual—in terms of his behaviour, emotional state, drive and ability to relate to others—that give to him both a resemblance to others and an individuality of his own. The concept of abnormal personality is important in psychiatry, since it provides a way of explaining and understanding persistent modes of behaviour and emotional experience that puzzle society and distress the patient and his family. Some people behave in an odd way from childhood, and their oddities may cause problems, especially if they offend moral codes or break the law in a relentless way that is not affected by punishment or 'treatment'. If they are antisocial they are called *sociopaths* or *antisocial psychopaths*. The important point is that the abnormality starts early and persists, unlike illness, which is clearly a change in feeling or behaviour. Persistent abnormality tends to be regarded as something like illness because it is inexplicable and not mere wilfulness which is unresponsive to treatment. Abnormal personalities are classified in various ways, some are quite arbitrary, others liken the disorder to psychiatric syndromes. In Britain the term *psychopath* is used to identify people who show persistently antisocial conduct, but the original use of the term related it to personality disorder pure and simple.

A popular definition is Schneider's: '. . . psychopaths are those abnormal personalities who suffer their abnormality or cause society to suffer.'

Types of abnormal personality include:

1. Inadequate personality.
2. Schizoid personality.
3. Obsessional personality.
4. Paranoid personality.
5. Histrionic personality (immature or hysterical).
6. Antisocial personality—psychopathic personality.

Inadequate Personality

This applies to people who cannot cope with life at any level. They are usually passive and submissive with a history of repeated failure at school, in work and in relationships. They drift from one job to another, are easily led and deceived. Often they are vaguely but persistently hypochondriacal and attend their doctor very frequently. They are usually feckless and may drift into minor criminality or the abuse of alcohol or drugs. Their lives are a catalogue of repeated mistakes and well-intentioned failure. They fill the ranks of recidivist offenders and often find a haven in institutional life, be it hospital or prison. Mood disturbance is labile.

Schizoid Personality

The schizoid personality has been likened to an abortive form of schizophrenia; this is offset by the fact that only 50 per cent of schizophrenics have a premorbid personality that could be fairly described as schizoid. Schizoid people are inward looking and tend to be shy, quiet, self-absorbed and withdrawn. They have usually been 'model' children, being quiet, obedient and bookish. They cannot relate easily with others and this reinforces a tendency to be seclusive and aloof. A schizoid person is emotionally cool and detached and makes a poor and unloving spouse. On the other hand their dreamy detached intellectualism may be advantageous and many go through life unscathed. If schizoid traits are marked then the person becomes a borderline psychotic who may pursue a cause with fanatical zeal and only get into difficulty if he neglects himself or adopts a crankish diet or takes hallucinogenic drugs in a search for cosmic revelation.

Obsessional Personality

Obsessional people are excessively perfectionistic and over-conscientious. Obviously to be conscientious is a valuable social trait but the obsessional personality tends to possess these traits to a degree that imposes handicap, since his exalted standards of perfection can never be attained. A moderate degree of obsessionality is useful in any professional or skilled person but when excessive it becomes a hindrance. Obsessionals make good subordinates but bad leaders. They tend to be indecisive and glum and over-concerned by bureaucratic trivia. They are often rigid in a wearisome and amusing way but are unimaginative and moralising and have little sense of fun. Their humour is dry and laboured and they suffer from guilt and self-doubt. Conscientiousness may be carried to absurd lengths; everything is listed and checked in a stultifying way. They are prone to depression and hypochondriasis, are easily upset by changes in routine and are usually loyal, diligent but rather dreary people. Their talk is larded with qualifying phrases and apology. They usually come from families where one parent has shown similar traits and where the family climate is strict with undue emphasis on self-control and keeping feelings out of sight.

Paranoid Personality

The paranoid personality is unrealistic often to the extent of being near deluded. He is suspicious, touchy and over-sensitive, and over-reacts to criticism, real or fancied. Criticism is borne hardly, something that his family or friends may sum up as a 'chip on the shoulder'. This makes it hard for him to settle in a job or relate with other people. Paranoid personalities often channel their basic sense of injustice into the support of a 'cause', but can prove to be an embarrassment to their associates by becoming fanatical. The paranoid tendency to over-value ideas and resent criticism can build up into bitter, even violent feeling. In their most extreme forms certain paranoid personalities have influenced world history in a disastrous way.

Histrionic Personality (hysterical or immature personality)

The criteria of maturity include stability, the ability to adjust to change and the ability to handle relationships in a sensible undemanding way without having to manipulate others to meet some pathological need. Mature people can accept success, failure, frustration and disappointment with relative equanimity. Immaturity is a state of emotional childishness. Children react stormily to frustration and the failure to achieve gratification of immediate needs. Growing up and maturation modify this response and encourage a state of independent self-reliance. Some never grow out of this infantile response pattern and become egocentric immature adults. They are often labelled as hysterical personalities, but the term histrionic is better since it avoids the implied but inaccurate correlation with conversion hysteria.

Histrionic people are usually emotionally labile—sudden bouts of desperate gloom pass quickly and are replaced by some capricious infatuation or enthusiasm which is dropped as quickly as it is taken up. Behaviour tends to be dramatic and the person is importunate and cannot tolerate frustration. The emotions are shallow—effuse demonstrations of feeling mean nothing and relationships with others are never stable. Sexual behaviour is often flirtatious with a façade of empty provocative eroticism.

Antisocial Personality—Psychopathic Personality

The antisocial personality presents society with many problems, mainly because of repeatedly antisocial behaviour. The psychopath seems unable to control his impulses, learn from mistakes or show any foresight about the consequences of his actions. This type of personality disorder is regarded as a form of 'sick' behaviour though it hardly conforms to a general theory of illness. The impulsiveness of the psychopath is like that of a child who flies into a rage when an immediate wish is not granted. The failure to learn from experience suggests arrested emotional development—a failure in social learning. Many have commented on the youthful appearance of certain psychopaths and on the presence of immature patterns in the E.E.G. This does not apply to all psychopaths, but suggests that at least some of them are people who have a constitutional abnormality. Another important feature of the psychopath is emotional shallowness which can extend to callous brutality.

In general the antisocial psychopath is unreliable and untruthful, with no regard for any consideration beyond his own needs. This means that he disregards laws and moral codes with a nonchalance that society finds inexplicable and sick in the sense that it requires psychiatric treatment—a dubious definition of illness. Family studies of psychopaths suggest an interplay of genetic and environmental factors. There is an increased incidence of parental alcoholism, psychosis, criminality and neglect in such families. Truancy, early institutionalisation and early delinquent behaviour all add up to a background that breeds psychopathy.

Treatment. The antisocial psychopath presents the biggest problem because of his effect on society. There is good evidence to suggest that even severe psychopathic offenders improve as they grow older. Group therapy in prison or in hospital may help the patient to some awareness of the impact of his acts on others. Also regular supervision by probation officers can provide a stabilising influence. Other personality disorders can be helped by simple psychotherapy and guidance through periods of crisis.

ANOREXIA NERVOSA

The first English description of anorexia nervosa was in the late 19th century by Sir William Gull in his observations on weight loss, food refusal and amenorrhoea in young girls.

Clinical Manifestations. Anorexia nervosa is a syndrome characterised by food refusal, severe weight loss and amenorrhoea. It is almost entirely confined to girls though cases in young men are described. It is important to stress the term 'food refusal' because usually the anorexic patient has a normal appetite, it is merely that he or she refuses to eat and adopts numerous devices to avoid it. These range from the obvious such as hiding food or throwing it away to the less obvious such as self-induced vomiting and the use of excessive purgation. Weight loss can be severe and extremely rapid leading in extreme cases to severe electrolyte depletion with dehydration and dangerously low potassium levels. The patient usually refuses food because she wants to remain as slim as possible whilst retaining an ordinary appetite but also indulging in episodic gorging. Associated with the malnutrition there may be secondary hormonal changes producing amenorrhoea and a growth of fine hair over the shoulders and back of the neck. Anorexic patients are often extremely manipulative and use every possible means to avoid eating, also they may have labile mood disturbance.

Aetiology. All the available evidence suggests that anorexia nervosa is not a unitary disorder. In rare cases there may be an underlying schizophrenic illness, a severe obsessional disorder or a depression. The majority of patients are young girls who indulge in straightforward food refusal based on a fear of being fat. Their self-image is one in which they see themselves as much fatter than they are. This can be demonstrated quite simply using linear analogue scales. It is suggested that the condition is on the increase, on the other hand it may be that it is being more readily diagnosed. Certainly it seems highly likely that there is a real increase in its incidence and a likely explanation for this is the fashionable preference for slim people. Presumably in an appropriately vulnerable individual ordinary conventional slimming gets carried to extremes ending up in a full-blown anorexic syndrome. In the past a good deal of attention has been paid to the possibility that the syndrome might be related to unconscious fears of adult female sexuality and also to conflicts with parents so that the illness becomes a way of showing barely concealed aggression towards over-bearing parents. There is no doubt that in a high percentage of cases disturbed relations with one or both parents are common but it should be realised that by the time the patient is in hospital the whole topic of the patient's food refusal has become a matter of anxiety and concern within the family so that the parents will have over-reacted to an admittedly dangerous situation. Hence it is true that Sir William Gull's original advice that the patient should be separated from the parents during treatment remains sound.

Management. A wide range of treatment methods have been tried. The main object is to overcome the patient's food refusal and get her back to a reasonable weight which she can tolerate. In severe cases the patient may require intravenous fluid and electrolyte replacement particularly when potassium levels are low. Also in severe cases feeding via a narrow nasogastric tube may be life saving. This is nowadays easily accomplished without any sort of trauma and without creating the unpleasant atmosphere of old-fashioned tube feeding. However, in the majority of cases neither of these measures is required and the basic approach to the patient consists in feeding aided by as much interaction with the nursing staff as possible. Long-term studies have quite definitely demonstrated that of all the various treatment methods tried, supervised feeding with good support and encouragement from the nursing staff the patient is the soundest treatment. Psychotropic drugs may be used to relieve tension and of these chlorpromazine is probably the most useful.

Behavioural methods have been tried with modest success. The patient is admitted to a hospital room which is stripped of everything except a bed, she is not allowed up for any reason, is presented with ordinary meals and is given a series of goals e.g. being allowed up, receiving visitors, having a radio, etc., all of which she can only achieve by eating a standard meal within a certain period of time. If the meal remains unfinished it is removed and there is as little contact between the staff and the patient as possible. Despite the extremely barren nature of this regime it has had some success but as yet it has not been shown to be superior to conventional supervised feeding with involvement of patient and understanding nurses.

Prognosis and Outcome. This is a condition with a mortality of approximately 4 per cent and the physician looking after anorexic patients has to be prepared for frequent readmissions after speedy relapses. It is customary to work out an acceptable target weight for the patient to attain and then work towards that. What is surprising is that the anorexia patient will tolerate the behavioural type regime previously mentioned with great nonchalance whereas one would expect the patient to discharge herself the same day!

PSYCHOSEXUAL DISORDERS

Introduction

Until comparatively recently doctors have been remarkably ignorant about psychosexual disorders. For no particular reason they were regarded as outside the province of the general practitioner and were left either to bewildered psychiatrists or endocrinologists. However, in recent years increased research into, and awareness of, the extent of these disorders has led the undergraduate medical student to a better understanding of them. Doctors are studying them with more interest under the impetus of research, such as that of Masters and Johnson, stimulated it may be added by public demand. The management of psychosexual disorders is not primarily a medical or psychiatric matter but one in which a variety of expertise should be available involving specialised help from psychologists with a particular interest in the problem and also by social workers and others who can offer sensible practical counselling and encouragement. However, the doctor is often the first person consulted about these problems and there are a number of basic psychosexual dysfunctions that doctors should be able to recognise—even talk about and try to treat!

The commonest psychosexual disorders are:
    (1) Erectile failure or impotence in the male
    (2) Premature ejaculation in the male

(3) Failure to achieve orgasm in the female (often unhappily in the past referred to as frigidity—an unkind term that should be dropped).

Erectile Failure

The common cause of erectile failure is straight anxiety which may have arisen through ignorance, fear, lack of experience or a first and disastrous sexual encounter. Unhappily one or two failures can make the condition become seemingly totally established thus giving the sufferer the idea that the disorder is incurable. Ninety per cent of men with erectile failure develop this because of anxiety but it should be remembered that there are important neurological causes; the most important are diabetic neuropathy and spinal cord lesions. Erectile failure from endocrine reasons also is rare but should be borne in mind. It should be mentioned that nowadays psychotropic drugs are so widely taken and many of these cause erectile failure. The list includes most of the hypnosedatives such as the barbiturates, and the commonest hypnosedative of all, alcohol taken to excess, also the benzodiazepine tranquillisers and most if not all of the tricyclic anti-depressant drugs. It can also be caused by heavy amphetamine taking and anti-hypertensive medications.

Management. It should be realised from the outset that it is quite impossible to treat erectile failure without the total co-operation of the sexual partner and in this respect most contemporary therapists start by advising both sexual partners to abstain for a set period and thereafter the male sexual potency will be regained by a wide range of techniques all having as their basis the gradual re-learning of sexual activity in a non-stress situation so that the anxious male loses his anxiety, regains his sexual drive and erectile potency. Patience is of the essence. At first encounter both partners are usually mutually resentful, distressed and very unhappy.

Premature Ejaculation

Premature ejaculation is the most treatable of the male psychosexual disorders. Here again the co-operation of the sexual partner is absolutely essential and the most successful techniques to date employ the comparatively simple method of the female partner compressing the glans penis just prior to ejaculation thus inhibiting it. In this way it is found that ejaculation can be delayed.

Failure of Female Orgasm

This used to be considered an extremely difficult topic beset as it was by terms such as frigidity, which implied in the female a sense of failure to achieve some highly idealised variety of sexual climax that left literally millions of women disappointed at what they had missed. Unhappily this sense of failure was compounded by ill-informed psychiatric opinion based on speculation. The work of Masters and Johnson and others showed that female orgasm was primarily achieved through clitoral stimulation and this simple finding has cleared the way for better management of this disorder which created a great deal of unhappiness but now, fortunately, given a good therapist and good co-operation between both sexual partners it can be relatively easily treated. Oral stimulation and mechanical aids are also important.

Sexual Deviations

Sexual deviations are hard to define. Traditionally both male and female homosexuality were regarded as sexual deviations but contemporary researches suggest that this is not so and most therapists regard male and female homosexuals as normal variants. On the other hand it is conceded that people whose sexual orientation is entirely towards their own sex frequently endure much unhappiness, as a result of guilt and fears of condemnation by society. Therefore they need sympathetic and sensible counselling to help themselves to live with their problem particularly when they are under pressure; this is especially true of the male homosexual since in the United Kingdom male homosexuality was illegal whereas female homosexuality was not. However, times and laws change, and indeed for that matter so do public attitudes. Homosexuality, i.e. a definite homosexual orientation, should be distinguished from homosexual behaviour, i.e. sexual behaviour which occurs in special situations such as in one-sex communities of one sort or another. Adolescents may experience problems of sexual identification and need delicate and sensible handling since often they suspect that they are entirely homosexual in orientation when they are not.

Fetishism is commonly regarded as a variety of sexual deviation. This means a state where a person is only able to achieve orgasm whilst stimulated in various ways beforehand. The stimuli may range from dressing up in black rubber raincoats, etc., to more bizarre garb.

Sexual deviations including the infliction of pain and cruelty on others and/or having this inflicted on the self, namely *sadism* and *masochism* are another matter altogether and are problems to be dealt with by therapists with particular interest and experience.

Transvestism or cross-dressing as it is sometimes called, implies the urge, usually in the male, to wear female clothing as a method of obtaining sexual gratification or as a preamble to sexual gratification. It is really hard to know whether this is a condition that requires treatment. At a pragmatic level one may comment that probably the criterion that determines a need for treatment is if the person is complaining about it or if the person's sexual partner finds it intolerable.

Transsexualism, that is the wish to be a person of the opposite sex, is another matter altogether. It has led to people undergoing complicated surgery, amputation of the penis, creation of an artificial vagina, breast implants, etc. Psychiatrists cannot really claim to have any great success in persuading transsexualists to change their minds. In fact one of the most striking things about the genuine transsexualist is that he, and it is usually a male, will not tolerate attempts to divert him from his chosen goal. It is to be questioned whether the extensive superficial changes that can be achieved are beneficial or ethical. No-one has as yet published a long-term follow-up of such patients. The author's experience is that transsexualism often overlies a degree of personality disorder and may also overlie a psychosis. The general practitioner will be wise to refer such patients elsewhere for further guidance and counselling.

Conclusion

In general then, psychosexual disorders are more freely spoken about nowadays than formerly. Their existence is more readily acknowledged and attempts are made to give the sufferer help. But still it must be conceded that it remains difficult for the male with erectile failure or premature ejaculation to find help but the prevalent impression is that perhaps this help is becoming more readily available.

THE DOCTOR AND MARITAL BREAKDOWN

It may seem strange to have a section entitled 'Marital Breakdown' in a textbook of medicine but it should be realised that the extent of medical practice reaches beyond the diagnosis and recognition of various obviously physical or psychological disorders. Increasingly doctors are expected, and rightly, to be able to offer advice, comfort and even counselling to people whose lives have become troubled and unhappy not only through illness of whatever sort but also where their unhappy state is related to some disharmony in their relationships within the family; clearly it is in the case of married couples and the break-up of marriage that the doctor can play a useful part. No-one is suggesting that every doctor could or should be a marriage guidance counsellor. There are well trained professionals and non-professionals whose job this is. But nevertheless, any doctor who claims to practise whole-person medicine should have more than a passing knowledge of some of the common problems in marriage that may effect the physical and psychological health of the patient.

In the first instance, marital breakdown in the United Kingdom is on the increase, the divorce rate is rising quite dramatically and particularly at risk are those people who get married between the ages of 17 and 19. Increasingly people with marital problems will consult their doctor.

The reasons for the increased rate of marital breakdown are no doubt a matter for speculation but some factors are obvious; early marriages are quite definitely at risk but after this one finds that straight incompatibility of temperament between the spouses is probably as common a cause of breakdown as any. If we add to this, boredom with the other person, failure of any sort of reasonable communication and move on towards the crises that tend to occur in the middle years of life, we have all the ingredients for the break-up of a marriage. Very often these crises of middle life may encompass on the one hand for the husband an excessive preoccupation and involvement with his work, leading him to neglect of wife and family or even his using his work as a way of avoiding a wife for whom he has grown to have little regard. On the other hand a wife may have perhaps over-identified with the rearing of the children and diverted less time and affection to her husband. More commonly than this, however, it may be that the wife is suffering from plain over-work and exhaustion in raising a family and performing all the tasks traditionally expected of the housewife even in a more liberated age. If we add possible fall-off in sexual life, backed up by sexual problems that may have existed previously, it can be seen that the middle years of marriage can be extremely threatening in terms of a potential breakdown. Another important point too is that alcohol abuse and alcoholism in men commonly reach their peak in the 40s and 50s and this disorder is probably one of the most potent wreckers of a marriage that one can recognise.

If the doctor is consulted by one or other marital partner seeking advice about marital disharmony, his course is obvious; he needs to have a full and frank discussion with both partners if possible and find out exactly what is going on. Unhappily, however, it is often the case that one marital partner consults the doctor, often initially with a complaint which may be apparently physical or psychological, but does not reveal that there is any marital problem except after some time or after direct questioning. It is often amazing the personal unhappiness and real distress that a persecuted wife may conceal from the doctor whilst repeatedly complaining about headaches, pains and aches of one sort or another, and this is something that every sympathetic doctor should constantly bear in mind. Once a patient has revealed that there are problems within the marriage, then the doctor's best course is to try and interview both marital partners to establish what exactly is the extent of their problem and preferably refer them for advice to an organisation such as a marriage guidance council. One or other marital partner may be receiving psychiatric treatment in which case it is important to ensure that the psychiatrist and social worker dealing with the family are fully aware of the marital state. In theory they should be but this is not necessarily always the case. There is one area of marital discord where the doctor's duty is very clear and definite indeed, and this is where a husband or wife has a spouse who is morbidly jealous. Morbid jealousy is a syndrome which may have an origin in paranoid psychosis but usually has an origin in paranoid personality disorder where the morbidly jealous spouse constantly accuses the other partner of fancied infidelity, usually over a period of years, and may persecute the partner in a relentless frightening way, including interrogation, physical violence and assault. It is vitally important that whenever a doctor is consulted by the victim of such persecution that he establishes as fully as possible what the extent may be since all too commonly these patients are in danger of their lives from a paranoid spouse. It is recommended that in such cases, psychiatric consultation is sought as a matter of urgency and the doctor has a direct obligation to advise the threatened spouse to take refuge away from the home when he genuinely feels that the victim's life is in danger.

MENTAL SUBNORMALITY

The basic defect of the mentally subnormal is that their intelligence level is sufficiently below the mean to prevent them from being able to lead an entirely independent existence. Like so many other words 'intelligence' is hard to define but it is generally agreed to cover innate ability, nourished by the environment. This ability encompasses learning, memory and comprehension as well as verbal and numerical ability. The diagnosis of subnormality is mainly but not entirely based on the intelligence quotient (I.Q.) which is estimated by using standardised tests of ability which have been given to representative samples of populations properly stratified by age. The average I.Q. is assumed to be 100, and scores are based on deviations from the mean scores achieved by people of similar age. Thus the I.Q. distribution follows a normal curve with the bulk of the population achieving mean scores, with geniuses at the upper end and severely subnormals at the lower end. But the I.Q. score is influenced by many other factors besides innate ability. Social and cultural deprivation are important influences as well as the emotional handicap imposed by the subject's awareness of his own deficiencies.

Bearing all this in mind, it may be difficult to see why mental subnormality is included under the rubric of psychiatry at all. The reasons are mainly historical and to some extent practical, since the mentally subnormal may develop behaviour disorders that call for psychiatric understanding. More important than this is the fact that the mentally subnormal are *frequently affected by associated disorders*. The proper recognition of this is leading slowly to the realisation that the care of the mentally subnormal is not a matter to be dealt with by herding large numbers of patients in under-staffed institutions, thus effectively cutting off any chance of improvement, but rather to be treated in a multi-disciplinary way calling on the skills of paediatricians, educational psychologists, social workers, etc., all with the object of finding out as fully as possible what may be the range of defect of the mentally subnormal.

The list of associated defects is large and includes *physical handicap*, e.g. cerebral palsy, congenital heart disease, defective vision, deafness. *Neurological* defect must also be considered, and this can range from epilepsy and pareses to specific disabilities such as dyslexia which can mimic subnormality or may be associated. *Learning disability* may be the prime handicap in subnormality—in other words the task of learning is that much more difficult for the patient. There is experimental evidence to confirm this.

Diagnosis of mental subnormality is made then after a comprehensive examination of the child.

Treatment should cover all the possible associated defects as mentioned, and in the case of a child, the general trend is to keep the child in the community using a full range of community services for the mentally handicapped—day and educational facilities and so on. Institutional care is recommended only when it offers a better chance of education, etc., which would outweigh the disadvantages of being away from home, and when the family is suffering as a result of the continued presence in the home of a severely subnormal child. The most severely handicapped subnormal patients are, however, a minority so that given adequate community resources it ought to be possible to provide local facilities for the treatment and care of the subnormal, with possibly longer stay facilities attached to district hospitals.

The Aetiology of Subnormality

Knowledge of this has expanded enormously since the discovery that Down's syndrome (mongolism) is caused by an extra autosome, i.e. trisomy 21. The list of known syndromes, caused by genetic inheritance and associated with mental subnormality, grows at such a pace that specialist works on the subject are the only source of adequate information.

Birth injury may contribute to subnormality as well as epilepsy. But after all the genetic and other causes have been excluded, there remains the bulk of the subnormals who are normal variants. Their handicap is in many ways the hardest to accept, since they are disadvantaged as it were by chance in a society that measures success by achievement and earning power. They deserve the same from society as their more fortunate fellows, and given good learning facilities and sensible consideration they can be helped to live a decent and satisfying existence.

PSYCHIATRY AND MEDICINE

It is easy to pay lip service to the notion of 'whole person' medicine, but difficult to practise it, since medical training correctly emphasises the importance of recognising and treating lethal physical illness. For this reason the psychosocial aspects of medicine tend to be studied as an afterthought. At its worst this leads to psychiatry being used as a refuse collection depot for unstudied disorders. Emotion colours all illness and emotion affects all doctors whether they care to admit it or not. Some illnesses seem to have an ill-comprehended emotional aspect and are called *psychosomatic*—a bad term which implies that any illness not so defined has no psychological aspects. Often the illnesses that have been labelled psychosomatic appear to have received the label on the rather dubious grounds that chronicity and recurrence *must* imply psychological causality. These illnesses have included rheumatoid arthritis, peptic ulcer, asthma, ulcerative colitis and hypertension. No one would deny that all of these are affected by feelings, but it is taking an unjustifiable step to assign prime importance to emotional causes. Much of medical practice is concerned with minor and self-limiting illnesses and emotional disturbances, and the effects on health of social disadvantage such as poverty, bad housing and poor education. The general population could improve their health overnight by stopping smoking, eating less, drinking less alcohol and taking more exercise. At the same time the doctor has to look out for early signs of serious illness in his patients. The conflict set up by this confusing role makes many doctors frustrated since they feel that the illnesses that were emphasised at Medical School have a higher status than common minor illness. A sharper emphasis on the psychosocial aspects of medicine will no doubt help to ease this situation.

Psychiatric Emergencies

Acute Excitement. This is a clinical situation that may occur in the home or in hospital. It is important always to establish as speedily as possible whether the cause is:

An organic brain syndrome.
Schizophrenia.
Mania.
Hostile 'acting out' by a psychopath usually intoxicated with alcohol or drugs.

There is not usually time to permit extensive examination of the mental state beyond finding out whether the patient's consciousness is clouded or not. This is vital, since it at least tells us whether or not the patient has an organic brain syndrome. All organic excitement responds to treatment of the basic illness, but in the meantime the patient needs sensible management to avoid exhaustion, etc. The patient should be approached in a calm and quiet manner and medication used effectively. Sedatives such as the barbiturates should not be used as they disinhibit the patient and make matters worse. The best medications to use are the neuroleptics such as chlorpromazine and thioradazine given by mouth or by injection. These are effective in all excited states. Nowadays it is usual to start with a tranquilliser such as diazepam by injection; this calms the patient and the neuroleptics can be given thereafter. In cases of delirium, chlormethiazole is especially valuable and is the treatment of choice in alcoholic or barbiturate delirium. Feeding and fluids plus good nursing complete the management. Saturation with vitamins—multivitamin preparations such as parentrovite—is also valuable. The acutely disturbed schizophrenic or manic patient may need to be transferred to a psychiatric unit—this is easier than formerly since more hospitals have psychiatric units or wards.

Suicide and Attempted Suicide. Successful suicides tend to be male, over forty-five, and have a history of depression and/or alcoholism, bereavement and divorce. Suicide attempts, nowadays called 'self-poisoning' tend to correlate with youth, female sex, social isolation and personality disorder. Admissions for self-poisoning are the commonest medical emergency under age thirty. Is the patient a suicidal risk? This is a common clinical problem. Assessment of a suicide risk should be left to the psychiatrist, but the student should be aware of the following:

(a) Most suicides give warning.
(b) Hypochondriasis, depression and living alone are a bad combination.
(c) Depressives with severe early-morning waking are at high risk.
(d) Alcoholism is a bad-risk condition.

Puerperal Psychosis. These are not specific psychoses but psychoses which happen to start after childbirth, and are either affective or schizophrenic. They always respond very well to neuroleptics and E.C.T.

Post-operative Psychosis. These may be organic delirious states, and if so, respond well to treatment as already outlined. Occasionally an acute affective or schizophrenic psychosis can be triggered off by surgery.

Termination of Pregnancy. The Abortion Act has ensured that unwanted pregnancy is rarely a psychiatric emergency but more a matter of psychosocial urgency. Psychiatric opinion is divided: some psychiatrists believe that there are no psychiatric grounds for terminating pregnancy and that the patient should get better with treatment and be supported through pregnancy. This is a minority view. The majority view is that termination is a reasonable way of dealing with the distress of unwanted pregnancy, particularly when there is severe mood disorder or psychosis.

Psychiatric Disorders in the Elderly

No one looks forward to growing old. The physical aspects, loss of elasticity, muscular weakness and stiffening joints are hard enough to bear. The increased risk of poor health or serious illness when for the average person good health is taken for granted is another burden of old age. In addition to this there are psychological changes in old age which do not make for a happy life. As people grow older they tend to become more rigid in outlook, tend to lose the range of emotions and drives that formerly had kept them going, and this tends to produce an impatient and intolerant reaction amongst younger people so that it is easy for the elderly person to feel progressively more lonely and rejected. Medical advances have not benefited the old as much as the young beyond the dubious advantage of prolonging life without improving its quality. In addition to this the older person is forced into senescence by having to quit work at a time when he may well be able to go on. Add to this the loss of a spouse and the departure of children, etc., and there are all the ingredients for emotional disturbance based on real loss of role and function plus relative poverty for most.

Important points to remember include:

(a) Organic cerebral syndromes in the elderly, whether caused by arteriosclerosis or senile dementia, may present as a subacute delirious state.

(b) Affective disorder is common and may be misdiagnosed as dementia, especially where the picture is one of apathy and slowness. Elderly depressives respond very well to antidepressant treatment, either E.C.T. or drugs.

(c) Paranoid states are fairly common. These may be due to late-onset schizophrenia (paraphrenia), affective disorders with paranoid colouring, or they may be paranoid reactions in a lifelong eccentric. The response to phenothiazines and anti-depressants is very good.

(d) Neuroses in the elderly are often overlooked. This group of patients too easily miss out on sympathy and understanding let alone psychiatric treatment.

ALCOHOLISM AND DRUG DEPENDENCE

Human beings have an enormous capacity for damaging themselves in the pursuit of pleasure, whether through alcohol, drugs, riding fast motor cycles or smoking heavily. In the case of alcohol and drug abuse and dependence the doctor is presented with a condoned toxin (alcohol) and a proscribed group of toxins, namely 'drugs'. The position is made more difficult by the fact that large numbers of people take drugs to excess but do not offend society, i.e. the thousands admitted to hospital annually with aspirin-induced bleeding and the thousands dependent on sedatives and tranquillisers.

Alcohol

Alcohol is condoned by society and is potentially very dangerous, but at the same time provides revenue as well as profit. Chronic alcoholism is a state in which a person is unable to control the amount he drinks and so develops physical, psychiatric and social handicap in consequence. Physical defects include malnutrition and vitamin deficiency which can cause *Wernicke's encephalopathy*, *hepatic cirrhosis*, *pancreatitis* and *gastritis*. Psychiatric disorders associated with alcoholism include depression, paranoid reactions, delirium tremens and alcoholic dementia. Severe alcoholism is not hard to diagnose, but many doctors still have a blind spot for someone whose drinking is getting out of control—a sign of impending alcoholism that is important to recognise. The signs include telling lies about alcohol intake, avoiding the topic and becoming preoccupied with having enough drink available at home on social occasions. At the same time the drinker who is losing control starts drinking earlier in the day and always has an excuse for a drink. Impending physical dependence on alcohol is established as a clinical fact when the patient experiences memory gaps and is sick and dizzy on getting out of bed. Soon he needs 'liveners' to get going in the morning and then the picture of total alcohol dependence is complete. Tolerance for alcohol varies, so that there are individual differences in dose resistance, but inevitably large amounts of alcohol taken daily have their effect and a person becomes dependent.

Drugs—Non-medical Uses

Non-medical use is a term which distinguishes casual drug abuse and dependence from therapeutic drug abuse and dependence. The former is related to the use of drugs for pleasure or to relieve distress while the latter is related to the 'accidental' discovery by a patient that a drug makes him 'high'. Drug abuse means taking a drug in a way that exceeds its proper medical use. Dependence means the development of a state in which a person has to go on taking a drug (or alcohol—itself a drug!) because he needs to get high on it or because he becomes sick if he stops. There is no need to distinguish too severely between physical and psychological dependence, except in two instances that are clinically important. The first is in the case of opiate drugs, where physical dependence usually is severe, though it presents no hazard to life. The second is in the case of alcohol/barbiturate dependence, where chronic dependence produces a state of intoxication in which acute withdrawal can cause fits which can be fatal, e.g. if vomit is inhaled.

Types of Drug Dependence

These are usually classified according to the type of drug involved. This is currently unhelpful, since the last ten years have shown that multiple drug use is likely to be the rule. A simple way of classifying the problem is to classify it as follows:

	Physical dependence	Psychological dependence
Central stimulant dependence	nil	severe
Opiate dependence	severe	severe
Alcohol/barbiturate dependence	dose-related—severe	usually severe
Hallucinogenic	nil	may be severe

Treatment of Alcoholism and Drug Dependence

In both cases the objectives are the same, namely abstinence and normal social functioning. In alcoholism, withdrawal is relatively easy and abstention is encouraged by social pressures and by the use of drugs such as disulfiram which cause severe symptoms if alcohol is taken. Patients should be encouraged to join AA (Alcoholics Anonymous), which promote abstinence through self-help and the recognition that alcohol has defeated the individual. In the case of drugs, the principles are the same except that in the case of opiate dependence physical dependence is often so bad that maintenance prescription of the drug is necessary as a social measure aimed at limiting an illicit drug traffic. With barbiturates and central stimulants (e.g. amphetamines and cocaine) prescribing the drug is quite useless and should never be practised. Withdrawal from drugs is best carried out in hospital; thereafter abstention is best encouraged by persuading the patient to enter a drug-free therapeutic community where former drug users can help him to a more realistic life style, and above all to the acceptance that a useful and satisfactory life can be lived without resorting to mind-altering drugs as a barrier between himself and reality.

PSYCHIATRY: FORENSIC ASPECTS

Law and psychiatry interrelate in many ways. Laws are made to regulate society, to control criminality and to guarantee equity and justice for all citizens. Psychiatric aspects of the law that students should know about include civil and criminal responsibility, the Mental Health Act and testamentary capacity.

Responsibility

In law it is assumed that a man is sane and responsible for his actions—he intends their result and must bear responsibility for their consequences. This is true for both criminal and civil matters. In criminal acts the law bases responsibility on *actus reus* (the guilty act) and *mens rea* (the guilty mind). Responsibility implies liability to punishment. The prosecutor has to prove the guilty act and the defence has to prove that there is no intent, i.e. no *mens rea*. Age is important—a person may be too young to form intent. Or intent may be said to be absent by reason of mental disorder. This used to be governed by the M'Naghten rules. M'Naghten was a schizophrenic who killed Sir Robert Peel's secretary, thinking he was Sir Robert, whom he believed was persecuting him. The rules said insanity was a defence if the accused was 'labouring under such a defect of reason from disease of the mind as not to know the nature and quality of the act; or if he did know it, that he did not know that what he was doing was wrong'. The rules were hard to apply and led to the legal concept of Diminished Responsibility for Homicide stated in the Homicide Act 1957, whereby a person is not convicted of murder if he 'was suffering from such abnormality of mind . . . as substantially to impair his mental responsibility'. Such a plea, if accepted, reduces the charge to manslaughter.

Civil Responsibility. Sanity and responsibility are assumed—an anomaly here is that a drunk man can make a valid will, sign a valid contract or get married as long as he is not so drunk that he does not know what he is doing.

Absolute Liability. For some offences liability is determined by scientific tests, e.g. a blood alcohol over 80 mg. per cent means unfitness to drive and loss of licence.

The Mental Health Act 1959

This is a model law which defines mental illness, subnormality and psychopathy and provides safeguards for the mentally ill against illegal detention and also guards their rights and property. Compulsory treatment is provided for in a fair and humane way. The student should be familiar with the sections dealt with in the table.

The Mental Health Act defines mental illness, psychopathic disorder and mental subnormality. Section 26 on compulsory treatment can be used only for the above, and in the case of psychopathic disorder this is only applicable under the age of 21. The Act repeals all previous laws and encourages informal admission as the ideal with compulsion as something only to be used as a last resort.

Section	Purpose	Application made by	Medical recommendation	Comment
25	Admit for observation	Nearest relative or Mental Health Officer	Two doctors, one recognised as having special experience under S.28 of Act	Lasts for 28 days
26	Compulsory treatment	As above	As above	Lasts for 1 year. Patient and family may appeal to Review Tribunal
29	Emergency admission	As above	Any doctor	Lasts for 3 days
30	To detain a patient in *any* hospital for observation		Hospital doctor (consultant)	
60	Provide compulsory treatment for offenders		Two doctors: usually prison M.O. and hospital consultant	Order is made by judge. Hospital doctor has right to discharge. Judge may recommend restriction of discharge under S.65
136	To provide facility for examination of persons 'deemed' of unsound mind in public by police officer		Police may take such a person to a 'place of safety' to be examined by M.W.O. and doctor	

Testamentary Capacity

Any one can make a valid will as long as he is of 'sound disposing mind'. Incapacity may be in question in cases of mental illness, especially organic states. The criteria for capacity are that the person should know the implications of the act of making a will, and know the extent of the estate and the likely beneficiaries. His judgement should not be impaired. Severe mental illness such as schizophrenia or dementia does not automatically make someone incapable, since there are often large islands of lucidity.

Doctors should never witness a will made by a patient, over and above the obvious bar to witnessing a will of which the doctor is a beneficiary.

PSYCHIATRIC TREATMENT

Psychiatric disorders are a collection of syndromes in which aetiology is at best only partly understood. This means that treatment is symptomatic and directed towards relief of distressing symptoms and supportive to the extent of helping the patient to adjust to his disorder and achieve the best possible social and personal functioning. In the past 20 years, there has been an enormous development in the field of psychopharmacology, i.e. the study of mind-altering drugs which have altered the whole face of psychiatry. Treatment will be reviewed under the following headings:

Psychopharmacology.
Other physical methods.
Psychological methods.
Social methods.

Psychopharmacology

Psychopharmacology is a relatively new science which is concerned with the structure and mode of action of drugs that alter the mental state. These drugs can be broadly classified as *psychotropic* drugs in that they alter feeling, behaviour and perception without any significant change in consciousness, unlike sedatives and hypnotics which produce an altered mental state by dulling consciousness. The study of psychopharmacology has opened up many questions about the relationship between brain biochemical activity and behaviour.

The study of the *biochemical aspects of psychiatric disorders* is not easy, mainly because the methods involved are relatively crude; nevertheless psychotropic drug activity has stimulated enquiry and suggested such possibilities as the **cerebral amine theory of depression.** Central transmitting substances in the brain appear to play a definite role in affective disorder. The substances concerned are the cerebral amines, noradrenaline, 5-hydroxytryptamine (5HT or serotonin) and dopamine. These amines are found in high concentrations in the hypothalamus and brain stem and are also stored in central neurone endings. The theory is that amine depletion causes depression and excess causes mania. Tricyclic antidepressant drugs probably act by blocking the reabsorption of free amines while monoamine oxidase inhibitors (M.A.O.I.'s) probably act by preventing oxidative deamination, thus increasing amine concentrations.

Schizophrenia. It is postulated that an abnormal transmitting substance —possibly hallucinogenic—could be produced in people with a constitutional biochemical defect, and thus lead to a self-perpetuating psychosis.

Deficiency states as in *myoedema, vitamin* B_{12}, *pellagra* (niacin and its precursor tryptophan) and *Wernicke's encephalopathy* (thiamine) are all examples of deficiency states that can cause a wide range of psychiatric symptoms.

Electrolyte disturbance may well play a part in affective disorder where change in sodium transfer across cell membranes may trigger off mania or depression.

Hallucinogenic and Amphetamine drugs can all produce psychoses, often severe and very similar in form to schizophrenia.

The main **psychotropic** drugs include

Neuroleptics: Antipsychotic drugs—used to calm psychotic agitation and hallucinosis.

Tranquillo-sedatives: Tranquillisers or anxiolytic drugs.

Antidepressants: These act on the biochemistry of depression.

Lithium: This is used in affective disorders.

Psychedelic drugs, e.g. hallucinogenic drugs. Rarely used in treatment but have stimulated research into the biochemistry of schizophrenia.

Neuroleptics. Interest in this large group of drugs started in 1952 when Delay and Deniker demonstrated the antipsychotic activity of chlorpromazine. In general the neuroleptics slow psychomotor over-activity, damp down feeling and block hallucinosis. This is probably related to their ability to diminish C.N.S. arousal via the reticular activiting system. There is little or no alteration in consciousness, and for these reasons the neuroleptics are most valuable antipsychotic drugs. They include:

- (a) Phenothiazines.
- (b) Rauwolfia derivatives.
- (c) Butyrophenones.
- (d) Thioxanthines.

There are many drugs in the neuroleptic group. Here only the most commonly used will be included.

(a) *Phenothiazines*

Drug	Dose (daily or as stated)	Side effects	Comment
Chlorpromazine	75–400 mg.	Rashes, hypotension, dizziness, dry mouth. Extrapyramidal symptoms. Jaundice. Blood dyscrasias.	The most widely used neuroleptic.
Thioradazine	30–600 mg.	Similar to chlorpromazine but less common.	Has an antidepressant effect.
Pericyazine	20–90 mg.	Extra-pyramidal effects common.	Valuable in aggressive behaviour. Also in chronic pain when combined with amitryptiline.

| Trifluoperazine | 3–40 mg. | Restlessness and extra-pyramidal symptoms. Insomnia. | Has an alerting effect. Used in inert schizophrenics. |
| Fluphenazine Decanoate | 25 mg. once a month by injection | Extra-pyramidal symptoms. Depression. | Very useful for patients difficult with medication. |

The phenothiazines are most effective in the treatment of schizophrenia, in which they calm excitement and enable the patient to remain in better contact with reality. They are also useful in calming organic excitement and in alcohol and drug withdrawal. They should not be used to render a patient so inert that he is deprived of feeling.

(b) *Rauwolfia Derivatives*
Reserpine is a potent antipsychotic drug but its use has been discarded in favour of the phenothiazines because it tends to cause intractable depression among other side effects.

(c) *Butyrophenones*
Haloperidol is the most widely used drug in this group. It is quickly absorbed and slowly excreted so that a twice daily dose is effective (up to 15 mg. daily). Extrapyramidal side effects are common. It is mainly used to calm manic excitement.

(d) *Thioxanthines*
These are a relatively undeveloped group of antipsychotic drugs—Chlorprothixene is the most widely used.

Tranquillo-sedatives (Anxiolytic or minor tranquillisers). This group is the most widely used psychotropic medication. They calm the anxious patient very effectively, though their precise indications and activity have not been so clearly demonstrated as compared with the neuroleptics and antidepressants.

The most widely used are the benzodiazopenes:

Chlordiazepoxide	15–100 mg. daily.
Diazepam	6–40 mg. daily.
Oxazepam	45–120 mg. daily.

They are believed to act on the limbic system. They cause little drowsiness and have valuable anti-convulsant effects. Excessive doses cause drowsiness, ataxia and dysarthria, and fits can occur in abrupt withdrawal. They are widely used in anxiety, in alcohol and drug withdrawal and in psychosomatic disorders. Intravenous diazepam is the treatment of choice in status epilepticus and in any state of wild uncontrolled behaviour.

Antidepressants

Tricyclic Antidepressants. These are the most widely used, the safest and the most effective antidepressants. Their use has all but replaced E.C.T., which is now given only to suicidally depressed patients. The most common tricyclics are:

Name	Daily dose	Comment
Imipramine	75–150 mg.	The first tricyclic. Imipramine and amitryptiline are the most effective tricyclics so far.
Nortryptiline	75–150 mg.	Some stimulant action.
Protryptiline	15–45 mg.	Some stimulant action.
Iprindole	45–90 mg.	Some stimulant action.
Amitryptiline	75–200 mg.	Sedative action.
Trimipramine	75–150 mg.	Sedative—often given in one dose at night.
Dothiepin	75–150 mg.	

General Comments on the Tricyclics

(a) They tend to take up to three weeks to act, though iprindole may act more quickly.

(b) Sedative or stimulant side effects may be used appropriately depending on whether the patient is anxious or anergic.

(c) They can impair concentration—patients should thus be warned.

(d) Atropine-like side effects are common, viz. dry mouth, constipation and delayed micturition. Use cautiously in old people. Contra-indicated in glaucoma and prostatic enlargement.

(e) Recent research suggests that adequate blood levels can be achieved with a once-daily dose.

(f) There is no merit in using two tricyclics at once. They should not be combined with M.A.O.I.'s.

(g) Interaction with hypotensive drugs and sympathomemetic agents.

Monoamine Oxidase Inhibitors. These were the first anti-depressants. There are probably a number of monoamine oxidases. This accounts for their uncertainty of action. Widely used in phobic anxiety and neurotic depression. They include:

Isocarboxazid	20–30 mg. daily.
Phenelzine	30–45 mg. daily.
Tranylcypromine	20–30 mg. daily.

Side effects. These can be serious and limit their usefulness.

(a) They potentiate sedatives, alcohol, narcotics and anaesthetics.

(b) Hypertensive crises occur if the patient eats foods that contain tyramine. The resulting flood of noradrenaline causes severe headache, collapse and intracerebral haemorrhage. The prohibited foods include cheese, yeast and beef extracts, broad-bean pods and certain red wines.

Lithium. Lithium has a mood-stabilising activity, and is used in manic-depressive disorders. It should only be used by experts since it is highly toxic; serum lithium estimations are the only way of monitoring therapy.

General Remarks on Psychotropic Drugs

(a) All psychotropic drugs are powerful. Dosage levels should always be kept at the minimal effective dose.

(b) Interaction with alcohol is common—patients should be warned of this.

(c) A good rule is to use one drug at a time, rarely two and never three.

(d) Patients on M.A.O.I.'s should carry a card with the drug dose and a list of food and drugs to avoid.

(e) Weight gain on tricyclics can be very heavy—this puts people off taking them.

Other Physical Methods

Electroconvulsive treatment or E.C.T. consists of inducing a fit by passing a 100 volt A.C. current across the head. This is done using thiopentone anaesthesia and muscle relaxants to avoid muscle or bone damage. It is used in affective disorders, where it can be life saving, and to a limited extent in schizophrenia.

Psychosurgery involving leucotomy, i.e. dividing connections between the frontal lobes and the thalamus, tends to be used in cases where patients are in states of chronic tension either through chronic depression or obsessional disorder.

Psychological Methods

Psychotherapy. All psychotherapy is based on the assumption that free communication between therapist and patient will encourage the relief of pent-up feelings and the uncovering of areas of conflict that will help the patient to solve problems and achieve a better level of self awareness and insight. Psychotherapy may be individual, i.e. on a one-to-one basis, and here the relationship between therapist and patient is of prime importance, since the patient will come to invest the situation and the therapist with a good deal of feeling which the therapist will have to handle in a mature and sensible way.

Group therapy is used increasingly, particularly in alcoholism and for personality disorders, since the group provides a good situation for people to learn to accept responsibility for themselves and their actions. In a sense psychotherapy remains the model of psychiatric treatment, since the term implies at least an acknowledgement that one person can influence another's behaviour and feelings beyond reassurance, counselling and advice. The philosophical assumption that underlies this notion has been questioned by those who envisage the human being as a set of mechanical systems driven by chance more than by choice and motivation, and this theory is no doubt given much support by the fact that patients improve spontaneously and under the influence of psychotropic drugs. On the other hand the equation drug+patient = recovery, is likely to be drug+patient+therapist = recovery, so that no doctor should undervalue the power of suggestion plus simple kindness as being potent therapeutic influences in recovery. Any doctor who attempts to practise medicine as a purely intellectual exercise neglects this aspect to the detriment of his patients.

Behaviour Therapy. The behaviour therapy model of treatment starts from the assumption that neurotic disorders and possibly psychotic disorders are learned maladaptive responses which can be relieved by a process of re-education based on Pavlovian theory.

In practice this means that maladaptive responses, i.e. neurotic symptoms, are removed by a process that involves desensitising the patient from the trigger stimulus. In these theoretical terms symptoms have no symbolic nor dynamic significance. This means that symptom removal removes the disorder. Behaviour therapy has to date been found to be of most value in the treatment of phobic states.

Social Methods. Psychiatric disorders do not exist in a social vacuum. The impact of social factors in colouring illness and in triggering it off are only being more clearly appreciated. The simplest example of this is the effect of prolonged institutionalisation on chronic mental hospital patients who become docile, passive and inert under the influence of custodial care which denies them freedom of choice and responsibility for their actions under the guise of concern for their welfare—a sort of benign dictatorship of the sick and ineffectual. The recognition of this has led to a greater awareness of the potent effect of social forces on people who are too weak or too disadvantaged to resist them. The psychiatric social worker is a therapist who sees mental illness in terms of sociological theory, and ideally should be a member of a therapeutic team who functions on terms of professional parity with the psychiatrist. The same is true, in an ideal situation, of the psychologist—too many medical students still are led to believe that the psychologist functions as a tester of mental function. There is to date no corner on expertise in the treatment of people whom society judges to be mentally ill, the doctor's only area of absolute expertise is in the recognition of and treatment of organic cerebral syndromes—in itself the most useful contribution that the doctor can make to a multi-disciplinary approach to the treatment of people who present with a wide range of distressing symptoms.

FURTHER READING

Freedman, A. M. and Kaplan, J. L., *Comprehensive Textbook of Psychiatry,* Williams and Wilkins, 2nd edition Baltimore, 1975.

Masters, William H. and Johnson, Virginia E., *Human Sexual Response* (1966), *Human Sexual Inadequacy,* Little, Brown and Co., Boston, 1970.

Slater, E. and Roth, M., *Clinical Psychiatry,* 3rd edition, Baillière Tindall and Cassell, London, 1969.

CHAPTER THREE

THE ALIMENTARY SYSTEM

SYMPTOMS OF ALIMENTARY DISORDERS

1. Pain

There is still no general agreement either about the mechanism of abdominal pain or its classification. Following the observations of Kellgren, who showed that human volunteers could distinguish only two types of pain, a superficial variety elicited by stimulation of the skin and subcutaneous tissues and a deep variety felt when any structure deep to the subcutaneous tissues was stimulated, doubt has been cast on the validity of the traditional classification of abdominal pain into visceral and somatic types. Furthermore, the description of pain given by patients with visceral and somatic lesions, such as carcinoma of the stomach and retroperitoneal sarcoma, often fails to provide any distinguishing clue.

Nevertheless, certain types of pain are sufficiently characteristic to be of great value in diagnosis. *Colic*, originally pain arising in the colon, is a term now applied to painful spasm in any hollow muscular viscus, usually due to partial or complete obstruction of its lumen. Intestinal colic is a spasmodic pain, coming in a succession of waves which rise to a peak of intensity and then subside; renal and biliary colic, however, may persist at a steady and very severe level for an hour or more. The patient doubles up or writhes about when it is at its height and warmth applied to the abdomen helps to relieve it. There may be associated vomiting. Colic is usually poorly localised, but small intestine spasm is felt mainly in the centre of the abdomen, large intestine colic in the lower abdomen, renal colic in the loin radiating to the groin and testicle on the same side, bilary colic in the right upper quadrant or epigastrium sometimes radiating through to the back, and uterine colic in the lower abdomen.

Pain due to inflammation of the parietal peritoneum, on the other hand, is a sharp steady severe pain accurately localised over the site of the inflammation. Pressure on the area causes tenderness and reflex spasm in the overlying muscles (guarding or rigidity) and since the pain is aggravated by movement the patient usually lies quite still.

Patients with acute appendicitis provide a good illustration of these two types of pain. In the early stages when there is obstruction and consequent spasm in the appendix the patient has colicky pain vaguely referred to the area around the umbilicus, and he frequently vomits at the outset; but in a few hours, when inflammation has developed in the appendix and spread to involve the parietal peritoneum, the pain becomes sharper and shifts to the right iliac fossa directly over the site of the lesion.

Pain and tenderness occur in the liver only when its capsule is acutely stretched by sudden distension of the organ, as in congestive cardiac failure; and in the spleen when there is inflammation in its peritoneal covering, as by an infarct extending to the surface. The mechanism of pain in peptic ulcer is considered on p. 68.

2. Vomiting

Vomiting is produced by compression of the stomach between the muscles of the abdominal wall and the diaphragm, with simultaneous relaxation of the cardiac sphincter and reverse peristalsis in the stomach and oesophagus. The causes are very numerous, but fall into a few main groups:

(a) When due to *intra-abdominal disease* it is usually preceded by nausea. In pyloric obstruction the vomiting may be projectile, the gastric contents being ejected from the patient's mouth with great force, and frequently very large quantities of vomit are produced containing recognisable food taken many hours previously. In intestinal obstruction the reverse peristalsis throughout the gut may eventually cause faeculent vomiting.

(b) *Cerebral vomiting* occurs in patients with raised intracranial pressure and there is often no preceding nausea. Labyrinthine disturbances are also common causes of vomiting, as in patients with acute vertigo or travel sickness.

(c) *Psychological vomiting* is also common. Some people vomit from sudden fear or horror, as for example if they see an accident in the street; others do so for less obvious and more deep-seated psychological reasons. Repeated persistent vomiting without loss of weight is nearly always of this type.

3. Heartburn

A burning pain behind the sternum is a symptom common in many alimentary disorders and is therefore not very helpful in diagnosis. It is perhaps most commonly found in patients with peptic oesophagitis due to gastro-oesophageal regurgitation; these patients may also have *acid regurgitation*, complaining that from time to time a bitter-tasting fluid rises up into the throat.

4. Waterbrash

Waterbrash is filling of the mouth with a tasteless fluid (saliva) and nearly always indicates the presence of a duodenal ulcer.

5. Diarrhoea

(a) *Acute diarrhoea* is usually due to dietetic indiscretion, food poisoning, infections such as bacillary dysentery, or an exacerbation in one of the causes of chronic diarrhoea.

(b) *Chronic diarrhoea* occurs:

(1) after operations such as gastrectomy and vagotomy,
(2) from lesions of the small intestine such as regional ileitis (Crohn's disease) and the malabsorption syndromes,
(3) in diseases of the colon, such as carcinoma, diverticulitis, amoebiasis and ulcerative colitis.

Apart from alimentary disorders such as the above, chronic diarrhoea may be due to general causes, such as thyrotoxicosis or anxiety neurosis.

6. Constipation

Many men and nearly all women when asked about their bowels reply that they have always tended to be rather constipated. They mean that instead of having a daily bowel action, which the patent medicine advertisements have taught them is essential for normal health, their bowels move only once every two or three days. They have therefore fallen into the habit of taking a purgative every day or once or twice a week, and they believe that continuing with this ritual is essential to their well-being. In fact, however, variations in the normal rhythm of the colon are quite wide, and to evacuate the bowel twice a week is not constipation; it may be just as normal and healthy as to evacuate it twice a day. On the other hand, the taking of regular evacuants seldom does any actual harm and when a patient with a lifelong dependence on one of them comes into hospital with an organic complaint, undoubtedly the most sensible plan is to continue prescribing his usual laxative. The time is not appropriate to attempt re-education of bowel function, which in any case would be most unlikely to succeed.

Normal regular movement of the bowels is not to be expected in febrile dehydrated patients who are taking little or no solid food and a dose of cascara or senna or a simple enema every few days is all that is needed. Greater care must be taken to ensure a regular evacuation in weak, elderly patients, in whom impaction of a mass of faeces in the rectum tends to occur.

Dyschezia is constipation due to functional sluggishness of the bowel, due mainly to persistent failure to answer the call to stool. It is treated by patient re-training of a regular bowel habit, helped in the early stages by a mild aperient such as senna or by glycerine suppositories.

THE MOUTH AND THROAT

Inspection of the mouth and throat in a good light is an essential part of every medical examination for, apart from purely local conditions which will not be discussed here, it occasionally reveals evidence of some general disorder.

Furring of the tongue is too common to be of much help in diagnosis and is often seen in smokers who are in good health. The 'black hairy tongue' due to alteration in the normal flora of the mouth is mainly seen in patients who have been treated with broad spectrum antibiotics. The thickly coated tongue and uriniferous breath of the uraemic patient contrast sharply with the clean dry tongue and sweetish ketotic breath of the severe diabetic.

Atrophy of the filiform papillae of the tongue, making the normal velvety surface smooth and shiny, is seen in *iron deficiency*, when it appears first round the edge of the tongue; in *vitamin B_{12} deficiency*, when it is usually first seen on the dorsum; in *riboflavin and nicotinic acid deficiency*, in this country usually the result of some intestinal disorder and sometimes associated with cracking at the angles of the mouth; and occasionally after the oral administration of antibiotics.

Brown pigmentation on the lips and on the buccal mucosa lining the cheeks is an important sign of Addison's disease, but is also seen in normal people of mixed racial origin.

Sloughing ulceration of the mouth and throat is an important sign of agranulocytosis and acute leukaemia and in the monocytic variety of the latter disease there may also be swelling and infiltration of the gums and occasionally of the tongue.

THE OESOPHAGUS

Peptic Oesophagitis

The squamous epithelium of the oesophagus is not designed to resist the digestive action of acid gastric juice and it frequently becomes inflamed and eroded in patients with gastro-oesophageal reflux. Such reflux occurs particularly, but not exclusively, in association with hiatus hernia. It should be noted too that other patients with hiatus hernia, with or without radiologically demonstrable reflux, suffer no ill-effects whatever.

Two important *symptoms* may arise from peptic oesophagitis. The commoner is *substernal pain*, similar in quality and distribution to angina pectoris; it is brought on, however, not by effort but by positions which encourage gastro-oesophageal reflux, mainly lying flat and stooping after a meal. The second symptom is *bleeding*, rarely presenting as haematemesis but sometimes causing severe and at first obscure anaemia.

Diagnosis. *Barium meal* examination in the Trendelenburg position demonstrates the gastro-oesophageal reflux and usually an associated hiatus hernia and the inflammation and erosion of the oesophageal mucosa can be confirmed by *oesophagoscopy*. Reproduction of the pain by introducing 0·1N hydrochloric acid into the lower oesophagus (*Bernstein's test*) or even by drinking a hot cup of tea is useful confirmatory evidence.

Treatment. (1) *Medical.* Most patients can be treated successfully by a simple regime designed to minimise gastro-oesophageal reflux and to neutralise any gastric acid which finds its way into the gullet. These ends are achieved by sleeping in a 'head up' position, either well propped up on pillows or with the head of the bed blocked, by avoiding stooping, and by taking small frequent meals. A tablet of Gaviscon chewed and washed down with water after meals and at bedtime helps by forming a mechanical barrier to reflux at the cardia.

(2) *Surgical* repair of the oesophageal hiatus in the diaphragm usually gives excellent results in those patients in whom severe symptoms persist in spite of a reasonable trial on the above regime.

Achalasia of the Cardia

Achalasia of the cardia is due to a disorder of motor function of the oesophagus. Essentially there is an absence of peristalsis through the lower two-thirds of the oesophagus and a failure of the cardia to relax. Normal peristalsis may be replaced by slow ring-like contractions. The oesophagus becomes dilated and its muscle wall is hypertrophied. Because it cannot empty properly the oesophagus may contain food residue. In severe cases these residues may spill over into the lungs to produce recurrent attacks of pneumonia.

Achalasia of the cardia is due to degeneration of the cells of Auerbach's plexus. This is most marked in the dilated portion of the oesophagus and results in denervation of the oesophageal muscle. At the cardia some innervation appears to persist, but it seems likely that the nerves which cause relaxation of the cardia have disappeared.

Clinical Features. Achalasia of the cardia may occur at any age, but is more common in middle age and in women. The chief symptoms are *dysphagia* and *regurgitation*. They may be gradual in onset or may start suddenly, sometimes following an emotional upset. The dysphagia is often worse when the patient is emotionally upset or worried. In the early stages of the disease radiographic examination with a barium swallow will show delay at the cardia and often considerable oesophageal activity in the form of spasm and ring contraction, but no proper peristalsis. Some patients complain of discomfort behind the sternum when the oesophagus becomes distended with food. X-ray of the oesophagus in advanced cases shows it to be grossly dilated and filled with food residue; when the level of barium in the oesophagus reaches a certain level the cardia opens momentarily to let a little through into the stomach. It is at this stage that spill-over into the lungs occurs and the patient develops recurrent attacks of pneumonia which may finally lead to severe lung damage. Other complications include the development of carcinoma of the oesophagus and of multiple arthritis. In the early stages of achalasia of the cardia the patient's general health remains remarkably good and there is no weight loss. When the condition becomes more severe weight loss may occur.

Treatment. Inhalation of octyl nitrite relaxes the cardia, but this effect lasts for only one or two minutes and treatment giving more permanent relief is always needed. Dilatation with an instrument such as the Starke dilator, which causes forcible rupture of muscle fibres at the cardia, is often very effective. If this fails, or if the gullet is obviously dilated, cardiomy-otomy (Heller's operation) should be performed. Results are excellent except in patients with gross dilatation and tortuosity of the gullet who require more extensive surgical procedures.

Carcinoma of the Oesophagus

This condition, which is much commoner in men than in women, should be suspected in any patient of middle age or beyond who develops dysphagia. The growth may occur in any part of the oesophagus and usually, though not invariably, the patient can indicate fairly accurately the level at which his food appears to stick. The dysphagia is steadily progressive, so that whereas at first there is difficulty only in swallowing solid food such as meat, within a month or two semi-solids and eventually fluids are affected also. The other striking symptom is rapid loss of weight.

Diagnosis. Barium swallow shows an area of narrowing which is rigid and may be irregular. Oesophagoscopy enables a biopsy to be taken for histological confirmation of the diagnosis.

Treatment. In general the prognosis is extremely bad, but carcinoma at the lower end of the oesophagus can occasionally be successfully resected. Alternatively, a Mousseau-Barbin tube, inserted at operation, may delay complete obstruction in swallowing for a month or two. Radiotherapy is usually ineffective, but occasional palliation of symptoms occurs after use of the supervoltage techniques available with the linear accelerator or cobalt unit.

THE STOMACH AND DUODENUM

Acute Gastritis

Acute gastritis is due to an irritant such as excessive alcohol or food poisoning, or occasionally to an acute specific infection such as influenza. The symptoms are loss of appetite, nausea, vomiting and abdominal discomfort; diarrhoea often occurs too, due to an associated enteritis. The vomited material is occasionally blood-stained. The symptoms subside spontaneously within a few days and usually all that is needed in the way of treatment is to keep the patient warm and comfortable and avoid any further irritation of his stomach. Occasionally, however, severe haematemesis necessitating transfusion occurs from acute superficial gastric erosions; sometimes these follow the taking of aspirin, of which even the soluble forms are common causes of minor gastric bleeding, but more often the aetiology is unknown.

Chronic Gastritis

Although chronic gastritis is a diagnostic label frequently attached to middle-aged and elderly patients with dyspeptic symptoms, it has no clear-cut pathology or clinical picture. The best-known variety is that due to chronic alcoholism. The patient complains of loss of appetite and nausea, particularly in the early morning, and frequently vomits mucus which has collected in the oesophagus and stomach during the night. He does not feel well until he has had another drink or two and so the vicious circle goes on. The only treatment of any value is complete and permanent abstention from alcohol.

PEPTIC ULCER

Peptic ulcers may be acute or chronic. They occur in the lower oesophagus, stomach or duodenum, or occasionally in the upper jejunum or at a gastro-enterostomy stoma.

Acute ulcers cause little in the way of symptoms and are seldom diagnosed unless they cause serious bleeding or perforation. They usually heal rapidly but often recur. Aspirin is a gastric irritant and may cause superficial gastric erosions which bleed.

Chronic peptic ulcers nearly all occur in the stomach or duodenum; when they co-exist the gastric ulcer usually develops second. A hereditary factor in gastric and duodenal ulcer has long been suspected from their frequent occurrence in several members of a family; furthermore, both types of ulcer have a higher incidence in persons of blood group O and are also more common in those who are unable to secrete their blood group substances in the saliva and gastric juice. This is a genetically determined factor; non-secretors number about 20 per cent of the general population and 30–35 per cent of the ulcer population.

Patients with duodenal ulcer as a group have twice as many parietal cells in their gastric mucosa as healthy people or patients with gastric ulcer and in general the further an ulcer is from the cardia the more hydrochloric acid is secreted by the stomach. Patients with duodenal ulcer also secrete more pepsin and have a tendency to nocturnal hypersecretion of acid. Gastric ulcers on the other hand tend to be associated with a low or normal acid secretion and with a gastric mucosa affected histologically by chronic gastritis; whether the latter is cause or effect is not known.

Chronic peptic ulcers occur at any age but are particularly common in middle life; gastric ulcers tend to arise in rather older people than duodenal ulcers. The sex incidence of gastric ulcers is almost equal; duodenal ulcers are 3–4 times more common in men than in women. In Western countries gastric and duodenal ulcers now seem to be significantly more common in poor people. There is no firm evidence to show that psychological factors, physique or personality are important in the cause of ulcer, but anxiety, overwork and stress of various kinds often lead to exacerbation of symptoms.

The increased incidence of duodenal ulcer in patients on renal dialysis is probably due to defective removal of circulating gastrin, and in patients with hyperparathyroidism to increased gastrin release induced by hypercalcaemia.

Oesophageal peptic ulcers arise in patients with hiatus hernia and gastro-oesophageal reflux. **Stomal ulcers** are particularly common in patients with gastro-enterostomy in whom no procedure to reduce acid secretion, such as

vagotomy, has been performed. **Upper jejunal ulcers,** usually at the duo-
deno-jejunal flexure, are associated with gross hypersecretion of gastric
juice, which is produced continually at a maximal rate. This is the Zollinger-
Ellison syndrome (p. 76).

Clinical Features. The principal and often the only symptom is *pain*,
which is usually accurately localised to the centre of the epigastrium. It has
two very characteristic features. The first is its *time-relation to food*:
duodenal ulcer typically causes a hunger pain, which comes on when the
stomach is empty and is relieved by the taking of food; in gastric ulcer
the timing is often less regular, but the pain tends to come on about half to
one hour after meals. The pain of duodenal ulcer often wakes the patient
up about 2 a.m., but curiously there is seldom pain before breakfast.
Though typically localised to the epigastrium, the pain is occasionally
referred to the lower abdomen, to the chest or to the back. The second
very characteristic feature is the *periodicity*. Apart from treatment the
history invariably tells of remissions, with complete freedom from symptoms for weeks or months, and subsequent relapses which are particularly
liable during the winter months.

Mechanism of the Pain. For many years there has been debate between
those who believe that the pain is due to spasm and those who ascribe it to
irritation of the ulcer by acid, but neither of these theories is entirely
satisfactory. It has been shown that pain is dependent on the presence of
acid in the stomach, but it is also dependent on inflammation in the ulcer.
From time to time a chronic peptic ulcer becomes inflamed and sensitive
and at these times the action of acid, and other stimuli, cause pain; at other
times they do not, even though the ulcer is still demonstrable by X-ray or
gastroscope. The cause and mechanism of these episodes of inflammation
constitute one of the basic unsolved problems of the disease. It is clear,
however, that the state of tone in the stomach and duodenum and the
acidity of their contents are largely incidental in the production of pain
and that the administration of antispasmodics and antacids at times when
the ulcer is in a quiescent phase is unlikely to serve any useful purpose.

Other symptoms including vomiting, a common event in patients with
severe pain, when it is followed by relief, and in those with pyloric obstruction from either spasm or cicatricial stenosis; and waterbrash, or the filling
of the mouth with tasteless watery saliva.

Physical signs are of minor importance. The 'pointing sign' is probably
the most helpful: the patient when asked where his pain is places his finger
tip on the centre of the epigastrium. There may also be some epigastric
tenderness.

Diagnosis depends on *barium meal* screening of the patient by an
experienced radiologist. The great majority of gastric ulcers occur in the
middle third of the lesser curvature and are quite easily demonstrated
in profile as a niche projecting from this aspect of the stomach. Ulcers
occur only in the first part of the duodenum, referred to by the radiologist
as the duodenal bulb or cap, and are much more difficult to demonstrate,

being identified with certainty in little more than half the cases. They are more often seen *'en face'* than in profile, appearing as a round pool of barium a millimetre or two in diameter surrounded by a clear halo, and sometimes mucosal rugae can be seen radiating from this area. Frequently, however, the only signs are irregularity, irritability and tenderness of the duodenal cap.

Endoscopy. With a modern instrument employing fibre-optics, ulcers (or other lesions) in the stomach or duodenum can be directly seen, and if necessary a biopsy may be taken, so that this is a very helpful examination when the diagnosis remains in doubt.

Tests for occult blood in the stools are usually positive in patients with active peptic ulcer.

Complications

(1) **Haemorrhage.** Slight bleeding always takes place from the raw surface, but if the ulcer is a deep one it may erode into an artery in the wall of the stomach or duodenum and lead to massive haemorrhage. The patient may vomit a large quantity of blood (this is a *haematemesis*) and it is obvious at once that serious bleeding is in progress, but if the blood goes the other way down through the intestines the diagnosis must be made first on the signs of internal haemorrhage and later on the appearance of a large amount of altered blood in the stools making them black and tarry. The latter event is a *melaena*. Internal haemorrhage should be suspected in any patient who complains of sudden faintness and is found on examination to be pale and sweating, with a fast thready pulse and a low blood pressure.

(2) **Perforation** is the most dangerous complication and is almost confined to men. The discharge of acid gastric or duodenal contents into the peritoneal cavity causes severe generalised abdominal pain and board-like rigidity of the abdominal muscles. The patient lies quite still, because any movement aggravates his pain, and he shows signs of shock (pallor, sweating, fast pulse and low blood pressure). The diagnosis is usually easily made from this striking clinical picture and emergency operation to close the perforation should be done without delay.

(3) **Pyloric stenosis** is a complication of ulcer in the duodenum or rarely in the pyloric canal itself and results from contraction of scar tissue laid down in the base of the ulcer. In many patients, however, the syndrome of pyloric obstruction is due mainly to spasm in association with an active ulcer and clears up as the ulcer heals. Obstruction at the pylorus leads to distension of the stomach, which is evacuated from time to time by vomiting, which is often copious and projectile; and if the vomit contains recognisable articles of food, such as tomato skins, known to have been eaten many hours previously, this provides clear evidence of delay in gastric emptying. Patients with pyloric stenosis lose weight and become dehydrated and the alkalosis resulting from loss of hydrochloric acid may lead to tetany, either overt (carpo-pedal spasm) or latent (positive Chvostek and

Trousseau's signs). The only satisfactory treatment for pyloric stenosis is gastro-enterostomy.

(4) **Hour-glass stomach** is the result of scarring from a chronic lesser curve ulcer and is usually simply an incidental X-ray finding. It is nearly always seen in women and is now rare.

Treatment of Peptic Ulcer
(1) Medical Treatment

(a) **Gastric Ulcer.** Bed-rest in hospital and giving up smoking have both been shown to accelerate healing of gastric ulcers. A similar effect has been shown in ambulant patients treated with carbenoxelone 100 mg. t.d.s.; this drug may cause fluid and salt retention, however, and these patients, particularly if elderly, should have their blood pressure and weight checked weekly. An increase in weight of 2 kg. or more is an indication for adding a thiazide diuretic and Slow K to the regime.

Milky diets and antacids do not promote ulcer healing, but may help to relieve symptoms. There is no known way of reducing the incidence of relapse.

(b) **Duodenal Ulcer.** Symptoms nearly always clear up after a few days of bed rest, but whether rest also promotes healing remains unproven. It seems wise to prohibit smoking, even though improved healing of duodenal ulcer has not been shown. Special diets do not influence the course of the disease, but when symptoms are severe the patient will be more comfortable if he takes small meals (avoiding items which he knows from experience are likely to upset him) and has a milky drink last thing at night and half-way between the main meals.

The histamine H2 receptor antagonist cimetidine may become the drug of first choice for duodenal ulcer; it gives symptomatic relief and promotes healing. It is given in doses of 200 mg. t.d.s. with 400 mg. at bedtime for at least one month and subsequently 400 mg. may be given at night to prevent relapse.

Anticholinergic drugs may be given to reduce gastric acid output; they do not promote healing, but some physicians believe they help to reduce pain and possibly the relapse rate. Poldine (Nacton) is a satisfactory preparation, the initial dose of 2 mg. four times daily being slowly increased until slight dryness of the mouth occurs; this indicates that an effective therapeutic concentration has been achieved.

After Care. The great majority of ulcers heal on the above regime, but few escape subsequent relapse. Although there is no known way of preventing recurrence, it is probably wise for the ulcer subject to continue having small regular meals and particularly to avoid long spells of work without food. He should abstain from smoking if he can do so without too much distress. Perhaps even more important, he should make a point of having two or three days in bed, with two-hourly milky feeds, at the first indication of recurrence of his pain, as this may prevent a major relapse.

The Treatment of Massive Bleeding. A patient who has had a large haematemesis or melaena is always an anxious and difficult problem in treatment. In the hope that the bleeding will stop spontaneously he must be kept as quiet as possible; an injection of morphine 15–20 mg. is therefore given on admission and repeated in a few hours if restlessness returns. Blood is taken for grouping and for haemoglobin estimation and an hourly pulse and blood pressure chart is started. The haemoglobin level does not reflect the severity of the bleeding until several hours later, so that the pulse and blood pressure give a better immediate indication. *Transfusion* may not be necessary if the patient is young and the haemorrhage relatively slight, but an elderly patient who has bled severely must be given at least two pints of blood without delay. For a patient whose bleeding is thought to have stopped transfusion at the rate of one pint in four hours is satisfactory, but the blood must be run in much more quickly if the bleeding is continuing. In addition to the obvious immediate risk to life, two serious hazards of failing to replace lost blood may be mentioned: in the elderly, severe anaemia may lead to cardiac failure by inducing an increase in cardiac output; and very occasionally recurrence of bleeding in a severely anaemic patient leads to permanent blindness. A good rule to follow is: 'When in doubt, transfuse.' At one time these patients were given only ice to suck, in the mistaken idea that this would rest the stomach. An empty stomach is in fact much more active than a full one and it is wiser to give the patient a *diet* corresponding to the first stage of the usual ulcer regime as soon as he can take it. *Cimetidine* 200 mg. I.V. 6 hourly should be given and a change made to oral administration when possible. Emergency *operation* may be needed if the bleeding continues or recurs, but carries a high mortality in these severely ill patients; the decision whether to operate, and when, calls for a high degree of clinical judgment on behalf of both physician and surgeon and cannot be made according to any hard and fast rules.

(2) Surgical Treatment

Surgery is very frequently demanded by the patient himself, who naturally thinks that if only he can have his ulcer cut out that will be the end of it and he need have no more tedious weeks in hospital and irksome diets. Unfortunately, however, the matter is not as simple as this. Partial gastrectomy may be performed for either gastric or duodenal ulcer, though for the latter many surgeons now prefer vagotomy with a drainage operation on the stomach. Many patients do very well after these procedures, but a proportion have persistent diarrhoea after vagotomy or various ill-effects (listed below) after gastrectomy. Severe post-gastrectomy syndromes are particularly common in young adults and the operation should seldom be performed before early middle age. With this proviso the *indications for surgery* may be stated as:

(1) Failure of the symptoms of a duodenal ulcer to remit, or failure of a gastric ulcer to show radiological evidence of healing, after an adequate period of efficient medical treatment.

(2) Pyloric obstruction.

(3) Severe bleeding, particularly if this has recurred and the patient is above middle age.

(4) Doubt whether a gastric ulcer be malignant. Duodenal ulcers are never malignant.

(5) Enormous ulcers and those invading the pancreas.

(6) Perforation is of course an immediate indication for operation.

Post-Gastrectomy Syndromes

(1) Malnutrition

(a) Most patients either lose weight or fail to gain weight. This may be partly due to inadequate food intake, the stump of the stomach being able to accommodate only a small meal, but some patients also develop steatorrhoea, in part due to poor mixing of food with pancreatic juice and possibly also to intestinal hurry and to bacterial contamination of the small bowel, which is normally sterile.

(b) Iron deficiency anaemia develops in about 20–30 per cent of the patients and may require parenteral iron therapy for its correction. Macrocytic anaemia is less common; usually due to folic acid deficiency.

(c) Very occasionally vitamin B_{12} and C deficiency develops.

(2) Post-prandial Attacks. These are of two types:

(a) *The Dumping Syndrome.* Symptoms start either during a meal or within half an hour, with abdominal fullness and sensations of 'rolling' or 'churning', nausea, palpitations, dizziness, and faintness. Soon afterwards the patient usually complains of weakness, fatigue, or exhaustion which may persist for up to three hours. Severe attacks may be precipitated by large meals or less often by sweet foods and drinks. The symptoms are probably the result of excessive jejunal stimulation: they can be reproduced by various abnormal jejunal stimuli such as the entry of iced water, hypertonic solutions, or distension by a balloon. Barium meal shows precipitate gastric emptying, the meal leaving the stomach within 10 minutes. Inadequate handling of a glucose load, with a lag type of glucose tolerance test and a reduction in plasma volume have been demonstrated and sodium tolbutamide 0·25–1·0 g. ten to thirty minutes before meals may help to prevent attacks. Dry meals rich in protein and poor in carbohydrate and lying down after eating are other helpful measures.

(b) *Late hypoglycaemic attacks* are due simply to functional postprandial hyperinsulinism. The patients are frequently rather nervous unstable people who have been subject to similar but milder attacks even before the operation. They require treatment by reassurance, correction of malnutrition if necessary, and should take small frequent meals with a low carbohydrate content.

CARCINOMA OF THE STOMACH

Carcinoma of the stomach is the third commonest cancer in the U.K. (after breast and bronchus) and occurs twice as often in men as in women.

Clinical Features. Early diagnosis is of the utmost importance if the patient is to have any chance of radical cure, and to this end the possibility of malignant disease of the stomach should be borne in mind when a patient of early middle age or beyond develops for the first time dyspeptic symptoms which persist for more than two or three weeks. The symptoms are very variable, but the most common are anorexia and epigastric pain which usually does not show the clear-cut relation to food seen in patients with peptic ulcer. Within a few months most patients show obvious loss of weight and anaemia, though occasional very slowly growing gastric cancers may cause only very vague symptoms for as long as two years. Frequently a good deal of bleeding occurs from the surface of the carcinoma, and the vomiting of altered blood which looks like coffee grounds is a characteristic feature. On the other hand, negative tests for occult blood in the stools do not exclude this diagnosis, for the infiltrating type of growth (causing the 'leather-bottle stomach') may extend widely in the wall of the stomach without causing surface ulceration. Some patients develop symptoms and signs of pyloric obstruction; less often a fundal tumour obstructs the cardia and the patient complains that his food appears to stick at the lower end of the gullet. In some unfortunate patients the earliest symptoms are those due to metastases in the liver or elsewhere.

Physical signs are usually present only in patients whose disease has advanced beyond the reach of curative surgery. Common findings at this stage are a hard fixed mass in the epigastrium and evidence of secondary deposits; important among the latter are an enlarged irregular liver, a hard lymph-node above the clavicle (described by Virchow), deep-vein thrombosis in the leg (Trousseau's sign), or on rectal examination bilateral Krukenberg tumours in the ovaries or a hard mass in the rectal pouch from trans-coelomic spread. The only sign sometimes found in early cases is slight epigastric tenderness.

Diagnosis depends mainly on the *barium meal* examination, which classically shows a filling defect and failure of peristaltic movements over the affected part of the stomach. It is now thought that not more than about 1 per cent of peptic ulcers of the stomach undergo malignant change; in this group a very large ulcer and a suggestion of filling defect at one end of it are signs arousing suspicion of carcinoma. A leather-bottle stomach is small, indistensible and inactive and the barium runs straight through it into the duodenum. Biopsy of the lesion by *endoscopy* leads to histological confirmation of the diagnosis. There is usually a *hypochromic anaemia* and a raised *sedimentation rate* but both of these may also be found in patients with simple gastric ulcer.

Treatment. Radical surgery provides the only opportunity for cure, but the prognosis is among the worst for all forms of carcinoma and five-year survivals are below 10 per cent. Even in advanced cases the primary growth should be resected whenever possible, for apart from possible prolongation of life symptomatic relief makes the procedure worth while.

DISORDERS OF THE INTESTINES

The Malabsorption Syndromes

These disorders are characterised by failure of absorption of essential food factors by the small intestine, with consequent chronic diarrhoea and malnutrition. All somewhat rare, the more common members are coeliac disease in children, idiopathic steatorrhoea, and tropical sprue. Similar effects may result from resection of part of the small gut, especially when a blind loop has been formed, from Crohn's disease, from pancreatitis, from drugs such as neomycin or phenindione and from the very rare Whipple's disease (intestinal lipodystrophy).

Tropical Sprue

Sprue is endemic in certain countries in the Far East, notably India, Sri Lanka, Indo-China, and the East Indies. It occurs also in the West Indies but is apparently rare in Africa. It particularly affects Europeans living temporarily in an endemic area, though usually not until after many years' residence. The gut shows abnormal or atrophic villi but the cause of the disease is obscure; at present the most popular theory for the failure of intestinal function is an alteration of the normal bacterial flora following recurrent dysenteric infection.

Gluten Enteropathy (Idiopathic steatorrhoea)

This is the adult counterpart of coeliac disease (which will not be described here) and sometimes the symptoms can be traced through a series of remissions and exacerbations back to childhood. It was noted in Holland after the second world war that children with coeliac disease who had been making good progress under conditions of near starvation during the German occupation began to deteriorate when wheat and rye were introduced into the diet. Further investigation soon confirmed that there was an intolerance to gluten, the protein part of the wheat or rye germ, but curiously enough not to the glutens in other cereals. It is probable that intolerance to wheat and rye glutens is also the cause of idiopathic steatorrhoea. The cause of this intolerance is probably deficiency of the enzyme which normally hydrolyses the toxic peptide part of the gluten.

Clinical Features. There is usually an insidious onset of looseness of the stools, general weakness, and loss of weight. The diarrhoea is persistent, though most patients have exacerbations from time to time followed by remissions in which the stools become temporarily almost normal. During exacerbations the stools typically are pale, bulky, frothy, and greasy; but they may be fluid and not obviously fatty, though analysis will usually reveal an excess of fat. Flatulence is usually severe and the distension of the abdomen contrasts with the progressive emaciation of the rest of the body. Clubbing of the fingers occasionally develops. Other symptoms and signs result from failure of absorption of essential food factors:

Factor Deficient	Clinical Effect
Iron	Hypochromic anaemia
Vitamin B_{12} ⎱ Folic acid ⎰	Macrocytic anaemia

(The anaemia is usually of mixed type)

Vitamin B complex 　aneurine (thiamine)	Peripheral neuritis (rare)
riboflavin ⎱ 　nicotinic acid ⎰	⎰ Glossitis ⎱ Stomatitis
Vitamin D ⎱ Calcium 　⎰	⎰ Tetany ⎱ Osteomalacia
Vitamin K	Haemorrhagic tendency
Potassium	Weakness, apathy, and mental disturbance

Diagnosis. Confirmation of malabsorption of fat is essential but analysis of a casual stool specimen for fat is useless. On a ward diet which contains about 70 g. of fat per day a 3–5 day collection should be made; a loss greater than 6–7 g. (more than 18 mmol.) daily is abnormal. If this is done a formal fat balance is usually unnecessary. The radio-active iodine labelled fat excretion test is not so accurate probably because the isotopic label becomes detached from the fat in the small bowel. Glucose tolerance test shows a flat blood sugar curve, but has been replaced by the xylose tolerance test in which impaired absorption of xylose is revealed by reduced excretion in the urine. Barium follow through, using 350 ml. of a flocculable barium sulphate suspension, shows a typical small intestine pattern; the mucosal markings are thickened and the barium is clumped in elongated masses. In gluten enteropathy and tropical sprue peroral small intestinal biopsy with a special capsule reveals that the normal epithelium with slender villi has been replaced by a flat or ridged mucosa; this is almost diagnostic. Occasionally a radio-active B_{12} absorption test or estimations of serum B_{12} and folic acid provide helpful additional data.

Treatment of gluten enteropathy. Although most patients respond completely to a strict gluten-free diet within a few weeks, some require supplements of iron, vitamin B_{12}, folic acid, calcium or vitamin D. A few continue to have diarrhoea or relapse, usually from failing to keep to the diet; it should be made clear from the onset, therefore, that wheat gluten will probably have to be avoided for life. In the U.K. gluten-free foods are prescribable under the N.H.S. (on EC 10), and patients derive help and moral support in keeping strictly to their diet by joining the Coeliac Society. If the patient is severely ill prednisolone may be given in addition to a gluten-free diet and usually causes improvement in the general condition and in the mucosal lesion.

Complications. There is a high incidence of lymphoma of the small bowel in these patients, most often reticulum-cell sarcoma of the jejunum. They are also more prone to carcinoma of the gastro-intestinal tract and even in other parts of the body.

About 60 per cent of patients with dermatitis herpetiformis have a gluten enteropathy. The reason for this association is not known.

Treatment of Sprue. Europeans who develop sprue in the tropics usually recover spontaneously when they return to a temperate climate. Sometimes a course of tetracycline, 250–500 mg. six-hourly for five days, is of benefit, probably by altering the bacterial flora of the gut. It is usual to give a diet rich in protein and vitamins and low in fat and roughage. Vitamin B_{12} is given intramuscularly, starting with 100 μg. on alternate days and gradually increasing the interval between injections during recovery. Folic acid 10–20 mg. three times daily is given by mouth. Other vitamin and mineral deficiencies are corrected as necessary.

Other Causes of Malabsorption

Obstructive jaundice impairs the digestion of fats and in long standing cases the resulting steatorrhoea may lead eventually to osteomalacia. In *chronic pancreatitis* lack of pancreatic digestive enzymes impairs the digestion of fat and protein and leads to steatorrhoea and heavy loss of nitrogen in the stools; absorption of glucose, iron, folic acid, and vitamin B_{12} is usually normal.

Extensive resection of the small gut may be followed by malnutrition, but in organic disease of the small intestine malabsorption results not from loss of absorbing surface but from bacterial activity. The normally sterile small gut may be invaded by coliform organisms, as a result of stasis, either above a *stricture* (as in Crohn's disease) or in a *blind loop* formed by a fistulous communication or surgical bypass, or as a result of direct access through a *gastro-colic fistula*. In the very rare *Zollinger-Ellison syndrome*, probably as a result of gastrin secretion by the pancreatic tumour always present, there is heavy and continuous outpouring of gastric juice and the usual clinical presentation is severe and intractable peptic ulceration, but sometimes the contents of the small intestine are rendered acid and steatorrhoea results from inactivation of the pancreatic enzymes. Another very rare cause of steatorrhoea and progressive wasting is *Whipple's disease* or intestinal lipodystrophy; the cause is unknown and the diagnosis can be made with certainty only by biopsy of the small intestine to show large foamy macrophages, filled with an unidentified glycoprotein, in the tunica propria, and lipogranulomatosis in the mesenteric lymph-nodes. The disease is progressive, but temporary remission of symptoms may be induced by corticosteroid therapy.

Disaccharide Intolerance

Digestion of disaccharides such as lactose, sucrose and maltose takes place within the mucosal cells. If one of the enzymes lactase, sucrase or maltase is lacking the corresponding disaccharide accumulates and may cause diarrhoea and malabsorption. Patients with *lactase deficiency* may give a history of diarrhoea after drinking milk; the diagnosis is supported by demonstrating a flat blood sugar curve after a loading dose of lactose. The deficiency may be an inborn error or the result of various diseases affecting the small intestine. Symptoms are relieved by a milk-free diet.

Crohn's Disease

In this disease of unknown aetiology there are single or multiple sharply demarcated areas of intestine, mainly in the lower ileum and in the colon, which become grossly thickened by lymphoid hyperplasia, ulceration, oedema, and secondary infection. Complications include cicatricial stenosis of the bowel, localised perforation, abscess, and the formation of fistulae. The sex incidence is approximately equal and symptoms usually begin in the twenties or thirties.

Clinical Features. Symptoms usually develop very gradually and there are often long natural remissions so that the history commonly extends over several years by the time the diagnosis is made. Most patients present with attacks of colicky pain round the umbilicus or in the right iliac fossa, with associated mild diarrhoea and general weakness. Loss of weight is usual and there is often low fever. The most helpful and important *physical sign* is a tender fixed mass, usually in the right iliac fossa, and the *barium 'follow through'* examination demonstrates gross filling defects and narrowing of the lumen of the affected segments of intestine. The blood count shows anaemia and some leucocytosis and a high sedimentation rate. Fistulous *complications* may lead to peri-anal abscess and fistula-in-ano, dysuria and passage of wind *per urethram* from ileo-vesical fistula or abscess in the abdominal wall. An associated granular proctitis is common.

Systemic Complications. Transient arthritis, usually confined to one large joint, is common; about 5 per cent of patients have ankylosing spondylitis; and about 20 per cent have symptomless sacro-iliitis, revealed by X-ray. Erythema nodosum is commonly seen, particularly in women; more serious is pyoderma gangrenosum, a term applied to deep ulcers with a sloughing base seen mainly on the legs, but sometimes on the face, thought to be a result of vasculitis. Iritis, episcleritis and conjunctivitis are important ocular complications. There is a high incidence of both gallstones and kidney stones. Cirrhosis of the liver is a rare association.

Treatment. The patient should be confined to bed during febrile exacerbations and should be advised at all times to avoid exhaustion from either physical or mental overstrain. Improvement does sometimes seem to follow the resolution of emotional problems and worries, but in the individual patient it is seldom that any useful action can be taken in this connection. Sulphasalazine is given as for ulcerative colitis (q.v.) to reduce the incidence of relapses and exacerbations. Rapid relief of symptoms often follows treatment with steroids, but the improvement is not always maintained and it is probably wise to reserve steroid therapy for the control of exacerbations. A suitable course would be prednisolone 40–60 mg. daily for a few days until the fever and other symptoms have subsided, then a maintenance dose of about 20 mg. daily for two or three weeks, after which the dosage should be gradually tailed off. Operation should be avoided if possible during the stage of active ulceration but frequently becomes necessary for the relief of complications such as perforation, cicatricial obstruction or fistulae. Resection of the affected segment of bowel is the treatment of choice.

Ulcerative Colitis

This is a serious and chronic disease of the colon and although temporary remission of symptoms is common, relapse nearly always follows after a variable interval of months or years and complete recovery is very rare. The cause of ulcerative colitis is unknown. Its acute stage is very similar to bacillary dysentery, which suggests that an infection might be responsible, but no specific organism has ever been isolated. Some authorities have been very struck by the characteristic personality of many of these patients, who are said to be fussy, tidy, meticulous people, emotionally immature and showing an abnormal dependence on one or other parent, and by the fact that the onset of the illness or exacerbations in its severity quite often appear to be precipitated by an emotional crisis associated with marriage, childbirth, or the death of a parent or near relative. It has therefore been suggested that the changes in the bowel are secondary to some psychological disturbance. Controlled psychiatric studies on small groups of patients have not supported this theory.

Clinical Features. It usually starts in early adult life and is slightly more common in women than in men. The principal symptom is *diarrhoea*, which continues in some degree throughout the whole course of the illness. During acute relapses the stools are greatly increased in number and contain *blood and mucus*, abdominal pain is often severe, the temperature is raised and the patient becomes very weak, anaemic and emaciated; in remissions the general health becomes more or less restored, but there is nearly always some persistent looseness of the stools. The severity of the disease varies greatly in different patients. There is an acute fulminating variety which renders the patient gravely ill, even moribund, within a few weeks; at the other end of the scale is a mild type which causes only relatively trivial inconvenience; and between these extremes the majority of patients require admission to hospital from time to time over many years and are always more or less severely disabled by their disease.

Physical signs are few, though there is usually some tenderness over the affected part of the colon. The blood count reveals *anaemia* which is sometimes severe and usually a *leucocytosis*. The *sedimentation rate* is very high during relapses and seldom falls completely to normal even during remissions. *Sigmoidoscopy* shows a very red, granular, bleeding, and superficially ulcerated mucosa. The *barium enema* in moderately severe or advanced cases shows the affected bowel to be shorter and narrower than normal and to have a rather fuzzy outline devoid of the normal haustral markings; these appearances are particularly helpful in assessing how much of the colon is involved. The double-contrast technique involves insufflation of air into the bowel after most of the barium has been removed and provides better definition of mucosal lesions.

Complications. Stricture of the bowel, peri-anal abscess, toxic dilatation of the colon, perforation leading to abscess or peritonitis, severe haemorrhage and the development of carcinoma in the diseased colon are complications particularly to be feared in the younger patients with severe ulcerative colitis. Opinions differ about the frequency of malignant change, but it certainly occurs sufficiently often in patients who have had a severe form of the disease for ten years or more to be a powerful argument in favour of treatment by colectomy. Increasing dilatation of the colon is a serious complication seen in very ill patients and is an indication for immediate operation.

The various *systemic complications* of Crohn's disease (p. 77) are also seen in patients with ulcerative colitis.

Treatment. There is no specific therapy and during the acute stages undoubtedly the most important measure is a period of complete *rest* in bed, The *diet* should be high in protein and in total calories; a milk-free diet may be worth trying in patients with persistent mild symptoms. Vitamin supplements should be given. For the relief of anaemia fresh *blood transfusion* is the most effective treatment and in addition often seems to be of benefit to the patient's general condition. *Iron* is indicated too and should be given parentally (see p. 508 for details) if oral preparations appear to aggravate the diarrhoea. To control the diarrhoea tab. codeine phosphate 30–60 mg. three or four times daily or diphenoxylate (Lomotil) 2 tablets three or four times daily are the most useful preparations and propantheline 15–30 mg. three or four times daily may help to relieve colic.

It is now usual to give oral *sulphasalazine*, which has been shown to reduce the incidence of relapses. The initial dose is 0·5 g. after food and is doubled in a few days unless the patient has side-effects such as headache, dyspepsia or malaise. Later toxic effects include rashes and haemolytic anaemia. This treatment must be continued over many months or years. In addition, many patients improve greatly after a course of prednisolone (Predsol) suppositories b.d. or retention enemas at night. Only if severe symptoms persist in spite of these measures, or for a very acute fulminating form of the disease, should systemic steroid therapy be instituted. *Prednisolone* is given by mouth in initial daily dosage of 40–60 mg. which is gradually reduced as soon as improvement in the patient's condition permits; a gratifying remission of symptoms is often induced, but all too often relapse quickly ensues when the drug is withdrawn. The immunosuppressive drug azathioprine may be tried in patients failing to respond to the above regime, but careful supervision with regular blood counts to detect early bone-marrow suppression is essential; the dose is 2–2·5 mg./kg. daily.

Many patients need surgery but there is no general agreement about the *indications for operation*. The procedure employed is total colectomy, and although it is occasionally possible to join the ileum to the rectal stump, most patients are left with a permanent ileostomy. With modern techniques, however, patients with this disability are able to lead almost normal lives. The present tendency therefore is not to regard surgery as the final desperate gamble for an almost moribund patient, but to advise operation after a reasonable trial of medical treatment. The improvement in health is usually well worth the price of the ileostomy and, as mentioned above, the risk of malignant change and other complications is a further incentive to relatively early surgery.

Protein-losing Enteropathy

In some gastro-intestinal diseases, notably ulcerative colitis, regional ileitis, idiopathic steatorrhoea and carcinoma of the stomach, exudation of plasma occurs into the lumen of the gut. The faecal nitrogen is not increased, since most of the plasma is digested and reabsorbed; but hypoproteinaemia and resulting oedema may develop in view of the liver's limited reserve capacity to synthesize albumen.

Diverticular Disease of the Colon

This expression is now preferred to the older terms diverticulosis and diverticulitis. Two varieties are recognised.

Diffuse diverticular disease becomes very common after middle age and is found in most elderly people. Diverticula with short necks and wide mouths occur throughout the colon and are probably the result of muscular atrophy without any increase in intraluminal pressure. Usually there are no symptoms, but occasionally a diverticulum perforates or leads to massive haemorrhage from the bowel; indeed, this is the commonest cause of the latter symptom.

Localised diverticular disease is most common in the sigmoid colon; it is thought that a rise in intraluminal pressure, due to irregular contraction of the hypertrophied muscle, forces diverticula through the thickened bowel wall so that their necks are often long and narrow. At first there may be obstructive symptoms such as distension, flatulence, and colicky pains, but later inflammatory changes may cause more persistent pain with fever and a tender mass may become palpable. A fistula between the colon and either the bladder or vagina should be suspected if the patient develops frequency of micturition or vaginal discharge. **Treatment.** Diverticular disease does not occur in parts of the world where a high-residue diet is eaten, and the addition of miller's bran to a Western diet, a tablespoonful two or three times daily, is usually effective in relieving symptoms. Appropriate surgical treatment may be needed for inflammatory complications.

Irritable Bowel Syndrome

This term is applied to the many patients who complain of disordered action of the bowels, usually diarrhoea, often with abdominal pain, distension and flatulence, in whom thorough examination and investigation fail to reveal any evidence of organic disease. Formerly such patients were often said to have a 'spastic colon'. Symptoms usually start before the age of 30 and may date back to childhood; it is unwise to make this diagnosis in patients presenting after the age of 50.

Treatment. Increasing dietary fibre by giving miller's bran, 1 tablespoonful three times daily, is often helpful; and dramatic improvement may follow the recognition and treatment of underlying anxiety or depression. Supportive follow-up is also beneficial.

JAUNDICE

Definition. Jaundice is an increase in the amount of bilirubin in the blood resulting in yellow discoloration of the sclerotics of the eyes, the skin, mucosae, and certain body fluids.

Physiology of Bile. After circulating in the blood for about 120 days red corpuscles are removed and broken up by cells of the reticuloendothelial system, mainly in the liver, spleen, and bone marrow. The haemoglobin is split into two fractions, an iron-containing part which is returned to the bone marrow for re-synthesis into haemoglobin and an iron-free porphyrin fraction from which the pigment bilirubin is derived. When liberated into the blood for transport to the liver this bilirubin is insoluble in water; it is therefore unable to pass into the urine and it gives an indirect van den Bergh reaction. The bilirubin is taken up by the liver cells, where it becomes conjugated through its carboxyl groups with glucuronic acid to form water-soluble bilirubin-glucuronides which give a direct van den Bergh reaction. In this form bilirubin passes down the bile duct to the duodenum, where it is converted into stercobilinogen, the pigment responsible for most of the normal colour of faeces. Some of this is absorbed (as urobilinogen) from the small intestine into the portal bloodstream; and though nearly all of this fraction is removed again by the liver cells and returned to the biliary passages, traces of it usually escape through the liver into the general circulation and are excreted in the urine.

Causes of Jaundice. It is obvious that jaundice may result either because too much bilirubin is liberated into the blood from excessive breakdown of red corpuscles (*haemolytic jaundice*) or because too little bilirubin is removed from the blood in its passage through the liver. The latter disorder can occur in two ways: the function of the liver cells may be deranged, so that they cannot take up the bilirubin from the blood (*hepatic jaundice*); or obstruction in the common bile duct may dam the flow of bile, so that the bilirubin-glucuronides excreted by the liver diffuse back into the blood (*obstructive jaundice*).

Haemolytic Jaundice. This is the least common of the three main types of jaundice and the yellow discoloration of the skin and other tissues is seldom more than slight. The *urine* contains *no bilirubin* since the bilirubin in the blood is insoluble in water; but as more bile pigment than normal is being produced and consequently an excess of urobilinogen is formed in the duodenum, more of this pigment is absorbed into the portal bloodstream than the liver cells can remove and an *excess of urobilinogen* passes through into the urine. The stools retain their normal colour and chemical analysis shows that they too contain an excess of urobilinogen (sometimes called stercobilinogen in this context). The causes of haemolytic jaundice are discussed under haemolytic anaemia (p. 512).

Obstructive Jaundice. When the common bile duct is obstructed the rising pressure in the biliary system causes bile to flow back into the perilobular lymphatics and by this route into the bloodstream. The bile salts produced in the liver also accumulate in the blood and are probably responsible for the pruritus and bradycardia often found in patients with obstructive jaundice. As explained above, the *bilirubin* in these patients is soluble in water and when its concentration in the blood rises above the renal threshold of about 34 μmol./l. *it passes freely into the urine*; the latter contains *no urobilinogen*, however, since none is being formed, and for this reason too *the stools are very pale*. Liver function tests which depend on qualitative changes in the serum proteins (and which are therefore manifestations of hepatocellular damage) are negative; these include the thymol flocculation, thymol turbidity, and colloidal gold tests. The level of the serum alkaline phosphatase, however, is raised and usually continues to rise in parallel with the level of the serum bilirubin, and in long-standing cases there is often a rise in the level of the total serum cholesterol.

The common causes of occlusion of the common bile duct are gallstones and carcinoma of the head of the pancreas or of the ampulla of Vater; see *A Short Textbook of Surgery*, 4th edition, Hodder and Stoughton Educational, 1977. A rare cause is chronic pancreatitis (p. 92).

Hepatic Jaundice. In this group the jaundice is due primarily to difficulty in the transport of bilirubin through the hepatic cell, and possibly in its conjugation; but the pattern of bile-pigments in the serum is in fact identical with that which follows occlusion of the bile duct, and the jaundice must be due partly to regurgitation from the bile canaliculi. In addition, diminished red cell survival is found in all these patients and adds a haemolytic component to the jaundice. There is usually a stage in the disease in which the stools are pale and the urine contains bilirubin but no urobilinogen, as in obstructive jaundice; there may also be a misleading rise in the serum alkaline phosphatase. Positive empirical liver function tests (such as the thymol flocculation, thymol turbidity and colloidal gold reaction) which depend on serum protein changes, and raised serum transaminase levels, are the characteristic biochemical findings. The total serum cholesterol is usually decreased.

Cholestatic jaundice is the condition in which the clinical and biochemical picture of obstructive jaundice is found in the presence of patent bile-ducts, and liver biopsy reveals stasis of bile in the liver cells and canaliculi. It is seen as a toxic effect of certain drugs, notably chlorpromazine (incidence 1 per cent), less commonly promazine, trifluoperazine, P.A.S., chlorpropamide, thiouracil, nitrofurantoin and methyl testosterone. A similar picture is seen in the rare recurrent jaundice of pregnancy, which appears in the third trimester and clears up in the puerperium. All patients in this group have a good prognosis, with the occasional exception of those with so-called primary biliary cirrhosis.

Familial Hyperbilirubinaemia

This condition, of which a number of varieties have been described in recent years, causes few if any symptoms and is usually detected on routine blood examination, so that in published cases there has been a high incidence in doctors and other hospital workers. The most common type is that described by *Gilbert*; there is a defect in the transport of bilirubin to its site of conjugation in the liver cell and non-conjugated (water-insoluble) bilirubin accumulates in the blood. Liver function tests are normal, needle biopsy shows normal hepatic structure, there are no complications and prognosis is excellent. The importance of the condition lies in distinguishing it from haemolytic jaundice and progressive hepatic disease. In the rarer *Dubin-Johnson* variety the hold-up occurs after conjugation and the clinical picture is that of obstructive jaundice; liver biopsy reveals a dark brown pigment in the liver cells. Diagnosis is important so that these patients may be reassured that they are not suffering from serious liver disease.

DISEASES OF THE LIVER

Infectious Hepatitis

There are two strains of virus causing acute hepatitis and differing mainly in their mode of transmission and incubation period. Virus A has an incubation period of about a month (20–40 days) and is present in the patient's stools, being transmitted by faecal contamination of food or water. Where hygienic standards are high only sporadic cases are seen, but where large groups of people live under relatively primitive conditions in a warm climate widespread epidemics may occur. Thus, during the war there were large outbreaks among troops in India and the Middle East. Under these conditions flies are important agents in the spread of the infection.

Virus B hepatitis and usually called serum hepatitis, has an incubation period of about three months (60–160 days) and is found only in the patient's blood. Some healthy people harbour this virus in their blood for prolonged periods (perhaps indefinitely) and people found to be B virus positive should be excluded from service as blood donors. Transmission to susceptible individuals occurs through transfusions or injections containing plasma, or even from the use of inadequately sterilised syringes or needles. Patients presenting with infectious hepatitis should therefore always be asked if they have been given any injection during the preceding four months. B virus hepatitis is a particular hazard in dialysis units treating patients with chronic renal failure.

After recovery the patient usually has lifelong immunity, but only to infection with the same strain of virus. Furthermore, there is some evidence that the virus of infective hepatitis causes only a mild gastro-enteritis in young children and that those who acquire the more severe illness in adult life are those who have escaped childhood infection and consequent immunisation. This is known to apply to some other virus infections, such as poliomyelitis, which are more serious in adults than in children.

Clinical Features. The illness starts with fever, general malaise, aching in the back and limbs, nausea, and loss of appetite; arthralgia and urticaria are common prodromal symptoms of serum hepatitis not seen in infectious hepatitis. *Anorexia* is a very constant symptom and its occurrence for a few days before the appearance of icterus is one of the most important points distinguishing hepatitis from other causes of jaundice. Clinical jaundice usually becomes manifest within a week and about the same time the temperature settles and the patient starts to feel better. At this stage the liver is usually somewhat enlarged and tender and in about 20 per cent of patients the spleen can be felt too. In the pre-icteric phase the *urine* usually contains an excess of urobilinogen; then when intrahepatic biliary obstruction occurs the urobilinogen disappears, bilirubin is found in the urine (which is consequently dark in colour) and the stools become pale; and finally during recovery after bilirubin has disappeared from the urine there may be a temporary return of urobilinogen in excess before the urine reverts to normal. The great majority of patients are jaundiced for only a week or two and then make a complete recovery. Very occasionally, however (less than 0·5 per cent), fulminating infection may cause death even before the appearance of jaundice; or, equally rarely, recovery is incomplete and slowly progressive hepatic damage leads eventually to cirrhosis. Very mild cases never develop clinical jaundice (infective hepatitis sine ictero) and usually escape recognition except during epidemics. Raised serum transaminase levels are a sensitive index of hepatocellular damage; they are found even in anicteric patients (and are helpful in tracing the course of an epidemic) and if persistent indicate the need for further bed rest and observation.

A long convalescence is advisable after this illness, since depression and tiredness are often rather persistent and it may be some months before the patient recovers his full mental and physical vigour. Abstention from alcohol for about three months is also a wise precaution.

A small number of patients with chronic hepatitis have been found to carry the B virus antigen in the blood. These patients are clinically similar to those with chronic active hepatitis (see below) but do not usually have evidence of multisystem disease. This finding suggests that chronic liver damage can occur as a result of the persistence of the B virus.

Treatment. There is no specific treatment for infective hepatitis. The most important measure undoubtedly is rest and as a general rule the patient should be kept in bed until the temperature has settled, his appetite has returned, biliburin has disappeared from his urine and his liver is no longer tender. Particular care should be taken in the disposal of excreta and the washing of hands after attending the patient. Diet should be regulated by the patient's appetite rather than the physician's fancy.

A short course of prednisone, starting with 40–50 mg. daily and tailing the dosage off over about a week, may be tried in patients who continue to be deeply jaundiced after six weeks or more and sometimes appears to hasten recovery. If the patient is so ill that he cannot tolerate 1,000 Calories by mouth the regime for acute hepatic failure (p. 88) should be instituted. Human gamma-globulin 0·06–0·12 ml. per kg. body weight, given not later than 6 days before the onset of symptoms, modifies the disease and its administration may be considered for specially debilitated patients at risk.

Active Chronic Hepatitis (Lupoid Hepatitis)

In some patients, usually but not invariably young women, hepatitis may persist and may proceed ultimately to a lobular cirrhosis. This type of hepatitis is frequently associated with disorders of other systems including renal tubular acidosis, Sjøgren's syndrome, arthropathy, alveolitis, and colitis.

Investigation may show impaired hepatic function; in addition the plasma gamma globulin is usually increased and in about half the patients antinuclear factor and antibodies to smooth muscle are found in the plasma. Liver biopsy shows liver cell necrosis with infiltration by lymphocytes and plasma cells.

Most patients die within five years. Treatment with steroids particularly if started early in the disease may induce a remission and there is evidence that it may prolong life.

Cirrhosis of the Liver

The word cirrhosis means tawny and was introduced by Laënnec because of the slightly icteric tinge sometimes seen in the livers of patients who have died of this disease. Later it became realised that a much more character-istic feature than the tawny colour is the presence of a great deal of fibrous tissue and cirrhosis has come to mean diffuse hepatic fibrosis. This may be the result of a number of different pathological processes, so that cirrhosis should be regarded as analogous with pulmonary fibrosis rather than as a disease entity.

Clinical Features. *Laënnec's cirrhosis* occurs most often in the forties and fifties and the alcoholic variety is commoner in men than in women. The disease is usually brought to light by the discovery of splenomegaly, hepatomegaly, jaundice, gastro-intestinal bleeding, or ascites. In alcoholics there is usually a history of epigastric discomfort, loss of appetite—particularly for breakfast—and morning sickness with vomiting of mucus, symptoms attributable to alcoholic gastritis; but patients with idiopathic cirrhosis have frequently had no symptoms up to the time of diagnosis. Furthermore, in about one third of cases seen at autopsy the disease has been unsuspected in life.

The clinical features arise from two main causes, hepatocellular failure and portal hypertension:

Hepatocellular failure may have many different effects. *Low-grade fever* often with leucocytosis is seen in about half the patients. More common is the development of *vascular spiders*, each consisting of a central dilated arteriole from which a number of tiny vessels radiate; these appear on the face, neck, upper half of the trunk and upper limbs. Their cause is not known; it is probably not the high blood oestrogen level, as once thought. Erythema of the thenar and hypothenar eminences and of the pads of the fingers ('*liver palms*') is also common. Mental and physical *fatigue, loss of weight* and vague *indigestion* are the rule. *Foetor hepaticus*, which can be detected in the breath and urine is a common sign; it is presumably due to a substance from the gut which is normally detoxicated by the liver. It is a sweetish somewhat faeculent smell which is usually likened to that of a freshly opened corpse. It is a grave sign, often quickly followed by hepatic coma, in patients with severe hepatocellular failure, though in patients with extensive porta-caval venous anastamoses it may be present intermittently for quite long periods and does not necessarily imply such a bad prognosis.

Hepatic coma is probably related to failure of the liver to convert ammonia to urea and the blood ammonia level is raised. It is more com-mon in patients with porto-caval connections and may be precipitated by a high protein diet, by the taking of nitrogenous compounds, or by gastro-intestinal haemorrhage, intercurrent infection or the rapid removal of ascitic fluid. Coma is preceded by a stage of lethargy with mental confusion, irrational behaviour and a typical 'flapping' tremor of the outstretched hands.

Jaundice in cirrhosis, due to failure of the liver cells to excrete bilirubin, is not very common and usually slight; when present it implies a bad prognosis.

Portal hypertension in cirrhosis is due to the combined effect of diminution in the portal vascular bed, the result of both fibrosis and the pressure of regenerating nodules of liver tissue against small portal venous radicles, and of the increased transmission of hepatic arterial pressure to the portal venous system. It leads to congestive *splenomegaly* and to the opening up of porta-caval anastamoses. The two situations in which these distended veins are of clinical importance are:

(a) the abominal wall, since here they are readily seen and are helpful in diagnosis. Portal blood passes to the umbilicus through the para-umbilical veins to reach collaterals of the caval system. There are usually only one or two distended veins, the classical 'caput medusae' being rare, but it can be demonstrated that the flow of blood is radially away from the umbilicus. This helps in the distinction from inferior vena caval obstruction in which the blood in the distended abdominal veins always flows from below upwards.

(b) Varicose veins in the *oesophagus and fundus of the stomach* are the most dangerous effect of portal hypertension, since bleeding from this source is always serious and often fatal. They may be demonstrated by barium swallow, using a thin emulsion to delineate the delicate mucosal pattern, though negative findings on X-rays do not exclude their presence. The spleen is almost invariably palpable in patients with portal hypertension and, as in any condition associated with splenomegaly, *pancytopenia* is frequently found in the peripheral blood (see hypersplenism, p. 518).

Ascites develops in cirrhosis from the combined effect of portal hypertension and the reduced plasma osmotic pressure which follows hepatocellular failure and diminished albumen synthesis. Accumulation of fluid in the peritoneal cavity reduces the effective body fluid volume and compensatory mechanisms to retain fluid in the body come into operation and lead in turn to increase in the ascites; they include increased secretion of anti-diuretic hormone from the neuro-hypophysis and of aldosterone from the adrenal cortex.

Clinical features of obscure origin, sometimes seen in cirrhosis, include *clubbing of the fingers, gynaecomastia,* and *scanty or absent body hair.* In acute hepato-cellular failure the circulation is overactive, as shown by a rapid collapsing pulse, high pulse pressure, warm extremities and increased jugular venous pressure. The *diagnosis* of cirrhosis is difficult to establish in the early stages. The first biochemical test to show abnormal results is usually the bromsulphalein (B.S.P.) retention test; later the serum albumen is reduced, the globulin raised and the serum transaminase levels elevated. Sometimes the serum bilirubin level is slightly raised. In early cases the diagnosis can be made with certainty by needle biopsy, but the indications for this procedure must be carefully assessed for each patient as it incurs a slight risk of haemorrhage which is occasionally serious.

Treatment. Whatever the aetiology of the cirrhosis the patient must abstain completely from alcohol for the rest of his life. An adequate mixed diet is important, but there is no advantage in giving protein supplements. Special indications are as follows:

(a) For **oedema and ascites** give a diet containing no added salt, frusemide 40 mg. daily and spironolactone 100 mg. four times daily with potassium supplements to reduce the danger of inducing hepatic coma. Paracentesis should be avoided if possible.

(b) **Haematemesis and/or melaena.** Many cirrhotics have a duodenal ulcer and the cause of the bleeding must always be considered and an emergency barium meal done if necessary. Bleeding from varices is usually better controlled by intravenous pitressin than by the inflatable balloons of a Sengstaken tube. If bleeding continues emergency operation (porto-caval anastomosis, or Tanner's operation if the portal vein is not patent) may be considered unless there is hepato-cellular failure or gross ascites.

(c) **Coma** from **acute hepatic failure.** Neuro-psychiatric symptoms of incipient coma are an indication for reducing the protein content of the diet. In established coma enough calories must be given as intravenous glucose, if necessary by intracaval catheter, to minimise endogenous protein catabolism; ammonium absorption from the gut is reduced by giving oral neomycin 1 g. four times daily and if necessary pitressin to cause evacuation of melaena stools; paracentesis, thiazide diuretics and sedative drugs must be avoided; and it may be necessary to give potassium if the serum level is reduced due to secondary aldosteronism.

Special Types of Cirrhosis

(1) **Obstructive Biliary Cirrhosis.** Some patients with chronic extra-hepatic cholestasis, usually due to stone in the common duct, carcinoma of the head of the pancreas, compression from peri-biliary lymph-nodes or surgical injury to the common duct, eventually develop diffuse hepatic fibrosis which in turn may lead to portal hypertension and hepato-cellular failure. This sequence of events occurs particularly in patients with long-standing partial or recurrent obstruction complicated by cholangitis and the clinical course is often punctuated by bouts of rigors and pyrexia (Charcot's 'biliary remittent fever'). The only effective treatment is surgical relief of the obstruction.

(2) **Primary Biliary Cirrhosis.** In this rare disease the primary disorder appears to be diffuse intra-hepatic biliary obstruction of unknown cause. Most of the patients are middle-aged women. Insidious onset of itching of the skin is slowly followed by the appearance of jaundice of obstructive type without fever or abdominal pain. The spleen is palpable at an early stage and later the liver becomes greatly enlarged; eventually signs of portal hypertension and hepato-cellular failure develop. Pigmentation and skin xanthomata are quite often seen. The prognosis is better than in Laënnec's cirrhosis; some patients recover and others run a very prolonged downhill course. A remission sometimes follows treatment with peni-

cillamine and this may be given a trial in patients who seem to be doing badly.

(3) **Haemochromatosis.** The primary lesion is probably an inborn metabolic defect which results in the absorption of a slight excess of iron. There is no mechanism by which this extra iron can be eliminated from the body and it is laid down in various tissues and organs, where eventually functional and structural changes may be induced. Symptoms rarely appear before early middle age. The disease is extremely rare in women (5–10 per cent of cases) and in them appears at a later age than in men, probably because the loss of iron in menstruation and pregnancy delays or prevents the clinical expression of the disease. Cirrhosis is a constant feature and the diagnosis should be considered in patients found to have a very enlarged firm liver and greyish pigmentation of the skin, notably over exposed parts. Impotence and general weakness are early symptoms and testicular atrophy with absent or scanty body hair are found much more commonly than in other forms of cirrhosis. Diabetes develops in about two-thirds of the patients. Death usually results from hepato-cellular failure or heart failure, the result of impregnation with haemosiderin of the liver cells and of the myocardium. The *diagnosis* may be confirmed by serum iron studies; the combination of a raised serum iron level with complete or almost complete saturation of the serum iron-binding capacity is almost pathognomonic. If any doubt remains needle biopsy of the liver will settle the matter. *Treatment* is by regular bloodletting; in most patients a pint a week can be taken for many months before early signs of iron deficiency appear in the blood picture. Thereafter a pint should be removed every month or two to prevent reaccumulation of iron in the tissues.

(4) **Syphilitic cirrhosis** (hepar lobatum) is now extremely rare but may be suspected in patients with hepatomegaly and gummata elsewhere in the body. Serological tests for syphilis are positive and the diagnosis is confirmed by the favourable response to anti-syphilitic treatment.

(5) **Cardiac Cirrhosis** (see p. 112).

(6) **Hepato-lenticular Degeneration** (Wilson's disease; see p. 465).

Drug Induced Liver Damage

There are a variety of drugs which may produce liver damage.

(1) **Toxic Hepatitis.** Certain substances including the *chlorinated hydrocarbons* (*carbon tetrachloride*) *benzene derivatives* (*trinitrotoluene, dinitrophenol*) are liver poisons and will produce necrosis of liver cells. This is probably due to direct action of the toxic agent on the liver. Industrial workers exposed to such hepatic poisons should be examined regularly for enlargement or tenderness of the liver and the urine should be tested weekly for bilirubin or urobilinogen.

Other substances only occasionally produce liver necrosis, which when it occurs however may be severe and fatal. This group includes some of the mono amine oxidase inhibitors and *paracetamol* overdose. The cause for this type of change is unknown but it may be some form of hypersensitivity reaction.

(2) **Cholestasis.** This produces a picture resembling obstructive jaundice without evidence of extra-hepatic biliary obstruction. Examination of the liver shows dilation of the bile canaliculi and sometimes inflammation in the portal area.

This type of liver damage is found most commonly with *chlorpromazine, methyl testosterone* and *thiouracil.* Uneventful recovery is the rule.

Acute Yellow Atrophy of the Liver

This term is applied to any very severe, usually rapidly fatal, variety of acute hepatic necrosis, whether of infective or toxic aetiology. Rapid onset of hepatic insufficiency and shrinkage of the liver are characteristic. Deep jaundice with purpura and bleeding from mucous surfaces and into internal organs are soon followed by hepatic coma and death.

Liver Function Tests (See Table on p. 91).

(1) **Their Use in the Differential Diagnosis of the Cause of Jaundice**

In the following table are listed the typical findings in patients with hepatic jaundice and obstructive jaundice. It must be emphasised, however, that in many jaundiced patients a clear distinction cannot be based on the biochemical findings alone and that not infrequently results are obtained which appear to conflict with the rest of the clinical evidence. These anomalous findings may be partly due to the fact that in many patients with a primarily hepatic jaundice there are a number of complex factors leading to the raised serum bilirubin levels found (p. 84); and partly because in longstanding obstructive jaundice liver cell damage may eventually develop. A clearer picture of the course of events is obtained if the tests are repeated several times during the course of the illness. It is unwise to perform laparotomy on a patient with obstructive jaundice if serum transaminase levels are grossly and persistently raised and the alkaline phosphatase level is more than 210 u/l.

(2) Assessment of Liver Damage in Cirrhosis

In patients with jaundice the severity of liver cell damage is indicated by the height of the serum bilirubin level, the degree of reduction in the serum albumen and of rise in the serum globulin levels, and elevation of the serum aspartate-amino-transferase level (normal <35 u/l).

In patients without jaundice the *bromsulphalein* (B.S.P.) *retention test* is an accurate index of the severity of liver damage. 1 ml. of a 5-per-cent solution per 10 kg. body weight is injected intravenously and 30 minutes later a sample of venous blood is taken from the other arm; normally the serum at half-an-hour contains only 0–10 per cent of the injected dose. This test can also be used as an accurate index of recovery after infective hepatitis; it cannot be used, however, when the serum bilirubin is above $35\,\mu$ mol/l.

Thrombosis of the Portal Vein

Cirrhosis accounts for about half the cases of portal vein thrombosis, but it is a rare complication seen in only about 1 per cent of cirrhotics,

Test	Normal Range	Hepatic Jaundice	Obstructive Jaundice
Serum bilirubin	Up to 17 μmol/l.	Raised	Raised
Serum albumin	30–46 g./l.	Reduced	Normal
Serum globulin	20–38 g./l.	May be raised	Normal
Serum aspartate-amino-transferase	Up to 35 u/l.	Raised	Normal or only slightly raised
Serum alkaline phosphatase	7–106 u/l.	Usually less than 200 u/l.	Usually over 200 u/l. Also raised in bone disease
Serum 5 nucleotidase	0–13 u/l.	Usually normal	Raised (but not in bone disease)
Urobilin in urine	0 to trace	Increased in early hepatitis	0
Bilirubin in urine	0	Often present for a few days after the stage of urobilinuria	Present
γ gluteryl transpepdidase	<40 u/l.	An index of enzyme induction. Raised in alcholic liver disease and also raised in obstructive jaundice	

Other causes are malignant disease, portal phlebitis secondary to cholangitis, pancreatitis, or appendicitis, and increase in blood platelets (thrombocytosis) such as occurs in polycythaemia vera and after splenectomy. The clinical features are abdominal pain, splenomegaly, haematemesis, and ascites and distinction from intrahepatic portal obstruction is difficult. Absence of hepatomegaly and signs of hepatic failure are sometimes helpful but the diagnosis can be established with certainty only by splenic venography (which can be performed by percutaneous injection of the dye). The only practical importance in recognising the condition is that it precludes porta-caval anastamosis.

Hepatic Vein Thrombosis (Budd-Chiari syndrome)

This very rare condition is usually a complication of renal or hepatic carcinoma, thrombophlebitis migrans or polycythaemia. It causes sudden vomiting, enlargement of the liver, slight jaundice and ascites which is very resistant to treatment. Anticoagulant therapy should be instituted, but it is difficult to be sufficiently sure of the diagnosis for this to be done. The prognosis is very bad.

DISEASES OF THE PANCREAS

Acute Pancreatitis

The cause of this relatively common disease is not known, but about half the patients also have disease of the biliary tract and many of them are alcoholics or morphine addicts. An acute attack may occur during or soon after an alcoholic bout. It is thought that the characteristic lesions are produced by pancreatic enzymes which have escaped from their normal channels. They include necrosis and haemorrhagic oedema of the gland and plaques of fat necrosis on the mesentery and peritoneum as well as on the pancreas.

Clinical Features. The main symptom is extremely severe and persistent pain in the epigastrium or left upper quadrant of the abdomen passing through to the back, with vomiting and sometimes profound shock. There is deep epigastric tenderness and frequently some abdominal distension. A serum amylase level of 900 u/l. or higher (normal range 70–300 u/l.) is practically pathognomonic of the disease, though smaller increases in the level may be the result of spasm of the sphincter of Oddi induced by morphine and are occasionally found in other intra-abdominal diseases.

Treatment. Unless there is doubt about the diagnosis laparotomy should be avoided as it incurs a high mortality. If pethidine 100 mg. intramuscularly every few hours fails to relieve the pain, morphine 15–20 mg. may need to be given in spite of its tendency to cause spasm of the sphincter of Oddi. Shock must be combated by restoration of normal fluid and electrolyte balance, antibiotics such as penicillin 500,000 units with streptomycin 0·5 g. twice daily are given to prevent secondary infection of the damaged pancreas, and pancreatic secretion is minimised by giving nothing by mouth and administering a vagal blocking agent such as atropine sulphate 0·6 mg. intramuscularly every three or four hours. Aprotinin (Trasylol) is said to inhibit trypsin and may be of value if given in the first 24 hours. A million units are given I.V. followed by 100,000 units hourly for 3–4 hours.

Chronic Pancreatitis

Chronic pancreatitis is the term applied to the extensive fibrosis and atrophy of the acinar and islet tissue which may follow repeated attacks of acute or subacute pancreatitis and which may lead eventually to pancreatic insufficiency and diabetes mellitus. The condition is usually seen in middle-aged men. The *clinical history* starts with recurrent episodes of upper abdominal pain as described above; a stage may then be reached in which attacks recur every week or two or pain may become almost continuous and extremely demoralising; and finally diabetes mellitus and/or pancreatic insufficiency may develop. Occasionally the final stage may be reached without any history of severe pain. Pancreatic insufficiency is characterised by loss of weight and the passage of bulky fatty stools. Calcification of the pancreas seen on X-ray strongly favours chronic pancreatitis. More precise diagnosis can be made by radiological demonstration of the pancreatic ducts (E.R.C.P.), abdominal ultrasound and analysis of the pancreatic juice obtained after a secretion test. Estimation of the serum amylase level is less helpful than in the acute disease, though it is usually somewhat raised.

Treatment. The fat content of the diet should be restricted to 70 g. or less, but enough protein and carbohydrate must be given to ensure an adequate calorie intake. Strong Pancreatin powder B.N.F. 0·25–2 g. should be given with each meal together with cimetidine to reduce gastric acid. Alcohol should be forbidden. In patients with severe intractable pain sphincterotomy or even partial or complete resection of the pancreas may have to be performed, but no operation gives consistently good results and the mortality is high. Diabetes if present is controlled in the usual way.

FURTHER READING

Sherlock, Sheila, *Diseases of the Liver and Biliary System*, 5th edition, Blackwell, Oxford, 1975.

Truelove, S. C. and Reynell, P. C., *Diseases of the Digestive System*, 2nd edition, Blackwell, Oxford, 1971.

Bouchier, I. A. D., *Gastroenterology*, 2nd Edition, Baillière, London, 1977.

CHAPTER FOUR

THE CARDIOVASCULAR SYSTEM

INTRODUCTION

Diseases of the cardiovascular system are the commonest cause of death. With an ageing population it seems likely that there will be further increases in the incidence of those varieties of cardiovascular disease which occur in both middle and advanced age, namely coronary artery disease and hypertension.

THE EXAMINATION OF THE CARDIOVASCULAR SYSTEM

(1) Cyanosis

The colour of a part in terms of its redness or pallor depends on the amount of blood in the capillaries of that part and the thickness of the overlying tissues—where that tissue is thin, e.g. lips and conjunctivae, the colour may be very deep. The colour of blood depends on its haemoglobin and therefore the state and amount of the haemoglobin also influence the colour of the part.

When the capillary blood contains an excess of reduced haemoglobin, it looks blue and produces a blue shade in the skin and mucosae. This is cyanosis. Five grams of reduced haemoglobin per 100 ml. are required to produce detectable cyanosis.

Cyanosis may be of two kinds:

    (a) *Peripheral cyanosis*, which is due to stagnation of blood in the capillaries, is best seen in the extremities and the lips and is often associated with coldness of the part. It may be abolished by warming the part. It is not seen in the tongue or mouth. It may occur in heart failure or be due to local causes such as poor circulation in the hands or feet. Normal people who are 'blue with cold' have this type of cyanosis.

    (b) *Central cyanosis* is due either to inadequate uptake of oxygen in the lungs secondary to pulmonary disease or to a right to left cardiac shunt which results in deoxygenated blood bypassing the lungs and passing directly to the systemic circulation. It is characterised by cyanosis which affects the mouth and tongue as well as the extremities, which are warm.

(2) Temperature of the Extremities

Coldness of the extremities is due to vasoconstriction or obstruction of the superficial blood vessels so that the blood supply to the skin is reduced.

In heart disease it is often due to the peripheral vasoconstriction which follows a fall in cardiac output. Conversely, in conditions with a high cardiac output the peripheral vessels are dilated and the skin is very warm.

(3) Clubbing of the Fingers

Clubbing of the fingers may occur in cardiac disease. In congenital cyanotic heart disease it is related to the degree of cyanosis and is often very marked, the fingers having a drumstick-like appearance. It is also seen in patients with cor pulmonale and in infective endocarditis. The possibility of other causes, including chronic lung suppuration, carcinoma of the bronchus, ulcerative colitis, the malabsorption syndrome, and cirrhosis of the liver, must not be forgotten.

(4) The Arterial Pulse

The pulse rate and rhythm as usually determined by feeling the radial pulse.

(a) *Rate.* During the first year of life the normal pulse rate is about 100–110 per minute. As the child grows up the pulse becomes slower and by puberty it has slowed to the adult rate, which is usually between 65–85 per minute. Athletes, however, may have a resting rate of 50 per minute or less. Increase in pulse rate is called *tachycardia* and may be due to emotion, exertion, fever, thyrotoxicosis, bleeding, intrinsic heart disease, paroxysmal tachycardia, atrial flutter or atrial fibrillation. Sleep eliminates emotion and exertion and therefore the sleeping pulse rate may be a valuable observation.

Undue slowing of the pulse is called *bradycardia* and is much less common; it may be due to sinus bradycardia as in hypothyroidism, obstructive jaundice or raised intracranial pressure and is quite commonly found in young fit people; it may also be due to disorders of the pacemaker or conducting system of the heart. It may also result from overdosage of digitalis or β blockers.

(b) *Rhythm.* Abnormalities of rhythm are considered on page 117.

(c) *Tension.* Measurement of the systolic blood pressure by digital compression of the pulse is misleading. It can only be accurately measured by the use of a sphygmomanometer.

(d) *Volume.* The pulse volume is dependent on the pulse pressure. It is better appreciated at the carotid artery than at the wrist. A small pulse volume means a small stroke volume and is often associated with peripheral vasoconstriction or with severe heart disease. A large pulse volume is usually associated with a large stroke volume and a low peripheral resistance.

(e) *Pulse Wave.* There are a number of variations in the pulse wave which may be helpful in diagnosis. They are best appreciated by feeling a large artery, for example the carotid rather than the radial.

(1) *Collapsing Pulse* (*Water hammer pulse*). This is detected by

lifting the patient's arm and grasping the wrist with the whole hand, when the pulse wave can be felt as an abrupt but forcible tap. It is associated with a wide pulse pressure with an abrupt rise and fall in the pulse wave. It is found most markedly in free aortic incompetence and may also be present in patients with patent ductus arteriosus, peripheral arteriovenous aneurysms, or a rigid atherosclerotic aorta.

(2) *Plateau Pulse*. This type of pulse is characterised by a wave which is slow rising, flattened, and more prolonged than normal. It is found in severe aortic stenosis.

(3) *Pulsus Bisferiens*. Pulsus bisferiens is a double pulse wave and is found in patients with combined aortic stenosis and regurgitation or in pure aortic regurgitation.

(4) *Pulsus Alternans*. Pulsus alternans consists of alternate weak and strong pulse waves. It may be appreciated on palpation of the pulse, but is more easily shown with the sphygmomanometer. It is found in left ventricular failure.

(5) *Pulsus Paradoxus*. Pulsus paradoxus is found in constrictive pericarditis and pericardial effusions. Normally inspiration sucks blood into the right ventricle with a corresponding rise in right ventricular output to fill the expanded pulmonary vascular bed. If the right ventricle cannot expand due to rigidity or a surrounding effusion, this compensating rise in right ventricular filling cannot occur and cardiac output falls. It can also occasionally occur in asthma where there is a sharp fall in intrathoracic pressure on inspiration.

(5) The Venous Pulse

The neck veins should be examined in the recumbent patient with the head and shoulders raised 30° from the horizontal. At this angle the column of blood in the jugular system should reach the level of the clavicle. The normal jugular venous pressure is measured with reference to the sternal angle and is usually recorded in cm. of blood. In normal individuals the range is between +3 and −6 cm. with the subject horizontal. Where precise measurement is required a catheter may be introduced into the atrium for continuous monitoring of pressure which is then sometimes called *central venous pressure*, but which really indicates right atrial pressure. On elevation of jugular venous pressure is found in *heart failure* and in certain conditions associated with a high cardiac output. It is also raised in superior vena caval obstruction when pulsation is absent. Finally minor degrees of elevated venous pressure may occur in conditions with increased intra-abdominal pressure such as pregnancy. The external jugular veins may be compressed as they pass through the cervical fascia; it is therefore best to observe the right internal jugular vein.

With the normal jugular *venous pulse* it is possible to observe 'a' and 'v' waves. The 'a' wave is caused by contraction of the right atrium and coincides with the first heart sound. It is followed by the 'x' descent due to relaxation of the right atrium. Pressure recordings in addition show a notch on the 'x' descent which is called the 'c' wave and is probably due to transmitted carotid pulsation. Following the 'x' descent the 'v' wave represents the rise in pressure which occurs when the right atrium fills with the tricuspid valve closed; it coincides with the second heart sound. Finally the tricuspid valve opens in ventricular diastole causing a fall in atrial pressure which is seen in the venous pulse as the 'y' descent.

Large 'a' waves are seen in tricuspid stenosis or when there is increased rigidity of the right ventricle due to hypertrophy such as occurs in pulmonary stenosis or with pulmonary hypertension. Very large 'a' waves or *cannon waves* are seen when the right atrium contracts against a closed tricuspid valve due to atrial and ventricular contractions being nearly synchronous. This occurs regularly in nodal rhythm and nodal tachycardia, and irregularly in complete heart block and rarely with ventricular ectopic beats. The 'v' wave is increased in right ventricular failure.

Large waves corresponding to ventricular systole occur in tricuspid incompetence due to the systolic pulse being transmitted to the right atrium.

A deep and abrupt 'y' descent is found in constrictive pericarditis and is due to the ventricular walls being sprung apart early in ventricular diastole. It may also occur in right ventricular failure due to rapid ventricular filling early in diastole.

(6) The Liver

With a rise in venous pressure such as occurs in congestive cardiac failure the liver becomes congested and enlarged. It may be painful and tender on palpation if the enlargement is rapid. Expansile pulsation in the liver is found in tricuspid incompetence. Chronic congestion may lead to some interference with liver function and result in slight jaundice and even cardiac cirrhosis.

(7) Hepatojugular Reflux

Continuous pressure over the liver or abdomen increases the filling of the right atrium and ventricle; in the normal heart this can be accommodated without raising jugular venous pressure but in right ventricular failure the neck veins become distended.

Dyspnoea, orthnopnoea, and *oedema* are discussed on page 108.

THE BLOOD PRESSURE

Introduction. The intermittent rise and fall of pressure within the arteries depends on the ejection of blood from the left ventricle. The peak pressure developed is called the systolic pressure and the lowest pressure the diastolic pressure. The difference between systolic and diastolic pressures is called the pulse pressure.

The height of the blood pressure depends on the cardiac output and the peripheral resistance to blood flow. An increase in cardiac output causes a rise in mean blood pressure, the systolic pressure being more affected than the diastolic pressure. A rise in resistance to flow or a rise in pulse rate causes a rise in mean blood pressure, the diastolic being more affected than the systolic pressure.

The rise in blood pressure which occurs on exercise or with emotion is predominantly due to a rise in cardiac output and this may often be associated with a fall in peripheral resistance. In essential hypertension, however, the cardiac output is normal and the elevated blood pressure is due to increase resistance to blood flow.

Another factor which modifies the blood pressure is the elasticity of the arteries. In youth when the arteries are elastic the pulse pressure tends to be low, even in the face of a high peripheral resistance. With increasing age the arteries become less elastic and the pulse pressure increases and may result in the development of so-called benign systolic hypertension of the aged, with a blood pressure in the region of 200/90 mm. Hg. This type of raised blood pressure may be of less significance than that due to an increased peripheral resistance.

Measurement of Blood Pressure. When measuring the blood pressure the subject must be at rest both physically and mentally as both recent exercise and anxiety may cause a transient rise. It is customary to take the blood pressure in the right arm, although, except where there is obstruction to the arterial supply to one limb, there is not usually more than a few millimeters of pressure difference between the two arms. It is important to ensure that the sphygmomanometer cuff is firmly and evenly applied. The cuff is fully inflated and then deflated and the pressure at which the brachial pulse returns is determined by palpation. This gives a rough guide to the systolic pressure. The cuff is then reinflated and the stethoscope applied over the brachial artery. The *systolic blood* pressure is the pressure at which sounds appear. The *diastolic* pressure is taken as the pressure at which there is a change from loud clear sounds to muffled sounds.

As the sphygmomanometer cuff is deflated, there is sometimes a pressure range between the systolic and diastolic pressures when no sound is heard. This is called the 'silent gap' and if the blood pressure is being measured by the auscultatory method, the return of sounds at the end of the silent gap may be mistaken for the true systolic pressure. This mistake is avoided if the systolic pressure is first determined by palpation.

THE HEART

Inspection. The apex beat may be visible and its position should be noted. A search should be made for other pulsations. A characteristic 'lift' can sometimes be seen between the apex and the left sternal border in patients with right ventricular hypertrophy, and if the pulmonary arteries are dilated this may extend up to the second or third left intercostal spaces. Aneurysm of the first part of the aorta produces pulsation in the second right intercostal space.

Palpation. The position of the *apex beat* should be confirmed; if it is difficult to locate, palpation should be carried out with the patient sitting forward and expiring fully. Normally the apex beat is in the 5th intercostal space just internal to the midclavicular line. It may be displaced either by shift of the mediastinum or by cardiac enlargement. In left ventricular hypertrophy the apex beat is displaced downwards and to the left and is of of a characterically localised and thrusting nature. Sometimes in left ventricular failure a double impulse starting in late diastole can be felt at the apex. This is due to forceful atrial contraction followed by left ventricular contraction (see Heart Sounds, below). If hypertrophy is combined with dilatation the apex beat feels more diffuse. With right ventricular hypertrophy a forceful impulse can be felt just to the left of the lower end of the sternum; if hypertrophy is minimal but there is a large flow through the right ventricle as in atrial septal defect the impulse has a tapping character.

Careful examination must be made for *thrills*. These are vibrations which may be appreciated by the hand and are really palpable murmurs. Systolic thrills can be felt in the appropriate areas in both aortic and pulmonary stenosis and in mitral incompetence. A systolic thrill can also be felt over ventricular septal defects and aortic aneurysms. A diastolic thrill may be felt in mitral stenosis. The presence of a definite thrill is always abnormal, and must be distinguished from the slight vibrations which may be felt over a forcibly beating heart.

Occasionally it may be possible to feel valve closures. For instance, the loud first sound in mitral stenosis due to forcible closure of the mitral valve may be actually palpable.

Percussion. It is doubtful whether percussion affords any more information than can usually be found on palpation, but it is customary to percuss out the left and right borders of the heart. By this means the cardiac area can be roughly outlined and percussion may occasionally be useful in the diagnosis of a pericardial effusion or of an aneurysm of the ascending aorta.

Auscultation. Auscultation must be carried out over the whole praecordium and not merely in the classical mitral, aortic, pulmonary, and tricuspid areas.

(A) **Heart Sounds.** There are four groups of heart sounds.

    (1) Sounds produced by valve closure—namely the first sound, caused by closure of the tricuspid and mitral valves, and the second sound from closure of the aortic and pulmonary valves.

    (2) Sound produced by valves opening—namely the opening snap of the mitral valve.

    (3) Sound produced by rapid ventricular filling.

    (4) Extra-cardiac sounds.

Some of the sounds may be heard in both normal and abnormal hearts; others only occur in the diseased heart.

(1) *Sounds of Valve Closure.* The *first heart sound* is produced by the closure of the mitral and tricuspid valves. In health it is either single or closely split. In right, and left, bundle branch block the splitting may be quite wide due to the asynchronous closure of the mitral and tricuspid valves.

The *loudness* of the first heart sound depends on the position of the A-V valves at the beginning of ventricular systole. If they have been forced well down into the ventricular cavity by the flow of blood from the atria they have a long way to snap back when systole begins and the first

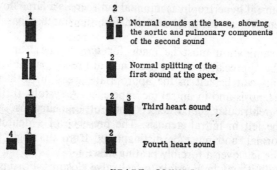

HEART SOUNDS

sound is therefore loud. This occurs particularly with a short P-R interval, and in mitral stenosis. In the latter condition it is probable that the rather prolonged blood flow through the stenosed mitral valve together with shortening of the chordae tendinae keeps the valve deep in the ventricle until systole starts. Loud first heart sounds are also heard in nervous people with tachycardia, in thyrotoxicosis and in anaemia and are due to the rapid ventricular contraction forcibly closing the A-V valves.

The *second heart sound* at the base of the heart is composed of the closure of the aortic and pulmonary valves. In most children and in many adults the second sound in this area can be heard to be closely split, the first element of the split being due to aortic valve closure and the second element to pulmonary valve closure. Normally this split increases with inspiration, probably due to a momentary increase in the stroke volume of the right ventricle with a prolongation of systole. In *right bundle branch block* the split is wide and widens on inspiration, in *atrial septal defect* the split is wide and fixed.

In *left bundle branch block* the splitting of the second sound may be reversed so that the aortic component follows the pulmonary component. In this case the sounds come closer together on inspiration.

(2) *Sounds produced by valves opening.* The most important of these sounds is the *opening snap of the mitral valve.* It is best heard between the

apex beat and the lower sternum. It is a sharp, high-pitched snap and occurs in early diastole. It is almost, but not quite, diagnostic of mitral stenosis; it is rarely heard in mitral incompetence.

Ejection clicks are high-pitched sounds occurring in early systole; they are found in valvar aortic or pulmonary stenosis and are due to sudden distension of the stenosed valve at the start of systole.

(3) *Sounds produced by rapid ventricular filling* (*Triple rhythm*). These extra sounds are probably produced by rapid distension of the hypertrophied and rigid ventricles. They are low pitched and can thus be readily distinguished from the high pitched sounds of valve opening and closure.

The *third heart sound* is produced by rapid ventricular filling with distension in early diastole. It is frequently heard at the apex in normal young adults, but in people over the age of 40 it is associated with increased rigidity of the ventricular muscle. It is heard best at the left sternal edge in right ventricular failure, and at the apex in left ventricular failure.

The *fourth heart sound* is produced by rapid filling of the ventricles associated with forceful atrial contraction and occurs just before the first heart sound in late diastole. It is best heard a little way inside the apex beat and is found particularly in hypertension and aortic valve disease. It does not necessarily mean that there is left ventricular failure but indicates left ventricular overload. It cannot be present if there is atrial fibrillation and may disappear if the overload is removed (i.e. if hypertension is treated). If the heart is beating rapidly the three sounds may assume the cadence of a horse's hooves when galloping. This is called *gallop rhythm*.

Sometimes both third and fourth heart sounds may be present and if the heart rate is rapid these additional sounds may blend to produce what is sometimes called a *summation gallop* or *canter rhythm*. It is always of serious significance and suggests gross failure of ventricular function.

(4) *Extra-cardiac Sounds.* These sounds are usually heard in the latter half of systole. They are of a scratchy or crunchy nature and often sound rather superficial. They alter in intensity with respiration and position. They have a variety of causes and are usually innocent.

A special type of extra-cardiac sound is the *pericardial friction rub*. It may be heard at the base or apex of the heart and may be systolic or diastolic in timing or sometimes both. It is a scratchy or crunchy sound. There is usually other clinical evidence to suggest pericarditis.

(B) **Heart murmurs** are caused by eddies set up in blood as it passes from a narrow to a wider channel. They may be caused by pathological narrowing of valves, by their incompetence, or by undue distension of channels. Eddies may also be produced by the unduly rapid passage of blood through the heart as in thyrotoxicosis. When describing murmurs the following points should be noted:

(1) Site and radiation.
(2) Timing.
(3) Loudness. This is usually graded 1–6 for systolic and 1–4 for

diastolic murmurs, grade 1 being very soft and grade 6 very loud.

(4) The pitch of the murmur.

(5) The presence or absence of a thrill.

Murmurs can be classified:

(1) Systolic murmurs.
(2) Diastolic murmurs.
(3) Continuous murmurs.

(1) *Systolic Murmurs*

    (*a*) *Ejection murmurs* are caused by the ventricles forcing blood through a narrowed orifice usually a stenosed aortic or pulmonary valve, or through a normal orifice into a dilated vessel such as an aortic aneurysm or a dilated pulmonary artery as in atrial septal defects. They can also be produced by rapid flow through a normal valve (see below).

    Characteristically this type of murmur commences after the first sound, rises to a crescendo in mid-systole and dies away before the second sound.

    (*b*) *Pansystolic murmurs* are due to incompetence of the mitral or tricuspid valves or to a ventricular septal defect. They last throughout systole up to the second sound, they are more or less constant in intensity with sometimes a late systolic crescendo.

    (*c*) *Late systolic murmurs* are found in coarctation of the aorta. Apparently normal subjects may occasionally have a *mid-systolic click* followed by a *late systolic murmur*. This is believed to be associated with various congenital abnormalities of the mitral valve, including elongated chordae or

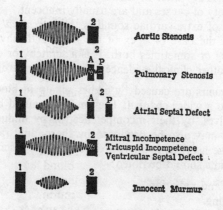

	Aortic Stenosis
	Pulmonary Stenosis
	Atrial Septal Defect
	Mitral Incompetence Tricuspid Incompetence Ventricular Septal Defect
	Innocent Murmur

SYSTOLIC MURMURS

voluminous valves. Occasionally late systolic murmurs are found in hypertrophic obstructive cardiomyopathy (see page 154) and are due to a combination of obstruction to the out-flow from the left ventricle and to mitral incompetence.

Systolic murmurs are usually high pitched.

Innocent Systolic Murmurs. A great many systolic murmurs are not due to organic disease. The cause of such murmurs is not fully understood but many of them may be associated with a high velocity of blood flow and can be considered to be attenuated ejection murmurs. They are particularly liable to occur with pregnancy, anaemia, or fevers. They are commonly heard along the left sternal border or at the apex and they are rarely very loud. Their timing varies but they are usually of short duration. They nearly always begin in early systole and finish by mid-systole. Their differentiation from organic systolic murmurs will depend partially on the character of the murmur and partially on the presence or absence of other evidence of cardiac disease.

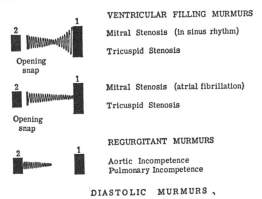

VENTRICULAR FILLING MURMURS

Mitral Stenosis (in sinus rhythm)

Tricuspid Stenosis

Mitral Stenosis (atrial fibrillation)

Tricuspid Stenosis

REGURGITANT MURMURS

Aortic Incompetence
Pulmonary Incompetence

DIASTOLIC MURMURS

(2) *Diastolic Murmurs*

(a) *Ventricular Filling Murmurs.* These murmurs are due to the flow of blood through stenosed mitral or tricuspid valves. They are separated from the second heart sound by a short gap of variable duration. In patients in sinus rhythm the murmur rises to a crescendo just before the first heart sound due to the contracting atria causing a momentarily increased rate of flow through the narrowed A-V valve. These murmurs are always low-pitched and rumbling.

The murmur of mitral stenosis is heard best with the patient lying on the left side. In mitral incompetence and ventricular septal defect there is increased blood flow through the mitral valve in diastole and although the valves are normal they may produce a low pitched diastolic murmur.

(b) The *Austin Flint Murmur.* This is an apical diastolic murmur heard in aortic regurgitation and is due to vibration of the anterior cusp of the mitral valve between the regurgitant flow from the aorta and the flow from the left atrium.

(c) *Regurgitant Diastolic Murmurs.* They are soft and high pitched and are due to regurgitation of blood through the aortic or pulmonary valves. They are heard best with the patient sitting forward and in full expiration. They start immediately after the second heart sound, are loudest at their onset and die away before the end of diastole.

(3) *Continuous Murmurs.* Certain murmurs continue throughout systole and diastole. They are found when there is blood flow between high and low pressure vessels, most commonly when a patent ductus connects the aorta with the pulmonary artery.

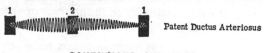

Patent Ductus Arteriosus

CONTINUOUS MURMURS

THE ELECTROCARDIOGRAM

The electrocardiogram records the electrical changes produced by the depolarisation and subsequent repolarisation of the heart muscle, associated respectively with systole and diastole. These changes are amplified and recorded on moving paper. The potential changes are recorded by electrodes attached in various combinations to the body. Each of these attachments is known as a 'lead'.

There are two main groups of leads, known as bipolar and unipolar.

Bipolar leads record the potential changes between two points of the body surface, the leads in common use being:

Lead 1—which records the potential difference between the right and left arm.

Lead 2—between the right arm and left leg.

Lead 3—between the left arm and left leg.

Unipolar leads record potential change at one position on the body's surface. This is done by connecting the leads from both arms and the left leg, the potential change from these three leads being zero. A further electrode is then placed at various positions on the body's surface and the potential changes at these positions recorded. The most usual positions are the chest leads which are numbered V1–6 and the limb leads which are designated a VR (which is the right arm), a VL (left arm) and a VF (left foot).

Tracings from all parts of the body have certain common characteristics. The first wave, which is usually upright, but may be inverted, is called the

P wave and represents atrial contraction. The next wave is a small downward deflection known as the Q wave and this is followed by an upright deflection, the R wave, and a further downward deflection, the S wave. This QRS complex represents ventricular contraction.

The P-R interval, measured from the beginning of the P wave to the beginning of the R wave, represents the time taken by the wave of excitation to pass down the bundle of His and should not exceed 0·2 second in the normal subject. The duration of the QRS complex represents the time taken for the wave of excitation to spread through the ventricle and should not exceed 0·1 second in the normal subject. The QRS complex is followed by a short interval and then by a deflection which is usually upright. This is the T wave and represents the recession of the wave of excitation through the ventricle. Changes in the S-T segment and T wave area are of importance in the diagnosis of damage to the heart muscle.

In normal people the basic deflection in each lead is of one of three types. This depends on whether the electrode faces the right ventricle, the left ventricle, or the ventricular cavity. If the heart is in the normal position, leads aVF and Vs 1 and 2 have complexes arising from the right ventricle. Leads aVL and Vs 4, 5, and 6 have complexes arising from the left ventricle and lead aVR has complexes arising from the ventricular cavities. The *right ventricular lead* is characterised by a small R and large S waves and the absence of Q waves, *the left ventricular lead* by a small Q wave followed by a large R wave and small or absent S wave. In the *ventricular cavity lead* the P wave is inverted, the QRS complex consists of a negative deflection and the T wave is also inverted.

If the heart is in an abnormal position, then of course the distribution of these complexes is changed.

In reading an electrocardiogram the following points should be noted:

(1) Heart rate.
(2) Heart rhythm.
(3) Nature and direction of the P waves.
(4) The duration of the P-R interval.
(5) The direction of the main deflection and general shape of the QRS complex.
(6) The width of the QRS complex.
(7) The size of the complexes.
(8) Any depression or elevation of the S-T segment.
(9) The direction and character of the T waves.

ECHOCARDIOGRAPHY

This is a method of investigation which is becoming increasingly important. It is non-invasive and harmless and can be carried out in a short time. Essentially it consists of recording the echoes obtained from a sound source of 1000 pulses per second. This shows the pattern of movement obtained from the pericardium, the interventricular septum and posterior wall of the left ventricle, the mitral, triscuspid, aortic and pulmonary valves and the left atrium. It is particularly useful in the diagnosis of:

(1) Left atrial myxoma (see page 155).
(2) Mitral valve disease.
(3) Left ventricular function.

The movements of the left ventricular wall and septum can be measured during systole together with the rate of change.

The thickness of the left ventricular septum can be measured and this can be useful in the diagnosis of hypertrophic cardiomyopathy.

(4) Pericardial effusion.

Echocardiography shows two echoes, one from the moving posterior myocardium and one from the inert pericardium.

RADIOLOGY OF THE HEART

The heart can be examined by chest radiography, by fluorescent screening or by introducing radio-opaque substances into the heart or coronary arteries which is then X-rayed.—this is known as angiocardiography.

In a plain radiograph of the heart, the right side of the cardiac silhouette is made up of the right atrium, the ascending aorta, and the superior vena cava. The left border is formed by the aortic arch, the pulmonary artery and the left ventricle. When the heart is examined by X-ray screening it should also be viewed in the left and right anterior oblique positions. If a little barium emulsion is swallowed the back of the heart is outlined and slight enlargement of the left atrium can easily be seen, especially in the right anterior oblique position.

Cardiac Enlargement. A general idea of the size of the heart can be obtained by measuring the maximum transverse diameter of the heart and the maximum transverse diameter of the chest; normally the heart diameter should not be more than half that of the chest.

Enlargement of individual heart chambers can also be demonstrated radiologically. Left ventricular enlargement causes rounding of the left lower border of the heart shadow on P.A. view, and in the L.A.O. position the left ventricle can be seen bulging backwards and overlying the spine. Right ventricular enlargement causes increase in the transverse diameter of the heart and there is often straightening of the left border of the heart caused by enlargement of the outflow tract of the right ventricle. Left atrial enlargement is best seen in the R.A.O. position when it can be seen to indent the oesophagus following a barium swallow. In the P.A. view the enlarged left atrial appendage appears on the left border of the heart, below the pulmonary artery. Right atrial enlargement produces a bulge at the lowest part of the right cardiac border.

A pericardial effusion also produces an increase in the cardiac shadow which is usually pear-shaped with clear-cut margins and the lung fields frequently appear clear. It is not always easy to differentiate between enlargement of the heart and a pericardial effusion so that aspiration may be necessary to settle the diagnosis.

By radiological methods it is also possible to assess the great vessels leaving the heart and to demonstrate calcification of the heart valves.

CIRCULATORY FAILURE

Failure of the circulation occurs when the heart is unable to maintain an adequate output. It can be of both acute and chronic forms which produce differing clinical pictures.

Acute Circulatory Failure

In this condition there is a sudden fall in cardiac output and blood pressure which is due to two causes:

Hypovolaemia—where there is inadequate venous return to the heart and thus a failure of output. This is commonly secondary to *haemorrhage, sodium deficiency* and *trauma*.

Pump failure—where the myocardium cannot maintain an adequate output of blood. It occurs commonly after *cardiac infarction* or *pulmonary embolism*.

Circulatory failure may also complicate *septicaemia* particularly by Gram negative organisms. The mechanism here is complicated. The clinical distinction between pump failure and hypovolaemia may be clear from the history and physical signs. In cases of doubt and to monitor progress, measurement of central venous pressure or better pulmonary artery wedge pressure (reflecting left atrial pressure) (see p. 109) can be useful. These will be low in uncomplicated hypovolaemia and raised in pump failure. However, it must be remembered that pump failure and hypovolaemia can coexist, in which case these pressures will be misleading.

Clinical Features. The picture is one of adrenergic overactivity with pallor and cold extremities due to vasoconstriction, sweating and tachycardia. The blood pressure is low. In severe cases perfusion of vital organs is impaired causing confusion, acute renal failure (see p. 388), and acidosis due to overproduction of lactic acid. *Shock lung*, in which there is increasing dyspnoea with hypoxia and bilateral shadows on X-ray, can develop and will require artificial ventilation.

Treatment. This depends on the cause. If the inadequate circulation is due to pump failure treatment is difficult and various agents have been tried to encourage the failing myocardium. Dopamine by continuous intravenous infusion in doses of 2–5 μg/kg/minute increases the cardiac output by an effect on the myocardium and also causes dilation of renal blood vessels and thus to some degree guards against acute renal failure. Dobutamine which acts largely on the heart is also used. Generally however, the prognosis is bad. In hypovolaemia, circulating volume should be restored by infusion of plasma expanders such as dextran (or blood if due to haemorrhage), using central venous pressure or pulmonary artery wedge pressure as an index of adequate replacement. Causative factors such as infection should be treated vigorously with antibiotics which may be combined with 500 mg. hydrocortisone I.V. six-hourly.

Heart Failure (Chronic Circulatory Failure)

Heart failure is a chronic failure of the ventricles to maintain an adequate output of blood for the needs of the body.

Cardiac Function in Heart Failure

The fall in cardiac output may be due to an increased work load from an obstruction caused by a valve lesion or hypertension, or to changes in the cardiac muscle such as may follow infarction. In response to the increased work load the cardiac muscle hypertrophies; at first this will compensate but in time myocardial contractility becomes impaired, and the increased mass of muscle becomes more rigid so that relaxation in diastole is limited. Diastolic filling is thus reduced with a fall in end-diastolic volume and a rise in end-diastolic pressure. Three factors may therefore be involved in the reduced stroke volume and the low output of cardiac failure.

(a) *Reduced contractility of the myocardium*, most frequently due to ischaemia.

(b) *Increased myocardial systolic tension* (*after load*), which is a reflection of the resistance to ventricular outflow. This will be raised in hypertension and in stenosis of the aortic and pulmonary valves. Cardiac failure itself causes a rise in peripheral resistance due to vasoconstriction and may thus potentiate the vicious circle.

(c) *Increased diastolic length of the myocardial fibres* (*pre-load*) which reflects endiastolic pressure and an elevated venous pressure.

These three factors are frequently interlocked so that one factor may potentiate the others. The resulting decreased cardiac output causes the signs and symptoms of heart failure.

(1) Oedema

(a) A fall in the blood flow to the kidneys leads to retention of sodium chloride and water which in turn causes a rise in circulating blood volume and the appearance of excess fluid in the tissue spaces; the distribution of this fluid is influenced by gravity so that it collects mainly around the ankles, or, if the patient is in bed, over the sacrum. It is known as dependent or cardiac oedema and characteristically pits on pressure. Sometimes ascites or pleural effusions develop.

(b) A rise in venous pressure (*vide infra*) at the venous end of the capillary further increases the amount of tissue fluids by preventing reabsorption.

(c) Increased production of aldosterone also leads to retention of salt and water.

(2) **Increased venous pressure.** The rise in venous pressure which is found in heart failure is due to:

(a) The rise in circulating blood volume.

(b) On the normal heart a rise in ventricular volume (preloading) at the end of diastole results in a rise in stroke volume and in cardiac output so that the diastolic volume is returned to normal. An essential feature of the failing heart is its inability to respond in this way. This impairment of ventricular function is reflected in the venous pressure so that in heart failure a rise in venous pressure is not followed by an increase in cardiac output as in the normal heart. The vicious circle of rising venous pressure and falling output can be broken either by increasing the output with digitalis or by decreasing blood volume and lowering venous pressure by diuretics, venesection or drugs which cause venous dilation.

(3) **Heart Rate**

A rise in heart rate leads to a rise in cardiac output. Tachycardia due to increased adrenergic activity is a compensating mechanism in heart failure. If this adrenergic 'drive' is removed by adrenergic blocking agents the heart failure is made worse.

(4) **Dyspnoea,** which is usually a prominent feature of cardiac failure, is due to a number of factors most prominent of which is oedema of the lungs which interferes with gaseous exchange. In addition the increased 'stiffness' of the lung due to oedema leads to an increased sensitivity of the lung stretch reflexes.

Patients with cardiac failure, except for a small group without pulmonary congestion, become dyspnoeic on lying flat (*orthopnoea*). This is due to the increase in amount of blood in the lungs which develops in the horizontal position and which leads in turn to an increase in pulmonary venous congestion. Changes in position may also affect cardiac output, but this probably plays a lesser part in the genesis of orthopnoea.

(5) **Cyanosis.** This is peripheral in type and results from the slowing of the circulation with consequent venous stagnation of blood.

(6) **Tiredness and weakness** are common symptoms associated with the low cardiac output and are due to poor periphereal perfusion.

(7) **Water and electrolyte disorder in heart failure.** In mild or moderate heart failure there is retention of sodium and water, so that although the total body content of sodium rises, the concentration of sodium in the blood remains normal. In severe and prolonged heart failure, particularly

if diuretics have been used vigorously, there is a tendency for the body to retain water rather than sodium and water so that the plasma sodium concentration falls. This is often associated with considerable potassium depletion due to both diuretics and possibly leakage of potassium from chronically hypoxic cells. The result is a patient who is oedematous due to extracellular overhydration and yet suffers from intracellular dehydration due to potassium deficiency.

It is customary and useful to divide heart failure into left and right ventricular failure for although in most cases of left ventricular failure the right ventricle will sooner or later fail as well, there is often at first only failure of one ventricle.

LEFT VENTRICULAR FAILURE

The chief causes of left ventricular failure are:

(1) Hypertension.
(2) Coronary artery disease.
(3) Aortic valvular disease.
(4) Mitral incompetence (*Rare*).
(5) Acute pulmonary oedema may also complicate mitral stenosis but is due to left atrial and not left ventricular failure.

The left ventricle may be called on to do increased work (after loading), either because an obstruction to output causes a rise in pressure (hypertension or aortic stenosis) or because there is an increased volume of blood to be handled (mitral or aortic incompetence). The ventricle hypertrophies and for a time is able to maintain an adequate circulation, but eventually it is unable to do so. A similar situation arises if the myocardium is diseased, usually as a result of cardiac infarction. In both cases the pressure rises in the left atrium (pre-loading) and pulmonary veins, leading to pulmonary venous pressure and ultimately to pulmonary oedema.

Clinical Features. Left ventricular failure may develop gradually or suddenly. When it is of slow onset the patient usually complains first of dyspnoea on effort. In addition, his sleep is disturbed. At first he is restless when lying flat and is relieved by two or three pillows (*orthopnoea*); later sleep is broken by *paroxysmal nocturnal coughing*, relieved by sitting up and hanging the legs out of bed; later still, *paroxysmal nocturnal dyspnoea* or *cardiac asthma* appears. Left ventricular failure of *abrupt* onset, almost invariably due to coronary thrombosis, may present with cardiac asthma without preceding symptoms. In the fully developed attack of paroxysmal nocturnal dyspnoea the patient goes to sleep and awakens an hour or two later in a state of great alarm, with a sense of suffocation and fighting for breath. He sits up and may throw open the windows. In severe attacks copiously frothy sputum is expectorated, which may be bloodstained and which is due to pulmonary oedema. After an hour or so the attack passes off and the patient sleeps until morning. Rarely does a first attack prove fatal.

It is not entirely clear why these attacks occur at night, but a number of factors including the recumbent position, which increase the extent of the pulmonary venous congestion, are operative.

Examination at the time of the attack may show evidence of left ventricular hypertrophy; if however left ventricular failure complicates myocardial infarction this may be absent. *Tachycardia* is usual and on auscultation *a third or fourth heart sound* may be heard. *Fine râles* from pulmonary oedema are heard at the lung bases, and there may be rhonchi from associated bronchospasm and bronchial oedema. If the attack is severe, there may be a fall in the systolic blood pressure. *Pulsus alternans* (p. 96) may be detected; when the difference in the systolic pressure exceeds 15–20 mm. of mercury, and particularly when the alternation persists after the tachycardia has subsided, it is of grave prognostic significance.

The *electrocardiogram* always shows some evidence of S-T or T wave changes over the left ventricle. A chest radiograph will show the hazy shadows of pulmonary oedema spreading out from each hilum into the lung fields.

Prognosis. It used to be said that the prognosis after an attack of cardiac asthma was poor, most patients dying within a year or two. With improved methods of treatment this is no longer entirely true and some patients may do quite well, particularly if the underlying disease, such as hypertension, is amenable to treatment.

RIGHT VENTRICULAR AND CONGESTIVE FAILURE

The chief causes of right ventricular failure are:

(1) Following left ventricular failure.
(2) Mitral valvular disease.
(3) Pulmonary heart disease.
(4) Certain types of congenital heart disease.
(5) Following pulmonary embolism.
(6) Thyrotoxicosis.

Tricuspid stenosis and constrictive pericarditis can also cause marked systemic venous congestion.

Clinical Features. Right ventricular failure is usually seen in patients who already suffer dyspnoea and orthopnoea from pulmonary congestion due to left ventricular failure or mitral valvular disease, and it is then often called *congestive cardiac failure*. When right ventricular failure occurs without pulmonary congestion or pulmonary disease, marked dyspnoea or orthopnoea is not usually a prominent feature although usually present to some degree. Other symptoms include tiredness, weakness, and loss of appetite.

The main signs of right ventricular failure are found in the systemic venous system. In a normal subject reclining at 30°, the neck veins are empty above the clavicles. In right ventricular failure, the *increased venous pressure* causes distension of the veins above this level. The pulsation in the distended veins can readily be distinguished from that of the carotids by the diffuse nature of the venous pulse, in which it is usually possible to distinguish at least two elements, and by the fact that the venous pulse can easily be obliterated by the finger. With severe right ventricular failure, there is stretching of the tricuspid ring leading to functional tricuspid incompetence and a consequent large systolic venous wave which can be seen in the neck and may be felt over the liver. It may disappear with treatment. Distension of the liver with blood, which follows right ventricular failure, may give rise to pain in the right hypochondrium. Palpation shows that the *liver is enlarged and tender*. If the congestion is of long duration the liver may be damaged, resulting in slight jaundice. Loss of appetite is common due to congestion of the stomach. Dependent *oedema*, for reasons already stated, occurs in right ventricular failure. If the oedema is severe it may be associated with ascites and pleural effusions. Muscle wasting is common but may be obscured by oedema. *Cyanosis* is common, partly due to poor oxygenation of the blood passing through the oedematous lungs and partly due to peripheral stagnation. Examination of the heart may show evidence of the disease causing the failure. In heart failure, the urine is usually diminished in volume, of high specific gravity, and may contain protein.

TREATMENT OF CARDIAC FAILURE

Acute Left Ventricular Failure

(1) The patient is best kept upright supported by pillows; if possible the legs should be dependent to allow as much oedema fluid as possible to drain away from the lungs.

(2) *Morphine* 15–20 mg. should be given intramuscularly. Its action in this condition is not fully understood, but its good effect is probably due largely to its sedative action which decreases anxiety and reduces hyperventilation. It is also a vasodilator and lowers venous pressure.

(3) Reduction in blood volume lowers venous pressure, relieves overfilling of the heart and leads to a rise in cardiac output and disappearance of oedema. It is usually achieved by a diuretic and *frusemide* 20 mg. I.V. is effective. Alternatively blood may be temporarily trapped in the limbs by means of cuffs inflated to just above the diastolic pressure.

(4) *Aminophylline* 250 mg. slowly intravenously is useful particularly if there is associated bronchospasm.

(5) Pure oxygen should be given if available.

(6) The patient may require rarely digitalisation but this is not usually an emergency measure.

With these measures it is usually possible to relieve the patient of an acute attack. Thereafter he should be treated as for congestive failure with rest and diuretics (see below). If the underlying cause is amenable to treatment, this should be dealt with. For the next few nights, many patients have difficulty in sleeping and a hypnotic (nitrazepam 5·0 mg.) is useful.

Right Ventricular and Congestive Failure

The essential steps in the treatment of cardiac failure are to reverse those disturbances of function which are responsible for the reduced cardiac output.

(a) Reduce the myocardial preload, i.e. reduce endiastolic pressure. This can be achieved by diuretics, some vasodilators and by rest.

(b) Increase myocardial contractility which can be achieved by giving digitalis although there is some debate on this subject (see digitalis).

(c) Reduce the myocardial afterload, i.e. reduce peripheral resistance. This can be achieved by vasodilator drugs or by relieving the valve stenosis by surgical means.

(1) *Rest* is extremely important in the treatment of heart failure. The patient is nursed in bed and may find breathing easier if he leans forward resting his arms on a bed-table. This upright position allows the oedema fluid to drain away from the lungs and relieves dyspnoea. If an adjustable bed is available the patient will be able to sit with his legs lowered which, by *reducing* the venous return to the heart, further relieves pulmonary congestion. An excellent alternative is a high-backed armchair; many patients find this very comfortable and so rest and sleep more easily. Every effort must be made to spare the patient unnecessary strain; all save the most gravely ill patients should be allowed up daily to the commode or toilet.

(2) *Diet* should be light and easily digestible. There is no reason to restrict fluid intake but salt should be reduced to 1·0 g. per day for at least the early stages of treatment. In severe or refractory cases it should be reduced to 0·5 g. per day, but at this level care must be taken that salt deficiency does not develop.

(3) *Digitalis* was the standard treatment for cardiac failure although with the introduction of effective diuretics it lost some of its importance. There is no doubt that it is highly effective in controlling heart failure complicated by atrial fibrillation. Its place in cardiac failure associated with sinus rhythm is less clear for although it can be shown to produce a positive ionotrophic effect at the start of treatment there is no evidence that this persists in the long term. Digitalis is obtained from the foxglove and there are several different preparations in use. They are all similar in their pharmacological action, but differ in the speed of onset and duration of effect and in the proportion of the oral dose which is absorbed. The following are the most commonly used preparations.

Preparation	Route of Administration	Maximum Effect	Duration of Half Life	Percentage Absorbed by Oral Route
Digoxin	I.V.	2 hours	40 hours	
	oral	6 hours		70%
Digitoxin	I.V.	6 hours	5 days	
	oral	12 hours		95%

After absorption, digitoxin is largely protein bound and is metabolised by the liver, so that accumulation does not occur in renal failure. Digoxin is excreted fairly rapidly by the kidneys, and retention occurs with impaired renal function.

Actions of Digitalis

In therapeutic doses digitalis has no effect on the normal heart but in heart failure the following occur:

(1) Increased force of contraction of the ventricles.

(2) Slowing of the heart by an effect on the sino-atrial node which is partly direct and partly mediated through the vagus.

(3) Depression of conduction in the bundle of His, so that in atrial fibrillation fewer impulses pass from the atria to the ventricles and the ventricular rate is therefore slowed.

These result in a rise in cardiac output and a fall in venous pressure. The increased renal blood flow causes a diuresis. Digitalis can be used in all types of heart failure. It is, however, not very helpful in the high output state which complicates anaemia and chronic lung disease nor in heart failure due to acute myocarditis, particularly diphtheria.

Dosage. There are many schemes of dosage of digitalis. They all aim at giving a loading dose fully to saturate the heart muscle with the drug followed by maintenance doses to replace the daily loss of the drug.

Two schemes of dosage are given below.

(a) Routine Digitalisation

The initial dose is 0·5 mg. twice or three times daily depending on the size of the patient. Thereafter the dosage is adjusted to keep the pulse rate between 70 and 80 per minute. The maintenance dose usually lies between 0·25 and 0·5 mg. daily.

Digoxin is excreted largely via the kidneys and for this reason patients with impaired renal function and especially the elderly are liable to accumulate the drug and develop signs of overdosage. Digoxin tablets containing 0·0625 mg. of the drug are available and may be useful in such cases.

Equivalent amounts of digitoxin can be used (tablets of digitoxin 0·1 mg. = digoxin 0·25 mg.).

The treatment's aims are relieving the symptoms and signs of heart failure and keeping the patient's resting heart rate at about 70 per minute.

(b) *Emergency Digitalisation.* This is rarely required and is not without risk. Digoxin 0·5 mg. is given *slowly* intravenously and is followed by digoxin 0·5 mg. orally after four hours and then digoxin 0·25 mg. t.d.s. until a satisfactory response is obtained.

Intravenous digoxin should not be given to a patient who has received digitalis within the last two months. Nearly as rapid a result can be obtained if the initial dose of digoxin is given orally.

Digitalis Blood Levels. It is possible to measure the concentration of *digoxin* in the blood. The therapeutic levels lie between 1·0 and 2·0 mcg/ml. Toxicity usually occurs at levels over 2·0 mcg/ml. There is, however, considerable variation with overlap between therapeutic and toxic levels and digoxin assays are not often necessary in controlling treatment.

Signs of Overdosage. The most important signs of overdosage are:

(1) *Coupled beats.* This is due to increased excitability of the ventricles leading to ventricular premature systoles which occur after every normal beat. If overdosage is allowed to continue ventricular tachycardia or fibrillation may occur.

(2) *Undue slowing of the pulse*—a resting pulse below 65 per minute suggests too much digitalis is being given.

(3) *Atrial tachycardia* with atrio-ventricular block may sometimes occur.

(4) *Nausea, vomiting,* and *diarrhoea.* Overdosage with digitalis can cause central vomiting—but it should be remembered that vomiting is sometimes a feature of heart failure itself.

(5) *Xanthopsia.*

It is usually sufficient to omit the drug for a day or two to abolish these effects.

Potassium and Digitalis. The presence of potassium ions decreases the effects of digitalis and vice versa. This means that overdosage of digitalis can be temporarily reversed by giving potassium salts. It will also be found that patients who are losing potassium ions (for instance, due to treatment with a thiazide diuretic or frusemide) may become more sensitive to digitalis and develop evidence of overdosage.

(4) *Diuretics* are extremely useful in patients with heart failure for they lead to decrease in extra-cellular fluid volume and lower venous pressure.

(a) *The Benzothiadiazines.* This group of diuretics prevent the reabsorption of sodium, potassium and water by the renal tubule. They are given orally. There are several drugs in this group with similar actions but differing in dosage.

Chlorothiazide	0·5–2·0 g.
Hydrochlorothiazide	50–200 mg.

Hydroflumethiazide	50–200 mg.
Bendrofluazide	5·0–10 mg.
Cyclopenthiazide	0·25–1·0 mg.

Their diuretic action lasts about twelve hours.

They are given usually orally each morning on a regular basis. Chlorthalidone in doses of 50–200 mg. is similar, but its action lasts up to forty-eight hours.

In the upper dose ranges these diuretics will produce some potassium depletion. This is important as it potentiates the effects of digitalis and may lead to signs of digitalis overdosage. Patients on diuretics should therefore receive potassium supplements (see below). The benzothiadiazines also have some blood pressure lowering action and therefore increase the effect of hypotensive drugs.

Side effects are not common, but benzothiadiazines cause some uric acid retention and may precipitate an acute attack of gout. Rarely they produce diabetes mellitus, which however usually recovers when the drug is withdrawn.

(b) *Frusemide* is a more powerful diuretic than the benzothiadiazines. Orally in doses of 40–120 mg. either daily or on alternate days it produces a diuresis lasting about six hours. It is also very effective intravenously in doses of 10–40 mg., producing an intense diuresis lasting about two hours.

Ethacrynic acid is similar to frusemide, and is given orally in doses 50–100 mg. daily. Both diuretics will produce potassium depletion and supplements will be required. Care must be taken when using these diuretics as they can cause such an intense diuresis that collapse may occur due to sudden salt and water loss. *Bumetanide* is also similar to frusemide with both its advantages and disadvantages.

(c) In addition *spironolactone*, which antagonises the action of aldosterone, has been used in patients with obstinate oedema. It acts on a different site in the renal tubules to the usual diuretics and can be useful. The dose is 100 mg. four times daily and it must be combined with another diuretic.

(d) *Triamterene* increases the excretion of sodium and water but reduces that of potassium. It is most effective when combined with one of the benzothiadiazines, the dose being 200 mg. daily. *Amiloride* is similar to triamterene but is rather more powerful. The dose is 10–40 mg.

Amiloride, spironolactone and triamterene can cause potassium retention and for this reason must be used with great care in renal failure.

(e) *Potassium supplements* will be required by patients on benzothiadiazines, frusemide or ethacrynic acid. Potassium chloride can cause ulceration of the gut, and Slow K (a slow-release preparation containing 8·0 mEq. K) in doses of three to six tablets daily is satisfactory.

(5) *Peripheral Vasodilators.* Drugs which cause arterial vasodilation lower peripheral resistance (i.e. afterload) and thus allow the myocardium to work more effectively. Likewise, drugs which dilate veins lower venous and thus endiastolic ventricular pressure (i.e. pre-load) and also help to raise the output in cardiac failure. Several drugs have been used for this purpose.

Nitroprusside	arterial and venous dilator	short acting and given by injection
Prazosin	arterial and venous dilator	long acting and given orally
Hydralazine	arterial dilator	long acting and given orally

When there is a fixed resistance to blood as occurs with valve stenosis vasodilators will not be effective and should not be used.

(6) *Sedation* is important in these patients as they are often restless and anxious. In the early stages a mixture containing chloral hydrate 1·0 g. and tincture of opium 0·6 ml. is useful last thing at night and later on a hypnotic such as nitrazepam 5·0–10 mg. can be used.

(7) *Oxygen* may be required in patients with severe heart failure and may be given either by a Ventimask or by an oxygen tent. The indications are marked cyanosis or distress.

(8) If the oedema is very severe, or if there are collections of fluid in the chest or abdomen, recourse must be made to tapping the chest or abdomen (*paracentesis*).

(9) Rarely it may be necessary to remove excess fluid by peritoneal dialysis.

Bed rest treatment should continue until the evidence of cardiac failure has disappeared. Thereafter the patient should be allowed gradually to return to activity, but his ultimate mode of life will be conditioned by the limits imposed by his disease.

ABNORMALITIES OF RHYTHM

(1) Extrasystoles (Ectopic Beats)

Extrasystoles, or more accurately premature systoles, are due to the cardiac impulse arising in an ectopic focus which may be in the atria, the atrio-ventricular node, or in the ventricles. As the contraction is premature the ventricles are only partially filled so that the resulting pulse wave is diminished or even impalpable at the wrist. The subsequent normal impulse falls in the refractory period so that no contraction occurs. During the pause more blood enters the ventricles than normal and the next beat is unusually forceful.

Extrasystoles are extremely common and most people have them at some time in their lives. Their incidence increases with age; they may occur only occasionally or may be as frequent as every alternate beat, this rhythm being known as pulsus bigeminus or coupled beats. They are often noticed when the patient is lying in bed at night, and though they disappear during exercise they may appear after exertion. They are often more frequent when the patient is tired or worried or during a feverish illness. In some people they may also be related to over-indulgence in tobacco, coffee, or alcohol. Extrasystoles may also occur in heart diseases.

Many patients fail to notice their own extrasystoles. Others complain of a thump in the chest which is due to the powerful contraction after the compensatory pause. Sometimes patients notice the compensatory pause and complain of a 'dropped beat'.

Extrasystoles can usually be diagnosed by the pulse, when a premature beat followed by a pause is felt. Multiple extrasystoles can be confused with atrial fibrillation; the former will, however, disappear on exercise, whereas atrial fibrillation will become more marked. Some confusion may also result if the extrasystoles cannot be detected at the wrist. They can, however, always be heard on careful auscultation of the heart.

Electrocardiogram. In atrial ectopics the E.C.G. will show a premature P wave followed by a normal QRS complex. In ventricular ectopics the E.C.G. shows a premature and abnormally wide QRS complex.

Prognosis and Treatment. Extrasystoles by themselves are of no significance. Their presence calls for a careful examination and if no abnormality is found reassurance should be vigorous. If extrasystoles are found at a routine examination in an otherwise normal heart it is usually best not to tell the patient.

Occasionally in subjects with heart disease multiple extrasystoles may herald the onset of a more serious arrhythmia; e.g. the occurrence of ventricular extrasystoles after a coronary thrombosis is sometimes followed by ventricular fibrillation (see p. 172). In those taking too much digitalis, ventricular extrasystoles cause coupled beats (**pulsus bigeminus**) and indicate that the drug should be discontinued for a day or two.

Drug treatment is rarely required for extrasystoles; reassurance and the avoidance of obvious precipitating factors are usually sufficient, and if the extrasystoles are very frequent and distressing, quinidine in doses of 200 mg. three times daily or propranolol 20 mg. three times daily will sometimes abolish them within a few days.

(2) Tachycardias

Paroxysmal tachycardia is classified as follows:
    Supraventricular
    Ventricular.

Supraventricular tachycardia is caused by rapid discharge from an atrial ectopic focus or more frequently from a circus movement involving the bundle of His. This becomes established if the impulse from a premature atrial beat reaches the A-V node while one pathway in the bundle is still refractory, the stimulus is conducted down another accessory pathway. By the time it reaches the ventricle the previously refractory pathway may have recovered so that the impulse is conducted back to the atria whence the whole cycle is repeated. In most cases the existence of such dual pathways in the bundle of His is not associated with any other apparent abnormality of the heart.

Supraventricular tachycardia may occur at any age but usually starts in youth and is only occasionally associated with heart disease. It is however a feature of the Wolff-Parkinson-White syndrome (see below).

The electrocardiogram shows a rapid rate with normal QRS complexes. Rarely there may be a functional bundle branch block with wide QRS complexes so that the tracing may resemble a ventricular tachycardia.

A more precise diagnosis of the conduction abnormalities and their relationship to the arrythmia can be obtained from electrocardiograms recorded directly from the conducting pathways (His electrocardiograms).

Ventricular tachycardia arises from an ectopic focus in the ventricles. It is nearly always associated with cardiac disease. The electrocardiogram shows a rapid rate with wide and abnormal QRS complexes.

Tachycardias when secondary to cardiac disease may complicate coronary artery disease particularly in the immediate post-infarction period, thyrotoxicosis and digitalis overdosage.

Clinical Features. An attack of paroxysmal tachycardia starts suddenly. The patient may remember the moment when his heart began to beat rapidly. The tachycardia may be described as palpitations or as a fluttering in the chest. It is always quite regular. Sometimes the attacks may start without warning and on other occasions they may be precipitated by a sudden movement or emotion. The attacks last any time from a few seconds to a day or two and then stop quite suddenly and normal rhythm is resumed; sometimes they are followed by extrasystoles. They may recur every few hours or only once or twice in a lifetime.

The degree of constitutional upset varies. Some patients are not disturbed by the attacks whereas others are anxious, feel faint or may complain of discomfort or even an anginal type of pain across the chest. Rarely patients may develop signs of heart failure during the attack, particularly if it lasts more than a day or so and more particularly if there is underlying heart disease.

Prognosis and Treatment. The prognosis in paroxysmal tachycardia, both of the acute attack and of subsequent events, depends on the presence or absence of underlying heart disease. If the heart is healthy the outlook is extremely good, though the paroxysms may cause a good deal of worry and distress.

In treating an attack of paroxysmal tachycardia it is important to know whether it arises from a supraventricular or from a ventricular focus. This is best determined by an electrocardiogram. Occasionally physical signs help. Rapid venous 'cannon waves' (p. 97) caused by the atria contracting against a closed atrioventricular valve, suggest a supraventricular tachycardia. Sudden slowing produced by carotid sinus stimulation suggest an atrial origin.

Supraventricular tachycardia can often be stopped by some trick which results in vagal stimulation, for example tickling the back of the throat, pressure on the eye-balls, or stimulation of one carotid sinus. If these manoeuvres fail and the heart is otherwise healthy it is often best to sedate the patient and wait for a spontaneous return to normal rhythm. If further treatment is required practolol intravenously (see below) may be successful. If these measures fail full digitalisation is effective but must not be followed by cardioversion, which is only indicated in resistant cases. Further attacks may be prevented by quinidine, disopyramide or digoxin.

In *ventricular tachycardia* intravenous lignocaine is the drug of choice. If this fails propranolol or phenytoin is sometimes successful (see below).

In patients who do not respond to drugs and in those where general condition suggests that rapid restoration of sinus rhythm is necessary electrical cardioversion should be used.

Drugs used to Decrease Cardiac Excitability

Class I (Membrane stabilisers).

Lignocaine is particularly useful in ventricular arrhythmias. It is given intravenously as a single dose of 50–100 mg. followed by an infusion of

4 mg./minute for 30 minutes
2 mg./minute for 2 hours
1 mg./minute thereafter.

Lignocaine is metabolised in the liver and when liver function is depressed as in cardiac failure or shock, the dose of lignocaine should be reduced. It may cause bradycardia and should not be used in heart block or when the heart depends on a low nodal or ideoventricular pacemaker.

Procainamide can be given orally in doses of 250 mg. q.i.d. to prevent arrhythmias. It can also be given intravenously, 250 mg. being injected over five minutes. It may cause considerable myocardial depression and hypotension and prolonged use may produce lupus erythematosus, which however is reversible on withdrawal of the drug.

Phenytoin is useful in both ventricular and atrial arrhythmias—either given orally in doses of 100 mg. t.d.s. or as a single intravenous dose of 125 mg. given over five minutes.

Quinidine is now rarely used in acute arrhythmias. It is sometimes effective in preventing arrhythmias in doses of 200 mg. t.d.s. by mouth.

Mexiletine is similar to lignocaine but can be given orally in doses of 400 mg., followed by 200 mg. t.d.s.

Class II (β blockers).

β adrenergic blocking drugs are used in cardiac arrhythmias. *Practolol* is a pure β blocker and most effective in atrial arrhythmias. *Oxprenolol* is

similar to *propranolol* in that it has in addition a direct (Class I) depressing effect on the myocardium which makes it particularly useful in ventricular arrhythmias. Drugs can be given intravenously—

Propranolol 2·0–5·0 mg.
Oxprenolol 20 mg t.d.s.

Given in this way they cause bradycardia, a drop in cardiac output and hypotension. These can be minimised by giving atropine 0·6 mg. I.V. β blockers can also be given orally to prevent attacks or where emergency treatment is not required.

Propranolol 10 mg. t.d.s. ⎫
Oxprenolol 20 mg. t.d.s. ⎬ and increased if necessary.

Propranolol and oxprenolol by reducing the adrenergic drive to the heart and by their depressing effect on the myocardium may exacerbate heart failure. They may also precipitate bronchospasm in the asthmatic. Practolol appears less likely to produce these side effects *but long term use may cause retroperitoneal fibrosis and sclerosis of the cornea.*

If antiarrhythmic drugs are given intravenously continuous E.C.G. monitoring is essential except in extreme emergencies.

Other Agents

Disopyramide is similar to quinidine but its side-effects are less common, it is particularly useful in ventricular arrythmias. The intravenous dose is 100 mg. given over 15 minutes, followed by 10 mg./hour. Orally the dose is 100–200 mg. q.i.d.

Verapamil may be particularly useful in ventricular tachycardias. The dose is 40–80 mg. t.d.s. orally, or 10 mg. as an intravenous bolus. *It must not be combined with β blockers as asystole may ensue.*

(3) Atrial Flutter

Atrial flutter is less common. It is nearly always associated with heart disease, commonly rheumatic, hypertensive, or coronary disease. The mechanism of flutter is not entirely settled. Until recently it was thought to be due to a wave of contraction circling round the atria, but more recently it has been suggested that it is due to an excitable focus in the atria, discharging at a high rate, usually between 210–300 per minute. The ventricles are unable to respond at this rate so that there is usually some degree of partial atrio-ventricular block, the ventricles only responding to every second, third, or perhaps fourth atrial contraction.

The *symptoms* of atrial flutter are variable. The patient may complain only of symptoms due to the underlying heart disease and the flutter may be found on examination. Sometimes there may be a complaint of palpitations of sudden onset. Examination may show little, especially when there is a considerable degree of heart block so that the ventricular rate is perhaps only 70 per minute. Sudden change in the degree of heart block resulting in doubling or halving of the pulse rate is characteristic of flutter. Halving of the pulse rate can sometimes be induced by pressing on one carotid sinus. In some patients, continuous variation in the degree of A-V block leads to complete irregularity of the pulse, which feels similar to that of atrial fibrillation. The rather unstable rhythm in atrial flutter may be troublesome to the patient and in most cases an effort should be made to induce a more stable rhythm.

ECG shows flutter waves at about 300 per minute which resemble the teeth of a saw. There is usually some degree of A-V block

Prognosis and Treatment. The prognosis of flutter depends largely upon the underlying heart disease and is, therefore, variable. Flutter is treated by giving full doses of digitalis; this usually converts the flutter to atrial fibrillation. If the digitalis is then stopped about 40 per cent of patients will revert to sinus rhythm. The remainder will either continue to fibrillate or return to flutter. The decision whether to continue digitalis indefinitely or to try to restore sinus rhythm (see below) depends on the underlying heart disease (see atrial fibrillation).

(4) Atrial Fibrillation

Atrial fibrillation is a common and important cardiac arrhythmia. Each small muscle bundle in the atria contracts independently at a rate between 400–500 per minute. These contractions can be seen as the 'f' waves in the electrocardiogram. The result of this disordered atrial activity is that there is no co-ordinated atrial contraction and the ventricles are stimulated in an irregular and often rapid fashion. This in turn throws a greater strain on the ventricular myocardium and may precipitate failure in an already damaged heart.

Atrial fibrillation is usually associated with heart disease, classically with mitral stenosis or thyrotoxicosis; it is, however, also quite common in coronary artery disease, in hypertension and it occasionally occurs in acute fevers. It may also be seen in constrictive pericarditis and carcinoma of the bronchus involving the myocardium. Sometimes it follows alcoholic excess or very heavy smoking and it is frequent after thoracotomy. Occasionally it occurs without any apparent cause. It may be paroxysmal or permanent. Atrial fibrillation is rare in aortic valve disease and in most forms of congenital heart disease.

Clinical Features. The onset of atrial fibrillation may pass unnoticed by the patient. More commonly he will complain of palpitations and may notice the irregularity of the pulse. Occasionally the onset is more dramatic, with fainting and collapse, and followed perhaps by acute cardiac failure. The *diagnosis* can be confirmed by feeling the pulse, which is characteristically completely irregular in force and rhythm. Exercise makes the arrhythmia more obvious (cf. extrasystoles p. 117). Further examination will usually show evidence of underlying heart disease.

Paroxysmal Atrial Fibrillation and Lone Atrial Fibrillation. Although atrial fibrillation is usually associated with heart disease, it is sometimes found when the heart is otherwise normal. These patients may either have paroxysms of atrial fibrillation or permanent fibrillation. Follow-up studies of these patients indicate that their prognosis is excellent, except for a number who develop the arrhythmia later in life and who may subsequently show evidence of underlying heart disease.

The electrocardiogram is characterised by complete irregularity of the QRS complexes and the disappearance of P waves with their replacement by small rapid fibrillation waves.

Treatment. The majority of patients with established atrial fibrillation have heart disease, perhaps with associated heart failure, and are best treated with digitalis. Occasionally the combination of a β blocker with digitalis will make control easier, but it must be used with care in patients with cardiac failure. Patients with mitral stenosis and atrial fibrillation should be anticoagulated to minimise the very real risk of systemic emboli. Patients with lone fibrillation and a slow ventricular rate often need no drug treatment.

In a small group of patients with atrial fibrillation an attempt should be made to restore sinus rhythm. This applies when there is no underlying heart disease, when thyrotoxicosis has been relieved and following a successful mitral valvotomy. Cardiac failure, any degree of cardiac enlargement or other evidence of severe heart disease are all contra-indications. The presence of atrial fibrillation for more than a few months is said to increase the risk of embolism when sinus rhythm is restored.

The method of choice in restoring sinus rhythm is cardioversion by direct current shock. Drugs are now rarely used.

Direct Current Shock for Cardiac Arrythmias. Cardiac arrythmias due to ectopic foci can be reverted to sinus rhythm in most patients by direct current shock. The widest experience is in treating atrial fibrillation. Cardioversion is performed under short duration anaesthesia, and the shock is delivered synchronously with the down stroke of the R wave of the electrocardiogram. It depolarises the heart muscle and allows the sino-atrial node to resume as the cardiac pacemaker. Although cardioversion is successful in some 80 per cent of patients, about 60 per cent of them relapse over the next year despite maintenance treatment with quinidine, procainamide or phenytoin. In patients with paroxysmal atrial fibrillation, attacks can sometimes be prevented by giving a β blocker or quinidine. If this fails and the attacks are troublesome the patient should be digitalised.

HEART BLOCK

A block in the conducting system may occur either between the S-A node and the atrium (sino-atrial block), or in the bundle of His, between the atria and the ventricles (atrio-ventricular block).

Sino-atrial Block. This is characterised by the disappearance of P waves and the subsequent QRS complexes, often at regular intervals. Treatment is with a parasympathetic blocking agent such as atropine, or with sympathomimetic drugs such as orciprenaline. If symptoms are troublesome pacing will be required.

Atrio-ventricular Block. There are three degrees of atrio-ventricular block:

(1) Prolongation of the P-R Interval

This degree of heart block can only be diagnosed with certainty from an electrocardiogram.

(2) Increasing P-R Interval with Dropped Beats (Wenckebach's Periods)

The P-R interval increases with each beat until finally a beat is dropped. With the next beat the P-R interval returns to normal and the cycle is repeated.

Clinically this type of block can be diagnosed by noting regular dropping of the heart beats. It requires electrocardiographic confirmation.

(3) Complete Heart Block

The atria and ventricles contract in complete dissociation, the stimulus to ventricular contraction arising in an ectopic focus which may be ventricular or nodal. This type of heart block is recognised by a slow pulse, usually between 30 and 40 per minute, and a wide pulse pressure; by dissociation between the atrial elements of the jugular venous pulse ('a' waves) and the carotid pulse; and by the presence of occasional 'cannon' waves in the jugular pulse which occur when the atrium contracts against a closed tricuspid valve. The heart is usually slightly enlarged. With careful auscultation it is sometimes possible to hear the sound produced by the contracting atria and the first heart sound varies in intensity owing to the varying intervals between the atrial and ventricular contractions (see p. 100).

Heart block may complicate cardiac infarction or occur as a result of a primary degenerative disease of conducting tissue. It may be associated with rheumatic fever, diphtheria and digitalis overdosage. In about 10 per cent of patients with complete block the disorder is congenital.

Clinical Features. Disorders of conduction may produce a variety of symptoms, usually as a result of bradycardia or transient cardiac arrest. These include attacks of dizziness, fainting or fits. They are particularly liable to occur in elderly patients whose cerebral circulation may be impaired.

Prognosis and Treatment. The prognosis of heart block depends upon the underlying causes. In congenital heart block the outlook is very good and it does not influence expectation of life. In patients developing heart block with pre-existing heart disease the prognosis should be guarded. Generally speaking, no treatment is required for heart block provided it is not producing symptoms. If it is associated with heart failure, digitalis can be used, but should be given with care as it may turn a partial into a complete block. Where the rhythm is unstable and particularly if there are attacks of dizziness or loss of consciousness artificial pacing is required.

Stokes-Adams Attacks. These are attacks of unconsciousness from cerebral anoxia resulting from circulatory standstill. Fifty per cent are caused by cardiac arrest, 25 per cent by ventricular tachycardia and 25 per cent by ventricular fibrillation. All cause effective pumping by the heart to cease.

When due to cardiac arrest they are associated with acquired heart block, particularly when the rhythm is unstable and is fluctuating between partial and complete block; circulatory arrest is due to a delay in ventricular contraction when complete block develops suddenly. In the attack the patient falls suddenly to the ground, blue and pulseless and breathing increasingly deeply; if the asystole lasts more than a few seconds convulsions occur. With the commencement of the heart beat, the patient develops a characteristic flush and consciousness returns.

Attacks may occur with varying degrees of frequency and any one may prove fatal.

Treatment

The Acute Attack (*Circulatory Arrest*). The following treatment is used in patients with heart block whose Stokes-Adams attacks are so prolonged as to threaten life. It should also be used when ventricular fibrillation or ventricular asystole complicates unstable rhythms, which are particularly liable to occur after cardiac infarction (p. 171).

The immediate signs of ventricular asystole or ventricular fibrillation are:

    (a) Loss of consciousness.
    (b) Absent pulses, the carotid being the best artery to palpate.
    (c) Cessation of respiration.
    (d) Dilated pupils, which occur within thirty seconds.

Resuscitation must be started at once as irreversible damage to the cerebral cortex may occur in two minutes. The immediate treatment is aimed at maintaining circulation and ventilation.

    (a) The patient must be laid supine on an unyielding surface and external cardiac massage applied by sharp compression of the lower end of the sternum about eighty times a minute.

    (b) The airway must be cleared and the lungs inflated. This can be done by either mouth to mouth respiration or better by an inflating bag (e.g. the Ambu bag) connected to air or oxygen.

    (c) As soon as possible 100 ml. of 8·4 per cent sodium bicarbonate should be given intravenously to reduce the rapidly developing acidosis, and repeated as required.

At this stage it is important to take an E.C.G. record to reveal whether there is asystole or ventricular fibrillation or whether normal rhythm has returned, but further resuscitation, if required, should not be delayed when no record is available.

If the heart is in ventricular fibrillation D.C. defibrillation at 200–300 joules may restore sinus rhythm but if the fibrillation continues after five shocks lignocaine 100 mg. I.V. should be given and defibrillation repeated.

When the heart is in asystole, the shock may restart it, but if asystole persists ventricular fibrillation should be provoked by giving 10 ml. of 1:10,000 adrenaline and 10 ml. of 10 per cent calcium chloride I.V. Sinus rhythm may then be restored with the defibrillator. If normal rhythm has not returned after ten minutes of maintained circulation recovery is unlikely.

Preventative. Stokes-Adams attacks can sometimes be prevented by giving slow release isoprenaline (Saventrine) 30 mg. eight-hourly by mouth, or ephedrine 30 mg. t.d.s. Prednisolone may occasionally be effective particularly in the period following a cardiac infarct, when it reduces oedema and inflammation around the bundle.

Generally however, the development of Stokes-Adams attacks is an absolute indication for a pacemaker, which is a much more reliable form of treatment. This can be temporary to tide the patient over a crisis, when the electrode can be wedged against the endocardium of the right ventricle by cardiac catheterisation, or permanent when it is implanted in the myocardium. The stimulating current is provided by a battery.

Bundle Branch Block

Until recently it was thought that the bundle of His divided into left and right branches which supplied the appropriate ventricles. It is now realised that the bundle divides into three branches, a left posterior division supplying the posterior part of the left ventricle, an anterior left division supplying the anterior and lateral aspects of the left ventricle and a right division. Each of these divisions can be damaged separately by disease processes.

Bundle branch block may occur acutely following cardiac infarction, it may be due to progressive disease of the conducting system of unknown aetiology and it is found with atrial septal defect. Right bundle branch block may also occur in normal hearts.

Clinical Features. Bundle branch block by itself produces no symptoms. Examination will show evidence of underlying heart disease if present and in addition, right bundle branch block causes a wide and fixed splitting of the second heart sound in the pulmonary area. Bundle branch block can only be diagnosed with certainty by an electrocardiogram.

Prognosis and Treatment. The prognosis depends on the underlying heart disease, often no treatment is required. The importance of recognising that the conducting system is trifasicular is that the electrocardiogram may show changes which suggest progressive damage to the system and give warning that complete block with its attendant risk of cardiac asystole is imminent. This is particularly important following cardiac infarction as asystole may be avoided by using a pacemaker.

The changes in the electrocardiogram which should be noted are:

    (1) Right bundle branch block causes widening of the S wave in lead 1 and in the left venticular surface leads and a wide R wave in lead 3.

    (2) Complete left bundle branch block causes widening of the R wave in lead 1, aVL and over the left ventricle and a wide S wave in lead 3.

    (3) Block of the anterior division of the left bundle leads to the development of left axis deviation of more than $-60°$.

    (4) Block of the posterior division of the left bundle leads to the development of right axis deviation of more than $+120°$.

The combination of right bundle branch block with either anterior or posterior left bundle branch block following cardiac infarction is usually considered to be an indication for pacing although the prognosis is poor whatever is done.

Isolated left or right bundle branch blocks do not usually require pacing unless for associated reasons.

Wolff-Parkinson-White Syndrome. This usually occurs in young subjects with otherwise healthy hearts. It consists of shortening of the P-R interval on the electrocardiogram with widening of the QRS complexes. It is due to an accessory bundle between the atria and the ventricles. Its main clinical importance is that it may be associated with recurrent episodes of atrial arrhythmias.

SICK SINUS SYNDROME

In this condition sinus bradycardia alternates with various atrial arrythmias, usually atrial tachycardia or fibrillation. It may occur as an acute phenomenon following cardiac infarction. In the elderly, it may present as a chronic disorder when it is believed to be due to fibrosis of the S-A node. The changes in cardiac rhythm are sometimes associated with transient loss of consciousness.

Treatment. Following cardiac infarction sinus bradycardia can sometimes be controlled by atropine, but if this fails a pacemaker is needed. In the chronic disorder a pacemaker is essential to prevent bradycardia, and the atrial arrythmia can be controlled by a β blocker.

HYPERTENSION

It is impossible to define the normal blood pressure for the term in this sense is without meaning. It is possible to find the average blood pressure for a group of healthy people and this average pressure is found to increase with age, being about 120/80 at the age of twenty, rising to 160/90 at the age of sixty. Within this apparently healthy group of people, however, is a wide range. For the purposes of life insurance and similar medical examinations 150/90 is usually taken as the upper limit of normal pressure, although this is probably a little high in the young and a little low in the elderly.

Causes of Hypertension. When a blood pressure which is above the usual level for the patient's age group is discovered the possible causes should be considered. They are the following:

(1) Essential hypertension (80 per cent).

(2) Hypertension associated with renal disease (20 per cent).

(3) Rare causes:

      (a) Hypertension associated with endocrine disease, i.e.:

            (i) Cushing's syndrome.

            (ii) Phaeochromocytoma.

            (iii) Primary Aldosteronism.

      (b) Coarctation of the aorta.

(4) A small proportion of women taking the contraceptive pill develop hypertension which is reversible when the pill is stopped.

The discovery of a raised blood pressure calls for full clinical examination, particular attention being paid to the cardiovascular system, including the femoral pulses, the retinae and examination of the urine. If there is any suspicion of a renal cause the urinary tract should be further investigated. Endocrine causes should also be remembered and can usually be diagnosed by specific tests.

ESSENTIAL HYPERTENSION

The cause of essential hypertension is unknown. There is at present a widespread opinion that patients with essential hypertension merely represent the extreme uppermost limit of normal variation in blood pressure in the population. There is little doubt that heredity plays a part and it is common to find evidence of hypertension in the patient's father or mother. Other factors which have been implicated are stress, salt intake and sympathetic overactivity but evidence is incomplete. It is however clear that the immediate physiological abnormality is a raised peripheral resistance.

Clinical Features. The blood pressure may remain raised for many years without producing any symptoms or signs; in fact if a blood pressure of over 150/90 is considered abnormal, quite a large proportion of the older people of this country have essential hypertension which in the majority of cases causes them no harm for many years. Many such subjects die in old age of some other complaint.

The symptoms and signs of hypertension are really due to the effects of the raised blood pressure on the cardiovascular system. These complications are particularly liable to occur when the diastolic pressure is high and when hypertension develops at a relatively early age; they are more common in men than in women. Other risk factors are smoking and hyperlipidaemia. The cardiovascular system and the kidneys are most commonly involved.

(1) *The Heart.* The heart is the organ most frequently affected by hypertension. The left ventricle must work against an increased resistance and may in time fail. The *symptoms* are those of left ventricular failure: dyspnoea on effort and paroxysmal dyspnoea at night. *Examination* in a fully developed case shows a full pulse with some thickening of the wall of the radial artery. The heart is enlarged and the apex beat is of the left ventricular type. In at least 50 per cent of patients there is a triple rhythm with a presystolic (atrial) extra sound best heard at the apex. Although the triple rhythm is common in the more severe hypertensives, it does not necessarily imply a failing left ventricle and is not of great prognostic significance. The aortic component of the second sound is loud. A systolic murmur either at the apex or base is quite common; it is usually due to flow through the aortic valve and only rarely to aortic stenosis or a functional mitral incompetence. Eventually the left ventricular failure may progress to congestive failure with raised venous pressure and peripheral oedema.

(2) *The Blood Vessels.* The increased pressure within the blood vessels leads to thickening of the walls of the medium-sized arteries and this change may be palpable in the radial artery at the wrist. Hypertension also predisposes to atheroma with an increased incidence of coronary artery disease. High pressures lead to fibrinoid necrosis of arterioles which further raises peripheral resistance and in the kidney may lead to renal failure (see below).

Hypertensive Retinopathy. The arteries of the retina may show a series of changes which have been subdivided:

Grade I.   Narrowing and increased tortuosity of the retinal arteries.

Grade II.   Arterial changes more marked and nipping of the veins at the arterio-venous crossing due to the thickened arterial wall pressing on the vein.

Grade III. Grades I and II with the addition of haemorrhage and/or exudates.

Grade IV. Previous grades with papilloedema.

Cerebral Arteries. The cerebral arteries are affected in hypertension. Microaneurysms will develop which may ultimately rupture, causing cerebral haemorrhage. Headaches are no more common in hypertensives than in the normotensive population, but with severe hypertension morning headaches may be a problem. In severe hypertension attacks of cerebral oedema occur, producing the clinical syndrome of *hypertensive encephalopathy* with blinding headaches, fits, unconsciousness, and transient palsies.

(3) *The Kidney.* In the majority of patients with essential hypertension there is no evidence of serious interference with renal function and death

from renal failure is rare. The urine may, however, contain a little protein, particularly in the more severe cases. In malignant hypertension (see below) there are marked changes in the blood vessels of the kidney, particularly fibrinoid necrosis of the afferent artery to the glomerulus, and in these cases there is a progressive decrease in renal function and death may occur from renal failure.

Investigation

Extensive investigation is not required in the majority of patients with hypertension as only about 1 per cent will reveal a removable cause. Chest X-ray and an electrocardiogram are useful to determine the presence of left ventricular hypertrophy. A blood urea and electrolytes to check renal function and plasma lipids are of some prognostic importance.

More extensive investigations including pyelography, estimation of urinary VMA and other tests of endocrine function are only required in the young hypertensive without a family history or where there is clinical suspicion of some underlying cause for the high blood pressure.

Malignant Hypertension (Accelerated Hypertension)

Malignant hypertension, which is relatively uncommon, may be regarded as the most severe grade of essential hypertension, although this view is not universally accepted. It is characterised by a high diastolic pressure (usually over 140 mm./Hg.), by marked arterial changes in the retina with papilloedema, and by progressive renal failure. It arises most commonly in men of early middle age.

Renin and Hypertension

Although renin will cause a rise in blood pressure via the angiotensin mechanism there is little evidence that excess renin is involved in the genesis of ordinary essential hypertension. Plasma renin levels in this disease are within the normal range and although β blocking drugs will decrease the blood pressure and lower the plasma renin concentration these changes do not appear to be causally related.

In patients with hypertension due primarily to renal disease and in accelerated hypertension there may be excessive renin release leading to *secondary hyperaldosteronism* and excess angiotensin. This may be a factor in still further increasing the blood pressure.

Prognosis of Hypertension

The prognosis of essential hypertension is very important for it largely determines the management of the patient.

Generally speaking the factors which influence prognosis are:

(1) Sex of the patient—women have a better prognosis than men.
(2) The height of the blood pressure. Both the systolic and

diastolic pressures are important. A diastolic pressure of over 130 mm. Hg. carries a bad prognosis.

(3) The degree of arterial change (particularly the retinal changes).
(4) The degree of hypertrophy of the left ventricle.
(5) Evidence of renal involvement.
(6) Plasma lipid levels.

It would seem that the majority of patients with mild or moderate essential hypertension, particularly middle-aged or elderly women, will live for ten or twenty years or longer, but even those with diastolic pressures of 100 will on an average have their life expectancy reduced by a few years. In those with high pressure and evidence of marked arterial or cardiac change the prognosis is considerably worse. Most patients with untreated malignant hypertension are dead within three years.

Treatment

General Measures. Most patients with hypertension require some *reassurance*. Their mode and tempo of life may require modification, but they should lead as normal a life as possible. There is no evidence that *diet* plays any part in the genesis of hypertension, but if the patient is overweight this should be corrected as loss of weight may cause some fall in blood pressure.

Because of the high incidence of coronary disease in these patients it is important to treat any associated hyperlipidaemia (p. 435) and the patient should stop smoking.

Sedation should be used in those patients who are unduly anxious. Diazepam 2·0 mg. three times daily is usually satisfactory.

Drug Treatment. It is now widely accepted that in severe hypertension treatment will reduce morbidity and mortality. The incidence of strokes and heart failure is diminished. Until recently lowering blood pressure did not appear to influence the risk of cardiac infarction but the use of β blockers may achieve this effect. There is as yet no drug which is entirely satisfactory and free from side-effects. Drug treatment is therefore usually confined to those with a blood pressure of over 170/105, although many experts would also treat the milder grades of hypertension, particularly in younger male patients. Generally speaking patients over 65 do not do very well with these drugs. If the blood urea is over 15 mmol./litre due to renal damage, lowering of the blood pressure may well precipitate acute renal failure.

The drugs available are:

(1) *Sympathetic Blocking Group*

(a) *Guanethidine* blocks the post-ganglionic fibres of the sympathetic system without affecting the parasympathetic system. The initial dose is 10 mg. daily and it may take several days until the full effect is seen. The dose is therefore increased every five days until a satisfactory fall in blood pressure is produced: the controlling dose is usually between 30–60 mg. daily. The fall in blood is postural so that the blood pressure must be measured both standing and lying.

Side-effects are:

(i) Diarrhoea is common and can be controlled by codeine phosphate 30 mg. b.d. or by combining guanethidine with a small dose of pempidine.

(ii) Other side-effects are nasal stuffiness, bradycardia, parotid pain, muscle tremors and failure of ejaculation.

(b) *Bethanidine* blocks the adrenergic neurone. The initial dose is 10 mg. b.d. which is increased until a satisfactory response is obtained. It is given up to four times a day as its duration of action is short. This means that a more flexible control is possible than with guanethidine.

(c) *Debrisoquine* is similar to bethanidine. It is relatively short acting. The initial dose of 20 mg. daily is increased as required.

(2) β Blockers

β blockers lower blood pressure but it may be several weeks before their full effect is seen. They can be divided into β_1 blockers (selective) which affect mainly the heart and $\beta_1 + \beta_2$ blockers (non-selective) which also affect the bronchi and arterioles. For lowering the blood pressure there is nothing to choose between these two groups but in the asthmatic a selective blocker is to be preferred though this may still cause bronchospasm.

		Initial Dose
Non-Selective	Propranolol	80 mg. b.d.
	Oxprenolol	80 mg. b.d.
	Sotalol	80 mg. b.d.
Selective	Metoprolol	100 mg. b.d.
	Atenolol	100 mg. daily

The dose is increased gradually until a satisfactory control of blood pressure is obtained.

Labetalol is both an α and β blocker although its α effect is not marked. It may well prove useful in patients who are resistant to simple β blockade. The initial dose is 100 mg. three times daily and this may be increased.

(3) Centrally Acting Group

Methyldopa lowers blood pressure by a central action. The initial dose is 250 mg. three times daily. The full effect is not seen for about five days, so dosage is increased gradually until control is satisfactory. (The usual dose is 1·0–1·5 g. daily.) Methyldopa is not as powerful as guanethidine and symptoms from postural hypotension are not common. Some patients complain of drowsiness early in treatment, also dry mouth and occasionally pyrexia. Water retention may occur but responds to diuretics.

(4) *Direct Acting Group*

(a) *Clonidine* lowers blood pressure by a direct effect on the arterial wall and by a central action. The initial dose is 50 μg. three times daily and is increased as required. It may cause depression in susceptible patients and it *should not be stopped suddenly as this may cause rebound hypertension.*

(b) *Hydralazine* has a direct effect on the artery. The dose should be kept below 200 mg. daily, or side-effects will occur. It causes tachycardia and can therefore be usefully combined with a β blocker.

(c) *Prazosin* is rather similar to hydrallazine, the initial dose being 0·5 mg. three times daily. *The initial dose may cause collapse due to a sudden fall in blood pressure.*

(d) *Diazoxide* is a direct-acting drug usually given intravenously It may produce a diabetic-like state.

(5) *Diuretics.* The benzothiadiazine group (p. 115) are satisfactory. Their mode of action is not clear. They produce a transient fall in blood volume but their hypotensive effects seems to depend on other factors. They are very effective when combined with blood pressure lowering drugs, particularly the sympathetic blocking group or β blockers, both of which may cause salt and water retention. Satisfactory diuretics are:

Bendrofluazide 2·5–5·0 mg. daily.
Chlorthalidine 50 mg. daily or on alternate days.

Potassium supplements are not normally required provided the patient is on a full mixed diet.

(6) *Rauwolfia.* The purified extract *reserpine* is usually used. It produces a mild hypotensive action which takes several days to appear and is probably due to a central action. The fall in blood pressure is not postural. The daily dose should not exceed 0·25 mg., and at this level side-effects including nasal stuffiness, bradycardia and most important, mental depression, are not usually troublesome. However it may cause an increased incidence of breast cancer.

(7) *Ganglion Blocking Group.* These drugs interfere with transmission at all autonomic ganglia, reduce the sympathetic tone of the arterioles and thereby diminish the peripheral resistance. Unfortunately there are several side-effects with this group of drugs, including postural hypertension, constipation, paralysis of accommodation, and difficulty with micturition.

The important ganglion blockers are:

Mecamylamine in doses of 2·5 mg. three times daily or *pempidine tartrate* in doses of 2·5 mg. three times a day increased until a satisfactory fall is produced.

Use of Hypotensive Drugs

Opinions differ as to the relative efficacy of these drugs in hypertension. In mild hypertension a diuretic alone may be sufficient. If this fails to control the blood pressure the diuretic may be combined with a β blocker or a β blocker is used alone. In more severe cases a diuretic can be given with either methyldopa or a sympathetic blocker such as debrisoquine. As an alternative a β blocker can be combined with a direct-acting vasodilator such as hydralazine or prazosin and a diuretic.

The more severe hypertensives will require admission to hospital for treatment, so that the blood pressure can be measured frequently while it is being brought under control. Mild hypertensives can usually be treated as out-patients.

In severe hypertension a reduction of blood pressure to about 160/100 is satisfactory, but in mild cases the aim should be to reduce it to 140/90 or lower.

Hypertensive Crisis

In very severe hypertension it may be necessary to lower the blood pressure rapidly. Diazoxide in a dose of 5·0 mg./kg. as an intravenous bolus will usually act quickly, the hypotensive effect lasting about three hours. As an alternative, hydralazine 15 mg. injected slowly intravenously is also effective.

RHEUMATIC HEART DISEASE

Acute Rheumatic Fever

Acute rheumatic fever is a disease affecting connective tissue, particularly that of the heart and its valves and the joints.

Aetiology. It is a disease of childhood and adolescence, about 90 per cent of cases occurring between the ages of eight and fifteen. It is common in temperate climates, as for example in the British Isles, and it affects the poorer classes, its incidence probably being increased by bad housing and overcrowding. The exact cause of the disease is unknown, but in many patients it follows about two or three weeks after a sore throat due to infection with haemolytic streptococcus (Lancefield Group A). It is possible that other organisms or viruses may play a part. There has been a sharp decline in the incidence of the disease in this country in the last fifty years, possibly related to an improvement in social conditions.

It seems probable that the heart and other organs and the streptococcus share a common antigen so that the antibody provoked by a streptococcal infection will have widespread effects.

Clinical Features. The attack of rheumatic fever nearly always follows seven to twenty days after a streptococcal throat infection. Typically but not invariably, the illness starts suddenly with fever, pain, stiffness, and sometimes swelling in one or more of the larger joints, namely the elbow, wrist, shoulder, hip, knee, or ankle. After a day or two the pain leaves the joint first affected and appears in another one; this *flitting from joint to joint* is unusual in other forms of arthritis and is a useful pointer to the diagnosis. Small joints are rarely affected. Skin rashes are sometimes seen in rheumatic fever; the most typical is *erythema marginatum* which consists of red rings of irregular size and shape which have slightly raised edges and normal centres. They tend to coalesce, and come and go rather quickly. In parts of the body where bones lie immediately under the skin, particularly shins, forearm, elbows, wrists, ankles, and scalp—*rheumatic nodules* may be felt. They are not tender, usually about the size of a pea and are not attached to the overlying skin.

In some children the rheumatic process takes a much milder and more insidious form which can easily be overlooked, though it is as likely as the more obvious type of rheumatic fever to be associated with active heart disease. Thus about half the patients who are later found to be suffering from chronic rheumatic heart disease give no history of rheumatic fever or chorea.

Evidence of Cardiac Involvement. The following findings may be taken as evidence of cardiac involvement:

(1) *Tachycardia.* Patients with active rheumatic carditis nearly always have a raised sleeping pulse rate and awaking pulse disproportionate to the degree of fever; that is more than 20 beats per minute rise per degree (C) of fever.

(2) *The Development of Cardiac Murmurs.* There are two types of cardiac murmur which indicate active rheumatic carditis. The *Carey Coombs murmur*, a short mid-diastolic murmur heard at the apex is the earliest indication of involvement of the mitral valve. When the rheumatic process resolves this murmur may disappear or if the valve is sufficiently damaged it may develop the typical presystolic accentuation of mitral stenosis. The typical rumbling murmur of mitral stenosis results from scarring of the valve, and takes two years at least to appear. The Carey Coombs murmur may be associated with a pansystolic murmur at the apex indicating mitral regurgitation.

Similarly the *soft early diastolic murmur* heard best down the left or right border of the sternum is typical of aortic incompetence and implies involvement of the aortic valve.

Isolated apical systolic murmurs are difficult to interpret in rheumatic fever because they are common in healthy children, but generally it can be said that the louder, rougher and more prolonged the murmur the more likely it is to indicate active carditis. It must however be emphasised that both systolic and mitral diastolic murmurs may disappear when healing of the rheumatic process occurs. The aortic diastolic murmur nearly always persists.

(3) *Cardiac Enlargement.* The development of cardiac enlargement indicates active carditis. It may be due to dilatation of the heart or to the presence of a pericardial effusion, or both.

(4) *Pericarditis.* The finding of a pericardial friction rub indicates active heart involvement.

(5) *Heart Failure.* The appearance of heart failure in acute rheumatic fever indicates a severe myocarditis. Rheumatic myocarditis may also be responsible for patients with established heart disease developing heart failure.

Laboratory Investigations. The blood shows a moderate leucocytosis with some anaemia and a raised E.S.R. The antistreptolysin titre in the blood is raised. A figure above 200 Todd units is considered significant, though it must be realised that this merely indicates a recent streptococcal infection and is not diagnostic of rheumatic fever. The electrocardiogram shows no specific abnormality, but there may be various conduction defects.

Treatment. The seriousness of this disease lies in the risk of carditis occurring at some time in the illness and resulting in chronic rheumatic heart disease.

The most important principle in the treatment is *rest*. The patient should be semi-recumbent on a firm mattress with two or three pillows. Sweating may be profuse. If the joints are very painful they may be supported by pillows and the pressure of bedclothes relieved by a cradle.

The specific drugs in the relief of rheumatic fever are the *salicylates*. High dosage is essential and should aim at producing a blood salicylate level of 30–35 mg./100 ml. Soluble aspirin 900 mg. to 1·5 g. four hourly for an adult should be given until symptoms are relieved or until deafness, tinnitus, nausea, and perhaps vomiting occur, when the dose should be slightly decreased. With this treatment the fever and joint pains should be relieved in two to three days.

Prednisolone 40 mg. daily is useful in the severely ill patient who is not responding to salicylates.

Whether the use of salicylates does more than relieve the symptoms of rheumatic fever is still open to doubt, but there is some evidence that adequate treatment with this drug does decrease the subsequent incidence of rheumatic valvular disease.

A course of *penicillin* should be given to eradicate any residual streptococcal infection, but it does not alter the course of an acute attack. It should also be used to prevent further streptococcal infections (see below).

Duration of Treatment

Complete rest must be enforced until all evidence of active disease has gone, which means the disappearance of all signs of infection and the return of the E.S.R. to normal. It must be remembered that high blood salicylate levels cause acceleration of the E.S.R.: conversely it is reduced if heart failure appears. Consequently the E.S.R. must be interpreted in the light of the whole clinical picture. It rarely requires less than six weeks to return to normal and patients may have to be confined to bed for many months. Thereafter a graduated return is made to normal activity, a careful watch being kept for recrudescence of acute rheumatism.

After-care. On return to normal life the child should not be fussed over, but exposure to cold and dampness should be avoided as much as possible. Because of the danger of further damage to the heart from relapses, streptococcal throat infections should be prevented by giving sulphadimidine 0·5 g. daily or phenoxymethylpenicillin 250 mg. twice daily, continuing until the age of 18 in childhood rheumatic fever or for five years if the disease starts after the age of 13.

Prognosis. Approximately half the children who have acute rheumatic fever develop rheumatic valve disease. About 70 per cent of those with a diastolic murmur will develop permanent valve damage but the prognosis with a systolic murmur is considerably better. The older the child at the time of the acute attack the less likely are the valves to be permanently affected. Some 95 per cent of those with no evidence of cardiac involvement when treatment is started have no residual heart disease. The incidence of permanent valve damage increases with increasing evidence of carditis and is more common after recurrent attacks.

RHEUMATIC CHOREA (Sydenham's Chorea)

Chorea may be considered as a manifestation of the rheumatic process in which the brain is affected. About 20 per cent of patients with chorea develop chronic rheumatic heart disease identical with that found after rheumatic fever. In a certain number of cases there may also be other manifestations of the rheumatic process. Chorea commonly occurs in childhood and adolescence, but a particularly severe though rare type of chorea is associated with pregnancy. It is commoner in girls.

Clinical Features. The child developing chorea is first noticed to be very restless and fidgety and some time may elapse before it is appreciated that her jerkiness and clumsiness indicate illness rather than original sin. All four limbs are usually affected though occasionally the disorder may be confined to one arm or leg or one side of the body (hemichorea). When the disease is at its height the *involuntary movements* are the most prominent feature. The child is constantly grimacing and making sudden, jerky, and ever varying movements of the limbs; these movements cease in sleep. In doubtful cases it is a useful test to ask the child to grasp one's hand, as she is unable to maintain a steady pressure and the intensity of her grip will be found to be always waxing and waning. The *muscles are weak* and have a *poor tone*, so that the joints can be moved through an abnormally wide range, and typically the outstretched hands are held with the wrists slightly flexed and the fingers hyperextended at the metacarpo-phalangeal joints. These movements must be differentiated from nervous tics, the most important points being that unlike tics they are not purposive and never repetitive. *Emotional changes* are common, consisting of depression, weeping, uncontrolled laughter, and hysteria. Examination of the cardio-vascular system may show evidence of cardiac involvement similar to that described under rheumatic fever. The E.S.R. is usually normal unless the heart is involved.

The average *duration* of the disease is about two months, though occasionally chorea may last up to six months or longer. After apparent full recovery odd choreiform movements may persist and be particularly noticeable when the child is under stress. These movements are often considered hysterical, but recently it has been suggested that they represent residual brain damage.

Treatment. *Rest* is the most important part of the treatment of this disease, in order to prevent or limit permanent heart damage. To achieve complete rest in this type of patient is not easy. Some children are happier in a single room, others prefer the company of a general ward. The cot or bed should have sides to prevent the child falling out and there should be padding to prevent injury. One or two pillows are satisfactory and great care should be taken of the child's skin and cleanliness. Feeding may be difficult and great patience will be required by the nurse or mother.

There is no specific treatment for chorea. Soluble aspirin 300 mg. t.d.s. and phenobarbitone 60 mg. t.d.s., during the day and a mixture containing chloral hydrate 0·3–1·0 g. at night is useful for sedating the patient.

Following an attack of chorea prolonged convalescence is required with efforts to improve general health as far as possible. About one-third of patients with chorea will have a further attack. *Prophylaxis* similar to rheumatic fever is recommended.

CHRONIC RHEUMATIC HEART DISEASE

Following acute rheumatic fever, the heart may return to normal; but in about half the patients the valves are so severely damaged that ultimately they will become deformed and scarred and will be unable to function properly.

The incidence of involvement of the various valves is approximately:

Mitral valve	80% of cases
Aortic valve	45% of cases
Tricuspid valve	10% of cases
Pulmonary valve	1% of cases
Mitral valve alone	50% of cases
Mitral and aortic valves together	20% of cases

The *natural history* of the condition starts with the acute rheumatism, usually between the ages of 8 and 15. There may have been one or several attacks. There is then usually an asymptomatic period of 15–20 years until the patient begins to notice dyspnoea.

By about the age of 30 many patients have had their first attack of congestive cardiac failure, which is often precipitated by the onset of atrial fibrillation or perhaps some extra strain such as ill-advised pregnancy. The attacks of cardiac failure become less and less amenable to treatment and death usually occurs in the mid-thirties. It must be realised that the foregoing account is merely an average course of events. In some patients the course is even shorter, whereas others may live to middle or even old age without developing any symptoms from their heart lesion.

ACQUIRED LESIONS OF THE HEART VALVES

MITRAL STENOSIS

Mitral stenosis is the commonest valve lesion and is nearly always due to previous rheumatic infection, although only about half the patients give a clear history of rheumatic fever. It is possible that a few cases may follow a viral endocarditis. It occurs more commonly in women than in men. It is probable that at the time of the acute rheumatic affection the mitral valves fuse at the point of insertion of the chordae tendinae. At first there may be little interference with the flow of blood from the left atrium to the left ventricle, but subsequently there is gradual contraction and narrowing of the mitral orifice and if the orifice is reduced below a size of about 1×0.5 cm. the passage of blood into the left ventricle is seriously obstructed. In addition there may be fibrosis and calcification of the valve cusps and thickening and shortening of the chordae.

There is thus a rise in pressure in the left atrium, which is transmitted back to the pulmonary veins, the pulmonary capillaries, and finally the pulmonary arteries, leading to pulmonary congestion. This passive rise in pressure is not very great, the pulmonary artery pressure being usually about 40 mm. Hg., but it would be sufficient to force fluid from the pulmonary capillaries into the alveoli and thus produce pulmonary oedema. This is prevented in two ways:

(1) There is a certain amount of thickening of the alveolar walls which become less susceptible to oedema.

(2) In a proportion of patients there is active vasoconstriction of the smaller branches of the pulmonary artery which 'protects' the pulmonary capillaries from the pressure developed by the right ventricle. The active pulmonary vasoconstriction, although lowering capillary pressure, causes a considerable rise in pulmonary artery pressure which is often about 80/40 mm. Hg.

Sometimes these protective mechanisms fail. This is liable to occur in the early stages of the disease when alveolar thickening has not developed and when the pulmonary artery vasoconstriction suddenly relaxes. Such patients develop attacks of *acute pulmonary oedema* which are always serious and may be fatal. In the majority of patients, however, the passive pulmonary congestion runs parallel with alveolar thickening. Such patients do not develop active pulmonary vasoconstriction or have attacks of pulmonary oedema. The *pulmonary congestion* does, however, lead to increased 'stiffness' of the lungs which plays a large part in causing dyspnoea which is a leading symptom of mitral stenosis. The changes in the walls of the alveoli also reduce oxygen uptake.

Finally the right ventricle fails and the fully developed picture of congestive cardiac failure emerges.

Clinical Features. *Dyspnoea* is the commonest presenting symptom of mitral stenosis and usually develops 10–20 years after the acute attack of rheumatic fever. It may be of two types:

(1) *Dyspnoea on effort* which becomes progressively more severe and is sooner or later accompanied by *orthopnoea*. This dyspnoea is due to increasing pulmonary congestion.

(2) A small proportion of patients with mitral stenosis present with attacks of *pulmonary oedema* similar symptomatically to those found in acute left ventricular failure. The mechanism of the oedema is considered above. These attacks frequently follow some undue excitement such as a dance or other unusual exertion; they may also be precipitated by pregnancy.

Pulmonary congestion is also responsible for two other symptoms of mitral stenosis, *bronchitis* and *haemoptysis*. The former is usually more marked in the winter but may be troublesome throughout the year. Haemoptysis may be confined to mere blood streaking of the sputum but sometimes takes the form of a frank haemoptysis presumably due to rupture of a congested blood vessel.

The low cardiac output which is often found with mitral stenosis of any severity is probably responsible for the general symptoms of *weakness* and *tiredness* which are found in the developed condition.

Sooner or later most patients with mitral stenosis develop *congestive cardiac failure*. This may occur insidiously, but common precipitating factors are:

(1) The development of atrial fibrillation.
(2) Intercurrent infection.
(3) Further acute rheumatic carditis.
(4) Infective endocarditis.
(5) Pregnancy.
(6) Anaemia.

Complications. There are three complications of mitral stenosis which are not uncommon and which may seriously affect the patient's prognosis. *Thrombi* commonly form in the left auricle of patients with mitral stenosis, particularly in the older patient with atrial fibrillation. In about 20 per cent of patients clots may break off from these thrombi and passing out into the systemic circulation obstruct arteries and produce a variety of symptoms and signs. Thrombi may also form in the deep veins of the legs leading to *pulmonary infarcts*; these are sometimes very intractable and precipitate cardiac failure which may be irreversible. Finally patients with mitral stenosis may develop *infective endocarditis*; this is, however, uncommon if atrial fibrillation is present.

Physical Signs. The patient with mitral stenosis typically, although by no means invariably, has a slight cyanotic flush on the malar region of the cheeks (*mitral flush*), which is due to the low cardiac output. If heart failure has supervened the patient will be orthopnoeic and slightly cyanosed. The pulse will be small and may show atrial fibrillation. The blood pressure is usually on the low side with a narrow pulse pressure.

Examination of the neck veins may show evidence of heart failure and in addition a small group of patients who are in sinus rhythm will show a large 'a' wave indicating pulmonary hypertension or co-existing tricuspid stenosis.

The *apex beat is tapping* and the lift of the *enlarged right ventricle* can be felt between the apex and the left border of the sternum. A *diastolic thrill* may be palpable at the apex.

If the mitral valve is still mobile the first heart sound is loud. This is due to the valve cusps being kept wide open by the prolonged flow of blood until the end of diastole. On ventricular contraction they close with a louder sound than normal valves, which are already half closed at this time. Careful auscultation at the lower end of the sternum will also show a sharp, clear sound following the second heart sound; this is the *opening snap of the mitral valve* and is due to the sudden opening of the anterior cusp of the mitral valve because of the high atrial pressure. It denotes a mobile valve. The pulmonary component of the second sound is loud and may even be palpable.

The typical *murmur of mitral stenosis* is a low-pitched, rumbling diastolic murmur, localised to the apex (ventricular filling murmur). It is best heard with the patient lying on the left side and is accentuated after exercise. It is due to the blood rushing through the narrowed mitral valve and if the patient is in sinus rhythm there will be a presystolic accentuation due to the left atrium contracting and forcing the last portion of the blood even more rapidly through the mitral valve. The presystolic accentuation usually disappears with atrial fibrillation. In severe mitral stenosis the murmur extends from the opening snap to the first heart sound; in less severe stenosis it is shorter. If severe pulmonary hypertension develops the mitral diastolic murmur may become brief and insignificant due to the associated low cardiac output.

Very rarely there may be heard a pulmonary diastolic murmur down the left border of the sternum (*Graham-Steell murmur*) due to pulmonary incompetence subsequent upon dilatation of the pulmonary artery; it must be stressed, however, that such a murmur is very much more commonly due to associated aortic incompetence.

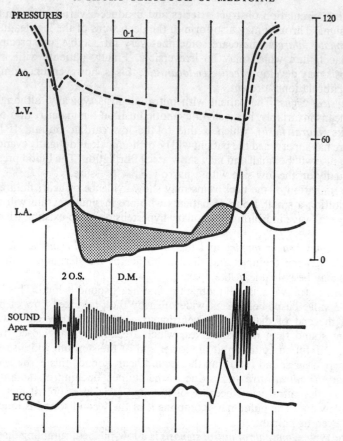

THE HAEMODYNAMICS OF THE DIASTOLIC MURMUR OF MITRAL STENOSIS WITH SINUS RHYTHM.

Mitral stenosis produces a persistent diastolic pressure gradient between the left atrium and ventricle. The gradient is represented by the shaded area in the figure. Note how, owing to the mitral obstruction, the gradient falls slowly in diastole and is sharply increased by atrial systole. The intensity of the diastolic murmur is related to the A-V pressure gradient, with a pre-systolic accentuation. The opening snap coincides with the opening of the mitral valve.

An *electrocardiogram* may show large wide P waves or atrial fibrillation; there may also be right ventricular hypertrophy. A *radiograph of the heart* may show some cardiac enlargement. The dilated left atrium forms a double contour above the right atrium on the right border of the heart. The left atrial appendage can be seen just below the left pulmonary artery. Screening in the right oblique position with barium in the oesophagus will show lesser atrial enlargement. Calcification of the mitral valves may be seen but this can also occur in mitral incompetence. The pulmonary arteries are often dilated. The lung fields will be congested if heart failure has supervened.

Normally the flow of blood through the lungs is higher in the lower than the upper lobes. In mitral stenosis there is constriction of the arteries to the lower lobe and thus a redistribution of the pulmonary circulation, so that pulmonary congestion affects both upper and lower lobes. In addition dilated lymph channels will show as fine horizontal lines in the costo-phrenic angles (*Kerley B lines*).

Left heart catheterisation is useful in that it allows the left atrial pressure and the gradient across the mitral valve to be measured. Right heart catheterisation is rarely necessary but gives information as to the pulmonary artery pressure and the pulmonary wedge pressure (indirect left atrial pressure).

Treatment. Minor degrees of mitral stenosis, producing no symptoms and without evidence of cardiac enlargement, are no contra-indication to leading a normal life, although extreme effort must be avoided.

Cardiac failure, with or without atrial fibrillation, should be treated as outlined previously (p. 113).

The risk of infective endocarditis can be greatly diminished by giving benzylpenicillin 1·0 mega unit just before dental treatment or tonsillectomy. followed by phenoxymethyl penicillin 250 mg. q.i.d. for five days. In patients sensitive to penicillin, erythromycin is an adequate substitute.

Anticoagulants are indicated after an embolism or in the older patient with atrial fibrillation.

The indication for operation is the onset of significant symptoms in particular dyspnoea, attacks of pulmonary oedema, or evidence of pulmonary hypertension. Mitral valvotomy also decreases the risk of systemic emboli. It is a mistake to wait until cardiac failure has developed.

If the symptoms, signs and investigations suggest the patient has pure mitral stenosis with a mobile valve, the closed operation is satisfactory, with a mortality rate of less than 5 per cent and about 80 per cent of patients obtain a satisfactory result. With calcified valves or with a significant degree of mitral incompetence open operation will be necessary, the mortality is higher and the results less satisfactory.

Restenosis can occur, probably in about 10 per cent of patients and its frequency depends on the state of the valve and the success of the previous valvotomy. Repeated emboli are best treated by valvotomy, but if this is impossible long-term anti-coagulation may be required.

Lutembacher's Syndrome

In this disorder, mitral stenosis is combined with an atrial septal defect. This results in a marked left to right shunt through the septal defect and the development of right heart failure without concomitant pulmonary congestion.

MITRAL REGURGITATION

Mitral incompetence may be due to dilatation of the mitral ring which is caused by general dilatation of the left ventricle and found in such conditions as aortic valvular disease or hypertension.

This group accounts for the loud apical murmur which may be heard with gross dilatation of the left ventricle and which will sometimes disappear when the associated heart failure is successfully treated.

It may also be due to rheumatic affection of the mitral valve and occur as the result of rupture of the chordae tendineae or damage to papillary muscle as in infective endocarditis, myocardial ischaemia or sometimes for no apparent reason.

RHEUMATIC MITRAL REGURGITATION

Rheumatic mitral regurgitation is slightly more common in men. The essential lesion is contraction and fibrosis of the chordae tendinae and thickening of the valve cusps so that the normal valve mechanism is unable to function. When the left ventricle contracts blood regurgitates into the left atrium so that the left ventricular stroke volume increases and the left ventricle dilates and hypertrophies. Left atrial pressure rises rapidly in ventricular systole but is not sustained and so pulmonary pressure is rarely as high as in mitral stenosis.

Clinical Features. Symptoms usually develop some years after the attack of rheumatic fever and generally a little later in life than in mitral stenosis. The presenting symptom is dysponea due to pulmonary congestion in which left ventricular failure will sooner or later play a part. The enlarged left ventricle may bulge into the right ventricle (*Bernheim effect*) producing some right ventricular obstruction and this may be partially responsible for producing the congestive failure which ultimately develops. The course is then usually rapidly downhill.

Sinus rhythm is more common than in mitral stenosis. The apex beat is hyperdynamic and suggests left ventricular enlargement. A third heart sound is often present. The first sound at the apex is not accentuated, the typical harsh pansystolic murmur is heard best at the apex and spreads towards the axilla, it is loud and may be associated with a thrill.

A short mitral diastolic murmur is quite common in mitral regurgitation. It is due to a rapid flow of blood through the rigid mitral orifice and is brief because pressure equalisation between left atrium and ventricle occurs rapidly.

Radiography shows left ventricular enlargement and often considerable dilatation of the left atrium, perhaps with expansile pulsation in ventricular systole; the valve may be calcified.

Treatment. The treatment is that of heart failure when it supervenes; infective endocarditis should be avoided as for mitral stenosis.

Surgical treatment consisting of valve replacement or refashioning has so far not proved very successful.

Other Types of Mitral Regurgitation

Rupture of a chorda or papillary muscle may precipitate cardiac failure or even death. The regurgitant murmur in this condition is often atypical in that it is short, being confined to mid- or late systole.

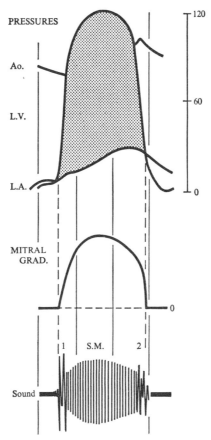

THE HAEMODYNAMICS OF THE PANSYSTOLIC MURMUR OF MITRAL REGURGITATION.

Aortic, left ventricular and left atrial curves, with phonocardiogram and pressure gradient across the mitral valve (not to scale). Note how the mitral pressure gradient and the regurgitant murmur last throughout systole.

MIXED MITRAL STENOSIS AND REGURGITATION

In many patients with rheumatic mitral disease there is a mixture of stenosis and regurgitation and the physical signs show features suggestive of both these lesions.

MITRAL VALVE PROLAPSE

This is due to myxomatous degeneration of the mitral valves. Sometimes there are no specific symptoms but on auscultation there is a midsystolic click which is often followed by a late systolic murmur. There is no treatment and the prognosis is good.

INNOCENT APICAL SYSTOLIC MURMURS

It must be clearly understood that the majority of apical systolic murmurs are not due to mitral valvular disease. A small proportion are transmitted from other areas: for example, they may be aortic systolic murmurs which can quite commonly be heard at the apex. The majority are benign murmurs due to a variety of physiological causes. These benign murmurs are not associated with other evidence of cardiac disease, such as cardiac enlargement or thrills, they may disappear at various phases of respiration, they alter considerably in intensity with changes in posture and they are usually neither harsh nor loud. If a murmur shows these characteristics it can usually be disregarded.

TRICUSPID VALVE DISEASE

Tricuspid Regurgitation

Tricuspid regurgitation may be due to dilatation of the tricuspid ring in association with right ventricular failure. It is common in the late stages of mitral stenosis and may occur in pulmonary heart disease and with various congenital lesions. Organic tricuspid regurgitation is usually rheumatic but may be part of the carcinoid syndrome (page 464) when cardiac involvement occurs.

Clinical Features. The patient will nearly always have the symptoms and signs of congestive heart failure. In addition, the effects of the direct transmission of right ventricular systole to the veins is apparent. Gross pulsation of the cervical veins is seen, both superficial and deep, so that if the neck is viewed from the front in silhouette it widens perceptibly with each beat. The lobes of the ears are moved by this forceful deep pulsation. Expansile pulsation of the liver may be felt, and even superficial veins in the back of the hands can be seen to pulsate (sign of Levine). If tricuspid regurgitation is not rapidly relieved then *cardiac cirrhosis* of the liver results, and prolonged renal congestion may cause heavy *proteinuria*. The combination results in markedly reduced serum albumen levels, with generalised oedema. There is a systolic murmur lasting throughout systole and best heard over the lower end of the sternum. It becomes louder during inspiration.

Treatment is along the general lines for congestive cardiac failure.

Tricuspid Stenosis

Tricuspid stenosis is nearly always rheumatic and is associated with rheumatic lesions of other valves.

Clinical Features. It is characteristic that these patients do not complain of much dyspnoea or orthopnoea, because the stenosed tricuspid valve guards the lungs against congestion. The main symptoms as the disease advances are weakness due to the low cardiac output together with peripheral venous congestion with liver enlargement and oedema.

There is a raised pressure in the neck veins and if the heart is in sinus rhythm a large presystolic wave ('a' wave) is present due to the right atrium contracting against the narrowed tricuspid valve and resulting in a sharp rise in pressure in the atrium and great veins. On auscultation a diastolic murmur similar to that of mitral stenosis can be heard over the lower each of the sternum. It is sometimes more marked on inspiration.

Treatment is along the usual lines for congestive cardiac failure.

AORTIC VALVE DISEASE

AORTIC STENOSIS

Aortic stenosis can be divided into valvar and subvalvar. Valvar stenosis may be congenital, may follow rheumatic fever or be due to atheroma of the valve. Although the commonest cause of isolated aortic stenosis is probably congenital, the exact frequency with which these three causes operate is still debatable because the end result, whatever the initial lesion, is a scarred, deformed valve, with deposits of atheroma, so that identification of the original aetiology is very difficult.

If, however, aortic stenosis is combined with mitral stenosis it can be presumed to be rheumatic and if it is diagnosed in infancy it is obviously congenital in origin.

Subvalvar stenosis may be due to muscle hypertrophy (see Cardiomyopathies, p. 154), or to a fibrous ring.

When the aortic valve orifice is reduced to about one-quarter its normal size the flow of blood is so restricted that the left ventricular pressure rises above the aortic pressure. This is followed by hypertrophy of the left ventricle and finally heart failure.

Clinical Features. Aortic stenosis may produce no symptoms, but in the majority of cases sooner or later the strain on the left ventricle produces first hypertrophy and then dilatation and failure. This may present as *dyspnoea on effort*, often with attacks of acute left ventricular failure causing pulmonary congestion with *paroxysmal nocturnal dyspnoea*. Once heart failure develops the downhill course is progressive and death usually occurs within five years.

The narrowed aortic valve reduces the cardiac output, which cannot be increased to meet the demands of the body on exercise. This may lead to *fainting after effort* and *angina of effort*. *Exercise syncope* is an important

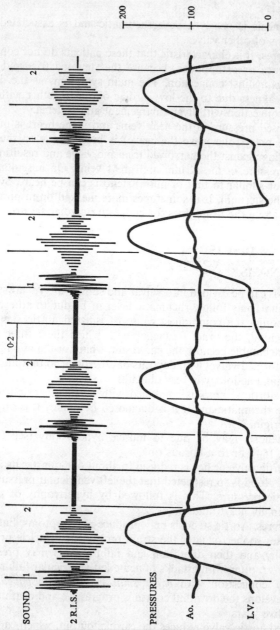

ALTERNATION OF THE INTENSITY OF THE EJECTION MURMUR IN AORTIC STENOSIS WITH LEFT VENTRICULAR PULSUS ALTERNANS.
Note the left ventricular pressure rising above the aortic pressure and the short diamond-shaped murmur. There is also pulsus alternans due to left ventricular strain. Sound is taken from the second right intercostal space.

symptom for it indicates severe stenosis and carries a poor prognosis. Sudden death may occur and is probably due to ventricular fibrillation.

The *pulse* in aortic stenosis is typically small, with a slow rise and a low pulse pressure; it may, however, be normal. In a fully developed case the heart shows evidence of *left ventricular hypertrophy* with a heaving apex beat. There is a *systolic thrill in the aortic area*. A *harsh systolic murmur* which is maximal in mid-systole (an ejection murmur) can be heard extending from the aortic area up into the neck and often also down to the apex. It is best heard in expiration. An ejection click may be noted between the first heart sound and the systolic murmur. This is due to tensing of the aortic valve. It is only heard if the valve is pliable, and is not heard in subvalvar stenosis.

A short blowing early diastolic murmur may be heard down the left border of the sternum; it is due to minimal aortic regurgitation and is caused by the damaged valves failing to close completely. The second sound at the base is absent or greatly reduced.

Not all patients with aortic stenosis show all the signs enumerated above. Sometimes the diagnosis may be suspected on the grounds of a harsh systolic murmur transmitted to the neck, without obvious abnormalities of the pulse or the presence or a thrill, but it must be remembered that innocent systolic murmurs at the base of the heart are very common and a diagnosis of aortic stenosis should only be made if the murmur is loud and quite characteristic and does not disappear with changes of posture or during different phases of respiration.

An *E.C.G.* shows left ventricular hypertrophy usually with a vertical heart. *Radiography* of the heart confirms the left ventricular hypertrophy and careful screening may show *calcification of the aortic valves*. The aorta may show post-stenotic dilatation, particularly in valvar stenosis.

Left heart catheterisation shows a considerable gradient across the valve often in excess of 50 mm. Hg.

Treatment. Asymptomatic cases of aortic stenosis with no evidence of left ventricular hypertrophy require no treatment except for the avoidance of undue physical effort; they may otherwise lead a completely normal life. Dental extractions and E.N.T. operations should be covered with penicillin as in mitral stenosis (p. 143). When heart failure develops it should be treated along the usual lines (p. 113).

Several surgical procedures are now available to relieve aortic valve disease. The indications for surgical treatment are:

    (1) Severe angina of effort.
    (2) Developing cardiac failure.
    (3) Syncopal attacks.

In aortic stenosis it may be possible to perform a simple valvotomy, but for severely damaged or calcified valves, or if there is aortic regurgitation, some form of valve replacement is required. This may be either a homograft aortic valve, or some form of prosthesis, of which the Starr-Edwards ball valve is probably the most satisfactory at the present time. In the best hands the operative mortality is down to about 10 per cent, although there may be a further 10 per cent of deaths within the next year. The principal postoperative complications are infection or thrombosis on the prosthesis, or residual valve leak with homografts.

AORTIC REGURGITATION

Aortic regurgitation may result from the following conditions:

(1) *Rheumatic valvular disease*, which commonly gives rise to a combination of regurgitation and stenosis.

(2) *Aneurysm of the ascending aorta* affecting the aortic valve ring, which becomes stretched and renders the valve incompetent.

(3) *Infective endocarditis*.

(4) *Rupture of an atheromatous aortic valve cusp*.

(5) A small proportion of patients with *severe hypertension*, especially those with coarctation of the aorta have some degree of aortic regurgitation.

(6) It may complicate *ankylosing spondylitis*.

(7) *Bicuspid aortic valves* may become incompetent when associated with infective endocarditis or with coarctation of the aorta.

If the aortic valve is incompetent blood flows back from the aorta to the left ventricle during diastole. This produces certain signs in the peripheral circulation and also imposes a strain on the left ventricle due to increased stroke volume. The freer the regurgitation the more striking are the peripheral signs and the greater the left ventricular strain. The rapid ventricular filling in diastole, due to the regurgitant flow, may cause premature closure of the mitral valves and thus limit ventricular filling from the atrium.

Clinical Features. The commonest presenting symptoms of aortic regurgitation are those of developing left ventricular failure, namely *dyspnoea on effort* and perhaps attacks of *cardiac asthma*; once heart failure develops the downhill course is usually rapid and death ensues within two or three years. Aortic regurgitation, particularly if due to rheumatic infection, can, however, exist for many years before heart failure develops.

Aortic regurgitation may be complicated by *angina of effort* because the low diastolic pressure found in this condition leads to poor filling of the coronary arteries. When angina occurs in aortic incompetence due to syphilitic aortitis an additional factor may be the involvement of the mouths of the coronary arteries by the gummatous process.

The *pulse in aortic regurgitation* is typically collapsing in nature, due to the rapid flow of blood forwards through the dilated peripheral arterioles and backwards into the left ventricle during diastole. It is best appreciated if the patient's wrist is grasped by the whole hand, when it can be felt as a distinct tap, which has been likened to a water-hammer. For similar reasons pulsation can sometimes be seen in the peripheral capillaries, particularly

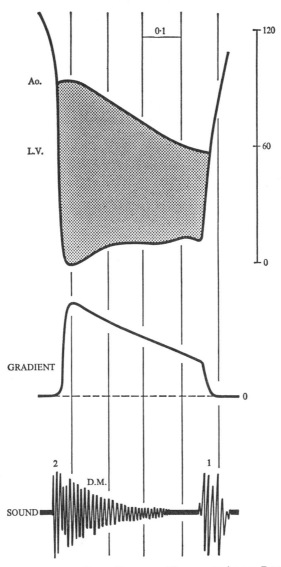

THE HAEMODYNAMICS OF THE EARLY DIASTOLIC MURMUR OF AORTIC REGURGITATION.

Simultaneous aortic and left ventricular pressure curves. The shaded area represents the gradient which is responsible for the regurgitant flow and murmur. The gradient is shown below (not to scale) and corresponds to the intensity of the murmur.

those of the nail bed, lips, and forehead. Marked pulsation can also be seen in the carotid arteries. There is a large pulse pressure, the systolic pressure being slightly raised and the diastolic very low. These peripheral signs are not present if there is only a slight leak back through the aortic valve.

The heart usually shows evidence of *left ventricular hypertrophy*, particularly if there is free regurgitation. The typical *aortic diastolic murmur* is soft and blowing and is not associated with a thrill. It is best heard with the patient sitting upright and with his breath held in expiration. It may be loudest down the left or right sides of the sternum or even at the apex. It is maximal immediately after the second sound and dies away through diastole.

There may in addition be an aortic systolic murmur, which is not due to aortic stenosis but to the greatly increased blood flow through the aortic valve.

If there is gross enlargement of the left ventricle it may be possible to hear a rumbling diastolic murmur at the apex, similar to that found in mitral stenosis. This may be due to blood passing through normal mitral valves into the dilated left ventricle or to eddies produced by the regurgitant stream of blood around the medial cusp of the mitral valve. It is known as *Austin Flint murmur*.

The chief complications of aortic regurgitation are heart failure and bacterial endocarditis.

Treatment. Surgical treatment for aortic disease is considered on p. 149. Complications should be treated as they arise. If the incompetence is syphilitic in origin, the syphilis should be treated, but this will not cure the leaking valve. Generally speaking the physical activities of patients with aortic incompetence should be limited. Penicillin must be used to cover dental extractions and E.N.T. operations.

ANEURYSMS OF THE AORTA

Aneurysms of the aorta are usually due to atheroma sometimes complicated by a dissection (see below). Syphilitic aortitis which was a common cause is now rare in the U.K.

Clinical Features. The substernal pain of *angina pectoris*, coming on when the patient exerts himself, and relieved by rest, is a common symptom of syphilitic aortitis. Other patients remain symptom-free until the strain imposed on the left ventricle by co-existing aortic regurgitation leads to *left ventricular failure* (p. 110).

When an *aneurysm* is present it may compress important structures which lie close to it in the chest and so produce groups of symptoms and signs. An aneurysm of the ascending aorta may erode the anterior chest wall, producing severe local pain and tenderness, and in addition may press on the superior vena cava causing obstruction.

It may be possible to percuss out the aneurysm to the right of the upper part of the sternum; and the aneurysm may finally appear on the surface as a pulsatile swelling which ultimately ruptures. It is common to find a harsh systolic murmur and thrill over the aneurysm. There may also be the typical murmur of aortic regurgitation.

An aneurysm of the arch of the aorta may compress the *trachea* and left bronchus causing a typical brassy cough and sometimes collapse of the lung, the *oesophagus* causing difficulty in swallowing, the *recurrent laryngeal nerve* causing paralysis of the left vocal cord and a hoarse voice, and the *sympathetic chain* causing Horner's syndrome (p. 264). When the aneurysm expands during systole it may push downwards on the trachea and left main bronchus causing a downward *tug on the trachea* and larynx which is best felt by standing behind the patient and palpating the cricoid cartilage. It may involve the origins of the great vessels and cause *inequality of the pulses.*

Aneurysms of the descending aorta rarely produce dramatic signs, but may cause *pain in the back and chest* wall by pressure and erosion of the spine and ribs. The fourth thoracic vertebra is most usually affected.

A radiograph will confirm the presence of aneurysmal dilatation arising from the aorta. Theoretically, on screening it should be easy to see expansile pulsation of the aneurysm, but this is not always so, partially because it may be confused with transmitted pulsation from the heart and partially because the sac of the aneurysm may be lined with blood clot which prevents pulsation. *Calcification* of the ascending aorta is suggestive of syphilitic aortitis.

Treatment is usually symptomatic but large aneurysms may be treated by surgery. If the aneurysm is due to syphilis 1 megaunit of benzylpenicillin should be given daily for 14 days.

DISSECTING ANEURYSM OF THE AORTA

This relatively rare complaint occurs in an aorta already damaged by *atheroma* or by *cystic necrosis* the cause of which is not known but it frequently complicates Marfan's syndrome. There is, however, an association with scoliosis. The blood forces its way between the layers of the aortic wall and splits it for a variable distance, often occluding various branches of the aorta. The blood in the false passage may re-enter the lumen, leaving the patient with a 'double-barrelled aorta', but more often it ruptures externally into pericardium, mediastinum, or retroperitoneal space and the patient does not long survive.

Clinical Features. The patient is seized by a sudden severe pain usually in the chest and often extending to the back. The attack is associated with collapse and may prove rapidly fatal. Examination usually shows a severely ill patient in great pain and a clue to the diagnosis may be provided by finding absent or unequal radial or femoral pulses. If the dissection involves the thoracic aorta it may produce acute aortic incompetence or a left-sided bloody effusion. Occlusion of the spinal arteries may cause focal neurological signs.

The E.C.G. shows no specific change. The diagnosis can be confirmed by aortography. If the patient survives the acute episode radiological examination shows widening of the aorta.

Treatment. Treatment consists of bed rest with morphine at frequent intervals to relieve the pain. Some patients can be helped by surgery and a surgical opinion should be sought. If the patient survives the acute attack the prognosis must be guarded as the process may recur, although there have been some remarkably long survivals. Treatment with β blockers may improve the long term prognosis.

ANEURYSM OF THE ABDOMINAL AORTA

An aneurysm of the abdominal aorta is nearly always due to atheroma. It may cause abdominal pain which is often quite severe and is due to pressure on the vertebral column and neighbouring organs. The diagnosis can be confirmed by palpation. Some such aneurysms can be treated by resection and replacement by an arterial graft. Death may occur from rupture of the aneurysm.

CARDIOMYOPATHY

Cardiomyopathy occurs in several diseases and affects primarily myocardium, although the endocardium or pericardium are also sometimes involved. It may complicate such generalised diseases as amyloidosis, scleroderma, systemic lupus erythematosus or leukaemia, or may appear as an isolated phenomenon. One well-defined variety is due to *endomyocardial fibrosis*, which is a common cause of cardiac failure in East Africa. Its aetiology is obscure.

There are two main types:

(1) *Congestive Cardiomyopathy*. This is essentially a dilatation of the heart with failure of the myocardium. The main clinical features are left ventricular failure rapidly followed by congestive failure. The heart is enlarged, often with a triple rhythm and sometimes functional mitral and tricuspid incompetence.

(2) *Obstructive Cardiomyopathy*. The essential feature is hypertrophy without dilatation. This leads to resistance to filling of the ventricles in diastole and to obstruction to outflow in systole producing a picture similar to aortic stenosis. The clinical course may be prolonged over many years but sooner or later congestive failure develops. Angina of effort may occur and sudden death is not uncommon.

Propranolol is effective in relieving the outflow obstruction and increasing diastolic filling; if this fails, removal of a segment of the hypertrophied muscle may be necessary.

Alcoholic Cardiomyopathy. Prolonged and heavy drinking can damage the heart muscle. Early symptoms are dyspnoea on effort and palpitation. There are no specific physical signs but tachycardia, ectopic beats, or atrial fibrillation may occur and the electrocardiogram may show T wave changes. At this stage the condition is probably reversible. If drinking continues, a state similar to beri-beri may develop with oedema and cardiac enlargement and with signs of a high cardiac output.

ATRIAL MYXOMA

This benign tumour usually develops in the left atrium and produces symptoms and signs similar to those of mitral stenosis. Peripheral emboli may occur. The treatment is surgical removal.

Echocardiography is particularly helpful in diagnosis.

THE HEART AND THYROID DISEASE

THYROTOXICOSIS

Thyrotoxicosis frequently affects the heart, particularly in the older age groups. The action of increased thyroid hormone is to raise the cardiac rate and output. In young subjects tachycardia with a full bounding pulse, high pulse pressure, warm extremities and an over-active heart are the chief signs in the cardiovascular system. In older patients these signs may be complicated by various arrhythmias, particularly atrial fibrillation, and by heart failure. The heart failure and atrial fibrillation of thyrotoxicosis are difficult to control adequately with digitalis and, the addition of a β blocker is useful. The thyrotoxicosis itself should be treated as quickly as possible; after this is relieved the heart usually returns to normal and if atrial fibrillation persists it can nearly always be easily reversed.

MYXOEDEMA

Myxoedema may also have effects on the heart. Bradycardia, sometimes extreme, is not uncommon. Patients with myxoedema have a high incidence of coronary artery disease. In addition, myxoedema is occasionally complicated by a pericardial effusion, the cause of which is not clear.

The *electrocardiogram* is characteristic, showing low-voltage QRS complexes in all leads, with flat T waves.

HEART DISEASE AND PREGNANCY

Pregnancy produces a number of changes in the circulation which throw an increased strain on the heart and which may be wrongly interpreted as evidence of heart disease.

These changes begin during the second month of pregnancy, increase until about the thirty-second week and then diminish. The chief changes are:

(1) An increase in cardiac output.
(2) Some retention of sodium and water.

Clinically there is tachycardia, a full pulse and warm, flushed and pulsating extremities. There may be some ankle oedema, although this may also be a sign of toxaemia. The apex beat is rather forcible and may in the later months of pregnancy be displaced a little to the left. The jugular venous pressure is slightly raised. The increased cardiac flow produces pulmonary and aortic systolic murmurs. A physiological third heart sound is not uncommon due to rapid ventricular filling.

Fitness for Pregnancy. The decision as to whether a patient with heart disease is fit for pregnancy is not always easy and when there is any doubt expert advice should be sought.

Generally speaking the following rules will be found useful:

(1) Patients with no symptoms or evidence of cardiac enlargement will usually go through a pregnancy without trouble.
(2) Patients who have had heart failure or who have severe effort intolerance should be advised against pregnancy; if they have already conceived, the pregnancy should be terminated in the first three months.
(3) The middle group present the main difficulty. This includes those with moderate dyspnoea on effort and some cardiac enlargement. Each of these cases will have to be judged on its own merits.

Cardiac Surgery and Pregnancy. If the patient has some lesion which can be corrected surgically this should be done before pregnancy or, if the patient is already pregnant, within the first three months.

General Management during Pregnancy. All patients with heart disease should be carefully observed by both physician and obstetrician.

Patients who have symptoms before pregnancy or those who develop some dyspnoea during pregnancy must have a full night's rest and in addition should rest during the afternoon. The earliest signs of cardiac failure are the development of pulmonary congestion causing cough and dyspnoea with râles at the bases of the lungs and X-ray evidence of congestion. Filling of the neck veins and the presence of slight ankle oedema are often misleading as these may occur normally in pregnancy.

If failure develops it should be treated in the usual way (p. 113).

Management of Labour. In most patients natural delivery assisted perhaps by forceps in the second stage is quite satisfactory. Caesarian section is rarely required except perhaps in coarctation of the aorta where there is a risk of rupture. During the period of labour and for four days afterwards ampicillin 500 mg. four times daily should be given as there is a risk of infective endocarditis.

Post-Partum Period. Rest is important in the post-partum period and the long-term problem of looking after a child and a home must be considered before embarking on a further pregnancy.

Mitral Stenosis in Pregnancy. The majority of patients with heart disease and pregnancy have rheumatic heart disease, usually mitral stenosis.

The main danger in these patients is the rapid development of pulmonary congestion with attacks of pulmonary oedema, which may be fatal. This usually starts early in pregnancy and is an indication for an emergency mitral valvotomy. In addition, atrial fibrillation may start in pregnancy and produce a rapid onset of cardiac failure.

With the fall in the incidence of rheumatic valve disease, congenital heart disease is relatively more common. Pulmonary hypertension, whether as part of Eisenmenger's syndrome or as an isolated phenomenon carries a bad prognosis for both mother and fetus and may well be an indication for termination of the pregnancy. In general expert guidance will be required for these patients.

Heart Disease and the Pill. Oral contraception should be avoided in patients with systemic or pulmonary hypertension, with coronary artery disease or with a history of venous thrombosis or pulmonary embolism.

CONGENITAL HEART DISEASE

Congenital heart disease may be classified as follows:

Acyanotic

Without shunt
Coarctation of the aorta
Dextrocardia
Bicuspid aortic valves
Pulmonary stenosis
Congenital aortic stenosis

With shunt (left to right)
Persistent ductus arteriosus
Atrial septal defect
Ventricular septal defect

Cyanotic

With right to left shunt
Fallot's tetralogy
Eisenmenger's Syndrome
Pulmonary atresia ⎫ Very
Transposition of the ⎬ rare
  great vessels ⎭

This list is by no means exhaustive, but covers the commoner congenital lesions. The diagnosis and management of congenital heart disease in infants and young children is a specialised subject and will not be considered here.

ACYANOTIC GROUP

COARCTATION OF THE AORTA

In coarctation of the aorta there is a narrowing of the aorta usually just below the origin of the left subclavian artery.

The narrowed aorta is partially bypassed by a collateral circulation between branches of the subclavian and axillary arteries and the intercostal and superior epigastric arteries.

Clinical Features. The condition may remain asymptomatic in early life and adolescence. It may present as hypertension; as heart failure, which usually develops between the ages of thirty and forty years; or as a subarachnoid haemorrhage due to rupture of a congenital berry aneurysm of the circle of Willis, which is a common (15 per cent) associated condition.

Examination shows a raised blood pressure in the arms; the mean blood pressure in the legs is usually normal, but with a low pulse pressure. The *femoral pulses* are either absent or feeble and delayed. There is often conspicuous *arterial pulsation in the neck*. The heart may show evidence of left ventricular enlargement and there is a widespread *systolic murmur* heard over the praecordium and at the back. This murmur is due to blood passing through the coarctation and also through the collaterals. A small number of cases are complicated by bicuspid aortic valves and these may have the characteristic murmur of aortic regurgitation. Careful examination will show pulsation in *collateral vessels*, particularly around the scapula. A radiograph of the chest will often show *notching of the ribs* due to erosion by the large and tortuous intercostal arteries.

Prognosis and Treatment. The prognosis is variable, but few patients with coarctation live beyond middle age. The possibility of resection of the coarctation should therefore be remembered when the abnormality is diagnosed, the optimum age for operation being between seven and fifteen years.

DEXTROCARDIA

Dextrocardia is often associated with transposition of the abdominal viscera. It is of no importance clinically except that if its presence is unrecognised it may lead to misdiagnosis.

BICUSPID AORTIC VALVES

These may remain symptomless throughout life, but are especially liable to severe atheromatous change and to infective endocarditis. They may be associated with coarctation of the aorta and may become incompetent.

CONGENITAL AORTIC STENOSIS

Congenital aortic stenosis is considered under aortic stenosis (p. 147).

PULMONARY STENOSIS

Simple congenital pulmonary stenosis is usually valvar and rarely infundibular.

Clinical Features. In mild pulmonary stenosis there may be no symptoms and the diagnosis is suggested by finding a *systolic ejection murmur and thrill* over the pulmonary artery, usually in the second or third left intercostal space. It may be associated with an ejection click.

Severe cases usually develop cardiac failure by early adult life. The venous pulse in the neck shows a large 'a' wave; there is evidence of right ventricular hypertrophy with a systolic ejection murmur and thrill in the pulmonary area. The second sound in the pulmonary area is usually single, because the pulmonary component is delayed and often inaudible.

If the foramen ovale is patent and the pressure rises in the right atrium during the course of severe pulmonary stenosis, there will be a shunt from the right to the left atrium with the subsequent development of central cyanosis.

An *E.C.G.* shows evidence of right ventricular hypertrophy, and an X-ray shows diminished vascularity of the lung fields with post-stenotic dilatation of the pulmonary artery.

Prognosis and Treatment. Severe cases of pulmonary stenosis rarely reach middle age and all cases run the risk of infective endocarditis. All but the mildest cases should be offered relief of the stenosis by valvotomy.

PERSISTENT DUCTUS ARTERIOSUS

The ductus joining the left pulmonary artery and aorta usually closes at birth or soon afterwards. If it persists, there is a shunt from the aorta to the pulmonary artery, with a consequent increase in pulmonary artery flow and in the output of the left ventricle.

Clinical Features. The condition is often symptomless when it is discovered. Infective endocarditis develops in about one-third of the patients who reach middle age. Cardiac failure is another complication which is found in the third and fourth decades, although in a proportion of patients with a large ductus it may occur even in infancy.

Examination may show a *collapsing pulse* with a low diastolic blood pressure. The apex beat is forcible and suggests some left ventricular hypertrophy. The *'machinery' murmur* which is characteristic of persistent ductus is best heard in the second left intercostal space. It is more or less continuous, starting in early systole, becoming louder in late systole and dying away towards the end of diastole. It may be associated with a thrill.

If the pulmonary artery pressures increase, the murmurs may be confined to systole when the pressure gradient is greatest.

In addition over a third of subjects with a persistent ductus have a *mitral diastolic murmur* which is presumed to be due to increased blood flow through the mitral valve.

A proportion of patients with a persistent ductus arteriosus develop pulmonary hypertension, with reversal of the blood flow through the duct and the development of peripheral cyanosis.

An *E.C.G.* may show some left ventricular hypertrophy and radiography some enlargement of the pulmonary vessels with a well-marked aortic knuckle.

Prognosis and Treatment. Persistent ductus arteriosus is amenable to surgical closure and this should be advised for all patients except those with pulmonary hypertension.

ATRIAL SEPTAL DEFECT

Atrial septal defect is commonly due to a failure of development of the septum secundum. More rarely the septum primum fails to fuse and this defect is usually accompanied by a deficiency in the mitral valve causing mitral regurgitation. Half or more of the blood which enters the left atrium passes through the defect into the right atrium and thus back through the pulmonary circulation. Usually the increased flow can be accommodated by the pulmonary circulation without a rise in pulmonary artery pressure. Rarely changes occur in the pulmonary vessels with a rise in pressure and a reversal of the atrial shunt.

Clinical Features. Atrial septal defect does not as a rule produce much in the way of symptoms until middle age when it usually presents as cardiac failure. *Examination* will show some right ventricular enlargement. The apex beat is not obvious and is sometimes described as 'tapping' in quality. The increased pulmonary blood flow may be detected as marked pulsation in the enlarged pulmonary artery, palpable in the second and third left intercostal space. The majority of patients have a *systolic murmur* in the pulmonary area due to increased blood flow from the right ventricle into the dilated pulmonary artery. The *second sound* in the pulmonary area is *widely split*. This split is not altered by respiration and is due to delay of the pulmonary element and is an almost constant feature of the disorder. Sometimes a diastolic murmur is present at the lower end of the sternum and is due to a very high flow rate through the tricuspid valve in diastole, and occasionally a pulmonary regurgitant murmur can be heard if pulmonary hypertension is present. In ostium primum defects there may be an apical pan-systolic murmur due to mitral regurgitation.

On a *radiograph of the chest* there is marked dilatation of the pulmonary arteries, which can be seen to pulsate on screening (hilar dance). The right ventricle is enlarged and the aortic knuckle is small.

The *E.C.G.* shows some evidence of right ventricular enlargement with characteristically an RSR pattern (right bundle branch block) in lead V1.

If pulmonary hypertension develops there may be reversal of the shunt through the defect leading to venous blood entering the left side of the heart and producing cyanosis.

Prognosis and Treatment. Most patients with atrial septal defect eventually develop cardiac failure, which should be treated along the usual lines. Surgical repair of the defect should be undertaken if possible.

VENTRICULAR SEPTAL DEFECT

The volume of the shunt between the left and right ventricles depends on the size of the defect and the pulmonary artery pressure and may vary considerably. It may be an isolated defect or may be complicated by other defects (see Fallot's tetralogy).

Clinical Features. *Small Defect* (*Maladie de Roger*). A small defect gives rise to no symptoms unless infective endocarditis supervenes. It is suggested by finding a *pan-systolic murmur and thrill* in the third or fourth left intercostal space.

The prognosis is good and the patient should live his normal span.

Large Defect. If the left to right shunt is large so that the pulmonary blood flow may be three or four times the systemic flow there is overloading of the pulmonary circulation and the output of the left ventricle is increased. Heart failure may present in middle age, or more commonly pulmonary hypertension may develop with reversal of the shunt and consequent central cyanosis. The heart is enlarged, with a forcible left ventricular type of apex beat. Marked pulsation over the pulmonary artery in the second and third interspaces will be palpable. A pan-systolic murmur and thrill in the third and fourth interspaces will be found, together with a functional mitral diastolic murmur due to the high flow rate through the mitral valve.

An E.C.G. may show evidence of some left ventricular hypertrophy and if pulmonary hypertension is present some right ventricular hypertrophy as well.

A *radiograph of the chest* may show dilated pulmonary arteries, which will be seen to pulsate on screening.

Prognosis and Treatment. Provided the disease is not causing symptoms and the pulmonary artery pressure is not rising, patients should be observed and spontaneous closure of the defect may occur. Otherwise surgical treatment will be necessary.

CYANOTIC GROUP

FALLOT'S TETRALOGY

Fallot's tetralogy is the commonest cause of cyanotic congenital heart disease. The tetralogy consists of pulmonary stenosis (valvar or subvalvar), ventricular septal defect, over-riding of the aorta so that it lies over both ventricles, and right ventricular hypertrophy. As a result of the obstruction of outflow from the right ventricle due to the pulmonary stenosis venous blood passes into the aorta. The size of the shunt will depend on the severity of the pulmonary stenosis and the pressure in the aorta.

Clinical Features. *Central cyanosis*, with polycythaemia and clubbing of the fingers, is usually present from birth or soon after. In severe cases the patient is under-sized. *Dyspnoea* is a prominent symptom. The patient often adopts a characteristic *squatting position* which decreases the right to left shunt by increasing the peripheral resistance and thus the pressure in the aorta.

The heart usually shows minimal right ventricular enlargement and the apex is tapping in quality. There is a *systolic murmur*, often accompanied by a thrill, in the second or third left intercostal space. The pulmonary second sound is single.

An *E.C.G.* shows marked right ventricular hypertrophy.

On *radiography of the heart* the cardiac apex is often elevated with a deep pulmonary bay, giving rise to the classical 'cœur en sabot'. The *lung vascular markings are much reduced*.

Prognosis and Treatment. Patients with Fallot's tetralogy rarely reach adult life. Operative treatment is now available, either the Blalock operation which aims at increasing the pulmonary blood flow by an anastomosis between a systemic artery and the pulmonary artery, or preferably by the Brock operation which directly relieves the pulmonary stenosis. More recently total correction of the deformity has been undertaken with relief of the stenosis and repair of the septal defect. This will probably become the treatment of choice ultimately.

There are a number of other causes of cyanotic congenital heart disease but they are rare and will not be discussed.

EISENMENGER'S SYNDROME

This group of disorders consists essentially of a right to left shunt coupled with pulmonary hypertension. The shunt is usually via a VSD, ASD or patent ductus, though more complicated congenital lesions may be involved. Whether the pulmonary hypertension is present at birth or is the result of the large pulmonary blood flow is not known.

Clinical Features. The age of onset of symptoms depends on the underlying lesion. With an ASD it is usually in middle age but with other lesions they may develop considerably earlier in life or even in infancy.

The patient is cyanosed with clubbing and complains of dyspnoea. The signs are those of pulmonary hypertension (page 182) with a systolic murmur from the shunt.

Treatment. There is no specific treatment and closure of the shunt is contra-indicated. Heart failure is treated in the usual way when it arises. Death usually occurs by middle age.

CONGENITAL HEART DISEASE AND INFECTIVE ENDOCARDITIS

Practically all forms of congenital heart disease are prone to develop infective endocarditis, but it is very rare in atrial septal defect. When, therefore, there is any risk of a transient septicaemia such as may occur with dental manipulation, extraction, or tonsillectomy, these patients should be given benzyl penicillin 1·0 mega unit just before operation followed by phenoxymethylpenicillin 250 mg. four times daily for five days.

ISCHAEMIC HEART DISEASE

The following conditions may cause cardiac ischaemic pain:

(1) Coronary artery disease.
(2) Aortic valve disease.
(3) Syphilitic aortitis.
(4) Severe anaemia.
(5) Paroxysmal tachycardia (occasionally).

CORONARY ARTERY DISEASE

One of the most striking changes in the twentieth century in the pattern of disease which affects the Western world has been the emergence of coronary artery disease as one of the most common causes of death, particularly amongst middle-aged men. The reason for this increase is not clear, but several factors may be involved, including a high intake of animal fat, lack of exercise, and excessive smoking.

Coronary artery disease starts with narrowing of the arteries by plaques of atheroma which contain cholesterol. Obstruction of the blood flow eventually becomes so severe that when exercise increases the oxygen consumption of heart muscle, not enough blood can pass through to supply it. The muscle, therefore, becomes ischaemic and produces the characteristic pain of angina of effort.

The next stage of the disease is the development of a thrombus on the plaque of atheroma, which cuts off the blood supply to an area of heart muscle and produces a cardiac infarct. This may be fatal, but often healing occurs with fibrosis and scar formation. If collateral circulation is good, however, the muscle will survive. It can be seen therefore that thrombosis is not necessarily followed by infarction, although the terms coronary thrombosis and myocardial infarction are often used synonymously.

It must be realised that some atheroma of the coronary arteries is present in all men and most women over the age of thirty and that the coronary circulation has great powers of opening collateral channels and thus circumventing narrowed arteries. Whether or not symptoms develop depends on the rate of progress of the atheromatous process and the ability of the coronary circulation to open up adequate collateral circulation.

The Background to Coronary Disease. It seems probable that clinical coronary disease is the result of a number of factors and processes. Many of these factors are now known, although the whole picture is not complete. A knowledge of these factors may be important in that some of them can be avoided, and therefore it may be possible to diminish the risk of developing coronary disease.

The most important factors so far discovered are:

(1) *Hyperlipidaemia.* Increase in blood lipids, both cholesterol and triglycerides, is associated with an increased incidence of coronary disease. The mechanism is probably a complicated one including both effects on the arterial walls and on coagulation. Hyperlipidaemia is essentially a disorder of lipoprotein metabolism but is considerably influenced by several factors in the diet. It is considered in detail on page 457. Communities living on a diet which includes a high intake of animal fat usually have a higher level of blood lipids than those whose fat intake is low. However in a community such as the United Kingdom with a high fat intake, and with a high incidence of coronary disease, the actual variations of fat intake do not seem so important. A high intake of sucrose has also been implicated, the excess carbohydrate being converted to triglyceride by the liver. Finally, a relative deficiency of unsaturated fatty acids (found in vegetable and fish oils) may also be a factor. How far these findings are applicable to the management of coronary disease is not clear. There is as yet no good evidence that lowering the serum cholesterol either by dietary means or by clofibrate improves the prognosis of patients with clinical evidence of coronary artery disease, except possibly when those with angina are treated with clofibrate. There is some suggestion that lowering the cholesterol levels in normal subjects may decrease the risk of developing coronary disease but the evidence is still incomplete. More recently the relative amounts of high density and low density lipoproteins have been considered important. A relative increase in high density proteins appears to protect against atheroma.

(2) *Hypertension.* A raised blood pressure carries with it an increased risk of coronary disease. The problems of treating hypertension are considered on page 131.

(3) *Cigarette Smoking.* There is a correlation between smoking and coronary disease, particularly in the younger age groups. The risk decreases if smoking is stopped.

(4) *Exercise and Obesity.* There is an increased incidence of coronary disease in the under-exercised and overweight.

Epidemiological studies suggest therefore that moderation in diet, avoiding excessive amounts of animal fat and sugar, regular exercise, weight control, and no cigarette smoking, plus lowering of a raised blood pressure if possible, should reduce the incidence of coronary disease, although proof of this is still incomplete. It would seem reasonable that they should also be applied to those who have had a coronary thrombosis.

ANGINA OF EFFORT (Angina Pectoris)

Clinical Features. The patient with angina of effort usually has few complaints apart from his pain. This is described as constricting, or as a heavy feeling, a pressing feeling, an ache or tightness. It is usually substernal and may radiate down the inside of the left arm or both arms or up into the neck or jaw. It may be felt only in the back. *It is brought on by effort and relieved within a few minutes by rest.* It is more easily provoked in cold weather, after a heavy meal, or with emotional upsets.

Anginal pain may be associated with some dyspnoea. This is believed

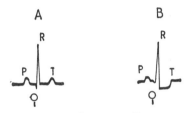

E.C.G. IN ANGINA OF EFFORT.
A: Normal at rest; B: Ischaemic changes on exercise.

to be due to temporary deterioration in left ventricular function with a rise in end-diastolic filling pressure.

The onset of the attacks of pain may be gradual or it may appear quite suddenly one day. A sudden onset of severe angina of effort should always raise the suspicion that the complaint has gone beyond a narrowing of the coronary arteries and that an actual coronary thrombosis with infarction has occurred. The course of the disease is variable. The symptoms may become progressively more severe, they may remain stationary or rarely they may improve. At any time a coronary thrombosis may supervene and this may be fatal.

Examination of the patient with angina of effort rarely shows any sign diagnostic of the disease. There may be evidence of associated hypertension but this does not help in the diagnosis, which depends entirely on an accurate history.

The *electrocardiogram* may be very useful in confirming the diagnosis. The following may be found:

(1) Some 50 per cent of patients with angina have a normal E.C.G. at rest. After exercise or pacing at a high rate with an elec-

trical pacemaker, the E.C.G. may show S-T depression. However, even a normal effort test does not exclude angina.

(2) The resting E.C.G. may show evidence of ischaemia with S-T depression or T wave inversion.

(3) There may be evidence of actual infarction.

Coronary angiography may be useful in showing the presence of an obstruction in the coronary vessels in cases where the diagnosis of angina is open to doubt. It should be remember however, that quite severe stenosis can exist in the coronery arteries without symptoms and that rarely ischaemic pain can occur without coronary artery disease showing on the angiograph. The other use of coronary angiography is to decide whether patients with ischaemic pain might benefit from a saphenous vein graft. If there is a single severe stenosis in the left main coronary artery and if myocardial function is good there is evidence that the operation improves the prognosis. With more widespread disease the evidence is less clear and further experience is awaited.

Prognosis and Treatment. Depression and anxiety often follow a patient's discovery that he has angina, which is understandable since the probability of sudden death at a relatively early age is common knowledge. Considerable reassurance is therefore required as many of these patients live full and useful lives for ten, fifteen or more years.

The patient's mode of life must be organised to fit both his disease and his temperament. Strenuous exercise must be prohibited, but moderate exercise is not harmful provided it does not produce pain and it may perhaps be beneficial. The patient should if possible continue in his occupation, but overwork or work which keeps him under continued pressure must be avoided. If he is overweight then weight must be reduced. Smoking undoubtedly reduces coronary blood flow and all patients with angina should be advised to abstain from it. Some patients improve remarkably on giving it up.

Nitrites are the most useful drugs for relieving the attacks of pain. *Glyceryl trinitrate* in doses of 0·5 mg. should be sucked or chewed and will relieve angina within two to three minutes. The drug should be used whenever the pain occurs but is more effective if used to prevent attacks of pain when some effort is required. Their most important effect is to lower blood pressure and thus cardiac work, rather than to increase coronary flow.

Long-acting coronary vasodilators can be used particularly in patients who have frequent attacks of angina; pentaerythritol tetranitrate 30 mg. is given three or four times daily.

β blockers are useful in angina for reducing the sympathetic drive to the heart. Propranolol (starting dose 10 mg. t.d.s.) or oxprenolol (starting dose 40 mg. t.d.s.) are satisfactory and the dose should be increased until symptoms are controlled.

There have been many attempts to improve coronary circulation by *surgical measures*. The introduction of coronary angiography has made possible better delineation of the extent of the coronary obstruction. Saphenous vein graft will certainly increase the coronary circulation and should be considered seriously in patients whose symptoms are not controlled by medical treatment, particularly if they are in the younger age group.

INTERMEDIATE CORONARY SYNDROME
(Acute Coronary Insufficiency)

A number of patients present with severe anginal pain, occurring at rest, lasting 20–30 minutes and not relieved by trinitrin. In such patients the E.C.G. may show transient depression of the S-T segment and T wave changes. The enzymes are not raised. In spite of the alarming symptoms, the prognosis is quite good. A small proportion of these patients develop a frank infarct, but in the rest the condition stabilises.

Treatment. These patients usually respond well to bed rest together with a β blocker given orally. When the acute symptoms are controlled the patients should be treated as for angina; some will require coronary angiography and possibly venous graft. Anticoagulants are not usually indicated.

PRINZMETAL'S ANGINA VARIANT

This type of anginal pain differs from the usual variety. It is commoner in women and may start at a relatively early age. The pain although similar in nature and distribution to classical angina is not related to effort, and is associated with elevation of the S-T segment on the electrocardiogram rather than S-T depression. In many patients particularly those in the younger age group, coronary angiography shows no evidence of obstruction. It has been suggested that the pain is due to ischaemia following a transient spasm of the coronary artery.

MYOCARDIAL INFARCTION

In subjects with coronary atheroma, there is always the danger that a clot may form on the atheromatous plaque, thus suddenly cutting off the blood supply to an area of heart muscle; in other words, a coronary thrombosis may occur leading to myocardial infarction.

When a large coronary artery is obstructed by thrombosis the patient may suddenly fall down dead; indeed this is the only cause of really sudden death. More often, however, the patient survives, and over the next few weeks the dead heart muscle is absorbed and replaced by a fibrous scar. This scar may be firm and strong, but occasionally, particularly if the infarct has been a large one, the scar may become stretched and produce an aneurysm of the heart wall. The functional ability of the heart may be near normal after recovery from an infarct; but sometimes after a large infarct, the loss of infarcted muscle so encroaches on the reserve power of the heart that congestive failure occurs, or the patient may be left with crippling angina of effort.

Clinical Features. A coronary thrombosis may occur at any time of the day or night, at rest or on exercise. The onset is usually sudden with severe substernal pain, of the same type and distribution as angina pectoris. It can be distinguished from angina by the fact that it often comes on when the patient is at rest, and, unlike angina, which is relieved by a few minutes' rest, it persists for several hours. Some patients will have noted that for a few days before the acute attack they have had mild and short-lived attacks of substernal pain, the so-called 'warning pains', while in other patients the only complaint may be the rather sudden onset of severe angina.

Rarely, other symptoms may overshadow the chest pain, for example sudden onset of left ventricular failure, abrupt loss of consciousness due to transient cardiac arrest or arrhythmia, or severe vomiting. These may all be presenting symptoms and only careful questioning will elicit a history of substernal pain. Generally speaking, however, the history is typical and the diagnosis obvious.

Examination in typical cases shows the patient to be anxious, pale, sweating, and with a rapid pulse and low blood pressure. In milder cases these signs may be missing and it is worth remembering that the blood pressure may not fall markedly for some hours after the acute attack. Cardiac arrhythmias of any type may occur with a coronary thrombosis, one of the most common being ventricular extrasystoles; these may herald the onset of a dangerous ventricular tachycardia or even ventricular fibrillation. Auscultation of the heart shows a triple rhythm in about half the cases. Sometimes it may be possible to hear transient apical systolic murmurs due to functional mitral regurgitation. If the heart is examined daily after the acute attack it is often possible to hear a pericardial friction rub on about the third or fourth day. Pericarditis should also be remembered as a cause of persistent chest pain after a cardiac infarct.

During the first week there is often a rise in temperature, a polymorphonuclear leucocytosis, and a rise in the sedimentation rate, all indications of the inflammatory reaction around the damaged myocardium.

The serum levels of glutamic oxaloacetic transaminase (aspartate aminotransferase S.G.O.T.) and creatine kinase (C.K.) are raised in most patients after an infarct. The enzymes are released by breaking-down heart muscle and the serum levels are elevated from the first to the fourth day after infarction. The upper limits of normal are:

S.G.O.T.	35 Karmen units/ml.
Creatine kinase	100 units/litre for men
	60 units/litre for women.

Serum levels of enzymes are raised in damage of other organs such as the liver, pancreas and skeletal muscle. The creatine kinase concentration is so sensitive to tissue damage that even an intramuscular injection can produce some elevation. A method is available to detect the appropriate isoenzyme of creatine kinase.

The E.C.G. should be used to confirm the diagnosis and define the position and extent of the infarct. The following changes may be found:

(1) *The Classical Picture of a Cardiac Infarct*

    (a) *Anterior infarction* produces a large Q wave and raised S-T segment in lead I and in the anterior chest leads with S-T depression in lead II. This changes during the next few weeks to a Q wave with marked T wave inversion in lead I and the anterior chest leads and the return of the S-T shift to the iso-electric level.

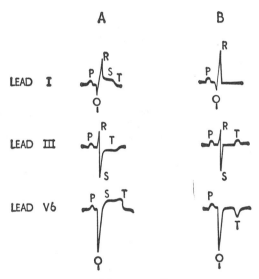

ANTERIOR MYOCARDIAL INFARCTION.
A: Immediate; B: After some weeks.

    (b) *Inferior infarction* with a large Q wave and raised S-T segment in leads II and III and aVF with S-T depression in lead I. This also changes in the next few weeks to Q wave with marked T-wave inversion, in leads II and III and aVF and return of the S-T shift to the iso-electric level.

    (c) *True posterior infarction* does not show pathological Q waves but may be identified by tall R waves combined with tall and symmetrical T waves in leads V1 and V2.

INFERIOR MYOCARDIAL INFARCTION.
A: Immediate; B: After some weeks.

(2) *Lesser Changes*

Symmetrical inversion of T waves without large Q waves or S-T segment shift.

A number of other minor changes in the electrocardiogram have been described which alone do not necessarily indicate myocardial infarction, but taken in conjunction with such a history as outlined above, are good enough evidence of an infarct.

It must be remembered that a full 12-lead electrocardiogram must be taken and must be repeated at frequent intervals as the changes after a small infarct may be confined to one lead and may be quite transitory.

Immediate Complications of Cardiac Infarction

(1) *Cardiac Failure.* It is quite common to find a mild and transient rise in venous pressure or some pulmonary congestion in the days following an infarct. It usually resolves rapidly but after a very large infarct the patient may be left in chronic failure. Rupture of a papillary muscle can lead to mitral regurgitation with failure.

(2) *Cardiac Arrythmias.* Some 80 per cent of patients develop some type of arrythmia after cardiac infarction. These may be transient and last no more than a few seconds, or may be prolonged and may seriously decrease cardiac output. The arrythmia may be of any type. They tend to disappear as the infarct heals, although atrial fibrillation and varying degrees of heart block may persist indefinitely.

(3) *Thrombo-embolic Phenomena.* Patients lying immobile after a coronary thrombosis are very liable to deep vein thrombosis in the calf veins with the attendant risk of pulmonary embolism. A thrombus may form on the endocardium over the infarcted area. A piece of clot may break off

and obstruct arteries in the systemic circulation, particularly those of the brain.

(4) *Hypotension.* Hypotension may complicate cardiac infarction; it may be due to a fall in cardiac output subsequent to extensive myocardial damage or sometimes to a prolonged arrythmia which interferes with cardiac function. The clinical picture is one of acute circulatory failure (see page 107) with peripheral vaso-constriction, cold extremities and mental clouding. If this state is prolonged oliguria will develop. Sometimes, however, the cardiac output may in fact be higher than normal, but the peripheral resistance is lowered by vasodilation. These patients usually have extremities of normal colour and temperature.

It is not uncommon for patients to develop vasovagal attacks with bradycardia, sweating, hypotension and nausea, and in some but not all such patients these symptoms appear to be precipitated by the administration of morphia.

(5) *Rupture of the Heart.* Sudden exertion in the week immediately after an infarct may cause a fatal rupture of the heart. This risk can be diminished by strict bed rest.

Treatment. In the early stages bed rest is important but need not be continued for more than four days for those with small infarcts, and up to ten days is usually sufficient for those with more extensive infarction. Thereafter the patient should make a gradual return to activity.

Severe pain is often a prominent feature immediately after the infarct and *morphine* 15–20 mg., according to the size of the patient, will be required to relieve the pain and mental anguish and may have to be repeated several times in the first twenty-four hours. Morphine may produce vomiting and hypotension, though this can sometimes be helped by combining it with prochlorperazine 12·5 mg. *Pentazocine* 30 mg. by injection is also used but can cause a rise in pulmonary artery pressure and thus further embarrass the circulation.

All unnecessary effort must be avoided, particularly in the first few days. If the patient is worried by constipation a small enema may be given after 48 hours and repeated every two or three days. If the patient is not too severely ill, a commode may be less exhausting than a bed-pan. To prevent thrombosis in the deep veins of the lower limbs, passive exercises should be given from the start. The diet should be light and easily digestible.

The value of *anticoagulants* after cardiac infarction has never been wholly accepted, and they are now used much less than they were. It is however common practice to give 5,000 units of heparin subcutaneously twelve hourly for the first few days after infarction to prevent venous thrombosis but with early mobilisation more prolonged treatment is not required. If full doses of heparin are only used for a few days dosage control is not necessary but if given for longer periods the Kaolin-Cephalin time (KCT) should be measured four hours after the injection of heparin and the dose modified accordingly.

Many patients are anxious and worried in the weeks following a cardiac infarct and sedation with diazepam 5·0 mg. three times daily may be useful. If cardiac failure, with or without atrial fibrillation, develops it should be treated in the usual way with digitalis and diuretics. Digitalis may somewhat increase the risk of ventricular arrhythmia developing and must, therefore, be used with caution.

Home Treatment or Hospitalisation. Opinions differ as to where patients should be nursed after a cardiac infarction. When there is no evidence of shock or cardiac arrythmias and the attack is not severe it is reasonable to treat the patient at home, providing the circumstances and facilities are suitable. It is still possible that such patients will develop a fatal ventricular fibrillation in the hours immediately after infarction but there is no clear evidence that any drug or other form of treatment, given when the doctor first sees the patient, will reduce the likelihood of this complication. Patients with serious infarcts or with arrythmias should be sent to hospital as quickly as possible so that they may be monitored for dangerous arrythmias and have the benefit of intensive care.

Monitoring, the Treatment of Arrhythmias and Hypotension. It is now realised that arrhythmias are a frequent cause of circulatory failure and death after cardiac infarction. If the patient is continuously monitored by E.C.G. in the two or three days after infarction, these arrhythmias can be diagnosed immediately and with appropriate treatment the mortality rate can be halved.

(a) *Prevention of Arrhythmias.* The use of various drug regimes to prevent the development of arrhythmias after infarction has not proved useful and at present it is best to treat arrhythmias as they arise.

(b) *Treatment of Developed Arrythmias*

> (1) Ventricular Ectopics. These are very common; if they are frequent or multifocal they should be treated with lignocaine 50–100 mg. intravenously, followed if necessary by infusion (see page 120). Oral phenytoin 100 mg. t.d.s. is also useful.
>
> (2) Ventricular Tachycardia. This should be treated by lignocaine as above. If this fails, D.C. conversion should be used (see p. 123).
>
> (3) Ventricular Fibrillation. Electrical defibrillation (see p. 125).
>
> (4) Atrial Tachycardia. Practolol 5·0 mg. intravenously is effective.
>
> (5) Atrial Fibrillation. The patient should be digitalised. The addition of a β blocker orally may be useful. D.C. shock may be required in resistant cases.
>
> (6) Heart block complicating an anterior infarct carries a poor prognosis and pacing will usually be required. In an inferior infarct heart block carries a better prognosis and pacing will only be needed if the rhythm is unstable.
>
> (7) Sinus Bradycardia. Atropine 0·6 mg. intravenously should be given.

(c) *Hypotension.* This may be due to vagal overactivity perhaps exacerbated by morphine, or to low cardiac output with circulatory failure. Vagal overactivity will respond to atropine (see above). In circulatory failure the foot of the bed should be raised provided this does not precipitate pulmonary oedema. Most of these patients have a low arterial oxygen saturation due to disorganisation of ventilation and perfusion in the lungs and should be given oxygen 2 litres/minute by M.C. mask (approx. 40–60 per cent). Vasoconstrictor drugs are rarely used for they raise the blood pressure at the expense of peripheral organ perfusion. Dopamine by continuous intravenous infusion in doses of 2–5 μg/kg./minute and increased as required is sometimes useful. Prolonged hypotension carries a bad prognosis.

Subsequent Management

When the period of rest has finished the patient is gradually allowed up, but should not return to work for at least three months after the acute attack. If possible the patient should return to his normal employment. If, however, his job is exceptionally heavy or if he is severely crippled by cardiac failure or angina of effort, then some change will be necessary. Overweight patients should be dieted until they reach normal levels. Heavy meals, especially those containing large quantities of fat, must be avoided. There is some evidence that long term treatment with a β blocker improves prognosis after an infarct particularly in the hypertensive subject.

In younger patients (under 55 years) there is a case for carrying out coronary angiography six weeks after the infarct, provided the myocardium is not compromised, the object being to discover any major stenosis (see page 166). Whether this will become routine practice remains to be seen.

Some patients will require considerable encouragement and support in the months following an infarct. They may become depressed, anxious, and irritable, and it is the doctor's job to show them that it is possible to lead a normal and useful life, even if they have had a heart attack.

In patients who are having recurrent infarcts the possibility of long-term anticoagulants should be considered.

Long-Term Complication of Cardiac Infarction

(1) *Post-infarction Aneurysm of the Ventricle.* This is an area of fibrous tissue in the ventricular wall which follows a transmural infarct, usually due to occlusion of the anterior descending branch of the left coronary artery.

Symptoms and Signs. The common symptoms are persistent left ventricular failure associated with dyspnoea and sometimes angina.

On examination it may be possible to feel the systolic thrust of the aneurysm and there may be a triple rhythm. The E.C.G. will show monophasic Q waves over the aneurysm and the S-T segment may remain elevated. X-ray of the heart usually shows cardiac enlargement and sometimes a bulge. The diagnosis is confirmed by left ventricular angiography with coronary arteriography and possibly by isotope scanning.

Treatment. In patients with marked symptoms relief can be obtained for the majority by surgery consisting of resection of the aneurysm and by-pass vein grafting of the coronary artery if possible.

(2) *Dressler's Syndrome.* In the month following an infarct a few patients develop pleural or pericardial pain and a friction rub may be heard. Similar symptoms may follow cardiotomy. The condition reponds to steroids or to aspirin.

Prognosis

Death from an acute attack usually occurs within the first 48 hours and the overall mortality is about 25 per cent. The prognosis is worse in old people and those with extensive infarct. Thereafter the mortality is around 7 per cent per year.

ENDOCARDITIS

ACUTE INFECTIVE ENDOCARDITIS

This usually occurs in the course of septicaemia due to organisms of high virulence. The endocardium is affected and the heart valves may be spared.

SUBACUTE INFECTIVE ENDOCARDITIS

Infective endocarditis is due to infection of the endocardium by organisms of moderate virulence. The most common infecting organism is the streptococcus viridans which is often an inhabitant of the mouth and throat of normal people. However, in recent years there has been an increase in infective endocarditis due to other organisms, particularly the streptococcus faecalis, the micro-aerophilic streptococcus, the staphylococcus and rickettsia.

Infective endocarditis starts on the heart valves, usually the aortic valve. It most commonly occurs on valves damaged by previous rheumatic fever. It may complicate various congenital lesions including ventricular septal defect, pulmonary and aortic stenosis, persistent ductus arteriosus and bicuspid aortic valves and may develop on various types of artificial valves. It is very rare in syphilitic aortitis and atrial septal defect. There is a group of patients, usually over fifty, who appear to develop infective endocarditis on an apparently normal heart. The infecting organism is frequently the streptococcus faecalis.

The starting point of infective endocarditis is often a transient bacteraemia. This may follow dental extraction or filling, when the organism is usually streptococcus viridans; or after operations on the urinary tract or bowel, when infection with streptococcus faecalis is more common. This emphasises the need for penicillin 'cover' if these operations are performed in a patient with damaged heart valves. The bacteria settle on the damaged valve, set up an inflammatory reaction which is followed by deposits of fibrin and the formation of a vegetation which often spreads from the valve to adjacent endocardium.

Clinical Features. The most constant clinical feature is a persistent *low grade fever*, and this diagnosis should be considered in any patient with rheumatic heart disease who develops a pyrexia for which there is no other obvious cause. Increasing *malaise, tiredness,* and *breathlessness* are common symptoms. In some patients sweating and vague point pains may suggest a recurrence of rheumatic fever. After the first week or two *anaemia* develops and the patient begins to lose weight. The fingers become *clubbed* and in patients left untreated generalised pigmentation occurs; this combined with the anaemia causes a characteristic coloration, sometimes described as the '*café au lait*' appearance.

The bacteraemia gives rise to antigen-antibody complexes which cause widespread vascular damage, which show as:

(1) Osler's Nodes. Small, tender, red round areas most commonly seen on the pads of the fingers and lasting 24–48 hours.

(2) Splinter Haemorrhages. Found under the nails.

(3) Purpura. Most commonly found on the chest and neck.

(4) Renal Damage. An increased number of red cells in the urine is a common feature. In addition, there may be widespread glomerular lesions which in time may progress to renal failure.

(5) Involvement of cerebral vessels which may give rise to neurological signs or even a confusional state.

In addition, emboli may break off from the vegetations on the diseased valves, and 30 per cent of patients will have major infarcts in the brain, liver, spleen, intestines, or limbs. Retinal involvement produces typical 'boat-shaped' haemorrhages.

The *spleen* is usually moderately enlarged, from the chronic septicaemia which is a feature of the condition. Infarction may lead to an acute attack of pain in the splenic area.

The *heart* shows signs of the underlying valve lesion, and rarely changes in the character of the murmurs can be detected. Heat failure may develop.

When infective endocarditis occurs in congenital heart disease with a left to right shunt such as a patent ductus arteriosus, the emboli are swept into the pulmonary circulation and lead to infarcts of the lung. This produces rather a different clinical picture, with recurrent episodes of fever, pleurisy, and patchy consolidation of the lungs, so that an erroneous diagnosis of recurrent pneumonia may be made.

Special Investigations. Examination of the blood reveals a moderate anaemia with a slight leucocytosis. The sedimentation rate is nearly always raised. The urine in the great majority of cases shows an increased number of red cells, although these may be only detected on microscopy.

The *diagnosis* is confirmed by isolation of the organism on *blood culture.*

At least four samples of blood must be taken for culture before antibiotic treatment is started and incubation should continue for three weeks. If organisms are isolated, their sensitivity to various antibiotics must be determined. It is best if blood for culture is taken at the height of the fever. If the patient is very ill and the diagnosis is suspected on clinical grounds, the blood cultures should be taken at short intervals so that the start of treatment is not delayed. There is rarely need to await the report on the blood cultures before giving antibiotics.

About 30 per cent of patients will have a persistently negative blood culture. In these patients a fungal or rickettsial infection should be considered, but it may be necessary to give a full course of treatment without the diagnosis being confirmed by a positive culture.

Complications. (1) *Rupture of a Valve.* The aortic valve may be weakened and finally rupture during the course of infective endocarditis. When this occurs it may lead to sudden death or to the rapid development of cardiac failure. Examination shows the characteristic, loud, regurgitant murmur (*cooing dove*).

Less commonly, mitral incompetence may develop as a result of a ruptured chorda, and both these complications are an indication for immedate surgery with valve replacement.

(2) *Mycotic Aneurysm.* Mycotic aneurysms may develop due to small emboli in the vessels supplying the walls of the large arteries. They may require surgical treatment.

Treatment. The patient must be in bed and be given full nursing care. The specific treatment will depend on the infecting organism.

(a) *Streptococcus Viridans.* 2·0 mega units of benzylpenicillin intramuscularly four times daily, is usually adequate if the organism is sensitive. If there is no response, or if the organism proves to be partially resistant to penicillin the dose can be increased to 20 mega units of penicillin or more daily. Owing to the bulk of the injection, it is necessary to give it by continuous intravenous drip. Blood levels can also be increased by giving probenecid 0·5 g. four times daily.

(b) *Streptococcus Faecalis.* 2·0 mega units of benzylpenicillin q.i.d., plus 0·75 g. of streptomycin b.d. The dose of antibiotics should be modified according to response and sensitivity tests.

(c) *Staphyloccocus Aureus.* The antibiotic programme will depend on sensitivities. Usually two antibiotics will be required and benzylpenicillin or cloxacillin plus streptomycin or gentamycin are useful combinations.

(d) *Patients with persistently negative blood* cultures should be treated with penicillin and streptomycin in the first instance.

Treatment should aim at abolishing the fever, stopping all embolic phenomena and restoring the E.S.R. and urine to normal. Blood cultures should of course be negative after treatment. The earlier treatment is started in the course of the disease, the better the chance of effecting a cure. Antibiotic therapy must be given for at least 6 weeks.

With these measures it is possible to eradicate infection in the majority of patients with subacute infective endocarditis. In spite of this mortality is still about 30 per cent. This is due to delayed diagnosis leading to extensive damage to the heart valves and chronic heart failure. In addition the production of immune complexes may cause widespread vascular disease particularly affecting the kidney. All patients must be carefully followed up as relapse or reinfection may occur.

PERICARDITIS

The following types of pericarditis may be encountered:

(1) Benign (probably visal).
(2) Rheumatic.
(3) Pyogenic.
(4) Tuberculous.
(5) Malignant.
(6) Subsequent to a cardiac infarct or cardiotomy.
(7) Associated with uraemia.
(8) Systemic lupus erythematosus.

Pericarditis may be dry or may be associated with an effusion.

DRY PERICARDITIS

Clinical Features. Dry pericarditis may occur from any of the above causes. Pain is a frequent, but not a constant, symptom. It may be praecordial or referred to the shoulder or neck region. It may be constant or made worse by movement or by respiration. The patient may also complain of symptoms which are related to the disease underlying the pericarditis.

Examination will usually show a pericardial friction rub; this may be either loud or soft; it usually sounds rough and rather superficial. It may be heard anywhere over the praecordium and may be either systolic and/or diastolic in timing.

E.C.G. Changes. In the early stages the electrocardiogram shows elevation of the S-T segment, the elevated segment being concave upwards. This is followed by the return of the S-T segment to the iso-electric line and flattening or inversion of the T waves. These changes, unlike those of cardiac infarction, can be recorded from both the anterior and posterior aspects of the heart at the same time.

PERICARDIAL EFFUSION

The symptoms and signs of a pericardial effusion depend on the underlying cause and on the size of the effusion. Small effusions may be indistinguishable from a dry pericarditis. When the size of the effusion increases rapidly the pressure within the pericardial sac rises, interfering with the venous return to the heart, a state known as *cardiac tamponade*. This in turn reduces the cardiac output and thus seriously interferes with cardiac function.

Clinical Features. The patient often appears restless and ill and complains of praecordial discomfort and dyspnoea. If the effusion is large, examination will reveal *pulsus paradoxus* (p. 96). The venous pressure will be raised, and the apex beat may be felt within the outer limit of cardiac dullness to percussion, which is increased. A pericardial friction rub can often be heard on auscultation, in spite of the presence of an effusion.

A radiograph of the heart shows a pear-shaped cardiac shadow with sharper margins than usual; this is because they have moved less during exposure of the film. *Echocardiography* is very useful for showing even small effusions.

Treatment. Effusions large enough to endanger life are rare. A high venous pressure and low arterial pressure are indications for tapping the effusion. It must be remembered that the high venous pressure found with pericardial effusions is necessary to maintain diastolic filling of the heart and attempts should not be made to lower venous pressure by venesection or by diuretics. Otherwise the treatment is that of the underlying condition.

Varieties of Pericarditis

Benign Pericarditis. Benign pericarditis can probably be caused by several viruses including coxsackie, mumps and influenza. It is most common in young adults and there is often a history of a recent upper respiratory tract infection. The onset is sudden with fever, malaise, and pericardial pain. Small effusions sometimes develop. Recovery is the rule within a few weeks, but a number of cases relapse.

Treatment is symptomatic.

Rheumatic Pericarditis. Pericarditis develops during the course of acute rheumatic fever in about 10 per cent of patients and provides definite evidence of cardiac involvement. It may or may not be associated with an effusion. Treatment is as for rheumatic fever.

Pyogenic Pericarditis. Pericarditis may occur as a complication of pneumonia or may complicate a septicaemia. It should be vigorously treated with antibiotics. Surgical drainage is rarely required.

Tuberculous Pericarditis. Tuberculous pericarditis is not common. It usually presents as a subacute pericarditis with effusion and some general malaise with evening fever. The effusion is a clear yellow fluid, occasionally bloodstained, and may be found on culture to contain tubercle bacilli.

Treatment consists of prolonged rest, with rifampicin, isoniazid, and ethambutol (see page 241).

If the effusion is large, aspiration may be required and streptomycin 0·5 g. should then be injected into the pericardial sac.

A number of patients subsequently develop constrictive pericarditis (see below).

Cardiac Infarction. A pericardial friction rub can often be heard transiently over the infarcted area within a few days of a coronary thrombosis.

Post Cardiotomy and Post Infarction (Dressler's Syndrome). Pericarditis may develop in the months after the occurrence. It responds to steroids.

Uraemia. A pericardial rub may be heard in the terminal stages of uraemia.

Malignant Pericarditis. Involvement of the pericardium by new growth may give rise to an effusion which may require tapping. This is a common terminal complication of bronchial neoplasms.

CHRONIC CONSTRICTIVE PERICARDITIS

Chronic constrictive pericarditis is due to previous tuberculous pericarditis or may follow viral or bacterial infection. The heart is encased in a shell of fibrous tissue which may be calcified, and as a result the heart is unable to expand in diastole and venous filling is greatly impeded.

Clinical Features. The patient is usually in adult life and complains of some dyspnoea on effort associated perhaps with oedema of the ankles and swelling of the abdomen. Orthopnoea is not a feature and the degree of dyspnoea is often slight in comparison with the evidence of gross venous congestion.

Examination sometimes may show a pulsus paradoxus and there often is atrial fibrillation. The venous pressure is high, but falls sharply during diastole (the y descent) when the tricuspid valves open. The heart is not usually much enlarged and auscultation may reveal a third heart sound or may be normal. Enlargement of the liver, ascites, and oedema of the ankles are often present. Long-standing disease may have caused chronic hepatic congestion sufficient to end in cirrhosis of the liver.

A radiograph of the heart usually shows a normally sized or slightly enlarged heart and calcification may be seen in the pericardium in about half the cases, provided lateral as well as postero-anterior radiographs are taken.

An *electrocardiogram* usually shows decreased voltage in the QRS complexes with widespread flattening or inversion of T waves.

Treatment. Treatment consists of surgical removal of the constricting pericardium. The operation is a major undertaking, but the results are usually satisfactory.

ADHERENT PERICARDIUM

Occasionally following rheumatic pericarditis the heart may become attached to surrounding structures. This may be diagnosed clinically by systolic retraction of the lower left ribs posteriorly (Broadbent's sign), fixation of the apex beat and systolic retraction of intercostal spaces. There is no evidence that an adherent pericardium has any effect on cardiac function and if heart failure supervenes in these cases it is due to the associated valve disease.

PULMONARY HEART DISEASE
PULMONARY EMBOLISM

A pulmonary embolus arises most commonly from deep-vein thrombosis in the leg or pelvis (p. 186). Rarely it may arise from an intracardiac thrombosis following atrial fibrillation or cardiac infarction. Phlebothrombosis in the legs occurs particularly in obese middle-aged or elderly patients who have been confined to bed, usually with heart disease, but also with other medical conditions, pregnancy, or after major surgical operations. Occasionally it occurs in apparently healthy people, particularly women taking an oral contraceptive.

Clinical Features. A large pulmonary embolism causes dilatation of the right ventricle with a drop in right ventricular output, and a rise in systemic venous pressure. This results in a fall in cardiac output which is accompanied by peripheral vasoconstriction. A massive embolism may cause sudden death but more commonly the patient complains of the abrupt onset of substernal tightness, or pain, dyspnoea and a sudden call to stool. He is sweating, pale and slightly cyanosed. The pulse is small and rapid, the blood pressure low, the cervical venous pressure is raised and frequently there is a gallop rhythm. X-ray of the chest may show a segment with diminished vascular marking and the diagnosis can be confirmed by pulmonary arteriography or lung scan.

The E.C.G. is variable. It may show a deep S wave in lead 1 with a Q or inverted T wave in lead III. The chest leads may show T wave inversion in lead V1–V3, or more rarely there may be a right bundle branch block pattern. The changes are usually transitory.

Smaller pulmonary emboli cause pulmonary infarction, the symptoms of which are often so slight that it is the most commonly overlooked serious respiratory lesion. When the infarct extends to the surface of the lung there may be acute pleuritic pain, and about 40 per cent of patients have a haemoptysis; but frequently the only clinical features are sudden shortness of breath or unexplained rise of temperature and/or pulse rate.

With a small embolus, X-ray may show a segmental shadow due to the infarct. If facilities are available a *perfusion lung scan* is often helpful in patients whose diagnosis is not clear.

It should also be remembered that repeated small pulmonary emboli may seriously obstruct the pulmonary vascular bed and lead to pulmonary hypertension and right ventricular failure.

Treatment. A patient who has had a pulmonary embolus should be nursed fairly flat in bed because the cardiac output and blood pressure may be low. In severe cases oxygen should be given by mask or by a tent. If the patient is in pain or distress a small dose of morphine 10 mg. can be given but there is a danger of respiratory depression. If morphine is used or if there is evidence of respiratory depression nikethamide 500 mg. intravenously can be given and repeated as required. Digitalis is not very helpful in the acute stage but if chronic heart failure ensues the patient should be digitalised and diuretics used (p. 113). *Anticoagulants* should be started with heparin 10,000 units six hourly intravenously. When heparin is given in this way for only forty-eight hours, control of dosage is not required. If however treatment is continued for longer periods the *kaolin-cephalin time* should be estimated before each dose to ensure that a progressive build-up of heparin is not occurring. Heparin may also be given by continuous infusion and this requires daily estimation of kaolin-cephalin time to determine and modify the dose. The anticoagulant effect of heparin is almost immediate.

At the same time treatment should be started with an oral anticoagulant. This group of drugs acts by suppressing the formation in the liver of pro-thrombin and factor VII, which are necessary for the coagulation of blood. Among those commonly used are:

Drug	Maximum Effect	Duration of Effect	Initial (1st day)	Dose Maintenance (daily)
Phenindione	24–36 hrs	48 hrs	200 mg.	12·5–50 mg.
Warfarin	24–36 hrs	48 hrs	30–60 mg.	5–10 mg.
Dicoumarol	36–48 hrs	72 hrs or more	300 mg.	25–100 mg.

The dosage of these drugs is controlled by estimation of the patient's prothrombin time which is kept between two and three times the normal.

The most important side-effect of these drugs is bleeding from over-dosage, a common site being the urinary tract. If this occurs the drug must be stopped. The coagulability of the blood can be restored by giving vita-min K_1 (mephyton) intravenously, it is important to use the smallest effective dose or there may be an abrupt fall in prothrombin time with further clotting. The dose usually lies between 10–50 mg.

Anticoagulants should rarely be used in the very elderly and in those in whom there is a risk of haemorrhage, e.g. from a duodenal ulcer.

The following drugs should not be combined with oral anticoagulants.

(1) Aspirin—risk of gastric bleeding.
(2) Liquid paraffin—enhances effect by blocking vitamin K absorption.
(3) Phenylbutazone, Clofibrate—enhance effect by decreasing plasma protein-binding.
(4) Barbiturates—enhance breakdown of anticoagulant in the liver.

The clot can be lysed by using *streptokinase*. However its control is more difficult, although a short course at the beginning of treatment may become widely used.

Anticoagulants are usually continued for at least six weeks, and many authorities consider they should be continued up to six months or longer, particularly if there is any evidence of recurrent embolism.

Rarely in patients with massive pulmonary embolism and where facilities are available *embolectomy* may be performed within a few hours of the acute episode.

PULMONARY HYPERTENSION

Physiology

In health the pulmonary circulation is a low pressure system (range = 15/5–30/15 mm.Hg.). It seems probable that at rest in the upright position the main blood flow is through the lower parts of the lungs. With increased flow as occurs on exercise, vasodilatation occurs and more blood passes through the upper zones. The pulmonary artery pressure rises only with flow rates above 15 litres per minute.

In man there is evidence that active vasoconstriction of the pulmonary arteries can occur, although its mode of production is unknown.

This may be in response to:

(1) Increased pulmonary blood flow.
(2) A rise in left atrial pressure.
(3) Hypoxia and perhaps hypercarbia.

Clinical Types of Pulmonary Hypertension

(1) Idiopathic (Primary) Pulmonary Hypertension

Idiopathic pulmonary hypertension is due to structural narrowing of the pulmonary arteries of obscure cause; it is probably often due to multiple small pulmonary emboli (see below).

(2) Secondary Pulmonary Hypertension

(a) Pulmonary hypertension may be due to progressive obliteration of the pulmonary arteries by repeated thrombosis or embolism. This often follows a phlebo-thrombosis in the puerperium. Early symptoms are dyspnoea on effort, cough and sometimes haemoptysis. Early diagnosis is important as at this stage the process may be reversible by anticoagulants.

(b) It may be secondary to increased blood flow through the lungs such as occurs in *atrial* or *ventricular septal defects* or with a *persistent ductus arteriosus*. In these conditions the pulmonary artery can usually accommodate the increased flow without a rise in pulmonary artery pressure. Sometimes, however, active constriction of the pulmonary arteries eventually develops and pulmonary artery pressure may even exceed the systemic pressure, with reversal of the shunt and the development of central cyanosis.

(c) In *mitral valve disease* there is usually a small passive rise in pulmonary artery pressure transmitted back from the left atrium. In a small proportion of cases there is in addition active pulmonary vasoconstriction with a considerable rise in pulmonary artery pressure.

(d) Pulmonary hypertension and heart failure may complicate *chronic lung diseases*, commonly chronic bronchitis or emphysema, or rarely pulmonary fibrosis due to silicosis, sarcoidosis or other causes. It is due to obliteration of the pulmonary artery bed by the lung disease; in addition there may be active vasoconstriction due to hypoxia and perhaps hypercapnia. The clinical features and management of *cor pulmonale* are considered on p. 182.

Clinical Features. Dyspnoea is common and other symptoms are cough and syncope. Early signs are evidence of right ventricular hypertrophy, a short systolic murmur and a systolic click over the pulmonary artery and a loud pulmonary element to the second heart sound. Later a giant 'a' wave in the jugular venous pulse, triple rhythm and cardiac failure with functional tricuspid incompetence may develop. The electrocardiogram shows right ventricular hypertrophy and strain.

Treatment. With repeated pulmonary emboli, long-term anticoagulant therapy may reverse the process. In mitral stenosis, relief of the stenosis will frequently release the vasoconstriction.

In those with increased pulmonary flow repair of the shunt with reduction of flow has proved disappointing.

DISEASES OF THE ARTERIES

Diseases of the peripheral vasculature may be subdivided into:

(1) Chronic obliterative arterial disease due to
    (a) Atherosclerosis.
    (b) Buerger's disease.

(2) Acute obstruction to the arterial circulation by embolism or thrombosis.

(3) Venous thrombosis, which may affect either the superficial or deep veins.

(4) Raynaud's syndrome.

(5) Acrocyanosis.

PERIPHERAL VASCULAR DISEASE
ATHEROSCLEROSIS

This occurs most commonly over the age of fifty and may complicate diabetes or hypertension. The areas of narrowing or occlusion are often first found in the femoral artery below the profunda femoris branch. Less commonly they develop in the iliacs or lower aorta. In more advanced cases the areas of narrowing can be found throughout the arterial tree of the leg. The arms are very rarely affected.

Clinical Features. When the femero-popliteal vessels are involved the earliest symptom is *intermittent claudication*, a cramp-like pain usually in the calf or more rarely in the thigh, causing the patient to limp. It may be bilateral or unilateral, but is usually worse on one side. It is brought on by walking and quickly relieved by rest. The degree of disability is variable. With obstruction of the lower end of the aorta (*Leriche's syndrome*) pain may be referred to the thighs and buttocks, there may be muscle wasting, and in men failure of penile erection may occur.

With more advanced disease pain may occur at rest and may be particularly troublesome at night when it may become almost unbearable.

When the circulation to the limbs is severely impaired, areas of gangrene may appear. They often start following trauma, particularly round the nail bed and over the heel. In the most severe cases, gangrene of a whole foot or even of extensive areas of the leg, may occur.

Examination shows absent or reduced pulses in the limbs and in advanced cases coldness of the limbs with failure of the vasodilatation which normally occurs on warming. If the limb is elevated it blanches unduly rapidly, and cyanosis on dependence may be extreme. Both these signs indicate reduced arterial blood supply.

There is an increased incidence of coronary artery disease in those with symptoms from peripheral atherosclerosis. This is a reminder that the disease is always general, not central or peripheral alone.

Prognosis and Treatment. For the majority of patients with intermittent claudication the condition is relatively benign and symptoms may last for years without progression and without the development of gangrene. In some patients symptoms may actually improve due to the opening up of collaterals. For the elderly patient with a mild to moderate disability, treatment should be conservative. Patients should be told to avoid trauma to the feet and the assistance of a chiropodist should be enlisted to help with care of the toe-nails and to deal with callouses, etc. Undue heat or cold should be avoided as far as the feet are concerned, but the body should be kept warm to produce as much reflex vasodilatation as possible. Various vasodilator drugs are used to try and improve the peripheral circulation; tolazoline 25 mg. t.d.s. is popular but there is no evidence that it has a therapeutic effect. Alcohol may be of value in moderate doses.

Tobacco reduces peripheral blood flow and should be avoided by all patients with vascular disease.

Indications for Surgery

Femoro-popliteal Obstruction. Surgery in this group is disappointing; patients under 60, with apparent unilateral disease and severe or progressive symptoms should have an arteriogram and if the disease is proved to be unilateral and limited, and if they are in good general health, operation, usually a by-pass graft is justified.

Aorto-iliac Obstruction. Patients in this group do better with surgery, and it should be offered to those with severe symptoms.

In a few patients, lumbar sympathectomy may be successful, but it is difficult to predict which patients will be helped by this operation. Finally, severe rest pain or gangrene may make amputation necessary.

BUERGER'S DISEASE

Buerger's disease is very rare. It occurs almost exclusively in men and usually starts between the age of twenty-five and forty-five, and is associated with heavy smoking. The lesions begin in the small arteries in the feet and lead to progressive obliteration from the periphery of the arteries of the lower limbs. Involvement of arteries in the arms and elsewhere is very rare.

Clinical Features. The disease usually starts in the foot with recurrent arterial thromboses. In addition, superficial venous thrombophlebitis develops in the legs and sometimes in the arms. The disease is slowly progressive.

Treatment. Treatment consists of care of the extremities, giving vasodilator drugs, and avoiding tobacco. Anticoagulants should be used for acute thrombophlebitis. Sympathectomy may produce prolonged relief of symptoms, particularly in the earlier stages of the disease. Amputation may be necessary in advanced cases.

ACUTE ARTERIAL OCCLUSION

Acute arterial occlusion may be caused by an embolus arising from the left side of the heart, usually in a patient with mitral stenosis or subacute infective endocarditis. Mural thrombi overlying infarcted areas may similarly become detached. Alternatively, thrombosis on an atheromatous plaque may occur *in situ* as a complication of chronic obliterative arterial disease.

Clinical Features. The onset is sudden with severe pain, pallor, coldness, loss of sensation, and weakness in the affected limb. The arterial pulses disappear below the level of the obstruction.

If the obstruction is due to a thrombus in situ the patient should be treated conservatively. Full anticoagulant therapy should be given; the limb should be kept cool to reduce its oxygen requirements to a minimum; the rest of the body must be kept warm; and a careful watch must be maintained for the appearance of gangrene. Amputation may sometimes be required. When obstruction is due to an embolism, embolectomy as soon as possible is the treatment of choice.

RAYNAUD'S SYNDROME

This is produced by spasm of the digital arteries. It may be the result of a variety of causes.

(1) *Idiopathic Raynaud's disease*, believed to represent hypersensitivity of the digital vessels to cold and responsible for about 50 per cent of cases.

(2) *Auto-immune disorders*, especially systemic lupus erythematosis and scleroderma.

(3) *Occupational* in butchers, fishmongers, and people handling vibrating tools.

(4) *Other arterial diseases*, atheroma, Buerger's disease.

(5) *Blood disorders*, polycythaemia vera, haemolytic anaemias.

(6) *Thoracic outlet syndromes*, cervical ribs, prefixed plexus.

(7) *Diseases of the nervous system*, syringomyelia.

(8) *Phaeochromocytoma*.

(9) *Drugs* including β blockers and methysergide.

Clinical Features. The idiopathic form is common in young women. It begins distally and spreads proximally. First the fingertips, then the fingers and even the hands become cold, white, and pulseless, and sensation and fine movement are impaired. Recovery is in the reverse order, and causes painful paraesthesiae in the affected areas, which become patchily discoloured red, white and blue. It may be followed by reflex vasodilatation, so that the hand is red and warm, and the pulse bounding. Rarely the nose and more frequently the toes may be affected. Early in the disease there is no evidence of permanent changes but after some years gangrene of the tips of the fingers may develop.

Treatment. The patient should avoid exposing the hands to cold and the whole body should be kept as warm as possible to promote reflex vasodilation. Vasodilator drugs are sometimes useful and tolazoline, 25 mg. t.d.s., is the most satisfactory. Sympathectomy is indicated if medical treatment fails but relapse usually occurs after a few years.

ACROCYANOSIS

This is a condition of unknown cause found in young people, characterised by painless cyanosis of the hands and feet, sometimes with swelling. The condition is harmless and treatment is unsatisfactory.

VENOUS THROMBOSIS

Deep Vein Thrombosis (Phlebothrombosis)

There are many factors which lead to a deep vein thrombosis, including venous stagnation, dehydration, and the rise in platelets which follows operation. It is particularly liable to occur after operation or during the course of a severe medical illness. Studies using phlebography and measuring the uptake by the thrombus of ^{125}I-labelled fibrinogen suggest that up to 35 per cent of patients have venous thrombosis after major surgery, although nearly all of them show no clinical evidence of disease. It may be symptomatic of a hidden neoplasm (particularly carcinoma of the pancreas or bronchus) or of Buerger's disease. It is more likely to develop in women on 'the pill'. Rarely it occurs for no apparent reason. The danger of a deep vein thrombosis is that a portion of the clot may break off and be swept through the right side of the heart to the lungs to produce a pulmonary infarct (p. 180).

Clinical Features. The symptoms of a deep vein thrombosis are often slight. There may be a slight rise of temperature with a leucocytosis and the patient may complain of pain in the calf. Examination will show perhaps slight swelling of the ankle, tenderness of the calf and dorsiflexion of the ankle will be painful (Homan's sign). Sometimes a pulmonary embolism will be the first indication of a deep vein thrombosis. With obstruction of the main venous return from the leg, the whole leg will become swollen and occasionally gangrene of the toes develops, thus leading to an erroneous diagnosis of arterial block.

Physical signs may be unreliable, but the following methods of investigation are available.

(1) *Ascending Venography.* This is most accurate but not entirely suitable for widespread routine use.

(2) *Injection of* ^{125}I *labelled fibrinogen* which becomes incorporated with the thrombus and can thus be detected.

(3) *Doppler ultrasound effect.* This measures the rate of flow of blood in the femoral vein on compressing the calf. It will only detect obstruction in the femoral vein and not in the calf.

Treatment. The patient and the affected limbs should be rested. Active movements are best avoided in the early stages in case a clot is dislodged, but gentle passive movements are allowed to prevent stagnation of blood. As soon as the acute stage has settled a crepe bandage should be firmly applied to the leg and the patient should be encouraged to walk.

Anticoagulants should be given and continued until one week after all the signs have disappeared and the patient is ambulant. If there is gross oedema of the leg the position of the obstruction should be defined by venography, and the thrombus removed. This must be done within 24 hours of the onset of symptoms.

Prevention. It would obviously be most satisfactory to prevent the development of phlebothrombosis, particularly in patients at risk following surgery. Intermittent stimulation or compression of calf muscles during operation may be helpful. Although early leg exercises in the post-operative period are widely used, there is no good evidence that they are effective. Heparin 5000 units subcutaneously before operation and then twice daily for seven days has been shown to be effective.

Superficial Vein Thrombosis

Thrombosis may occur in the superficial veins, particularly of the lower limbs. The vein becomes painful and on examination the thrombosis can be palpated as a tender cord. The skin over the thrombosis may be red. Superficial vein thrombosis may occur as a result of injury or as a complication of varicose veins. It should be remembered that it occasionally indicates a deep-seated neoplasm. There is little risk of pulmonary embolism.

Treatment consists of firmly bandaging the limb and allowing the patient to walk as much as is comfortable. Phenylbutazone in doses of 100 mg. three times daily for a few days will often reduce inflammation and discomfort.

Iliac Vein Compression

Obstruction of the venous return from the lower limbs by the right common iliac artery has recently been recognised as an occasional cause of swollen legs. Usually in such patients the left common iliac vein is compressed (68 per cent) but the lower end of the inferior vena cava (16 per cent) and the right common iliac vein (16 per cent) may also be affected. The condition is twice as common in women as in men, and is believed to be a major factor in the occurrence of acute venous thrombosis after childbirth or surgical operations (p. 186), which may be followed by lifelong oedema of one or both limbs. In other patients no such acute episode is recorded, the patient presenting with aching and swelling of one or both legs.

Swelling occurs three times as commonly on the left as the right, and the whole of the affected limb is swollen. Pain in the limb on exertion is the rule, and has been termed 'venous claudication'. It differs from arterial claudication (p. 184) in that it takes longer to appear and is less quickly relieved by rest. It usually affects the calf, but may spread to the thigh. Sometimes there are recurrent episodes of thrombosis, and chronic varicose ulcers may occur.

The diagnosis is proved by combined phlebography and arteriography, and treatment is surgical.

Thrombosis of the Axillary Vein

This occasionally occurs in young, fit adults, particularly following trauma to the vein such as produced by carrying a rucksack. There is a swelling of the arm and the axillary vein is tender. An embolism is rare and the arm should be rested until the condition subsides.

FURTHER READING

Cantwell, J. D., *Modern Cardiology*, Butterworth, London, 1977.

Wood, P., *Diseases of the Heart and Circulation*, 3rd Edition, Eyre and Spottis-woode, London, 1968.

Pickering, Sir George, *High Blood Pressure*, 3rd edition, J. & A. Churchill, London, 1974.

Oram, S., *Clinical Heart Disease*, Heinemann, London, 1971.

Krikler, D. M. and Goodwin, J. F., (Eds.), *Cardiac Arrhythmias*, W. B. Saunders, Philadelphia and London, 1975.

Schamroth, L., *An Indroduction to Electrocardiography*, 5th Edition, Blackwell Scientific Publications, Oxford, 1977.

CHAPTER FIVE

THE RESPIRATORY SYSTEM

ANATOMY AND PHYSIOLOGY

For descriptive purposes the respiratory system is subdivided into the upper respiratory tract, consisting of the nose, nasopharynx, and larynx, and the lower respiratory tract, comprising the trachea, bronchi, and lungs. The lining membrane of the air passages has a rich blood supply which enables it to warm and moisten the inspired air. A thin film of mucus covers the whole respiratory tract, and is kept continuously moving upwards away from the lungs by the sweeping action of the ciliated mucous membrane; this is a most effective filter for removing particles of dust from the air before it reaches the lungs. The irregularity of the nasal cavity and the accessory air sinuses which open into it increase the area of mucous membrane with which the air comes into contact, and so makes the warming and filtering more efficient; on the other hand, swelling of the mucous membrane readily obstructs drainage of secretions from the sinuses and so may predispose to sinusitis. Another important defence mechanism is the cough reflex.

ANATOMY OF THE BRONCHIAL TREE

A proper knowledge of the anatomy of the bronchial tree is essential to the understanding of the localisation and spread of many diseases of the lung. Many lung infections spread via the bronchi and the distribution of the infection is determined by the segments which these bronchi supply. Unless the anatomy of the broncho-pulmonary segments is known, the correct localisation of disease within the lung, whether by means of physical signs or radiography, is impossible. Finally, treatment by postural drainage requires a knowledge of the direction of the bronchi so that the patient may be correctly positioned.

Surface Markings of the Lobes

The upper and lower lobes of the left lung are separated by the oblique fissure. The right lung is composed of three lobes and the right oblique fissure separates the lower lobe from the upper and middle lobes. On each side the oblique fissure extends from the anterior end of the 6th rib and runs upwards and backwards round the chest wall, usually along the line of the 5th or 6th rib to the vertebral column. Its surface marking roughly corresponds to the position of the medial border of the scapula when the hand is placed on top of the head. The horizontal fissure separates the right upper lobe from the middle lobe. Its surface marking starts at the fourth right costal cartilage and runs horizontally around the chest to join the oblique fissure in the mid-axillary line. The segment of the left lung which occupies the position corresponding to the middle lobe is called the lingula, and it is part of the left upper lobe.

The Broncho-pulmonary Segments

The bronchi to the separate lobes of each lung arise from the main bronchi on their respective sides. The primary subdivisions of the lobar bronchi, together with the segments of lung which they supply, form the broncho-pulmonary segments. The segments of each lobe are named after their corresponding bronchi.

The Upper Lobes. The right upper lobe bronchus divides almost immediately into anterior, apical, and posterior branches. The anterior and posterior bronchi have axillary branches which supply the lateral part of the upper lobe.

The left upper lobe bronchus quickly gives origin to the lingula bronchus which runs downwards and forwards, subdividing into superior and inferior branches. It then gives off branches to the anterior, apical, and posterior segments of the lobe, but differs from the right side in having a common apico-posterior bronchus.

The Middle Lobe bronchus is only present on the right side and runs downwards and forwards dividing into lateral and medial divisions.

The Lower Lobes. The right lower lobe bronchus gives off an apical branch which arises opposite the middle lobe bronchus and runs backwards to the apical segment of the lower lobe. The basal bronchi consist of anterior, lateral, and posterior branches and, in addition, a medial basal (or cardiac) bronchus supplies a small segment on the medial aspect of the lower lobe.

On the left side the arrangement is similar, but the medial basal is usually insignificant or absent.

LOOKING AT THE CHEST X-RAY

A chest radiograph is an integral part of the examination of a patient suspected of lung disease, and indeed in many conditions radiological abnormalities are present long before the development of physical signs.

The film should be examined in a systematic, rather than haphazard, manner. Firstly it should be ensured that the film has been taken straight by observing that the medial ends of the clavicles are equidistant from the centre of the spine. Undue rotation can produce abnormal looking appearances of the mediastinum and the hilar shadows, as well as gross differences in the opaqueness of the two lungs. The trachea should be central; displacement may be due to rotation, shift of the mediastinum (see palpation, p. 201) or due to a superior mediastinal swelling (p. 258). The dia-

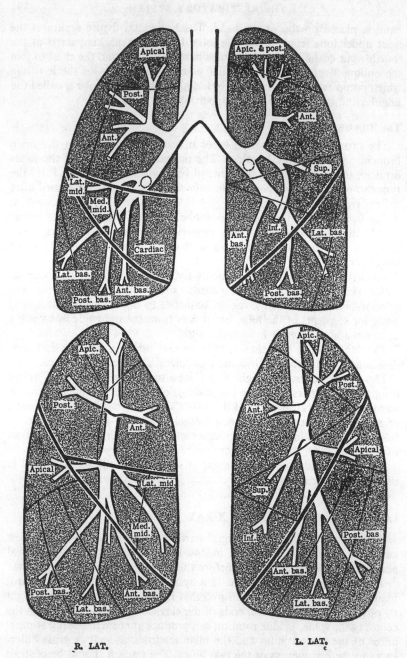

R. LAT.   L. LAT.

THE BRONCHO-PULMONARY SEGMENTS.

phragms should next be examined; flattening of the diaphragms occurs with over-inflated lungs and undue elevation of a diaphragm may be due to diminished lung volume on that side or to diaphragmatic paralysis. The right diaphragm is normally higher than the left and the costo-phrenic angle should be clear and at an acute angle, filling-in being due to fluid or pleural thickening. The lung fields are then examined by comparing one side with another; the apices of the lungs above the clavicles are first compared and then coming down the chest X-ray and using the anterior ends of the ribs as markers one interspace is compared with the other on the opposite side. In this way small focal lesions can be detected. In addition, the pulmonary vascular markings should be examined and an assessment made as to whether there is any diffuse shadowing in addition to the normal markings. The position of the horizontal fissure should be noted. The hilar regions should be examined; enlargement may be due to a prominent pulmonary artery, pathological enlargement of the pulmonary artery, enlarged lymph glands or hilar mass. Starting with the first ribs, and comparing one side with another, both the posterior and anterior parts of the ribs should be examined for abnormalities. A lateral chest X-ray will be necessary for full interpretation of a lesion and for correct anatomical localisation (see bronchopulmonary segments p. 191), and in addition a lateral film is essential for a suspected lesion in the left lower lobe as it may be obscured in the straight X-ray by the heart shadow.

RESPIRATORY FUNCTION TESTS

Tests of respiratory function aid the clinical assessment of a patient, for they provide a quantitative method of estimating the respiratory ability. They may be helpful, for example, when thoracic surgery is being considered and serial recordings are of value, both in assessing the effectiveness of a form of treatment and in following the progress of a disease. In addition, they may indicate the nature of underlying disease, either causing an *obstructive ventilatory defect*, as in asthma, chronic bronchitis and emphysema, or a *restrictive ventilatory defect*, as in fibrosing alveolitis and kyphoscoliosis.

Some tests are easy to perform and others require skill and complicated apparatus. Each has its limitations and it may be necessary to test several aspects of function before reaching a satisfactory conclusion. It is proposed to discuss the principles involved, rather than the technical aspects.

TESTS OF VENTILATION

The diagram, which is self-explanatory, illustrates the various subdivisions of the lung volume. The *Tidal Volume* is the volume of air breathed in or out at rest. The *Minute Volume* is the product of the tidal volume and the number of breaths per minute. They provide useful information in suspected cases of hypoventilation, as with respiratory depression from drugs. They are measured by the patient breathing through a small portable instrument called a Wright's 'Respirometer', which can also be connected to an endotracheal or tracheostomy tube.

The *Functional Residual Capacity* (FRC) is the resting expiratory volume of the lung and the *Total Lung Capacity* (TLC) is the maximum volume of gas in the lungs after a full inhalation. A full unhurried exhalation from the TLC gives the *Vital Capacity* (VC). A reduction in all of these volumes indicates a *Restrictive Ventilatory Defect*, and is a feature of many disorders of the lung, pleura and thoracic cage where there is stiffness, deformity or weakness.

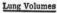

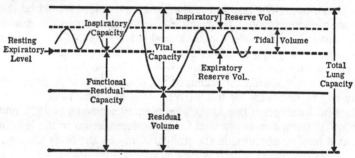

Tests of Pulmonary Ventilation

The *Residual Volume* (RV) is the volume of gas remaining in the lungs after a full unhurried inhalation and its proportion of the TLC is fairly constant. Up to the age of thirty years, it forms 20 to 25 per cent of the TLC but it then increases with age. The RV/TLC ratio is abnormally increased in those diseases where there is airflow obstruction, and consequently over-inflation of the lungs, as in asthma and emphysema. However, airflow obstruction is best measured when the vital capacity is determined with reference to speed. For this, the robust and portable 'Vitalograph' can be used. The *Forced Vital Capacity* (FVC) is the volume of a maximal exhalation carried out as rapidly as possible following a maximal inhalation to TLC. The volume expired during the first second of the FVC is termed the *Forced Expiratory Volume in one second* ($FEV_{1.0}$). The percentage of the FVC expired during this first second is termed the *Forced Expiratory Ratio* (FER) and is normally 75 per cent or more. A reduction in both the $FEV_{1.0}$ and FER occurs in those disorders with an *Obstructive Ventilatory Defect*. An improvement of the $FEV_{1.0}$ occurring five minutes after an inhalation of a bronchodilator, such as salbutamol, helps to distinguish a reversible airflow obstruction (asthma) from an irreversible airflow obstruction (as in emphysema or chronic bronchitis).

The *Peak Expiratory Flow Rate* is the maximal expiratory flow rate achieved during a maximal forced exhalation. It is measured with a Wright's 'Peak Flow Meter' which is small, portable and easy to operate. Although measuring rather different aspects of airflow, both the *Peak Flow* and $FEV_{1\cdot 0}$ are reduced in the diseases causing airflow obstruction.

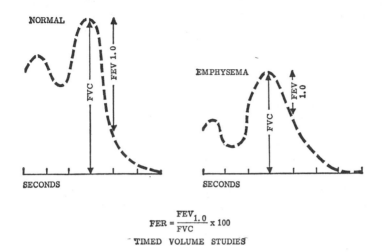

$$FER = \frac{FEV_{1\cdot 0}}{FVC} \times 100$$

TIMED VOLUME STUDIES

All the measurements described are determined by the patient's sex, age and size, being larger in males than females, increasing until adulthood, then declining with age. The predicted values for any individual have a large normal range. For example, for a man of 39 years, who is 5ft. 11ins. (1·79m.) tall, the normal ranges are:

Forced Expiratory Volume in one second	$(FEV_{1\cdot 0})$	2·9–4·7 litres
Forced Vital Capacity	(FVC)	4·0–6·0 litres
Forced Expiratory Ratio	(FER)	63–92 per cent
Peak Expiratory Flow Rate	(PEFR)	482–722 litres/minute

BLOOD GAS ANALYSIS

Measurements of the oxygen and the carbon dioxide tensions in arterial blood can be used to assess the efficiency of alveolar ventilation and also the matching between ventilation and perfusion of the lung. Normally the partial pressure of CO_2 ($PaCO_2$) and O_2 (PaO_2) in arterial blood are 40 mm.Hg (4·8–6·3 KPa) and 100 mm.Hg (11·9–13·2 KPa) respectively.

Alveolar hypoventilation leads to arterial oxygen desaturation and retention of carbon dioxide in the blood with a consequent rise in its arterial partial pressure ($PaCO_2$) and the development of a respiratory acidosis. This state of affairs may be **precipitated** by any complication producing severe impairment of ventilation, such as poliomyelitis or respiratory depression from drugs, or it may be **persistent** in patients with chronic chest disease.

'Mismatching' between ventilation and perfusion occurs when there is filling of the air space (as in pulmonary oedema or pneumonia), or with infiltration of the lung. In these conditions there are areas of the lung in which perfusion continues but ventilation is prevented. This effectively results in venous blood passing straight through the lung without being oxygenated, as in intra-cardiac right to left shunts. There is a resulting reduction in the partial pressure of arterial oxygen (PaO_2) but as carbon dioxide is about twenty times more diffusable than oxygen, there is no increase in the partial pressure of carbon dioxide ($PaCO_2$). Indeed, hyperventilation is often present at rest, which may produce an increased excretion of carbon dioxide by the lungs with a reduction in the $PaCO_2$, and the development of a respiratory alkalosis. At rest, the reduction of the partial pressure of arterial oxygen (PaO_2) depends on the severity of the condition, and the compensatory hyperventilation, but after exertion it falls sharply with perhaps a further reduction in $PaCO_2$.

In chronic hypoxic states, the respiratory centre depends on the hypoxia for its stimulation. Relief of severe hypoxia by oxygen therapy is an important part of the treatment of Cor Pulmonale for example, but this may release the respiratory centre from its 'hypoxic drive' and depress ventilation. The patient may thus be relieved from hypoxia, but the additional reduction in alveolar ventilation leads to further retention of carbon dioxide. Mental disturbance usually occurs when the arterial pH is less than 7·2 or the $PaCO_2$ higher than 100 mm.Hg, and coma usually supervenes with arterial levels of pH below 7·1 or the $PaCO_2$ above 120 mm.Hg. The serial estimation of the $PaCO_2$ from arterial puncture or the mixed venous blood by the Campbell rebreathing technique are thus valuable in ensuring the proper control of oxygen administration in such patients.

GAS TRANSFER

In certain conditions the predominant physiological defect is one of impairment of transfer of gases between the pulmonary capillaries and the alveoli. This occurs in such diseases as fibrosing alveolitis, asbestosis, infiltration of the lungs with sarcoid granulomata, carcinomatosis lymphangitis, and pulmonary oedema. The abnormality can be determined by measuring the *transfer factor* of the lung for carbon monoxide (TLCO). There are various methods for its measurements, but the most usual is to measure the uptake of carbon monoxide from the lung after a single full inhalation to TLC of a gas mixture containing a low concentration of carbon monoxide. In the above conditions, hyperventilation may be present even at rest, and the impaired gas transfer may be reflected in a lowered PaO_2 and a normal or low $PaCO_2$, these changes becoming more marked after exertion (see 'mismatching' between ventilation/perfusion in Blood Gas Analysis above). In the conditions described, in addition to the blood gas changes and reduced TLCO, if the pathological changes are sufficiently advanced, then there will be a restrictive ventilatory defect with reduction in FVC and FEV_1, but the FER and the PEFR are usually normal. In contrast, although the TLCO is lowered in emphysema, because the area of the alveoli available for gas transfer is reduced due to destructive dilatation of the alveoli, the FER and the PEFR are also reduced indicating the associated airflow obstruction.

THE WORK OF BREATHING AND COMPLIANCE

The measurement of the work involved in breathing requires the summation of various complicated physiological processess. These include such aspects as the oxygen requirements of the respiratory muscles and the mechanical effects of overcoming airway resistance, tissue resistance and lung elasticity. Most of these are difficult to test but lung elasticity, or *Lung Compliance*, can be measured fairly simply by recording the negative intrathoracic pressure through an oesophageal catheter, at the same time as ventilatory volumes. The lung compliance is the inspiratory volume which is produced by a change in negative pressure of 1 cm H_2O and in the normal is 0·09 to 0·33 litres/cm H_2O.

The normal values have been related to the Functional Residual Capacity (FRC) as they are influenced by the size of the lungs. The compliance is *reduced* in conditions which produce abnormally stiff lungs. Examples of such conditions are pulmonary venous congestion from *mitral stenosis* or *chronic left ventricular failure*, and *diffuse fibrotic or infiltrative lesions of the lungs*.

SYMPTOMS AND SIGNS OF LUNG DISEASE

Types of Cough and Sputum

A cough is a forced expiration against a closed glottis. A high pressure of air is built up in the trachea and bronchi and the sudden opening of the glottis is followed by explosive discharge, producing the characteristic barking noise. This removes collections of mucus and foreign particles from the air passages. The cough reflex is stimulated by irritation of nerve endings in the larynx, trachea, bronchi, and even the pleura.

In the early stages of respiratory tract infections, inflammatory swelling of the mucous membrane causes the cough to be dry and unproductive. With the later development of inflammatory exudate, the cough produces clear or whitish, sticky sputum. In *whooping cough* the exudate is particularly tenacious. The patient gives a series of quickly repeated coughs during one expiratory movement in an effort to dislodge the sputum, and this is followed by an inspiratory 'whoop' through a partially closed glottis. The cough typically occurs in paroxysms and is not always associated with a 'whoop'.

A yellow or greenish colour to the sputum signifies that it is purulent. This occurs with secondary pyogenic infection during respiratory tract infections. Purulent sputum is also expectorated in patients with *bronchiectasis*. With change of posture when waking in the morning, the patient coughs up the infected sputum which has collected in the dilated bronchi during the night. The quantity of sputum depends on the degree of infection and extent of the disease. It may amount to several ounces per day and is sometimes very offensive in smell due to the action of putrefactive bacteria. Purulent sputum tends to be more fluid than other types as enzymes from the pus cells liquefy the mucus.

The cough in *bronchial carcinoma* is at first persistent and unproductive due to invasion of the mucous membrane. With increase in size of the growth, secretions collect distal to the partially obstructed bronchus so that mucopurulent, often bloodstained, sputum is then produced.

In *pulmonary tuberculosis* there may be no sputum in the earlier stages of the disease. If sputum is produced it is clear or white and very sticky, so that it remains in separate lumps in the sputum mug (nummular sputum).

During the early stages of *pneumococcal pneumonia* the patient may cough up very viscid sputum tinged with blood which gives it a rusty colour.

Cardiac asthma (p. 110) is due to acute engorgement of the lungs with blood. In extreme cases oedema fluid exudes into the alveoli and the attack is associated with the expectoration of a large quantity of clear, frothy sputum, which is sometimes pinkish in colour due to the presence of red cells. In *bronchial asthma*, however, the sputum consists of firm, whitish pellets, which can sometimes be unravelled in water into spiral ribbons (Curschmann's spirals). These represent casts of the bronchial tubes in which they have formed.

Haemoptysis

The coughing up of blood must be distinguished from haematemesis, the vomiting of blood.

(1) Blood from the lungs is usually bright red, frothy, and mixed, with sputum. That from the stomach is usually dark in colour, having been altered to acid-haematin by the hydrochloric acid; it is often mixed with food.

(2) Many patients can state definitely whether the blood has been coughed up or vomited.

(3) Often there will be symptoms or signs which point to disease of the lungs or the alimentary tract.

The common causes of haemoptysis are:

Respiratory	Cardiovascular
Carcinoma of the bronchus	Pulmonary infarct
Pulmonary tuberculosis	Mitral stenosis

Acute or chronic bronchitis   Acute left ventricular failure
Bronchiectasis
Lung abscess

Although there may be an isolated haemoptysis in carcinoma of the bronchus, characteristically the ulcerated area leads to repeated daily blood-streaking of sputum. An early lesion of pulmonary tuberculosis sometimes presents with an haemoptysis of an ounce or more of bright-red blood, not associated with sputum. Blood-streaking of sputum is very common in respiratory tract infections and ulceration of the mucosa in bronchiectasis sometimes produces severe haemoptysis.

Every patient presenting with haemoptysis should be fully examined and have a chest radiograph, particularly to exclude bronchial carcinoma and pulmonary tuberculosis. A normal chest radiograph does not exclude an early bronchial carcinoma, and ideally bronchoscopy should be performed to exclude this possibility. However, unless there are good clinical grounds for suspecting a bronchial carcinoma, bronchoscopy is often not justified at this stage and it is sufficient for the patient to be followed-up carefully with fairly frequent chest radiographs. Cytological examination of the sputum for malignant cells can also be carried out. The majority of such patients do not develop any serious disease and in nearly half of all patients presenting with a small haemoptysis, no definite cause is found.

Pain in the Chest

Acute pleuritic pain from pleurisy is sharp and stabbing in character and aggravated by coughing or deep breathing. The pain is usually localised to the site of the pleurisy, but it may be referred to the abdominal wall and be confused with an acute abdominal condition. With diaphragmatic pleurisy the pain is referred to the tip of the shoulder, as the skin in this situation has the same sensory nerve supply (C3, 4, and 5).

Lesions of the chest wall, such as fractures or secondary deposits in the ribs, may cause severe local pain and tenderness. The aetiology of *Tietze*'s *syndrome* is uncertain, but it is a painful condition, usually involving one of the upper costo-chondral junctions. Chest pain may also be referred from the thoracic spine. The seventh cervical nerve supplies the pectoralis major and pain referred from this root may be felt in that muscle as well as in the arm. Intrathoracic structures, other than the lungs, can produce pain in the chest, common examples being the pain from coronary thrombosis and hiatus hernia.

Types of Respiration

Respiration in men is mainly diaphragmatic in type and in women it is mostly costal. Inspiration is a more powerful muscular movement than expiration, the latter depending on elastic recoil of the lungs and relaxation of the diaphragm and intercostal muscles. Obstruction to the large air passages produces a prolonged inspiratory phase with stridor, as inspiration is the more powerful movement. The bronchi and bronchioles normally dilate on inspiration and narrow on expiration, so that obstruction of the smaller air passages, as in asthma, leads to prolonged, wheezy, and difficult expiration.

Respirations in *pneumonia and pleurisy* are rapid and shallow, the inspirations being abruptly stopped, often with an audible grunt, as soon as the pleuritic pain is felt. Normally, expiration immediately follows inspiration and there is then a pause before the next breath. In pneumonia this rhythm is sometimes reversed, the pause taking place between inspiration and expiration.

The acidosis which occurs with uraemia and diabetic ketosis causes very deep breathing, known as *air hunger*, or *Kussmaul's breathing*, due to marked stimulation of the respiratory centre. *Cheyne-Stokes breathing* is a characteristic respiratory arrhythmia occurring when the respiratory centre has a diminished sensitivity to carbon dioxide in the blood. The amplitude of respiration progressively deepens until a maximum is reached and then diminishes until there is a period of apnoea. During the period of apnoea, the carbon dioxide in the blood rises to a level high enough to stimulate the respiratory centre. There is then an exaggerated response producing the period of hyperventilation, which washes the carbon dioxide out of the blood until the stimulus to respiration is removed and apnoea occurs. The whole cycle lasts two or three minutes and is then repeated. This type of breathing occurs with left ventricular failure and with various cerebral causes of depression of the respiratory centre.

Clubbing of the Fingers

The earliest change is a filling in of the angle between the skin at the base of the nail and the base of the nail itself, the skin becoming swollen and shiny. The base of the nail may be fluctuant. Later increased curvature of the nails occurs and finally the pulps of the fingers become enlarged. Clubbing has many unrelated causes:

Cardiovascular

(1) Infective endocarditis.
(2) Cyanotic congenital heart disease.
(3) Arteriovenous communications in the arm.

Respiratory

(1) Carcinoma of the bronchus.
(2) Chronic suppuration in the chest, such as bronchiectasis, lung abscess, and empyema.
(3) Chronic fibrosing alveolitis.

At times clubbing is familial and there is no underlying disease. More rarely it is associated with cirrhosis of the liver, steatorrhoea, or polyposis of the colon.

EXAMINATION OF THE CHEST

Inspection

(1) *The General Contours*

(a) *Kyphosis* and *kyphoscoliosis* may be developmental in origin. If gross, they may in later years give rise to severe impairment of lung function and heart failure. Abnormalities of spinal curvature may also occur secondary to intra-thoracic disease.

(b) *Funnel-shaped depression of the sternum* (pectus excavatum) may occur in varying degrees. Deep depression may displace the heart to the left and lead to the erroneous diagnosis of cardiac enlargement.

(c) *Over-inflation of the lungs,* such as occurs with asthma and emphysema, leads to increase in the antero-posterior diameter of the chest and the shoulders are held high.

(d) *Unilateral flattening* of the chest occurs with long-standing pulmonary or pleural fibrosis.

(2) *The Respiratory Movements*

(a) The respiratory rate is increased in many conditions, including acute and chronic lung disease, cardiac failure, and anxiety. It is decreased with depression of the respiratory centre, as in narcotic poisoning and with various cerebral lesions.

(b) The accessory muscles of respiration may be used if there is severe respiratory distress, as in an asthmatic attack.

(c) Decreased movement on one side of the chest indicates disease of the lung or pleura of that side.

(d) The respiration may have a special character (see p. 199).

Palpation

The position of the mediastinum is assessed by determining the position of the apex beat and the trachea. Shift of the mediastinum towards the side of the lesion indicates shrinkage of the lung due to collapse or fibrosis. Displacement away from the lesion occurs with fluid or air in the pleural cavity. Displacement of the trachea alone is more likely with contraction of an upper lobe and shift of the apex beat alone is a lesion of a lower lobe.

Tactile vocal fremitus (T.V.F.) is decreased with air or fluid in the pleural cavity and with pulmonary collapse. Increased tactile vocal fremitus occurs with conditions which also produce bronchial breathing.

Percussion

Normally the lungs are resonant to percussion and there are areas of dullness over the heart and liver. In emphysema and pneumothorax, hyperresonance is sometimes found and cardiac and liver dullness are either diminished or absent. Impaired resonance is found over consolidated,

Condition	Inspection	Palpation	Percussion	Auscultation
*CONSOLIDATION	Respiration rate increased. Movement decreased on affected side.	Mediastinum central T.V.F. increased over consolidation.	Dullness over consolidation.	Bronchial breathing ⎫ Bronchophony ⎬ Over consoli- W.P. ⎭ dation. Fine or medium rales.
ABSORPTION COLLAPSE	Movement diminished on affected side.	Mediastinum shifted to affected side. Absent T.V.F. over collapsed segment.	Dullness over collapsed area.	Breath sounds diminished or absent. Voice sounds diminished or absent.
FIBROSIS	Flattening of the chest and diminished movement on affected side.	Mediastinum shifted to affected side. Increased T.V.F. over fibrosis.	Dullness over fibrosis.	Bronchial breathing ⎫ Bronchophony ⎬ Over W.P. ⎭ fibrosis Frequent coarse rales due to concomitant bronchiectasis.
FLUID	Movement diminished on affected side.	If large, mediastinum shifted to opposite side. T.V.F. absent over fluid.	Stony dullness over fluid, the line tending to rise in the axilla with moderate effusions.	Absent breath sounds and voice sounds over fluid. Sometimes bronchial breathing, W.P., and aegophony above upper level of fluid.
PNEUMOTHORAX	Movement diminished on affected side.	If large, mediastinum shifted to opposite side.	Normal or hyper-resonant. Diminished cardiac dullness on the left and liver dullness on right.	Breath sounds and voice sounds diminished or absent. Sometimes if large, bronchial breathing, W.P., and positive coin sound.

* These signs are only heard over a considerable area of consolidation. With small patches of pneumonia, or when the pneumonic process has not reached the surface of the lung, signs may be scanty and are often confined to a small area of crackling rales.

collapsed, or fibroid lung, or with pleural thickening. A flat, dull note is found over pleural fluid.

Auscultation

(1) *The Breath Sounds*

The normal breath sounds are rustling, with a long inspiratory phase followed by a short expiratory phase. Over the lung roots the normal breath sounds take on a bronchial character. The breath sounds are diminished or absent with fluid or air in the pleural cavity and with impaired inflation of the lung, as in emphysema and collapse. In *bronchial breathing*, the breath sounds have a harsher quality and the expiratory phase is longer than the inspiratory, with a short gap between the two. Bronchial breathing is heard in the normal by listening with a stethoscope over the larynx or trachea. When bronchial breathing is heard over the lungs, it indicates a pathological process which is enhancing the transmission of the tracheal sound to the chest wall. It occurs with pneumonic consolidation, with fibroid lung (fibrosis plus bronchiectasis), and over a large cavity. It also occurs sometimes above the upper level of a pleural effusion and over a large pneumothorax, which acts as a resonating chamber. Bronchial breathing is always accompanied by whispering pectoriloquy and by increased T.V.F. and bronchophony.

(2) *The Voice Sounds*

Normally, when the stethoscope is placed over a peripheral part of the lungs the spoken voice comes through in a modified form so that the consonants are blurred and indistinct; the whispered voice cannot be heard at all. Transmission of the spoken and whispered voice in an unmodified bronchial form (such as can be heard in the normal subject by listening over the trachea, though it is not necessarily as loud as this) is called respectively *bronchophony* and *whispering pectoriloquy* (W.P.). They occur under the same circumstances as bronchial breathing.

Aegophony is the peculiar nasal quality to the voice sounds heard above the upper level of an effusion.

(3) *Rhonchi*

A rhonchus is a musical squeak due to air passing through a narrowed bronchus. It is low pitched if the bronchus is large and high pitched with small bronchi. Rhonchi are most marked on expiration and may be cleared by coughing. The narrowing is commonly due to bronchial spasm or mucosal swelling or exudate. A bronchial neoplasm may produce a persistent low-pitched rhonchus.

(4) *Râles*

Râles are popping noises due either to air bubbling through fluid or to the sound of alveolar walls opening. The râles are coarse if the fluid is in large bronchi and fine if the bronchi are small. *Crepitations* are very fine râles due to fluid in the bronchioles or alveoli. They are sometimes heard at the bases of the lungs in normal people who have been breathing quietly, when they are due to the noise of the partially closed alveoli opening, but they should disappear after a few deep breaths. They are persistent with pulmonary oedema or fibrosing alveolitis. If the râles are associated with bronchial breathing, they become very clear cut (*consonating râles*). Râles are most marked towards the end of an inspiration. There are coarse, crackling râles in bronchiectasis, medium râles in bronchitis, and crepitations in pulmonary oedema, pneumonia or fibrosing alveolitis.

DISEASES OF THE UPPER RESPIRATORY TRACT

HAY FEVER AND PERENNIAL RHINITIS

These are allergic disorders characterised by bouts of sneezing, profuse watery nasal discharge, and smarting and watering of the eyes. Hay fever is due to sensitivity to grass pollens and occurs during the months of May to August; perennial rhinitis is due to sensitivity to a variety of allergens, such as house dust, and may occur throughout the year.

Treatment. *Hay fever*: A course of desensitisation injections may be given if skin testing confirms pollen sensitivity (see asthma p. 217). At least three yearly courses are required for a prolonged effect. *Antihistamines* are of considerable value during an attack. Usually one preparation can be found to suit the patient. Among the most valuable are chlorpheniramine, 4·0 mg. twice daily or promethazine, 25 mg. once or twice daily; the latter often causes troublesome drowsiness. *Disodium cromoglycate* or *beclomethasone* inhaled into the nose are both valuable in the treatment of hayfever.

Perennial rhinitis: Precipitants such as house dust, pets, or feathers should be avoided. Skin testing is seldom helpful as the patient is often sensitive to many allergens. Antihistamines may be tried, but are not usually as successful as in hay fever. Good symptomatic relief may be obtained with *betamethasone* (0·1 per cent) nasal drops or with *beclomethasone* spray. Surgical treatment, e.g. submucous resection, should be avoided unless there is a very definite indication.

VIRUS INFECTIONS OF THE RESPIRATORY TRACT

The following are some of the viruses which affect the respiratory tract:

Rhinovirus
Adenovirus
Influenza virus
Parainfluenza virus
Respiratory syncytial virus
Coxsackie ⎱ Enteroviruses
ECHO ⎰

All the above viruses have a nucleic acid content of RNA, with the exception of the adenovirus which is DNA containing. An increasing number of serotypes are being identified with some of the above viruses; for example, there are more than 90 serotypes of the rhinovirus and 33 of the adenovirus. The enteroviruses, ECHO and Coxsackie A and B, also produce respiratory infections as well as other illnesses such as pericarditis and meningitis (p. 296). The influenza virus consists of types A, B and C; influenza A virus is the cause of pandemics and major epidemics, B virus causes smaller epidemics and is a less virulent type of infection and influenza C is principally endemic producing a fairly trivial respiratory infection. Major changes in the antigenic nature of influenza A virus occur about every ten to fifteen years, but minor changes may occur during the intervening years —the so-called 'antigenic drift'. For this reason effective vaccines against influenza should contain type B virus and the latest strain of type A, at the present time A/Hong Kong/68 (H3N2). The development of effective vaccines against the other respiratory viruses has not been possible because of the large number of viruses involved and because there would be no cross-protection between the different serotypes in the same group.

Generally speaking each type of acute respiratory illness can be produced by a number of different viruses. A cold, for example, can be caused by the rhinovirus and the adenovirus, and the latter virus may also be responsible for a sore throat, an influenza-like illness or pneumonia.

CORYZA (The Common Cold)

Coryza is an infection of the mucous membrane of the nose and nasopharynx. The majority of cases are due to infection with the rhinoviruses, but any of the other respiratory viruses may be responsible—in particular the adenoviruses. It is spread by droplet infection, particularly in crowded places such as buses, trains, and cinemas. There is a high level of endemic infection during the autumn and winter and chills and dampness seem to be predisposing factors. After sneezing and profuse watery nasal discharge for a few days, secondary bacterial infection often occurs and the secretions become thick and yellow. Infection may spread causing:

(1) *Acute sinusitis*, with fever, headache or pain in the face, and localised tenderness may be present over the frontal or maxillary sinuses. Chronic sinusitis may result.

(2) *Acute otitis media* with fever, deafness, and earache.

(3) *Tracheitis, bronchitis, or pneumonia.*

Treatment. A day or two in bed usually cuts short the course and prevents complications. It also helps to limit spread of the infection to others.

Soluble aspirin 0·6 g. six-hourly, often alleviates the minor discomforts. Inhalation of tinct. benzoin and menthol, one teaspoonful in a jug of hot water, may relieve the nasal congestion.

ACUTE LARYNGITIS AND LARYNGOTRACHEOBRONCHITIS

Acute laryngitis occurs with the common cold and in young children with parainfluenzal virus infection. Tracheitis and bronchitis often occur at the same time. The throat is sore, the voice is at first hoarse and then reduced to a whisper and there is a dry, painful cough. In small children, swelling of the mucous membrane of the larynx may cause serious obstruction, the condition known as 'croup'; breathing becomes noisy and laboured and alarming paroxysms of coughing occur.

Treatment. If feverish the patient should be in bed in a warm room where the atmosphere is not too dry. The dryness of central heating, electric and gas fires should be prevented by using a steam kettle. The patient must not talk, since the larynx needs rest. Smoking is forbidden. Steam inhalations containing tinct. benzoin co., one teaspoon to one pint of boiling water, given for ten minutes three times a day, often give great relief; hot gargles and frequent hot drinks make the throat more comfortable. Linctus codeine, 4·0 ml., will suppress an irritating cough.

CHRONIC LARYNGITIS

It is more common in men than in women and is particularly liable to occur with untrained over-use of the voice. Hence the term 'clergyman's throat', though costermonger's throat would be more apt, as excessive use of tobacco and alcohol are often predisposing factors. Chronic sinus infection may also play a part.

Clinical Features. The voice is hoarse and weak. Examination of the larynx shows congestion with thickening of the vocal cords, either generalised or confined to the posterior third.

Persistent hoarseness for more than three weeks demands expert examination of the larynx. It may be due to papilloma, carcinoma, laryngeal palsy, or more rarely tuberculosis or syphilis.

Treatment. Complete rest of the voice is important. The patient should not speak above a whisper for several weeks. Nasal infection should be treated if present and tobacco and alcohol forbidden.

DISEASES OF THE BRONCHI

ACUTE TRACHEITIS AND BRONCHITIS

Acute tracheitis and bronchitis may complicate colds, influenza, measles, and other virus infections, and are particularly liable to occur in cold, damp and foggy weather. After the first few days, secondary bacterial invasion commonly occurs. Broncheolitis in infants is due to the respiratory syncytial virus.

Clinical Features. Acute tracheitis causes a dry, painful cough with soreness behind the sternum. Spread of infection to the bronchi produces tightness of the chest, with wheezing and difficulty in breathing. At first there is a little sticky, mucoid sputum, but secondary bacterial infection soon makes it yellow and more profuse. The severity and duration of the fever and of the general malaise are very variable; usually the illness is a mild one, lasting a few days. It may be serious and lead to pneumonia in young children, in the elderly or debilitated, or in patients with chronic bronchitis.

The signs of acute bronchitis are moderate fever, raised respiratory rate, particularly in children or in those with underlying lung disease, widespread rhonchi and often râles.

Treatment. The patient should be kept in bed. The room should be warm and the atmosphere not too dry. A steam kettle or steam inhalations reduce the soreness and aid expectoration. A dry, troublesome cough is helped by linctus codeine 4–8 ml. t.d.s. or elixir diphenhydramine 4 ml.; the latter also aids sleep.

After a few days the fever settles and the cough disappears. Convalescence is advisable after an attack of acute bronchitis, as early return to work with exposure to cold and a smoky atmosphere may delay complete recovery. Antibiotics are not required in mild, uncomplicated acute bronchitis. They are required where the risks of bronchopneumonia are greater:

(1) In a patient with severe bronchitis.
(2) In children and in the elderly and infirm.
(3) In the presence of complicating disease, such as heart disease.
(4) In patients with chronic bronchitis or bronchiectasis.

In these circumstances ampicillin or tetracycline (250 mg. four times daily), or co-trimoxazole (Bactrim or Septrin) two tablets twice a day are usually effective.

CHRONIC BRONCHITIS

Great Britain has a higher mortality rate from chronic bronchitis than any other country in the world. It is a major cause of chronic disability and death, particularly in men over middle age. It is related to air pollution, cigarette smoking and the liability to viral respiratory tract infections, and is most common in outdoor manual workers in urban districts. It is a complication of the pneumoconioses (p. 245), and obesity is an aggravating factor.

In the early stages there is hypertrophy of the mucous glands of bronchi, even when there is no inflammatory cell infiltration of the mucosa. In addition goblet cells replace the normal peripheral bronchial epithelium. Later, inflammatory changes in the mucosa occur with micro-abscesses and ulceration of the alveolar walls. When the sputum is mucoid bacteriological study is unrewarding. With persistently purulent sputum, and in acute exacerbations of bronchitis, haemophilus influenzae and the pneumococcus are the most common pathogens isolated.

Clinical Features. The earliest symptom is probably the 'smoker's cough', with the early morning production of non-infected mucoid sputum. This causes no disability and the patient is unlikely to seek medical advice. Later the patient complains of a winter cough with sputum, often with wheezing. At first these symptoms may only occur in episodes after a cold, which is slow to clear. Later they persist throughout the whole winter and eventually during the summer as well. These is usually a moderate amount of sputum, which may be mucoid or purulent; the latter nearly always occurs during an acute exacerbation of bronchitis, but sometimes the sputum is persistently purulent. A large volume of sputum should arouse suspicion of concomitant bronchiectasis.

After some years increasing dyspnoea, due to progressive airways obstruction and the development of emphysema, becomes an even more urgent symptom. The patient becomes too breathless to work and finally becomes completely disabled. There is considerable variation in the degree of disablement as many patients go throughout life with chronic cough and sputum and little dyspnoea, whereas others may become complete respiratory cripples within a few years.

Examination shows generalised rhonchi due to narrowing of the bronchi by spasm, mucosal swelling and exudate. Râles may also be heard particularly at the bases. As emphysema develops it produces additional signs (p. 209). A *chest radiograph* in chronic bronchitis may show no abnormality until emphysema is present.

Treatment. This is generally disappointing, but in certain cases considerable symptomatic improvement can be achieved. The progress of the disease may be slowed by preventing, as far as possible, acute exacerbations of bronchitis and by treating them vigorously when they occur. This is more rewarding in the early case where lung destruction is not advanced and symptoms are minimal.

General Management. The smoky atmosphere of the city and dusty work should be avoided. This ideal is difficult to achieve as most patients, for financial and social reasons, cannot move to a healthier district or change their occupation. They can give up smoking and should be strenuously urged to do so. They should be advised to sleep in a warm bedroom, with the windows closed in the winter and they should stay at home in foggy weather and when they have a cold. A cold must be taken seriously, and the patient should be given a prophylactic antibiotic (see below) without delay.

Bronchodilators. Some degree of bronchospasm is often present and may be relieved by salbutamol, aminophylline inhalers containing salbutamol or orciprenaline.

Prednisolone may be tried in some severely disabled patients in whom persistent bronchospasm is thought to be an important feature. Eosinophils in the sputum and a family history of allergy may be useful guides.

This steroid therapy should be continued only if there is striking improvement within a week; it is then given on the same lines as for chronic asthma (p. 220).

Expectorant mixtures aim at loosening and aiding the expectoration of sputum. Pharmacological evidence suggests that in the dosage usually prescribed they have no effect on the volume or characteristics of the sputum expectorated. However, many bronchitic patients and doctors find such mixtures helpful and they continue to be prescribed. The reader is referred to the National Formulary for suitable prescriptions.

Sedative cough mixtures are used to suppress a troublesome cough at night, or to enable a patient to attend a social meeting in comfort. Examples are linctus codeine (N.F.) 4–8 ml. and linctus pholcodine (N.F.) 4–8 ml.

Prophylactic antibiotics do not prevent colds, but are used to prevent the secondary bacterial infection and to cut short, or prevent, acute exacerbations of bronchitis. In a small group of patients with persistent purulent sputum considerable improvement can be achieved by prolonged treatment with antibiotics, from November to March. However, the majority of patients are best treated by giving them a supply of antibiotics so that they can start a course, on their own initiative, at the first signs of a cold. As haemophilus influenzae and the pneumococcus are the common pathogens, tetracycline 1 g. daily, ampicillin 1–2 g. daily, or co-trimoxazole (Bactrim or Septrin) in a dose of two tablets twice daily, are preferred to penicillin.

Breathing Exercises, see p. 211.

Heart failure in chronic bronchitis is quite common; it may be due to concurrent hypertension or coronary artery disease, or to true cor pulmonale (p. 212), or to a combination of factors.

EMPHYSEMA

Emphysema may be defined as a condition of the lungs in which there is pathological enlargement of the distal air spaces either from chronic dilatation or from destruction of their walls. Emphysematous bullae, which are cystic spaces of varying size, may develop and at post-mortem the lungs appear bulky as they fail to deflate. The numerous pathological classifications of emphysema are both complex and confusing. There are two main types:

Pan-acinar emphysema. There is a dilatation or destruction of the acinus. This is the lung tissue distal to the terminal bronchiole and includes the respiratory bronchioles, alveolar ducts, atria and alveoli.

Centrilobular emphysema. The dilatation or destruction is more proximal and involves the respiratory bronchioles. The emphysema is present in the centre of the lobules with the more distal part remaining unchanged. Bronchiolitis is probably the main causative factor.

Aetiology. Emphysema most commonly occurs with long-standing disease of the bronchi, namely chronic bronchitis or chronic asthma, or a combination of the two. At times it may be related to an occupational cause such as exposure to dust, and in coal miners' pneumonoconiosis (p. 246) there is characteristically a centrilobular emphysema ('focal' emphysema). Occasionally it develops as a primary disease without any previous history of bronchitis and familial cases of mainly basal emphysema are now recognised where there is a deficiency of alpha-1-antitrypsin in the blood.

The actual mechanism of production of emphysema is debated; 'air-trapping' due to widespread narrowing of the bronchioles, and weakening of the respiratory bronchioles and the alveolar walls from inflammation are both likely factors. The proteolytic enzymes released from leucocytes in the presence of inflammation are more likely to be destructive to the tissues with deficiency of the principal inhibitor, namely alpha-1-anti-trypsin.

Effects on Lung Function. Emphysematous lung loses its elasticity and thus expiration requires a muscular effort on the part of the patient. Apart from the increased work involved, the forced expiration produces early closure of the diseased respiratory bronchioles and thus enhances the diffuse airflow obstruction already present. The chronic over-inflation of the lungs also leads to increase in the fixed volume of gas in the lungs, the residual volume, with the result that the mixing of inspired air in the lungs is less efficient. These two factors lead to alveolar hypoventilation. In addition, over-ventilation of the under-perfused alveoli (where there is atrophy of the pulmonary capillaries), under-ventilation of normally perfused alveoli (producing a right to left shunt) and reduction in the total surface area of the alveoli all lead to deficiency in the transfer of gases between alveoli and the pulmonary capillaries (p. 196).

It is now recognised that blood gas abnormalities and cor pulmonale are less likely in 'pure' emphysema ('*pink puffers*'), but do occur if there is accompanying chronic bronchitis, being a particular feature of this disease ('*blue bloaters*').

Clinical Features. The major symptom is dyspnoea. When emphysema is not too advanced there is likely to be only moderate shortness of breath on exertion. With progression of the disease the patient eventually becomes unable to walk more than a few steps. Quite frequently the breath is exhaled through pursed lips. The rate of progress of the disease is variable. Frequently it is slow, the patient reaching old age with only moderate disability. Sometimes it is rapid, the patient becoming a complete respiratory cripple by middle life. Occasionally the onset of severe disability is apparently sudden. This is usually precipitated by fog or a respiratory tract infection, the patient not admitting to significant symptoms beforehand.

With well-established emphysema, the chest appears over-inflated, with thoracic kyphosis, increase in the antero-posterior diameter of the chest, and horizontal ribs. Chest expansion is diminished, the chest being lifted up by the accessory muscles of respiration rather than expanded. The percussion note is hyper-resonant and the areas of cardiac and liver dullness are diminished. The breath sounds are faint, often with prolonged expiration. Rhonchi and râles may be present, indicating bronchial disease. Respiratory function tests show impaired ventilation with airflow obstruction (p. 194), increased residual volume (p. 194), and impaired gas transfer (p. 196). In advanced cases with associated chronic bronchitis hypoxia causes cyanosis, and the presence of cor pulmonale produces additional signs (p. 212).

The *chest radiograph* may be normal unless emphysema is well developed. In such cases the lung fields appear unduly translucent with atrophy of the peripheral vessels. The main pulmonary arteries are large and the heart thin and vertical. Bullae may be visible as localised areas of increased translucency. The ribs are horizontal and the diaphragm depressed and flattened.

Treatment

    (1) *To improve the airways and prevent progression of the disease.* Treatment of bronchial infection and bronchospasm are dealt with under chronic bronchitis (p. 207) and asthma (p. 217).

    (2) *To make full use of the remaining lung tissue.* This is best achieved by *breathing exercises*. Most subjects with emphysema breathe with the upper part of the chest and hardly use the diaphragm at all. Exercises teach the patient to use the diaphragm and lower ribs more efficiently.

    (3) *Heart failure from cor pulmonale.* For treatment see p. 213.

Compensatory Emphysema

When a section of lung contracts by fibrosis or collapse, or is removed surgically, the rest of that lung expands by over-inflation to fill the space. This is known as compensatory emphysema and is not usually associated with any defect of function.

Unilateral Emphysema

Unilateral translucency of a lung may be due to a large bulla or cyst, or be due to compensatory emphysema as a result of a totally collapsed lobe in the lung on that side. It also occurs when there is over-inflation of a lung due to partial obstruction of a major bronchus; this can produce a 'ball-valve' mechanism so that air enters on inspiration but is trapped in the lung on expiration. This is likely to be due to a bronchial neoplasm in an adult and to pressure from tuberculous glands in a child. *Unilateral emphysema* (Macleod's syndrome) may follow an obliterative bronchiolitis occurring in early childhood; this arrests development of the lung which normally proceeds until the age of 8 years. The affected lung has both diminished ventilation and poor perfusion; the chest X-rays shows attenuated vessels and an expiration film will show failure of the lung to deflate with shift of the mediastinum to the opposite side.

RESPIRATORY FAILURE

The function of the lungs may be so impaired by various diseases that oxygenation of the blood becomes seriously deficient; this is respiratory failure. It is associated with central cyanosis and with low oxygen and with high carbon dioxide tensions in the arterial blood, and with respiratory acidosis (p. 429.) It may be due to *depression of the respiratory centre* by poisons, drugs, anoxia or cerebral disease; to *failure of the respiratory muscles* as in poliomyelitis, acute infectious polyneuritis and myasthenia gravis; to *loss of functioning lung* as in extensive pneumonia, pulmonary collapse, pneumothorax or following surgical lung resection; to *obstruction of airways* as in status asthmaticus or severe bronchitis.

Patients with chronic lung disease are especially prone to respiratory failure with any of the above complications, which may occur separately or in combination.

Respiratory failure can occur independently of cor pulmonale, although it may precipitate it.

Treatment is directed at the underlying cause. *Respiratory stimulants* (p. 213) are indicated when there is depression of the respiratory centre. *Oxygen therapy* (p. 213) and some form of *assisted respiration* may be essential to maintain life. *Tracheostomy* may be required. It improves ventilation by reducing dead space and airway resistance and enables sputum to be sucked out of the air passages in a patient unable to cough adequately. It may be combined, using a cuffed endotracheal tube, with positive-pressure ventilation, but such treatment needs careful management and it is only feasible in specialised units. One of the disadvantages of assisted respiration is that it may not be possible to wean patients with chronic lung disease from the respirator or the tracheostomy.

COR PULMONALE

This is cardiovascular disease secondary to disease of the lungs. It occurs most commonly with chronic bronchitis and emphysema; also with chronic asthma and with diffuse fibrosis of the lungs due to such diseases as sarcoidosis and the pneumonoconioses. It may follow the long-standing deficient ventilation of severe kyphoscoliosis or gross obesity.

It is mostly precipitated by a respiratory tract infection, which increases the severity of respiratory failure causing *hypoxia* and carbon dioxide retention (*hypercarbia*). The abnormal blood gases produce impairment of renal function with retention of sodium and water, increase in blood volume and at first a rise in cardiac output. The systemic arterioles are dilated with warm extremities and bounding pulse, and dilatation of the cerebral vessels may produce headache and even papilloedema. The effect of the hypoxia on the pulmonary arterioles, however, is to produce active vasoconstriction. This, combined with obliteration of these vessels by disease and with the increase in cardiac output, produces pulmonary hypertension. It is only in the later stages of the disease, if pulmonary hypertension becomes severe or if the heart muscle is seriously affected by anoxia, that the cardiac output falls.

Clinical Features. The patient is cyanosed, with signs of chronic bronchitis and emphysema. The extremities are warm but cyanosed, and the pulse full. The venous pressure in the neck is raised, the liver enlarged and there is dependent oedema. The heart sounds are often difficult to hear due to the overlying emphysematous lung, but it may be possible to detect triple rhythm. With gross enlargement of the right ventricle a right ventricular heave may be palpable and the systolic murmur of functional tricuspid incompetence be heard, with systolic pulsation of the neck veins. Proteinuria and a raised blood urea may be present. If the cardiac output falls, the extremities become cold and the pulse small; venous congestion and oedema increase and signs of right ventricular hypertrophy and dilatation are more obvious.

An electrocardiogram shows the large sharply pointed P waves of right atrial hypertrophy and there may be signs of right ventricular hypertrophy. The heart is usually vertical.

Radiography shows dilatation of the main pulmonary arteries with cardiac enlargement. The lung fields may show evidence of emphysema.

Treatment is primarily directed at improving alveolar ventilation.

Bronchial infection is treated with an effective antibiotic, such as ampicillin or tetracycline 250 mg. four times daily.

Bronchospasm is best treated by aminophylline, either intravenously or by rectal suppository and a course of corticosteroids may be indicated.

Oxygen therapy is required for acute respiratory failure and highest concentrations can be achieved by using an oxygen tent or B.L.B. mask. However, in patients with cor pulmonale and chronic carbon dioxide retention the respiratory centre may depend on oxygen lack for its stimulation and treatment with high concentrations of oxygen may produce respiratory depression with increasing CO_2 retention, the patient becoming drowsy or comatose. For this reason it is best to use oxygen in a concentration of 28 per cent by a mask using the Venturi principle (Ventimask or a Venturi head tent), or by using a nasal catheter with a flow rate of 4 litres/minute. This method should produce a pO_2 level of above 50 mm.Hg., which is usually considered safe. Even this method of oxygen administration can cause increasing CO_2 retention during the first few days, and a watch must be kept for CO_2 narcosis; estimations of blood gases and pH are invaluable (see p. 195). If respiratory depression does occur, *respiratory stimulants* should be used. These arouse the patient, increase the ventilation and induce coughing. Nikethamide is effective, and is given intravenously, either by intermittent injections (2 ml.), or by continuous infusion; too large a dose may produce twitching or convulsions.

Physiotherapy is important to assist the patient to clear the air passages of secretions.

Assisted positive pressure ventilation with cuffed endotracheal tubes or with tracheostomy may be lifesaving for the patient with some chronic lung disease whose air passages fill with mucopurulent secretions due to an acute respiratory infection; they should seldom be employed for uncomplicated chronic lung disease, as it may be impossible ever to wean the patient from them.

Diuretics (p. 115) should be given for dependent oedema and may improve alveolar ventilation by eliminating pulmonary oedema. *Digitalis* is disappointing in cor pulmonale but is indicated if atrial fibrillation is present.

Polycythaemia. In patients who develop severe secondary polycythaemia with a PCV of 60 or more great clinical improvement can occur after adequate venesection to lower the PCV to normal levels. This is best done with simultaneous infusion of dextran or Hartmann's solution into the other arm so that there is little disturbance of the circulating volume at the time of the venesection.

Sedation. All hypnotics are potentially dangerous because of the liability of producing respiratory depression. Morphia is contra-indicated. Treatment should be directed at relieving anoxia which is the cause of restlessness and mental confusion. However, when these symptoms are severe chloral hydrate or intramuscular paraldehyde are the safest drugs.

BRONCHIECTASIS

The essential pathological change in bronchiectasis is dilatation of the bronchi. It usually results from pulmonary collapse or as a complication of various types of pneumonia. In many patients the disease follows an attack of pneumonia complicating one of the childhood fevers, particularly whooping cough or measles. Plugging of some of the bronchi by sticky mucus lends to absorption collapse and dilatation of the bronchi in the related portion of the lung. At this stage the process is reversible if the obstructing plugs of mucus are removed by vigorous physiotherapy, that is by firm percussion on chest wall combined with postural drainage and 'assisted' coughing. If the bronchial plugging is allowed to persist for any length of time, however, inflammatory changes develop in the walls of the dilated bronchi and lead to permanent bronchiectasis.

Bronchiectasis also develops distal to a chronic bronchial obstruction, such as bronchial carcinoma or bronchostenosis. Pressure of tuberculous nodes on a bronchus, from childhood primary tuberculosis (p. 237), may lead to bronchiectasis in later life. This most commonly affects the middle lobe, producing the *middle lobe (Brock) syndrome*.

Pulmonary infection which heals by fibrosis, particularly tuberculosis of the upper lobes, commonly leads to associated bronchiectasis.

Sometimes an infective bronchiolitis results in a progressive form of the disease in the absence of pulmonary collapse. A similar widespread bronchiectasis commonly develops from a suppurating bronchiolitis in patients with fibrocystic disease of the pancreas.

Clinical Features. The clinical features of bronchiectasis are variable and depend on the extent of the disease and the degree of infection in the affected bronchi.

(1) *Classical Bronchiectasis.* There is a history of recurrent episodes of pneumonia in childhood—the first often occurring after an attack of whooping cough or measles. The patient has a cough productive of a considerable volume of purulent sputum which may sometimes contain blood. In the winter there are exacerbations of the condition with increased cough and sputum and with fever, and recurrent attacks of pneumonia may occur. Examination shows a thin patient who looks ill. Dyspnoea and cyanosis are present if sufficient volume of lung is involved. The fingers are often clubbed. Examination of the chest usually shows signs of fibrosis (see p. 203) and of retained bronchial secretions over the affected lobe or lobes. The physical signs may be few, perhaps only an area of persistent crackles, if healthy lung separates the diseased segments from the chest wall. If the patient is encouraged to cough, large quantities of foul sputum are expectorated, and his breath may, in addition, always smell foul. Such is the picture of classical bronchiectasis which is nowadays rare, and the majority of patients with this disease present in less dramatic form.

(2) *Other Types of Bronchiectasis.* Some patients with bronchiectasis have no symptoms at all, particularly those with bronchiectasis of the upper lobes where drainage is continuous. Such bronchiectasis is frequently the result of old tuberculous infection. In others recurrent haemoptysis, sometimes profuse, is the only symptom. Sometimes infection occurs only in the winter following upper respiratory infection and for the rest of the year the patient is well. In such patients there may be no physical signs, or simply persistent crackles over the bronchiectatic lobes.

Complications of Bronchiectasis. Patients are prone to recurrent attacks of pneumonia either in the affected lobe or in another part of the lung due to 'spill-over' of infected sputum. Spread of bronchiectasis and lung fibrosis may follow. Lung abscess and empyema may also occur. Haematogenous spread, from infected thrombus in a pulmonary venous radicle, may lead to cerebral abscess. If infection has been extensive and prolonged, amyloid disease may develop, but is now rarely seen.

Diagnosis. The chest radiograph may show no abnormality; more commonly there is some increased striation in the bronchiectatic lobe due to bronchial wall thickening and crowding of the blood vessels and cysts with fluid levels may be seen. Abnormal shadowing will be present if there is much associated fibrosis, with compensatory emphysema in the surrounding lung. The diagnosis of bronchiectasis is confirmed and its extent determined by *bronchography*. Radio-opaque iodised oil is introduced into the bronchi to make them opaque to X-rays. The right bronchial tree is outlined first and both postero-anterior and lateral views are obtained. The left lung is then filled and an oblique view taken. The diseased bronchi appear dilated, their walls are often irregular and their outline blurred.

Treatment. Management depends on the careful assessment of the patient's history and the extent of the bronchiectasis.

Surgical Treatment. This is rarely indicated. Young patients with a history of severe chronic infection which is not controlled by medical means can be considered for surgical treatment. The disease should be confined to one lobe and complete bronchograms are required to exclude bronchiectasis in other parts of the lung. Surgery is contra-indicated if the disease is too widespread, if there is coincident asthma or chronic bronchitis or if there is impaired ventilatory capacity.

Medical Treatment. In many cases the disease is not severe enough to warrant surgical treatment. In others the bronchiectasis is too extensive for resection, or the remaining lung is too damaged by chronic bronchitis and emphysema. Sometimes the patient's age or general health make operation impossible. In such cases medical treatment is usually remarkably effective, though clearly it cannot be curative.

The symptoms can nearly always be satisfactorily controlled and the complications largely prevented by regular and competent *postural drainage*. The patient is taught the position in which secretions will drain from the bronchiectatic area towards the main bronchi and the trachea. This enables sputum to be coughed up. The lower lobes are affected in the majority of patients. Postural drainage for this lobe is achieved by leaning face downwards over the side of the bed with the hands on the floor. Alternatively the foot of the bed is raised on 18-inch blocks, the patient lying on his face or side, according to the segments affected. Postural drainage of the right middle lobe is achieved by placing the patient on his back with a pillow under the right side of the chest and the foot of the bed is slightly raised. With upper lobe bronchiectasis, drainage will take place if the patient is sitting up, leaning towards the unaffected side. The appropriate position must be adopted for at least 10 minutes twice a day, and forcible coughing should be continued until no more sputum will come up. Drainage of the secretions can often be improved by 'clapping' on the chest over the affected lobe. The physiotherapist or the nurse may carry out this procedure, but later the patient's relatives will have to be instructed. Postural drainage should be carried out first thing in the morning as sputum collects in the dilated bronchi during the night. It should also be performed before retiring to bed and it may be necessary to repeat it before the midday and evening meals. A hot drink given before each treatment may increase expectoration.

A course of ampicillin or tetracycline, 250 mg. six-hourly, for one or two weeks may be given if the purulent sputum becomes more profuse, particularly if the patient also has fever and malaise. Sometimes continuous antibiotic treatment over the winter months may be considered. In patients with foul sputum there is often infection with the anaerobic organisms of Vincent's angina (Vincent's spirillum and the fusiform bacillus) and penicillin is the antibiotic of choice. No treatment is necessary in patients whose bronchiectasis is symptomless and without evidence of infection.

ASTHMA

Patients with bronchial asthma suffer attacks of wheezing and difficulty in breathing, due to bronchial spasm and sticky secretions. The cause of the disease is complex, and in most patients several factors contribute to its development.

In *extrinsic* (allergic) asthma both heredity and allergic factors predominate, and the condition usually starts in earlier life. A type I (anaphylactoid) hypersensitivity mechanism operates; inhaled allergen combines with reaginic antibody fixed to cells in the bronchial mucosa and damage to the cells releases histamine and various other spasmogens. Reaginic antibody has been identified with the immunoglobulin IgE. *Intrinsic* (late-onset) asthma usually occurs in later life. Allergy is usually not important and the condition is more often associated with bronchitis and psychological factors.

(1) *Heredity.* When asthma starts in childhood or adolescence there is more likely to be a family history of an allergic disorder, such as hay fever, asthma or urticaria.

(2) *Allergy.* There are a large number of substances to which the asthmatic may become allergic. They may be inhaled from the atmosphere or absorbed from the gut. The inhalants are the most important. Common examples are pollen and spores from plants, moulds (such as *Aspergillus fumigatus* and dry rot) dust of various kinds (such as house dust which contains mites which live on scales of human skin) and animal hair. Ingested allergens are less often to blame, but champagne and aspirin are classical examples.

The history is the best guide to the part that allergy plays. Eosinophilia suggests that allergy is important but may also be present with intrinsic asthma. If attacks occur only in the spring and early summer it is reasonable to suspect that pollens are responsible; or attacks may be induced by a particular food, by a drug, such as aspirin, or by proximity to a cat or dog. Skin tests can also be done. A drop of a specially prepared solution of the suspected allergen is placed on the skin and a superficial prick made through it. The result is positive if a raised wheal appears within 15 minutes. A positive skin test does not necessarily imply that the asthma is related to the particular allergen, and is only of significance if it coincides with the history. Allergy is more important in asthma starting in early life.

(3) *Infection.* When asthma starts later in life it often appears to

be complicated by chronic bronchitis and allergy is much less prominent. Respiratory tract infections, however, often precipitate asthma in asthmatic patients in whom allergy is also much in evidence.

(4) *Reflex Factors.* The bronchi are supplied by the vagus nerve, and various stimuli may induce attacks by a reflex mechanism. Common examples are sudden exposure to cold air, laughing, severe exertion, and heavy meals.

(5) *Pharmacological Factors.* Beta-blocker drugs, given for angina or hypertension, may precipitate asthma. Exertional asthma is probably precipitated by some mediator, as yet unidentified, which can be blocked by anti-allergic drugs, such as disodium cromoglycate.

(6) *Psychological influences* play some part in nearly every asthmatic and quite often they appear to be mainly responsible, if not in starting the asthma, at least in maintaining it. Treatment is not likely to be satisfactory unless these influences are appreciated, and the patient may require specific treatment for anxiety or depression.

Clinical Features. An asthmatic attack usually starts fairly suddenly and lasts about an hour or so, but the duration varies a good deal. Many asthmatics have a bad spell lasting some weeks, when they may be continuously rather wheezy with frequent acute exacerbations, especially during the night. A severe attack lasting more than a day or so is known as *status asthmaticus*. During an attack the patient complains of tightness in the chest and difficulty in breathing. There is often cough, dry at first, but towards the end of an attack some sticky, tight little pellets of mucus are produced. The sputum is purulent when there is associated respiratory tract infection or when it contains large numbers of eosinophils. On examination the chest is over-inflated and there are widespread rhonchi, particularly on expiration. Respiratory function tests show impaired ventilatory capacity due to airflow obstruction, which improves after inhalation of a bronchodilator.

The structure and function of the lungs return to normal between attacks. However, patients with long-standing severe asthma often develop emphysema and are then persistently short of breath.

Treatment. (a) *During Attacks.* A patient can usually abort or cut short an attack of asthma by using a pressurised aerosol containing *salbutamol*. The patient must be carefully instructed in its use; after breathing out fully the vapour is then inhaled and the breath held for a short period to allow absorption to take place. Patients must be warned that frequent repeated use of an aerosol containing isoprenaline or related substances may be dangerous, particularly if the asthma is not being relieved. Another valuable drug for severe attacks is intravenous *aminophylline* 0·25–0·5 g. in 10–20 ml. sterile water.

Severe status asthmaticus which has failed to respond to these drugs is a potentially fatal illness. Although the patient is exhausted by sleeplessness and by the effort expended on breathing, on no account must morphine or any other opium derivative be given. The resulting depression of respiration is liable to cause death. Any hypnotic is best avoided, but if restlessness is increasing the exhaustion to a dangerous extent, diazepam 2·0–5·0 mg. may be given but even this drug can cause respiratory depression. *Steroids* may be life saving but this effect is not immediate. The most rapid response is obtained by giving I.V. hydrocortisone 200 mg. three-hourly. Oral prednisolone is also started, giving 60 mg. on the first day, 40 mg. the next day and 30 mg. subsequently. Improvement usually occurs within a day or so and it is best to tail off the steroids over a period of 8–10 days, as long-term treatment is best avoided unless really essential. Status asthmaticus is likely to be associated with infection, either as a precipitating factor or as a secondary feature, and an antibiotic, such as ampicillin, is indicated.

(b) *Between attacks* the treatment of each patient has to be planned after careful assessment of the various possible causative factors indicated above. The aim of treatment is prevention, for the longer the patient can be kept free of attacks the less likely asthma is to return.

The psychological handling of the patient is of the utmost importance. The doctor must be a good and sympathetic listener and an atmosphere of calm confidence must be preserved at all times.

It is advisable for the asthmatic to avoid contact with various substances to which he is or may become allergic; the bedroom should be bare and spartan, containing no cushions, curtains or other soft furnishings which harbour dust; feather quilts should be avoided, and sorbo rubber substitutes should be used in place of feather pillows and hair mattresses. The bedclothes should be changed frequently when there is sensitivity to housedust mite. When there is clear-cut allergy—for example, to pollen—specific desensitisation may be attempted. This is done by giving a series of 7–9 subcutaneous injections of the allergen (ALAVAC-P) at weekly or fortnightly intervals, starting with a very small dose and gradually increasing it until the patient is able to tolerate quite a large dose, or in other words has become desensitised. The patient must be kept under observation for at least half an hour after each injection. Syringes containing 1:1,000 adrenaline must be available, and an injection of 0·5 ml. of adrenaline and 10 mg. of chlorpheniramine given at once if the patient develops any reaction, such as wheezing or faintness. If a reaction occurs at the next injection the dose is reduced slightly, and then steadily increased again over the following weeks. Desensitisation against pollens must be completed before the end of April, as severe and even fatal reactions may occur if injections are given when pollens are present in the atmosphere.

Regular administration of *ephedrine* is helpful for the prevention of attacks, young children being given 15 mg. twice or three times daily and older children or adults a dose of 30–60 mg. Ephedrine has a cerebral stimulating effect and if used at bedtime it may be necessary to combine it with a hypnotic to ensure sleep. It may also cause difficulty in micturition in elderly men with prostatic hypertrophy. It is best to continue ephedrine for a month or two. Alternatively, oral salbutamol 2–4 mg. three or four times a day may be used. *Choline theophyllinate* 200 mg. four times daily is of value at times. A rectal suppository of aminophylline, 0·36 g., before sleep often prevents a troublesome attack at night. The allergy blocker *disodium cromoglycate* 1 to 4 capsules a day may be of great value in prophylaxis of patients with *extrinsic* (allergic) asthma. It is administered by inhalation using a Spinhaler. When emotional factors are important tranquilliser or antidepressants may be used.

All asthmatics should be taught *breathing exercises* which should be carried out regularly.

Some patients with chronic asthma, usually of late onset respond poorly to bronchodilators and are controlled only by continuous steroid therapy, and in them the dangers of such treatment are outweighed by the benefits. Initial dosage of 30–40 mg. prednisolone daily is gradually reduced to the minimum effective level, usually between 5 and 10 mg. Alternatively, the asthma may be controlled by using a corticosteroid aerosol, such as beclomethasone, two inhalations three times a day, thus avoiding systemic side-effects.

CARCINOMA OF THE BRONCHUS

This disease has become much more common in recent years. It is now the commonest type of cancer in men, in whom it occurs four or five times more frequently than in women. The reports from the Royal College of Physicians and others have emphasised the importance of cigarette smoking as a cause of bronchial carcinoma. There is also some evidence that the incidence is higher in those who live in the polluted atmosphere of industrial areas. An increased incidence is reported in miners exposed to dust from chromium, nickel, and radioactive ores, and pulmonary asbestosis is said to increase its incidence by fifteenfold. About half the tumours arise within an inch or two of the bifurcation of the trachea. The remainder are peripheral. Histologically they are squamous adeno- or anaplastic carcinomas (the latter group including the less common oat cell carcinoma).

Clinical Features. A dry cough is the commonest early symptom. Recurrent haemoptysis may result from ulceration and sometimes this is the presenting symptom. Mucopurulent sputum occurs as increase in size of the growth produces progressive bronchial obstruction, then distal infection and shortness of breath develop with collapse of the lung segment supplied by the affected bronchus. A persistent wheeze due to the narrowed bronchus and dull deep-seated pain are not uncommon symptoms. Some patients are symptom free when the disease is discovered by mass radiography or remain so until one of the **complications** occurs. These are:

(1) *Pneumonic Infection.* The segment of lung beyond the bronchial obstruction is particularly liable to infection. Patients may present with a segmental pneumonia, which either fails to resolve satisfactorily or recurs repeatedly in the same area of lung. Such events should always raise suspicion of an underlying carcinoma.

(2) *Collapse.* Complete obstruction of a bronchus by carcinoma produces collapse of the lung segment supplied by that bronchus. The collapsed lung may become infected causing fever and toxaemia, but there may be little or no sputum because of total bronchial obstruction. Collapse may be associated with a pleural effusion on the same side, with the result that there is no mediastinal shift.

(3) *Lung abscess* may develop in an area of pneumonic infection (see above). When the growth is in the periphery of the lung its centre may become necrotic and be coughed up. This produces a ragged abscess cavity with walls which are composed of carcinomatous tissue, and which characteristically are thick and irregular when seen on a radiograph.

(4) *Superior vena caval obstruction* may occur from pressure of a growth in this situation. The patient complains of fullness in the head and face and may be in acute discomfort. There is oedema of the face and upper limbs, with gross distension of the neck veins and anastomotic veins over the upper part of the chest. Other causes of this syndrome are aneurysm of the ascending aorta, malignant mediastinal glands, malignant thymoma and haemorrhage into a retrosternal thyroid.

(5) *Local Spread and Pleural Effusion.* Carcinoma cells may invade the mediastinal lymph nodes and the pleura, giving rise to a pleural effusion which is often, but by no means invariably, bloodstained.

(6) *Atrial fibrillation* may occur due to direct involvement of the atria and sometimes is a presenting symptom.

Spread of the growth to the pericardium may produce a pericardial effusion.

(7) *Distant Metastasis.* Bronchial carcinoma may metastasise to the liver, the bones, the suprarenals, the brain, the skin, and the lymphatic glands, the deposits causing symptoms and signs referable to the organs affected. When secondary neoplasm is suspected and the primary focus is not apparent, the lungs are a prime area of suspicion and the chest should be examined clinically and radiologically for carcinoma of the bronchus.

(8) *The Nervous System.* Tumours occurring at the apex of the lung may involve the first rib and the lower part of the brachial plexus producing Horner's syndrome (see p. 264) together with pain down the arm with weakness and wasting (Pancoast's tumour). Both laryngeal and diaphragmatic palsy may occur due to invasion of the recurrent laryngeal and phrenic nerves. Lung cancer may present with cerebral metastases, and a chest radiograph should always be taken when a cerebral tumour is suspected. Occasionally patients with carcinoma of the bronchus develop neuropathies or myopathies or cerebellar degeneration (p. 327).

(9) *Endocrine.* Rarely Cushing's syndrome may be caused by a tumour producing an ACTH-like substance; or the tumour may produce an 'inappropriate' secretion of anti-diuretic hormone (ADH) with water retention and hyponatraemia. Hypercalcaemia may occur because of extensive deposits in bone but may also be due to production of a parathormone-like substance. Acute adrenal insufficiency may result from destruction of the adrenal glands by secondary deposits.

Physical Signs. There may be no abnormal signs in the chest in spite of well-marked symptoms or obvious metastases. The changes when present may be those of collapse, pneumonia, lung abscess, or pleural effusion. A combination of effusion with collapse is common. Clubbing of the fingers is frequent and hypertrophic pulmonary osteoarthropathy sometimes occurs; this causes pain and swelling in the fingers, wrists and ankles which may suggest rheumatoid arthritis, but the radiograph shows typical subperiostial new bone formation. The condition regresses if the carcinoma is resected. A careful examination should be made for secondary deposits in the liver and the lymphatic glands, particularly cervical and supraclavicular.

Diagnosis. A patient presenting with any of the above features should have radiological examination of the chest. This will confirm the presence of collapse, consolidation, effusion, or abscess cavity, or may show a mass spreading out from the hilum, or a peripheral mass.

If the diagnosis remains in doubt the patient should be bronchoscoped, and a biopsy of the suspected lesion removed for microscopy. Biopsy of scalene nodes or of clinically enlarged glands may confirm the diagnosis. Bronchoscopy will be essential if surgery is contemplated in order to assess the extent of the growth and its operability. Expert examination of the sputum for cancer cells is positive in 80 per cent of cases.

Treatment. The main hope of cure lies in *surgical removal* of the affected lobe or lung. Unfortunately, many patients cannot be treated in this way, either because the carcinoma has already metastasised or is too extensive, or because the patient is not fit enough to withstand the operation. With successful removal the five-year survival rate is about 20 per cent.

Radiotherapy can be used to produce a remission in patients unsuitable for surgery, and for oat cell carcinoma it is probably just as effective as surgery. It is extremely unlikely to destroy the growth, although occasional cures have been reported. More commonly it is used to relieve symptoms. It is of value in patients with superior mediastinal obstruction, and in those with haemoptysis, persistent cough or severe pain from bone metastases. It is best avoided in patients generally ill with advanced disease, or with large tumours, as it is likely to make them worse.

Cytotoxic drugs, e.g. cyclophosphamide, may also produce a temporary remission.

The average survival time of patients without treatment is about nine months from the onset of symptoms.

ADENOMA OF THE BRONCHUS

Bronchial adenoma is a benign tumour either a true adenoma or more often a carcinoid tumour. It rarely undergoes malignant change. It is much less common than carcinoma of the bronchus and occurs more often in women. It may present as recurrent haemoptysis or as bronchial obstruction with lobar infection. Diagnosis is confirmed by bronchoscopy. The adenoma should be removed surgically, usually with the affected lobe.

HAMARTOMA

This benign tumour of the lung is composed of a mixture of tissues normally present in the lung, particularly cartilage. It usually produces no symptoms and is discovered on the chest radiograph as a rounded opacity with clear-cut edges, a 'coin' lesion. There may be areas of calcification, best seen on tomography, when it may be impossible to distinguish it from a tuberculoma. Calcified glands and calcified lesions in other sites of the lung will be in favour of tuberculoma. Otherwise the likely differential diagnoses are an isolated secondary deposit or a peripheral carcinoma of the lung. Surgical resection may be the only certain way of establishing the nature of the lesion.

THE PNEUMONIAS

Classification can be based both on the nature of the infecting organism and on the anatomical distribution of the pneumonia.

(1) *Lobar pneumonia* is pneumonic consolidation confined to one or more lobes of the lung. It is due to infection by specific organisms such as virulent *pneumococci* and *Friedländer's bacillus* (*Klebsiella pneumoniae*). Infections with *Staphylococcus aureus* and *M. tuberculosis* may produce lobular or lobar pneumonia.

(2) *Bronchopneumonia* is consolidation occurring in patches around infected terminal bronchi. It may be confined to a small segment of lung, or with widespread bronchial involvement the infection will be scattered throughout the lungs. It is most often caused by organisms such as *streptococci*, *Haemophilus influenzae* and non-epidemic strains of *pneumococci*. These are normally present in the upper respiratory tract and can spread down the air passages to infect the terminal bronchi. The very young, the elderly and the debilitated are particularly prone and it is often the terminal event in a seriously ill patient. Bronchopneumonia is often the result of secondary bacterial invasion following an acute viral bronchitis.

Influenza may at times cause a fulminating bronchopneumonia due to super-added infection with *Staphylococcus aureus*, or less frequently with the *pneumococcus*, *Haemophilus influenzae* or the *haemolytic streptococcus*. In the early stages, *tuberculosis* starts as a localised patch of bronchopneumonia, but widespread *tuberculous bronchopneumonia* may occur.

(3) *Acute Virus or Rickettsial Pneumonias.* Pneumonia associated with influenza or measles is usually complicated by bacterial infection. There is a further group of virus and Rickettsial infections including ornithosis, Q fever and others which cause a patchy pneumonia.

(4) *Inhalation Pneumonias.* These vary from a small patch of collapse-consolidation associated with a viral respiratory tract infection to severe suppurative infection following inhalation of infected material.

(5) *Pneumonias secondary to disease of the bronchi*, such as bronchial carcinoma (p. 220) or bronchiectasis (p. 214).

BACTERIAL PNEUMONIAS

Pneumococcal Pneumonia

Clinical Features. Pneumococcal lobar pneumonia may occur at any age; it is quite a common terminal event in the lives of the elderly or infirm, but it may equally attack people in the prime of life. It is more common in the winter months, and usually occurs sporadically. It is due to infection with virulent strains of pneumococci.

The onset is usually sudden with shivering or even a rigor and sometimes vomiting. The temperature rises abruptly and fever remains continuous. The face is typically hot and flushed and cyanosis may be marked. The respiration rate rises out of proportion to the temperature. An acute dry pleurisy develops over the affected lobe leading to severe pain on respiration, so that the breathing becomes rapid, shallow, and sometimes grunting. The development of herpes on the lips completes the classical picture. A painful cough is common at this stage of the disease and the sputum may have a 'rusty' tinge.

Examination of the chest at the onset usually shows little except diminished movement on the affected side together with reduced breath sounds, and perhaps some râles or a pleural rub. After the first 24–48 hours, the signs of consolidation appear; dullness, bronchial breathing, whispering pectoriloquy, and bronchophony over the consolidated lobe. There is a polymorphonuclear leucocytosis.

In the days before antibiotics were available recovery occurred by crisis at about the seventh day, the temperature falling quite rapidly and the patient's general condition taking a sudden turn for the better. Antibiotic treatment modifies the course of the disease and the patient's condition usually begins to improve within 48 hours of starting treatment. As the signs of consolidation disappear they are replaced by coarse râles due to the liquefying inflammatory exudate.

In the elderly, lobar pneumonia may not produce the dramatic picture outlined above. There may be little fever and the diagnosis depends on finding signs of consolidation.

Chest radiography confirms the presence of lobar consolidation.

Complications

(1) *Delayed Resolution.* The time taken for the lung to return to normal, with disappearance of physical signs and radiological clearing, varies a good deal in different patients. If resolution is delayed for more than two or three weeks the possibility of some underlying condition such as carcinoma or bronchiectasis must be investigated. Alternatively the pneumonia may be due to organisms resistant to the antibiotic in use, such as the tubercle bacillus. This will require careful and perhaps repeated examination of the sputum. Bronchoscopy and bronchography may be required. Pneumonia responds slowly to treatment in patients with diabetes, cirrhosis, chronic alcoholism, or nephritis.

There remains a small group of patients in whom the pneumonia instead of resolving proceeds to fibrosis and chronic suppuration. Postural drainage and inhalations should be used, but the affected lobe may require surgical resection.

(2) *Effusions.* Since the advent of chemotherapy, empyemata have become uncommon but serous pleural effusions appearing about one to two weeks after the onset of the pneumonia continue to occur. Treatment is by daily aspiration with infusion of 500,000 units of benzylpenicillin into the pleural cavity until the fluid subsides. The pleural fluid should be cultured for organisms and systemic antibiotics should be continued. The site of the aspiration is determined by the position of the physical signs and by radiography. The majority of serous effusions subside within a week or so of treatment.

(3) *Empyema.* In a small proportion of patients the effusion becomes purulent and the patient's condition deteriorates. Fever recurs and becomes remittent in type. The patient looks ill and suffers from anorexia, malaise, and drenching sweats. Examination of the chest reveals signs of fluid (p. 203). A white count shows considerable polymorph leucocytosis. The diagnosis is confirmed by aspirating pus from the pleural cavity. Empyema is considered further on p. 254.

(4) *Heart Failure.* Cardiac failure complicated perhaps by cardiac arrhythmia, particularly atrial fibrillation, may occur in elderly patients. For treatment see p. 113.

(5) *Other complications* include pericarditis, endocarditis, and meningitis. Certain patients have severe headache and some neck stiffness in the early stages of pneumonia, although the cerebrospinal fluid is normal. The syndrome is called meningismus.

Staphylococcal Pneumonia

Clinical Features. Staphylococcal pneumonia may occur at any age. It can occur as a primary infection but more commonly as a complication of influenza. It is often part of a staphylococcal septicaemia and there may be a history of a recent boil or some other staphylococcal infection. Pulmonary infarcts may be secondarily infected with staphylococci.

The onset is often acute with malaise, vomiting, anorexia, and rigors. Pleurisy may occur. The sputum is purulent and may be bloodstained. Fever is characteristically remittent.

The *physical signs* are variable and often inconspicuous. They are often bilateral with patches of impaired resonance, reduced breath sounds and râles. Bronchial breathing may be present. *Radiography* of the chest confirms the presence of consolidation which often cavitates to form an abscess. Alternatively thin walled abscesses may occur which are distension cysts typical of staphylococcal pneumonia, particularly when part of a septicaemia. Empyema and spontaneous pneumothorax may also occur.

It is often striking that a lung riddled with pneumonia and abscesses can resolve completely with antibiotic treatment, but residual areas of fibrosis and cyst formation are not uncommon. The lung abscesses and pleural infection rarely require surgical treatment.

At times staphylococcal pneumonia complicating influenza becomes a fulminating infection.

The *diagnosis* is confirmed by sputum culture. The sensitivity of the organism to various antibiotics should be determined, as it may be widely resistant.

Friedländer's Pneumonia

Clinical Features. Pneumonia due to Friedländer's bacillus (*Klebsiella pneumoniae*) is not common. It usually presents as lobar consolidation and the onset may be acute although often it is insidious. Friedländer's pneumonia has a tendency to progress to lung sloughing with abscess formation and fibrosis. The mortality rate is considerable. The diagnosis is confirmed by finding the organism in the sputum, by culture or more immediately by direct staining.

Treatment of Specific Bacterial Pneumonias

General. Severe pleuritic pain is best treated with an injection of intramuscular pethidine 100 mg. or subcutaneous morphine 15 mg. The beneficial effects of these drugs in promoting rest far outweigh the dangers of respiratory depression. A persistent unproductive cough may be relieved by linctus pholcodine co. 4–8 ml.

If the patient becomes cyanosed, oxygen should be given. An oxygen tent or mask may frighten or distress the patient and careful explanation and reassurance are important.

Most patients can be allowed up five to seven days after the temperature has become normal, but this will be influenced by the patient's age and the severity of the illness. Breathing exercises should begin when the temperature falls and should be continued through convalescence, the length of which depends on the occupation and the home environment.

Specific Treatment. In practice it is not always easy to be sure of the nature of the organisms and culture of the sputum takes time or may be impracticable.

Pneumococcal Lobar Pneumonia responds satisfactorily to treatment with ampicillin 500 mg. 6-hourly.

The patient usually responds within 48 hours, but treatment should be continued for one to two weeks. If clinical response is satisfactory the treatment can be changed to ampicillin 250 mg. 6-hourly.

Other antibiotics are occasionally required when the patient is sensitive to ampicillin or when the organisms are resistant, such as may occur in pneumonia complicating chronic bronchitis or bronchiectasis. In these patients it is often advisable to use a 'broad spectrum' antibiotic, such as tetracycline 250 mg. four times a day or co-trimoxazole tablets 2 twice-daily.

Staphylococcal Pneumonia. Quite frequently, infection is due to penicillin-resistant organisms and if the patient is severely ill, there is no time to await the result of sputum culture or the clinical response to benzylpenicillin. Under these circumstances cloxacillin 500 mg. intramuscularly six-hourly should be given. Subsequent antibiotic treatment will depend on the response of the patient and the result of sensitivity tests, and it is advisable to continue treatment for several weeks because of the liability to relapse. If clinical response is satisfactory, cloxacillin can be given orally.

Recovery is usual in these severe cases but when staphylococcal infection is associated with *fulminating influenzal pneumonia,* the outlook is grave (see below).

Friedländer's Pneumonia is resistant to penicillin but responds to gentamicin 40–80 mg. 8-hourly. Many strains of *Kl. pneumoniae* are also sensitive to trimethoprin-sulphamethoxazole, cephaloridine, cephalexin and chloramphenicol. The sensitivity of the organism to antibiotics should be determined whenever possible. If abscess formation or fibrosis ensures, surgical treatment may be required.

Tuberculous Pneumonia

Tuberculosis may rarely present with lobar pneumonia or widespread bronchopneumonia, associated with severe constitutional symptoms. It will fail to respond to penicillin. The sputum of every patient with pneumonia which does not respond to ordinary antibiotic treatment must be examined, and the diagnosis of tuberculous pneumonia will be established by finding the organism.

Treatment is along the usual lines for tuberculosis (see p. 241).

Pneumonia Complicating Influenza

Influenza is sometimes complicated by pneumonia; this is rare when influenza is sporadic, but may become common during epidemics and accounts for the majority of deaths which occur.

Any type of pneumonia may complicate influenza. The most common is a localised aspiration pneumonia (see p. 229) and staphylococcal pneumonia also occurs. Of particular importance is the severe infection called *fulminating influenzal pneumonia.* There is an overwhelming toxaemia due to a combination of infection with the influenzal virus and the staphylococcus aureus. *Haemophilus influenzae* has also been implicated as the secondary invader.

Clinical Features. The onset of severe pneumonia complicating influenza is rapid, often alarmingly so. The patient has a simple attack of influenza which appears to be progressing in the usual way when over a few hours the condition deteriorates rapidly. The respiration rate becomes rapid, cyanosis appears, sometimes with a typical greyish blue colour (*heliotrope cyanosis*). There may be evidence of circulatory collapse with rising pulse rate and falling blood pressure. Pleuritic pain is uncommon. Examination of the chest shows evidence of patchy consolidation with scattered râles and perhaps an occasional area of bronchial breathing. Leucopenia is common.

Treatment. In *fulminating influenzal pneumonia* treatment must be started before the results of sputum culture are available. Antibiotics are therefore used which are active against both the *staphylococcus* and the *Haemophilus influenzae*. Benzylpenicillin 1·0 mega units together with cloxacillin 500 mg. and ampicillin 500 mg. intramuscularly six-hourly should be given immediately and subsequent antibiotic treatment will depend on the response of the patient and the result of sensitivity tests. Alternatively the antibiotics may be given by I.V. drip. Most patients require nursing in an oxygen tent. Circulatory collapse with a falling blood pressure can be treated with I.V. hydrocortisone 200 mg. four-hourly until improvement occurs.

VIRUS PNEUMONIAS

Most cases of so-called virus pneumonia have, in fact, an area of collapse-consolidation occurring at the time of a viral respiratory tract infection. This is the result of blockage of a bronchus with sputum with superimposed secondary bacterial infection. Infections with viruses, such as the adenovirus and influenza can affect the lungs producing pneumonia, but the roles of primary virus infection and bacterial infection are often in doubt. In these circumstances it is reasonable to give antibiotic treatment as for bacterial infection.

Mycoplasma Pneumonia

The organism *Mycoplasma pneumoniae* has features of both a virus and a bacterium. Although it is small and has no cell wall, at the same time it does not require a living organism for culture and is sensitive to the tetracycline group of drugs. It is not sensitive to the penicillins as these depend on their action on the bacterial cell membrane for their antibiotic effect.

Clinical Features. The disease starts with the general symptoms of a virus infection, namely malaise, anorexia, headache, backache, and sometimes depression, followed within a day or two by cough and sometimes pleurisy.

Venous thromboses may occur. Examination of the chest usually shows only a patch of râles or perhaps an area of impaired resonance and bronchial breathing. Radiography reveals an area of consolidation having a rather ground glass appearance and of varying distribution. There is no leucocytosis and the blood contains cold agglutinins and will produce nonspecific agglutination of the streptococcus MG.

Treatment. Tetracycline should be given in full dosage of 500 mg. six-hourly for a few days followed by 250 mg. six-hourly.

Ornithosis (Psittacosis)

The organism (*Bedsonia*) occurs widely among many species of birds and is intermediate between a virus and a rickettsia. The illness is caught mainly from parrots, budgerigars and canaries. It is an influenza-like illness and the patient may develop patchy consolidation in the lungs. Splenomegaly is common and rose spots resembling those seen in typhoid fever may be found. At times a severe fulminating pneumonia with considerable mortality may develop.

In the early stages the organism can be cultured from the blood or sputum and at a later stage a rising titre of serum antibodies can be demonstrated.

Treatment. The organism responds to tetracycline which should be given in full doses of 500 mg. four times daily.

Q Fever

The organism (*Rickettsia burneti*) is known to infect domestic animals such as sheep, cows and goats. Human infection probably occurs through drinking raw milk, from inhaling animal dust or from ticks. It is characterised by fever, toxaemia, cough and 'atypical' pneumonia. Q fever endocarditis may also occur.

Treatment. Tetracycline in full doses is effective but response is slow. Treatment may have to be prolonged, particularly with endocarditis when it may have to be continued for six months to a year.

INHALATION PNEUMONIAS

The aspiration of infected material into the lungs may give rise to pneumonia. The distribution of the consolidation depends on the quantity of material inhaled and its nature. If large amounts of highly infected or irritating material are inhaled, as when an anaesthetised patient inhales vomit, a widely distributed and severe bronchopneumonia involving both lungs may result. If a smaller amount of highly infected material is inhaled into a segment of lung it will result in pneumonic consolidation of that segment and unless aspirated material is coughed up or sucked out and the infection controlled, the consolidation may proceed to abscess formation (see below). Recurrent attacks of inhalation pneumonia, perhaps with abscess formation, are sometimes seen in patients with oeso-phageal obstruction from achalasia of the cardia or stricture, and are due to spillover of material from the oesophagus to the bronchi when the patient is asleep.

Much more common is aspiration of infected material from the upper respiratory tract in patients with coryza, sinus infections, or other upper respiratory tract infections. This is sometimes called *aspiration pneumonia* or *pneumonitis,* and abscess formation is unusual.

Aspiration Pneumonitis

Clinical Features. This is the commonest type of pneumonia seen in general practice. It is due to bronchial obstruction by mucus, with subse-quent infected lobular or segmental collapse. The mucus is *aspirated* from the upper respiratory tract at the time of a cold or sinus infection, or it may have a bronchial origin at the time of a bronchitis. The clinical picture varies considerably depending on the nature of the accompanying bacterial infection. At one extreme the pneumonitis may be discovered by chance on radiography, there being no localised or constitutional symptoms. With virulent organisms, however, the clinical picture resembles that of the specific bacterial pneumonias. Most commonly, a few days after a cold or bronchitis, the patient's general condition becomes a little worse and there is malaise, cough, continuing fever and sometimes pleuritic pain. Usually the only physical sign is a patch of râles over the affected area. Radiography of the chest shows an opacity due to an area of segmental collapse and consolidation. *Treatment* with ampicillin 500 mg. four times daily combined with simple postural therapy is usually satisfactory.

LUNG ABSCESS

The *causes* of lung abscess are:

(1) *Inhalation of infected material* into the bronchial tree. This material usually comes from the upper respiratory tract, particularly gross paradontal infection. It is liable to be in-haled when the cough reflux is suppressed during sleep, or when the patient is in a coma or under anaesthesia. Infected pus and blood clots may also be inhaled at the time of dental extractions or tonsillectomy. The material is inhaled into a bronchopulmonary segment and leads to segmental pneu-monia which breaks down to form an abscess. The contents are coughed up leaving a chronic abscess cavity usually in-fected with a mixed group of organisms. If they include var-ious anaerobes such as Vincent's spirillum, the pus may be-come putrid and lung abscesses are classified into *putrid* and *non-putrid* on this basis. Sometimes the breakdown of lung tissue is very rapid and the state is sometimes called *gangrene*

of the lung. Inhalation of foreign bodies or vomit may also cause lung abscesses.

(2) Secondary to breakdown of peripheral carcinoma or to bronchial obstruction from carcinoma or other causes.

(3) Abscesses may develop in the course of various *specific pneumonias,* namely staphylococcal pneumonia, Friedländer's pneumonia and tuberculosis.

(4) Rare causes include extension of an amoebic abscess of the liver through the diaphragm, actinomycosis, infected hydatid cyst, and abscesses developing during the course of a pyaemia.

(5) In a small proportion of patients with lung abscesses, *no cause* can be found.

The site of the inhalation lung abscess is influenced by gravity. As the unconscious patient lies usually on his side or back the most dependent segments in these positions are those most frequently affected. These usually include the segments supplied by the axillary branches of the upper lobe bronchi and the apex of the lower lobe.

Clinical Features. These depend on the underlying cause of the abscess. With 'putrid' lung abscess, onset of symptoms is usually acute. There may be a history of coma or an anaesthetic in the presence of parodontal infection, or of dental extraction or some other operation on the upper respiratory tract one to three weeks previously. The patient complains of fever, shivering, night sweats, malaise, and anorexia. Pleurisy is quite common. There is usually a cough with mucoid sputum; after some days, the abscess discharges into a bronchus and the patient coughs up large quantities of foul purulent sputum. This may be preceded by a foul smell to the breath and is pathognomonic of lung abscess.

When the abscess has discharged, the patient's general condition may improve but unless adequate treatment is given he continues to cough up large quantities of purulent sputum sometimes mixed with blood. If the abscess is allowed to become chronic there is the risk of cerebral abscess, of blocking of the abscess cavity with rapid deterioration in the patient's condition, and amyloid disease. The abscess may rupture into the pleural cavity leading to an empyema.

Clubbing of the fingers develops. The *signs* over a lung abscess are variable. Usually there is impairment to percussion together with râles and sometimes bronchial breathing; a pleural rub may also be heard. Both postero-anterior and lateral chest radiographs must be taken; the exact segment of lung involved will then be apparent. In the early stages the affected segment is opaque, but when discharge of the abscess has occurred a cavity can be seen containing a fluid level and sometimes a slough. The radiograph of a breaking-down peripheral carcinoma is characteristic, the walls of the abscess cavity being thick and irregular.

The white count shows a polymorphonuclear leucocytosis. The sputum should always be examined bacteriologically as the lung abscess may be secondary to a specific bacterial infection, such as the *Staphylococcus aureus*, Friedländer's bacillus, or *M. tuberculosis*.

Treatment. Treatment is initially by antibiotics and correct postural drainage. It is usual to start with intramuscular benzylpenicillin 0·5 to 1 mega unit six-hourly, but this may have to be changed depending on the result of the sputum examination or if there is a poor clinical response. The position for postural drainage is determined by the site of the affected segment; treatment must be intense, 4–6 times daily, and the patient must sleep so as to give the abscess dependent drainage.

With this treatment the lung abscess usually resolves. When the response is not satisfactory or when drainage is not occurring freely, bronchoscopy is required to exclude any obstruction to drainage, such as a carcinoma of the lung. External drainage is rarely required.

In a small proportion of patients in whom the abscess fails to heal and who are left with a grossly damaged lobe, resection may be necessary.

PULMONARY COLLAPSE

Collapse of the lung may occur in two ways:

(1) *Absorption Collapse.* If a bronchus either to a whole lung or to a segment of lung becomes completely blocked, then the air in that segment is absorbed into the blood stream and the segment collapses to a smaller size. The space formerly occupied by the collapsed lung is filled by any combination of the following:

(a) The diaphragm is elevated.

(b) The mediastinum moves towards the side of the collapsed lung (see 'palpation' p. 201).

(c) The remaining lung becomes hyperinflated, a condition known as compensatory emphysema.

(2) *Pneumothorax and Hydrothorax.* If air or fluid is introduced into the pleural space then the elastic tissue in the lung will contract and the lung will collapse to a smaller size, the degree of collapse depending on the volume of air or fluid in the pleural cavity. The mediastinum may be displaced to the opposite side if the pneumothorax or effusion is large.

Absorption Collapse

Bronchial obstruction may be due to several causes; the more important are:

(1) *Bronchial carcinoma*, or rarely bronchial adenoma.

(2) *Foreign material* in the bronchial tree. Mucus or inflammatory exudate may collect following an operation, but is also found in asthma, bronchitis, bronchiectasis, measles, and whooping

cough. Sometimes foreign material may be inhaled, for instance blood clot from the mouth following dental extraction, or foreign bodies such as beads, peanuts, or pieces of bone.

(3) *Compression of the bronchus from outside* may occur from enlarged lymph nodes in tuberculosis, sarcoidosis or Hodgkin's disease, or occasionally may be due to aortic aneurysm.

Both bronchial carcinoma and external compression of the bronchus usually cause collapse of major segments of lung. Mucus may also cause collapse of a major segment, but if inhaled into the finer bronchi may cause multiple small areas of collapse. Absorption collapse is usually followed by some degree of infection and sometimes this may be severe enough to lead to abscess formation (see p. 230). If the lung is not re-expanded within a month, permanent changes occur and the lung does not return to normal.

Clinical Features. The symptoms of collapse depend on the extent of lung involved. They may also be overshadowed by the symptoms of the underlying lung disease.

Obstruction of a large bronchus usually gives rise to dyspnoea, sometimes severe, and to a feeling of tightness across the chest. If infection occurs, there will be fever. Examination shows an increase in the pulse and respiration rate and perhaps also some cyanosis. There will be mediastinal shift towards the lesion with dullness to percussion and absent breath sounds over the collapsed area. Smaller segments of collapse may give rise to little in the way of symptoms or physical signs and can only be diagnosed by radiography. The interpretation of radiographs in this condition depends on a knowledge of the anatomy of the bronchopulmonary segments; both postero-anterior and lateral films of the chest are required to localise the collapsed segment.

Treatment. This is directed towards relieving the bronchial obstruction and controlling any pulmonary infection. This in turn depends on the underlying pathology, for often it is due to carcinoma of the bronchus.

In those cases occurring with bronchitis or asthma, where bronchial obstruction is due to a mucus plug, the patient should be positioned so that drainage from the obstructed bronchus is aided by gravity. The chest wall over the collapsed lung should be percussed and the patient encouraged to cough. Using these methods the plug is usually dislodged. Rarely, aspiration through a bronchoscope is required.

Post-operative Absorption Collapse is due to blocking of a bronchus by a mucus plug. A number of factors render this likely to occur:

(1) It is more common after abdominal and chest operations, for these make coughing painful and interfere with the clearing of mucus from the bronchi.

(2) Infections of the respiratory tract, such as a cold or bronchitis, increase bronchial secretions.

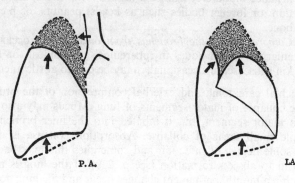

UPPER LOBE OF R. LUNG.

P.A.   LAT.

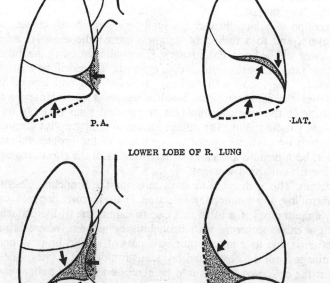

MIDDLE LOBE OF R. LUNG

P.A.   LAT.

LOWER LOBE OF R. LUNG

P.A.   LAT.

DIAGRAM OF RADIOGRAPHIC APPEARANCES OF LOBAR ABSORPTION
COLLAPSE

(3) The use of excessive amounts of atropine makes the sputum viscid and more difficult to clear from the bronchi.

Clinical Features. Post-operative collapse usually occurs within two or three days of operation. The symptoms and signs are those described under collapse (see p. 203).

The subsequent course will depend on the adequacy of treatment and the resistance of the patient, but if the condition is allowed to persist there is a danger of bronchiectasis and pulmonary fibrosis developing.

Treatment

Preventive

    (a) No subject with an acute respiratory tract infection should be given a general anaesthetic except in an emergency.

    (b) Patients with chronic respiratory infections should receive breathing exercises, postural drainage and in some cases, antibiotics, before a general anaesthetic. Smoking should be forbidden.

    (c) Infected teeth and sinuses should be treated before an anaesthetic.

    (d) Immediately after the operation the patient should be encouraged to clear sputum from the bronchi and his position in bed should be changed regularly to prevent stagnation of secretions in one part of the lung.

Curative

    (a) The patient should be postured so that drainage of the blocked bronchus is assisted by gravity.

    (b) Coughing should be encouraged. This causes pain from the operative incision which can be controlled by supporting the wound when the patient coughs, and by giving i.m. morphine 10 mg. The chest over the collapsed lung should be percussed rapidly and further coughing encouraged.

    (c) If these measures are not followed by improvement in the patient's condition over the next few hours, the mucus should be aspirated by bronchoscopy.

    (d) Oxygen must be given to those patients who are cyanosed and distressed.

    (e) Ampicillin 250–500 mg. six-hourly should be given to deal with any associated infection.

CYSTS OF THE LUNG

Cysts of the lung may be classified as follows:

(1) Congenital Cysts

Congenital cysts of the lung are due to maldevelopment of part of the primitive lung buds. They are lined with epithelium similar to that of the respiratory passages. They may be single or multiple.

Clinical Features. *In infancy* a single congenital cyst may have a valve-like connection with a bronchus so that air is sucked in during inspiration, but cannot be expired. The cyst expands until it interferes with respiration, causing distress and cyanosis. The situation can be temporarily relieved by inserting a needle into the cyst and connecting it by a rubber tube to a water seal. Further treatment is surgical.

Congenital cysts are also likely to become infected through their connection with the bronchial tree. Single cysts then present a picture similar to that of lung abscess and multiple cysts may be mistaken for bronchiectasis. Although antibiotics may control the infection and constitutional upset, postural drainage of the cyst is usually unsatisfactory due to inadequate bronchial connections; surgical excision of the infected cyst is therefore advisable when practicable.

(2) Acquired Cysts

These are much more common than congenital cysts of the lung. They have a variety of causes, but are basically due to stretching and breaking down of alveoli; they are not lined with respiratory epithelium. The chief causes are:

(a) *Acute lung infection*, particularly staphylococcal pneumonia (see p. 225).

(b) *Pulmonary tuberculosis* may lead to cavities with a stop valve connection with a bronchus. They become distended and take on the characteristics of cysts.

(c) *Emphysema.* Localised or generalised cysts of the lung may occur.

Clinical Features. Large bullae interfere with respiratory function, for they decrease the total alveolar surface of the lung, diminish mixing of respiratory gases and may interfere with the normal stretch reflexes arising in the lung.

Generally the alveolar over-distension and cyst formation are so widespread in both lungs that no specific treatment is possible, but bullae can occasionally be resected.

PULMONARY TUBERCULOSIS

General Considerations

Infection with the tubercle bacillus in a subject who has never previously experienced contact with the organism is called *primary tuberculosis*; re-infection after the primary lesion is called *post-primary tuberculosis*. The disease follows different courses in the two instances, the difference being attributed to the acquisition of antibodies in response to the primary lesion.

In Great Britain and the U.S.A., and most of the other countries of the

Western Hemisphere, infection is almost entirely with the human bacillus. In less economically developed countries milk still serves as a vehicle for infection with the bovine organism, and primary abdominal tuberculosis and its sequelae may occur.

The human bacillus is spread almost exclusively by droplet infection and lesions other than in the lung are uncommon. There is a wide range of susceptibility to the disease. Negroes, and dwellers in isolated communities, have little natural resistance. It is not a hereditary disease, but increased susceptibility may be inborn; if one of a pair of identical twins develops tuberculosis the other has a greatly increased chance of being affected, even if living in a totally different environment. Resistance may also be conditioned by such factors as malnutrition, overwork, and lack of sleep. The risks of infection are much increased by proximity, either from overcrowding of housing, or individual exposure, for example in dentists, and in doctors or nurses working in sanatoria.

Deaths from tuberculosis of all forms fell steadily in all civilised communities from the turn of the century. The rate of decline was so regular, with the exception of the war years, in the British Isles that it may be concluded that it was little influenced by any passing fancy in therapy and that the improvement was more likely to be due to public health measures. Since the introduction of effective chemotherapy death rates have declined precipitously.

PRIMARY TUBERCULOSIS

Characteristically the initial lesion is small and the local lymph nodes bear the brunt of the infection.

Pulmonary. A small pneumonic lesion (Ghon focus) may be situated in any part of the lungs. Lymphatic spread soon occurs and the local lymph nodes become enlarged. The radiographic appearance of a small shadow in the lung associated with hilar lymphadenopathy is known as the *primary complex*. It is accompanied by a change in the Mantoux reaction to positive (see p. 240). There is usually little upset in health and the natural tendency is to heal by fibrosis and calcification. In the past, primary tuberculosis commonly occurred in young people and up to 1950 over 95 per cent of urban dwellers had unknowingly healed such lesions before reaching adult life. Not all primary lesions heal spontaneously and without complications. As tuberculosis is now less common, an increasing proportion of children reach adult life without infection and it is these for whom protection is sought by vaccination with B.C.G. (see p. 243).

Complications. Sometimes the lung lesion increases in size to spread through the lobe, and rarely it may cavitate. This is more liable to occur in young adults, who are also prone to develop primary *tuberculous pleural effusions* (see p. 252).

In infants and young children particularly, the enlarged hilar lymph nodes may cause compression of a bronchus with segmental collapse, producing the radiographic appearance known as a '*hilar flare*'. This may lead to permanent bronchiectasis, such as in the *middle lobe syndrome* (p. 214). An infected lymph node may also rupture through the wall of a bronchus, the caseous material being discharged into the bronchial tree and causing a widespread *tuberculous bronchopneumonia* (p. 223). Alternatively, the lesions may erode blood vessels so that blood-borne tuberculosis may occur in such sites as bone, joints, kidney, epididymus, Fallopian tubes, brain, or meninges.

Miliary Tuberculosis

Miliary tuberculosis is due to widespread haematogenous dissemination. In primary tuberculosis it usually results from a caseous lymph node eroding a bronchial vessel, but it also occurs at times with post-primary lesions.

Clinical Features. The onset is usually insidious with general malaise, pyrexia, loss of weight, and sweats. Children often become listless and lose interest in their toys. Evidence of miliary spread through the lungs is not obvious early in the disease but later cough develops, with little sputum or dyspnoea. In some cases meningeal involvement is the most prominent feature and the patient presents with a tuberculous meningitis (p. 295).

Chest signs are either absent or confined to scattered fine râles. The spleen is often just palpable and careful examination of the retina may show choroidal tubercles. They are greyish-white lesions about one third the size of the optic disc. A chest radiograph shows the typical fine mottling of miliary tubercles throughout the lungs.

Treatment. This is along the usual line with chemotherapy (see p. 241). The prognosis is quite good provided meningeal involvement is not too advanced.

Primary Abdominal Tuberculosis

Bovine organisms gain access to the gut in infected milk. Small ulcers form in the small intestine and the infection spreads through lymphatics to the abdominal lymph nodes (*tabes mesenterica*). The nodes usually heal with calcification, but sometimes the infection spreads to the peritoneum (*Tuberculous peritonitis*). Miliary tuberculosis can result from involvement of abdominal blood vessels.

Tuberculous Cervical Lymphadenitis

The initial infection occurs in the tonsillar crypts and spreads to the cervical lymph nodes. These may become chronically enlarged and heal by fibrosis and calcification. They may undergo caseous necrosis, the pus tracking through the fascial planes to form a superficial cold abscess at some distance from the nodes ('*collar stud*' *abscess*).

Both the above are now uncommon in the U.K., except in immigrants.

POST PRIMARY TUBERCULOSIS

General Considerations. The infection is almost invariably pulmonary and usually occurs in the upper lobes or the apical segment of the lower lobe. The early lesion is a small area of tuberculous bronchopneumonia which radiographically appears as a soft shadow about 1 cm. in diameter. Spread is initially by direct extension to adjacent lung. Later *caseation* occurs and the necrotic centre of the lesion is discharged into a bronchus, producing a cavity in the lung, and cough with sputum. The infected sputum may be inhaled into other parts of either lung, producing new tuberculous lesions by *bronchogenic spread.* These may follow the same course. Peripheral lesions may cause *pleurisy,* which may progress to tuberculous *effusions* or empyema (p. 256). *Haemoptysis* occurs with erosion of blood vessels. *Tuberculous bronchitis* may produce a valvular obstruction to the bronchi draining a cavity, so that it distends to form a *tension cavity.* A *tuberculoma* is a blocked cavity with thick walls and full of inspissated material. It shows on the chest radiograph as a rounded opacity with clear-cut edges and may show areas of calcification.

The rate of progress of the disease is variable. It is rapid at times, but more commonly it is slow, the early lesion taking some years to develop into widespread tuberculosis. It depends on the extent and severity of the original infection and on the patient's resistance. The disease may become arrested at any stage, either permanently or temporarily, due to spontaneous healing by resolution, fibrosis, and calcification, or as the result of treatment. Alternatively widespread tuberculous bronchopneumonia, miliary tuberculosis, or metastatic tuberculosis may supervene. As opposed to *acute tuberculosis,* with infiltration and cavitation, a state of *chronic fibrocaseous* or *fibroid tuberculosis* may develop with gross fibrous contraction of the upper lobes and emphysema of the lower lobes. Respiratory reserve is then diminished and dyspnoea becomes a prominent symptom.

The expectoration of infected sputum may cause *tuberculous tracheitis, laryngitis,* or *tuberculous ulcers on the tongue.* Swallowed sputum may cause gastritis or tuberculous ulcers in the lymphoid patches of the *ileum.* The colon is usually spared, but tuberculous *fistula-in-ano* is common.

In patients with long-standing extensive disease, secondary amyloidosis may develop.

Clinical Features. Most patients with early tuberculosis of the lungs are free of symptoms but some present with haemoptysis.

The disease is usually well advanced by the time symptoms have developed. Classically they are chronic ill health, cough with mucoid sputum, low-grade fever, anorexia, tiredness, progressive weight loss, and night sweats. In advanced cases the patient appears ill, sweating and has lost weight, and the continual coughing up of infected sputum may spread infection and lead to further symptoms. Tracheitis causes retrosternal soreness, and laryngitis hoarseness and dysphagia. Tuberculous ulcers in the mouth, usually around the edge of the tongue, are extremely painful. Gastritis from swallowed sputum causes dyspepsia. As this may be a presenting symptom, pulmonary tuberculosis must always be considered in the differential diagnosis of dyspepsia. Tuberculous ileitis causes diarrhoea, and occasionally symptoms from bleeding, perforation, or obstruction. Fistula-in-ano causes a sero-sanguinous perianal discharge.

There are no abnormal signs from an early lesion. The first physical sign to appear is usually a small area of persistent fine râles at one or other apex, but by this time lung involvement is considerable. With more extensive disease there will be impairment to percussion, more widespread râles and sometimes areas of bronchial breathing if consolidation or cavities are near the chest wall. Fibrosis of an upper lobe leads to shift of the trachea towards the lesion, flattening and diminishing movement of the upper chest with impaired percussion note, bronchial breathing, and râles.

Signs of fluid will be present if there is an associated pleural effusion or empyema.

Investigations

Radiography is essential for diagnosis, to assess the extent and nature of the disease, to detect cavities and to follow progress. Both posteroanterior and lateral views are required at the start, and tomograms may be helpful to demonstrate cavities and delineate the extent of the lesion.

It is difficult to judge the activity of a lesion from a single radiograph. Cavitation means activity and soft fluffy opacities are usually of recent onset. Hard and calcified shadows suggest healing and inactivity. Serial films provide the best way of judging both the activity and progress of the disease.

There is no radiological appearance which is diagnostic of tuberculosis, although cavitating disease involving the upper lobes is extremely suggestive of it. Often the diagnosis depends on exclusion of other diseases or the confirmation of tuberculosis by sputum examination.

Sputum examination is essential in a patient suspected of having pulmonary tuberculosis. The finding of tubercle bacilli confirms the diagnosis and indicates that the disease is active and the patient infectious. Relatives and close contacts must be radiographed, sometimes repeatedly.

A random sample of sputum, stained by the *Ziehl-Neelsen technique*, may be examined by direct microscopy, or a 24-hour collection may be made, concentrated, and similarly examined. The sputum should also be cultured, as this increases the chance of finding tubercle bacilli and sensitivity tests to chemotherapeutic agents may be made. Guinea-pig inoculation is sometimes carried out, the animal being examined for tubercles after 6–8 weeks. Gastric washings, laryngeal swabs, and pleural fluid may be similarly examined. In general, the ease of finding the organism and the number found are indications of the extent of the disease.

Sedimentation Rate. A normal E.S.R. does not exclude an active lesion. A raised E.S.R. may be additional evidence of activity, and serial measurements are useful in following the progress of the disease.

Mantoux Test. Fixed antibodies to the tubercle bacillus develop in a patient with active tuberculosis, and persist after the infection has become inactive. There are rare exceptions to this; for instance, in some cases of overwhelming miliary tuberculosis. The antibodies can be demonstrated by injecting intradermally an antigen prepared from dead tubercle bacilli (tuberculin). An antigen-antibody reaction occurs in the skin, producing an area of redness and swelling and rarely ulceration. A *positive result* is judged as a papule larger than 5 mm. which appears within 2–4 days of injection. False positive results appear in the first 48 hours and last only a day or two. The test may be carried out by using a Tine skin prick test, or by hypodermic injection of a 1:10,000 solution of tuberculin; if this proves negative then in increasing strengths of 1:000 and 1:100 should be used. A positive result simply indicates the presence of antibodies and implies previous exposure; it is not a measure of activity. A negative result would indicate that a radiographic pulmonary opacity is not tuberculous.

Treatment. Active disease requires treatment, whereas healed disease only requires observation. It is not always easy to decide if a lesion is active, but it must be regarded so in the following circumstances:

(a) Clinical evidence of disease, i.e. fever and weight loss.
(b) Tubercle bacilli in the sputum.
(c) Radiological evidence of spread of the disease.
(d) The presence of cavities.

The *principles of treatment* are well established and include general measure to raise resistance, specific treatment, and local measures to the lung.

(1) **General.** With effective chemotherapy prolonged bed rest is no longer required, but the patient should be kept in bed if he is ill with fever or toxaemia. It need not be absolute for more than a week or two, after which most patients can be allowed to feed themselves, later to wash themselves and to visit the lavatory. Good food is essential. This means adequate, but not excessive calories, plenty of protein, with sufficient vitamin and mineral content. Iron and vitamins may be given as a supplement if necessary. The aim should be to regain, but not exceed, the normal body weight. Fresh air, bright surroundings and a cheerful atmosphere should encourage the patient towards recovery.

(2) **Chemotherapy.** Some general principles governing drug therapy may be stated:

(1) Chemotherapy is indicated if the disease is active.
(2) It should be continued for one to two years.
(3) No drug should be given alone. Combinations of the drugs should be used to avoid the emergence of drug-resistant strains of tubercle bacilli.

Treatment is started with three of the drugs to obtain a maximum therapeutic effect and to cover the possibility that the organism is resistant to one of the drugs. Sputum culture and tests of the organism's sensitivity to the drugs will subsequently determine this. For many years the three standard drugs in the treatment of tuberculosis have been *streptomycin,* *isoniazid* (INAH) and *para-aminosalicylic acid* (PAS). After about two months' treatment with these drugs, the streptomycin can be stopped and PAS and INAH continued as the long-term drug therapy. Streptomycin is given as 1·0 g. intramuscularly daily, although it is safer to give 1·0 g. on three days a week in patients over the age of forty because of the increased danger of vestibular damage. Similar care must be taken in patients with impaired renal function. INAH is given orally 300 mg. daily and PAS 12 g. orally daily. It is best to give these in a combined preparation, for otherwise if the patient fails to take one of the drugs (usually PAS) the organisms will inevitably develop resistance to the other drug. Both PAS and streptomycin are liable to produce hypersensitivity reactions, streptomycin may produce vestibular damage and PAS may cause intolerable gastro-intestinal upset. Under these circumstances, *rifampicin* or *ethambutol* can be used. In addition, these drugs are being used routinely as first-line drugs. Ethambutol may be used instead of streptomycin and is given in a single oral daily dose of 15 mg./kg. body weight and it is given for the first two months of treatment. It is also used for long-term therapy in combination with INAH. Optic neuritis has been reported when ethambutol was given in larger doses, when it was customary to check the visual acuity every four weeks; otherwise it is remarkably free of side effects. Rifampicin has an activity comparable to that of isoniazid and is being used more and more frequently as a long-term drug together with INAH, thus replacing PAS in the primary drug treatment of tuberculosis. Its major disadvantage is expense, and side-effects include cholestatic jaundice. It is given before breakfast as a single oral daily dose of 450–600 mg. (10 mg./kg. body weight), and is best given in a combined preparation with INAH (300 mg. daily).

Corticosteroids are of value in acute tuberculosis with severe toxaemia which is not responding quickly enough to chemotherapy alone.

(3) Local Measures

    (1) *Collapse therapy* for producing relaxation of the lung has been little used since the advent of effective chemotherapy. The procedures of introducing air into the pleural cavity (*artificial pneumothorax*) or into the peritoneum (*pneumoperitoneum*) have fallen into disuse. The latter was often combined with diaphragmatic paralysis, produced by crushing the phrenic nerve in the neck. Permanent collapse procedures have also been abandoned. These included the introduction of foreign bodies extrapleurally (*plombage*) and resection of ribs and allowing the chest wall to cave in (*thoracoplasty*).

    (2) *Postural Retention.* A tension cavity associated with bronchial disease can sometimes be closed by positioning the patient so that the cavity is dependent. Retention of secretions in the affected bronchus may change the bronchial obstruction from

being valvular to complete, with consequent closure of the cavity.

(3) *Resection.* Surgical resection and chemotherapy were both introduced at approximately the same time. It is now realised that with adequate longer-term chemotherapy, resection is usually unnecessary; it is reserved for certain selected cases.

  (a) Patients with localised cavitation which persists in spite of adequate rest and chemotherapy.
  (b) Some cases infected with tubercle bacilli resistant to chemotherapy.

The physician may be more inclined to advise resection in patients who will not persist with rest and chemotherapy, whereas such factors as extensive disease or the greater age of the patient will influence against the decision to resect. It should be performed while continuing chemotherapy and be followed by further rest and prolonged chemotherapy.

Treatment of the Minimal Lesion

A *minimal lesion* is a small area of infiltration without evidence of cavitation, which radiographically does not extend over more than one interspace. It is usually discovered on routine radiography and the patient is symptom free. Opinions on treatment vary, but it is probably best to admit the patient to hospital for a period, for rest, assessment of activity and institution of drug therapy. Thereafter the majority can be treated on an out-patient basis, leading sensible and well-ordered lives with adequate diet and rest. Chemotherapy is administered as on page 241, and rifampicin and INAH are the ideal long-term drugs, usually given for 9 to 12 months.

Prophylaxis

This includes measures to raise standards of hygiene and improve living conditions, and the detection of both early and infectious cases of pulmonary tuberculosis by routine radiography in countries where tuberculosis is still common.

Efforts have been made to increase individual resistance by vaccinating susceptible (Mantoux negative) subjects with an attenuated strain of the tubercle bacillus (Bacille Calmette-Guerin: *B.C.G.*). An intradermal injection of 0·1 ml. of the vaccine is made, and the appearance of a papule or ulcer at the site of injection within 10–14 days indicates a successful vaccination. It may be associated with enlargement of local lymph nodes and may take as long as three months to heal. Conversion of the Mantoux reaction to positive should occur between the 6th and 8th week after vaccination.

The World Health Organisation have used B.C.G. vaccination on an enormous scale in India, Africa, and some parts of Asia with few ill effects and benefits that are already apparent. It is available at chest clinics and infant welfare centres in the U.K.

OPPORTUNIST MYCOBACTERIAL INFECTION

Acid-fast bacilli distinct from *M. tuberculosis* may at times produce a lung infection which mimics an indolent form of tuberculosis. These different 'atypical' mycobacteria can be distinguished on cultures by their rate of growth and ability to produce pigment. *M. kansasii*, the commonest variety seen in this country, produces a yellow pigment when cultures grown in the dark are exposed to light.

Treatment. *In vitro* sensitivity tests invariably show these organisms to be resistant to streptomycin, isoniazid and PAS; depending on the results of the sensitivity tests, the infection is best treated with combinations of rifampicin, ethionamide and ethambutol. Response to drug therapy is slower than with tuberculosis and surgical resection may be indicated in some cases.

FUNGUS INFECTIONS

Histoplasmosis, coccidiomycosis and *blastomycosis* are fungus diseases of the lungs occurring in the U.S.A., but they are not endemic in this country.

Torulosis. Sporadic cases occur. It is due to infection with the yeast *Cryptococcus neoformans.* Pulmonary lesions may develop into cavitating granulomas, or into tumour-like masses. Infection may spread by the blood stream to the meninges mimicking tuberculous meningitis, even when the pulmonary lesions are small.

Treatment consists of surgical resection, where feasible, combined with intravenous amphotericin B. Cryptococcal meningitis has also been successfully treated with 5-fluorocytosine.

Aspergillosis. The fungus *Aspergillus fumigatus* is not pathogenic to the normal respiratory tract. It may infect pulmonary infarcts, and cysts or cavities which have resulted from such diseases as staphylococcal pneumonia, tuberculosis or sarcoidosis. A solid ball of fungus (*mycetoma*) grows free in the cavity. On tomography a crescent of air may be seen above the opacity, which can also be shown to move its position when the patient is tipped. Precipitins to aspergillus can be detected in the patient's blood. Recurrent haemoptyses may occur and the sputum may be thick and purulent.

A different and distinct syndrome results from hypersensitivity to aspergillus in the sputum. It produces asthma, recurrent areas of pulmonary collapse and increase of eosinophils in the blood and sputum.

Treatment. Inhalations of brilliant green or hydroxystilbamidine may be given; in severe infections I.V. amphotericin B or oral cotrimoxazole may be tried. In patients with asthma, corticosteroids are usually the only effective form of treatment. A mycetoma does not respond to this treatment; it is usually best left untreated, or in suitable cases resected surgically.

Moniliasis. The yeast *Candida albicans* is a normal saprophyte found in the respiratory tract and in the intestines. The administration of antibiotics may encourage its growth so that it may be abundant in the sputum but not necessarily pathogenic. It may, however, invade the mucosa, causing *thrush* in the mouth and pharynx, and at times in the oesophagus and in the trachea and bronchi; it may also cause diarrhoea and ano-genital pruritus. It is debatable whether monilial infection of the lung itself occurs. Rarely, in debilitated patients and in patients on treatment with antibiotics, steroids and cytotoxic drugs (with such diseases as leukaemia and reticuloses), blood stream infection and meningitis may occur.

Treatment. Nystatin by mouth, 4 ml. t.d.s. (100,000 units per ml.), is the drug of choice. Inhalations of nystatin or brilliant green may be used for bronchial moniliasis. In the rare systemic infections intravenous amphotericin B or oral 5-fluorocytosine may also be used.

DUST DISEASES OF THE LUNGS (The Pneumoconioses)

Silicosis

Silicosis is due to the inhalation of fine particles of free silica. It occurs in coal miners, and in the granite and sandstone industries, in metal foundries, in various grinding processes in which sandstone is used and in the pottery industry.

The earliest change is the development throughout the lungs of fine, fibrotic nodules around the particles of silica. As the disease develops these nodules increase in size and coalesce until finally there are large areas of fibrosis. Tuberculosis may complicate the picture.

Clinical Features. In the early stages there are no symptoms or signs and the diagnosis depends on the radiographic picture of diffuse mottling combined with a history of exposure.

The first symptom is dyspnoea on effort and later cough with mucoid sputum develops. Eventually the patient becomes severely disabled and death occurs from bronchopneumonia, tuberculosis or cor pulmonale.

Prevention consists of adequate exhaust ventilation, damping down the dust and personal protection by means of masks. All people exposed to silica dust should have regular chest radiographs.

Treatment. There is no specific treatment and those showing evidence of the disease must be removed from exposure to dust.

Asbestosis

The inhalation of asbestos fibres, which are silicates, causes a progressive diffuse fibrosis of the lungs, particularly the lower lobes. Blue asbestos (crocidolite) is more destructive than white asbestos (chrysolite). The chief symptoms are cough and dyspnoea and the clinical picture is that of fibrosing alveolitis (p. 249); *asbestos bodies*, formed of asbestos fibres and fibrin, can be found on microscopy of the sputum. Preventative measures are similar to those used in silicosis. Carcinoma of the bronchus is a common complication and malignant mesothelioma of the pleura also occurs. Calcified pleural plaques also occur in workers exposed to asbestos dust.

Coal Miners' Pneumoconiosis

A special type of pneumoconiosis affects miners who inhale coal dust, rather than rock dust which produces silicosis. In this country it is most prevalent in the South Wales coal-fields. There are two types:

(1) *Simple Pneumoconiosis*. Radiographically there is diffuse reticulation at first. Later scattered small nodules up to 5 mm. in diameter develop, often with surrounding emphysema. The disease is only progressive if the worker remains exposed to dust.

(2) *Progressive Massive Fibrosis*. Radiographically there are large dense shadows mostly in the mid and upper zones, with surrounding emphysema. It probably represents a massive fibrotic response to low grade inflammation. Although tuberculous infection or infection with atypical mycobacteria may be suspected, usually it cannot be proved. It is progressive even if the subject is no longer exposed to coal dust.

Clinical Features. There are no symptoms in the early stages. In the later stages of simple pneumoconiosis and with massive fibrosis dyspnoea on exertion is a prominent symptom. Cough and sputum, sometimes blackened by coal dust, develop and recurrent bronchitis is common. In advanced cases the patient becomes grossly disabled and death from cor pulmonale is usual.

Prevention. Of importance are adequate ventilation and reduction of dust by damping it down with water, by wet drilling and wet cutting. Masks are not very satisfactory as they interfere with the performance of heavy work. Chest radiographs at regular intervals should be carried out on all workers at risk, and those showing evidence of pneumoconiosis should be removed from further exposure to coal dust.

Byssinosis

Byssinosis is due to exposure to dust arising from the processing of cotton. It is believed to be an unusual allergic reaction of the bronchi to cotton dust. In the early stages of the disease the patient complains of dyspnoea, tightness in the chest, and cough which characteristically occurs on Mondays when the patient returns to work. Later the dyspnoea and cough becomes permanent and finally emphysema develops. Prevention is by adequate ventilation.

PULMONARY EOSINOPHILIA

There is a group of conditions characterised by a varying degree of constitutional upset, cough, transient infiltration of the lung and eosinophilia in the blood.

The *chief causes* of this syndrome are:

(1) *Worm and Parasite Infiltration.* Pulmonary infiltration and eosinophilia may result from the migration through the lungs of the larvae of *Ascaris lumbricoides* (see p. 573 or *p. 570 in Special Tropical Edition*).

(2) *Asthma.* Some patients may develop patchy areas of consolidation with eosinophilia during asthmatic attacks. Sometimes this is associated with the presence in the sputum of *Aspergillus fumigatus*, to which the patient has become sensitised. Skin test to *Aspergillus* is positive and antibodies may be detected in the blood.

(3) *Tropical Eosinophilia.* This is a well-defined clinical entity, occurring in tropical countries, particularly India and Pakistan, and probably due to microfilarial infestation. The symptoms may be acute or chronic with fever, cough, malaise, and attacks of dyspnoea. Radiography may show miliary mottling and there is always a high eosinophilia.

The condition usually responds to diethylcarbamazine in oral doses of 4·0 mg./kg. body weight, t.d.s. for four days.

(4) *Polyarteritis Nodosa.* Transient infiltration of the lung with eosinophilia, often with associated asthma, may occur in polyarteritis nodosa.

SARCOIDOSIS

Sarcoidosis is a disease in which epithelioid cell tubercles, without caseation, are present in all the affected organs. The older lesions become converted to hyalinised fibrous tissue. A similar granulomatous lesion is sometimes seen on biopsy, for example, of skin or lymph node, in quite unrelated conditions such as carcinoma or reticuloses. This *sarcoid reaction* must be distinguished from the disease sarcoidosis.

A few patients with sarcoidosis develop frank pulmonary tuberculosis. The aetiology of sarcoidosis is not known, but tuberculosis is favoured by some authorities in this country. There is also an immunological defect present, with depression of the delayed type of hypersensitivity response in most patients.

Clinical Features. The three commonest clinical presentations are:

(1) *Erythema nodosum* with *bilateral hilar node enlargement, fever* and often *polyarthritis.*

(2) *Routine chest radiography.* The patient is commonly symptom free and an apparently healthy young adult. The radiograph may show hilar node enlargement, or hilar nodes with pulmonary mottling, or mottling alone. If the patient is breathless it is likely that long-standing fibrotic sarcoid will be present.

(3) *Iridocyclitis*. This is commonly acute and transient. It may, however, be insidious and persistent with keratic precipitates forming in the anterior chamber, adhesion of the iris to the lens and obstruction of the angle of the anterior chamber leading to glaucoma. The choroid and retina may also be involved.

Other organs which may be involved include the *spleen, lymph nodes, liver* and *salivary glands*. *Skin lesions* are characteristically few, sharply defined, brownish in colour with a predilection for the face. They may persist for months or even years; they are benign, do not ulcerate and involute spontaneously, leaving either no trace or a pigmented or atrophic scar. *In the nervous system* a granulomatous basal meningitis may produce pituitary lesions or cranial nerve lesions. *Cystic bone change* may occasionally occur, usually in the heads of the metacarpals. *Hypercalcaemia* may be present and probably represents an abnormal sensitivity to vitamin D. Rarely the *heart* is involved, leading to congestive failure, or sudden death.

Investigations

Chest radiograph is essential. Pulmonary involvement is one of the main features of the disease, and it can only be assessed by following the changing radiological picture.

Tuberculin Reaction. A negative Mantoux reaction supports the diagnosis. However, as one third of the patients with proved sarcoidosis give a positive reaction to 10 TU (1:1,000 old tuberculin), a positive reaction does not exclude it. If a patient with sarcoidosis and a negative Mantoux reaction is treated with corticosteroids, the reaction then becomes positive; this is almost diagnostic of sarcoidosis.

Plasma Proteins. In approximately one third of cases there are raised α_2 and/or γ globulins present. This probably indicates activity of the disease.

Kveim Test. The intradermal injection of a saline suspension of sarcoid tissue obtained from spleen or lymph node of patients with active sarcoidosis is followed by the development of a nodule in the skin within the next six weeks. Biopsy of this nodule will show sarcoid histology. The test is positive in about 70 per cent of cases of sarcoidosis.

Biopsy of skin lesions or affected glands will confirm the diagnosis. Liver biopsy is positive in about 50 per cent of patients with sarcoidosis, even when there is no clinical evidence of involvement of the liver.

Respiratory function tests are only abnormal when there is marked pulmonary mottling, when the main defects are those of *compliance* (p. 197) and *gas transfer* (p. 196). In the later stages of pulmonary fibrosis impairment of *ventilation* may be marked.

Progress and Treatment

There is no evidence that anti-tuberculous chemotherapy influences the course of the disease.

Steroids are indicated in iridocyclitis because of the danger to sight, and local instillation of drops is usually sufficient. Steroids are also indicated with hypercalcaemia, because of the danger of renal failure.

Erythema nodosum and hilar node enlargement carries a good prognosis. With hilar node enlargement 70 per cent of patients improve spontaneously; the remainder develop pulmonary infiltration. With pulmonary infiltration 50 per cent of patients improve spontaneously; if this has not occurred within two years then it is unlikely to remit subsequently. The infiltration may then remain unchanged with little or no disability to the patient, but in a proportion it progresses to severe fibrosis with associated bronchiectasis and bullous change. These patients become respiratory cripples and eventually succumb to cor pulmonale (p. 212).

No specific treatment is indicated in patients with hilar node enlargement. Steroids are usually indicated in patients with pulmonary mottling showing no sign of resolution after a year. It often produces symptomatic relief and hastens resolution, and is aimed at preventing the development of severe fibrosis. Prednisolone 20 mg. daily is a satisfactory starting dose. A daily maintenance dose of 5 to 10 mg. may be required for several years, as relapse may occur if treatment is too short. Steroids have no effect on the lungs in the fibrotic stage but may help to relieve symptoms.

Once the disease has remitted it does not recur.

PULMONARY FIBROSIS

Generalised Pulmonary Fibrosis

This is relatively uncommon. The causes are:

(1) The pneumoconioses (p. 245).
(2) As an end result of infiltration of the lungs by a variety of pathological processes, including sarcoidosis (p. 247), and some of the generalised lipoidoses.
(3) Fibrosing alveolitis.

Fibrosing alveolitis (Chronic interstitial pulmonary fibrosis)

This is a generalised disorder of the alveolar walls in which inflammatory changes advance to progressive fibrosis. It may occur in association with the collagen diseases, such as rheumatoid arthritis and scleroderma, or be of an idiopathic variety with no known cause. Allergic forms of fibrosing alveolitis where inhalants produce a type 3 sensitivity reaction in the alveolar walls, are being more frequently recognised. *Farmer's lung* where there is sensitivity to spores in mouldy hay, and *Bird fancier's lung*, where there is a sensitivity to bird protein, are examples of this. In the latter cases precipitins to the protein of birds, such as pigeons and budgerigars, may be detected in the patient's blood.

Clinical Features. Dyspnoea is the leading symptom and cough, though usually present, is not associated with much sputum. Clubbing of the fingers is common in more advanced cases. Examination of the chest often shows fine râles, particularly at the bases, and late inspiratory rhonchi may be heard. The chest radiograph shows fine diffuse mottling most marked at the bases. Respiratory function tests indicate that the main defect is that of gaseous exchange across the alveolar membrane (see Gas Transfer, p. 196). The progress of the disease may at times be very slow, but the final outcome is death from hypoxia and right ventricular failure.

Treatment. If there are known or suspected allergens present these must be removed from the patient's environment; a course of steroids may be very effective in tiding the patient over an acute episode in the allergic variety. On the whole the treatment is not very satisfactory in the idiopathic variety or in those cases associated with collagen disease. Steroids may limit the fibrosis and relieve dyspnoea in some patients provided the fibrosis is not too advanced. Steroid therapy may have to be continued indefinitely in the smallest possible maintenance dose to maintain improvement, usually prednisolone 5 to 10 mg. daily, as severe relapse may occur when it is stopped. Advanced cases are helped by oxygen therapy in the home and by portable oxygen.

Localised Pulmonary Fibrosis

Fibrosis of the lungs is commonly localised to one or more lobes, or even a segment of a lobe. It is usually the result of inflammation and common causes are tuberculosis, unresolved pneumonia, chronic lung abscess and long-standing collapse. Bronchiectasis invariably develops in such fibrotic segments or lobes. Persistent infection is not common with fibrosis of the upper lobes because drainage is adequate.

Clinical Features. In some patients there are no symptoms, except perhaps the history of the original illness which led to the fibrosis. This is often the case with healed, fibrotic tuberculosis of the upper lobes, and no treatment is required.

In others the clinical picture is that of the accompanying *infected bronchiectasis*, both with regard to symptoms and complications (see p. 214). Diagnosis and treatment are also discussed under this section.

The physical signs of fibrosis include flattening of the chest overlying the lesion with diminished movement, impaired percussion note, bronchial breathing, whispering pectoriloquy, and bronchophony. The mediastinum is shifted towards the side of the lesion and coarse râles are present with associated bronchiectasis.

DISEASES OF THE PLEURA

PLEURISY

Inflammation of the pleura may be *dry* or associated with *effusion*, the former often proceeding to the latter.

DRY PLEURISY

It may be due to:

(1) *Pneumonia* either bacterial or viral.

(2) *Pulmonary infarct* (p. 180).

(3) *Tuberculosis*. This variety nearly always progresses to pleurisy with effusion.

(4) *Lung abscess*.

(5) *Epidemic pleurodynia* (Bornholm Disease). This is a Coxsackie virus infection which may occur in outbreaks. It affects the muscles of the chest wall and produces a primary pleurisy without lung involvement.

(6) *Injury* to the chest and lungs.

Clinical Features. The cardinal symptom of dry pleurisy is *pain*, described on p. 199.

On examination the respirations may be short and grunting, for severe pleuritic pain limits inspiration. The diagnosis is confirmed by finding a *pleural rub*, which is a superficial grating or crunching sound related to respiratory movements. It appears to arise just under the stethoscope, which indeed it does, and characteristically comes and goes. Occasionally a pleural rub may be heard in a patient who makes no complaint of pain.

Chest radiography may reveal underlying disease if present, but shows no specific sign of dry pleurisy. Screening may show diminished movement of the chest and diaphragm on that side.

Treatment. Bed rest and analgesics are required. Tabs. codeine co. 2 four-hourly, pethidine 50–100 mg. intramuscularly or hypodermic morphine 15 mg. may all be used, depending on the severity of the pain. Some patients obtain relief by applying a hot-water-bottle over the area. Specific treatment is that of the underlying lesion, and subsequent management will depend on this.

PLEURISY WITH EFFUSION

Fluid in the pleural cavity may represent a transudate or an exudate.

Transudates occur when the osmotic pressure of the plasma is reduced (the nephrotic syndrome or cirrhosis of the liver) or when the venous pressure is high (congestive cardiac failure or constrictive pericarditis). The fluid in a transudate is usually clear and of low specific gravity. It contains less than 2·0 g. protein per 100 ml.

Causes of pleural transudates are:

(1) *Cardiac failure*.

(2) *Nephrotic syndrome*.

(3) *Cirrhosis of the liver*.

Exudates occur in the presence of inflammation or neoplasm. They are of high specific gravity and contain more than 2·0 g. protein per 100 ml.

Exudates may be clear (tuberculous, neoplastic disease). Cloudiness may be due to blood (neoplasm, pulmonary infarct) or pus cells (pneumonia or lung abscess).

Causes of pleural exudates are:

(1) *Tuberculosis.*
(2) Complicating *pneumonia.*
(3) *Neoplasm.*
(4) *Subphrenic abscess,* and complicating other inflammatory lesions outside the chest.
(5) *Pulmonary infarction.*
(6) During the course of some *collagen diseases,* notably systemic lupus erythematosis.
(7) Complicating fibroma of the ovary (*Meigs' syndrome*).

Tuberculous Pleural Effusion

(1) **Effusion Associated with Primary Tuberculosis.** This is the common type of tuberculous effusion and usually occurs between the ages of fifteen and thirty and within a year of Mantoux conversion. It is believed that at this stage the tissues are sensitised to the tubercle bacillus, and if bacilli reach the pleura there is an acute inflammatory reaction with an out-pouring of fluid into the pleural cavity.

Clinical Features. The onset is variable. Sometimes it is acute with fever, malaise, sweating, and severe pleuritic pain. Other patients have little pain but complain of vague ill-health and dyspnoea on effort. Occasionally an effusion may be found on routine examination or chest radiograph in a patient with no symptoms.

Examination shows the typical signs of effusion (see p. 203). If it is large there is mediastinal shift to the opposite side, with flat dullness on percussion and absent breath sounds over the effusion.

Chest radiograph shows the effusion as an opacity at the base of the hemithorax. It obliterates the costophrenic angle and rises up into the axilla. The mediastinum may be displaced to the opposite side. It is unusual to see any intrapulmonary lesion.

Diagnosis is confirmed by aspiration of a sample of fluid. It is straw-coloured and contains cells, most of which are lymphocytes, although in the early stages polymorphs may predominate. Tubercle bacilli can be isolated from the fluid by culture or guinea-pig inoculation in about 50 per cent of cases.

The *course* is usually towards resolution. There is a potential danger of the infection spreading and occasionally miliary tuberculosis, renal tuberculosis, or tuberculous meningitis occurs. Slow absorption of a large effusion may lead to pleural fibrosis, with subsequent restriction of lung expansion and contraction of the chest wall. Before chemotherapy was available about 25 per cent of patients developed frank tuberculous lesions in the lungs within five years of an effusion.

Treatment. The aims are to eradicate the infection and to prevent serious residual pleural fibrosis by encouraging rapid clearing of the effusion.

Antitubercular drugs should be given for 12 months, starting with triple chemotherapy (p. 241). Unless the effusion appears to be disappearing rapidly aspiration should be carried out every 2 or 3 days until no further fluid can be removed. Half to one litre should be removed at each aspiration. Fluid should be removed without delay if there is much mediastinal shift or if the patient is short of breath. Effusions which do not resolve, or which keep reforming in spite of these measures, may be treated in addition with corticosteroids. The steroid therapy need not be prolonged and must be combined with chemotherapy; prednisolone 20 mg. daily reducing to a maintenance dose of 10–15 mg. daily for 6 weeks is satisfactory.

Bed rest should be continued until the effusion has cleared usually a month to 6 weeks. The patient should then make a gradual return to full activity and should remain off work for 3 to 6 months. Follow-up supervision with chest radiographs is essential as with other forms of tuberculosis.

Effusion with Post-primary Tuberculosis

Effusions may develop with post-primary pulmonary tuberculosis and usually indicate severe pleural tuberculosis. They resolve more slowly than effusions associated with primary tuberculosis, being more resistant to treatment and being liable to develop into tuberculous empyemata. They occurred as a complication of artificial pneumothorax, when this was used as therapy for tuberculosis.

Treatment. One pint of pleural fluid should be aspirated every other day until the pleural cavity is dry.

The subsequent management depends on the nature of the underlying lung disease, and will require bed rest and systemic chemotherapy (see p. 241).

Neoplastic Pleural Effusion

Malignant effusion is most commonly due to carcinoma of the bronchus. It also occurs with spread of extra-thoracic growth to the pleura, such as carcinoma of the breast, stomach, kidney, ovary, or testicle. Pleural effusions are not uncommon in Hodgkin's disease.

Clinical Features. The degree of general ill-health is variable and depends on the extent and nature of the primary neoplasm. The effusions are often of insidious onset, but as they usually become large dyspnoea is a common symptom. The fluid usually reaccumulates rapidly after aspiration; it is often blood-stained and may contain malignant cells.

Treatment. The patient must be kept comfortable by repeated aspiration; usually large quantities can be removed without danger. It is sometimes possible to prevent or slow down the reaccumulation of fluid by radiotherapy or by the introduction of nitrogen mustard into the pleural space.

Effusions associated with breast carcinoma may respond to hormone treatment.

Blood-stained Pleural Effusions

Blood-stained effusions are not uncommon. The chief causes are:

(1) Neoplasm, commonly bronchial carcinoma.
(2) Pulmonary infarct.
(3) Rarely tuberculosis.
(4) A haemothorax which has been diluted by a pleural exudate may have the appearance of a blood-stained effusion.

HAEMOTHORAX

Haemothorax may follow trauma to the chest wall. It also occurs with a spontaneous pneumothorax, presumably from rupture of pleural adhesions; it is then a haemopneumothorax. Rarely an aneurysm may leak into the pleural cavity.

Blood in the pleural cavity clots rapidly and fibrin is deposited on the pleural surfaces. Pleural reaction also occurs, with outpouring of further fluid. If the blood is left in the pleura, organisation with pleural fibrosis occurs with subsequent serious interference with lung function.

Clinical Features. If the pleural bleeding is large and rapid the patient will be shocked and collapsed, with rapid pulse and respiration. There may or may not be evidence of trauma to the chest. There are *signs* of pleural fluid (p. 203) or in those cases complicating a pneumothorax the signs are those of both fluid and air in the chest.

Diagnosis is confirmed by aspiration of blood from the pleural space. It is important to distinguish between a frank haemothorax and a blood-stained effusion.

Treatment. The general treatment for internal haemorrhage should be given. Morphine may be required, the patient's blood group should be determined and a transfusion given when necessary.

The effusion should be aspirated and the pleural space kept as dry as possible by further daily aspiration. Antibiotics should be given during the period of aspirations as there is a danger of secondary infection, usually staphylococcal.

Severe bleeding or serious damage to the chest wall will require surgical treatment. Thoracotomy is also necessary when the blood cannot be evacuated by aspiration.

EMPYEMA

Empyema may be defined as a localised collection of pus in the pleural cavity. It most commonly results from a pneumonia, usually pneumococcal lobar pneumonia. It may also be due to spread of infection from a lung abscess, from a subphrenic abscess, from mediastinal sepsis and from a chest wound. Empyema may also result from tuberculous infection of the pleural cavity (see p. 256). Infected serous fluid may collect in the pleural cavity during the course of a pneumonia (*syn-pneumonic empyema*). It is not localised and it usually resolves with adequate treatment. It may, however, progress to become purulent and localised, and by this time the underlying pneumonia has usually resolved (*meta-pneumonic empyema*). When an empyema becomes loculated in the fissures between the lobes it is known as an interlobar empyema.

Clinical Features. Empyema most commonly arises one to two weeks after the start of a pneumococcal pneumonia. Instead of the temperature falling and the patient recovering, the temperature begins to rise again and takes on a remittent character. The patient looks ill, has drenching sweats and complains of malaise and anorexia. Examination of the chest shows the signs of fluid; the mediastinum will be shifted if the collection of fluid is large, but this is not usual. There is dullness over the fluid; classically the upper limit of the dull area rises in the axilla, but this is not constant and often the dullness is largely posterior. Usually there are absent or diminished breath sounds over the fluid, although particularly in children it is sometimes possible to hear bronchial breathing which may lead to an erroneous diagnosis of unresolved pneumonia.

It is important to take both postero-anterior and lateral radiographs of the chest so that the fluid may be exactly localised. The diagnosis is finally confirmed by needling the chest and withdrawing turbid fluid. In the early stages, the fluid will be thin and serous, but if a true empyema develops it will become thick and purulent. The fluid should be cultured for organisms.

With correct treatment the *prognosis* in empyema is good except (1) when it is associated with a severe infection, (2) when the patient's resistance to infection is low due to debility, and (3) in young children.

Treatment

(1) *The Stage of Infected Pleural Effusion.* The patient should be at rest in bed, propped up on pillows. The diet should be light and fluids plentiful. The infected effusion must be aspirated daily to keep the pleural cavity as dry as possible; following aspiration, 500,000 units of benzylpenicillin should be injected into the pleural cavity. At the same time systemic antibiotic treatment should be continued; benzylpenicillin, 500,000 units six-hourly is satisfactory unless the infecting organism is resistant to penicillin, when the appropriate antibiotic should be used. With this treatment most effusions will subside. Sometimes, however, the infection is not controlled and the aspirated fluid becomes more and more purulent.

(2) *True Empyema.* Treatment at this stage is surgical. Resection of a portion of a rib and the insertion of a drainage tube into the most dependent part of the empyema cavity ensures the best possible drainage. The aim is complete obliteration of the empyema cavity with the minimum of pleural scarring and fixation of the lung. It is therefore essential, once a true empyema has developed, not to delay surgical drainage or the wall

of the abscess cavity may become so thick and rigid that it cannot be obliterated.

The drain is left in the empyema cavity until this space has disappeared. If the drain falls out before the cavity has been obliterated it must be replaced gently because of the danger of causing spread of infection to the brain (resulting in cerebral abscess). Breathing exercises are given to re-expand the lung and minimise fixation. Provided treatment is correctly carried out results are good. *Failure of the empyema cavity to close* is usually due to:

(a) too long a delay before drainage.
(b) inadequate drainage with pocketing of pus; it will be neces-sary to radiograph the cavity, outlined with radio-opaque material, to determine the correct site for drainage of the most dependent part of the cavity.
(c) failure to recognise that it is a tuberculous empyema.
(d) presence of an underlying neoplasm.
(e) a foreign body in the empyema cavity.

An empyema cavity which fails to close owing to undue thickness of its wall will require permanent drainage with a tube; or surgical decorti-cation of the lung can be performed with removal of the abscess cavity.

Tuberculous Empyema

Tuberculous empyema nearly always occurs in an effusion complicating post-primary pulmonary tuberculosis, and it is very rare in a tuberculous effusion associated with a primary infection. It was a recognised complica-tion of artificial pneumothorax, but this type of treatment for tuberculosis is not used now.

Clinical Features. The degree of constitutional upset varies. Some patients appear surprisingly well considering the chest is filled with tuberculous pus. Others have evidence of toxaemia with weight loss, sweating, and fever. If secondary infection occurs, particularly with the staphylococcus aureus, the patient becomes severely ill. This is especially likely to occur if there is a bronchopleural fistula, such as may result from the rupture of a pulmonary cavity into the pleura. The signs are those of fluid in the chest. If a pneumothorax is also present the signs are those of fluid and air in the chest: an area of dullness below due to the fluid, with resonance above. It may be possible by tilting the patient to demonstrate shifting dullness.

Treatment. The patient requires the usual general treatment for tuber-culosis, including a full course of antituberculous chemotherapy (see p. 241). The chest should be aspirated every other day until it is as dry as possible and streptomycin 1·0 g. should be instilled into the pleural cavity after aspiration. Unless full expansion occurs, decortication, thoracoplasty or resection of part or all the lung may be required.

SPONTANEOUS PNEUMOTHORAX

Air collecting in the pleural cavity as a result of some pathological process is known as spontaneous pneumothorax. The artificial introduction of air, which was used as a form of therapy for pulmonary tuberculosis, is known as an artificial pneumothorax.

The commonest cause of spontaneous pneumothorax is the rupture of a small vesicle under the visceral pleura which allows air to pass from the lung to the pleural space. This type of pneumothorax is common in young people and more common in men than women. It is not associated with any underlying lung disease. The patient is often slim with long fingers and high arched palate. In about 10 to 20 per cent of patients it recurs, sometimes repeatedly.

A spontaneous pneumothorax may also complicate lung disease such as emphysema and asthma. In addition, air may enter the pleural space from wounds of the chest wall or from a perforation of the oesophagus.

When the spontaneous pneumothorax is due to the rupture of a vesicle, the tear usually seals off rapidly and the air is absorbed from the pleural cavity over the next week or so. Occasionally a valve-like opening develops between the lung and the pleural space so that air can enter, but cannot leave the pleura; this leads to the accumulation of air in the pleural cavity and the development of a *tension pneumothorax*.

Clinical Features. The onset is usually sudden with pain in that side of the chest, and dyspnoea. The degree of constitutional upset is variable, but some patients may be quite shocked and collapsed. Occasionally the pneumothorax is found on routine examination and no history of chest pain can be elicited.

Examination of the chest may show diminished movement of the affected side. The degree to which the mediastinum is displaced away from the side of the pneumothorax is variable and depends on the size of the pneumothorax. Tactile vocal fremitus is decreased or absent. The note to percussion is either normal or hyper-resonant. On auscultation there are diminished breath sounds and absent voice sounds over the pneumothorax. An exocardial clicking sound may be heard over a small left-sided pneumothorax. A *coin sound* is sometimes present when their is a large or tension pneumothorax; this is a musical chiming heard through a stethoscope placed over the pneumothorax cavity when a coin laid on an adjacent part of the chest wall is tapped with another coin. The development of a *tension pneumothorax* is suggested by increasing dyspnoea, cyanosis, and distress. There will be signs of a pneumothorax with considerable mediastinal displacement. If the tension is not relieved, death may rapidly ensue.

Occasionally a spontaneous pneumothorax may be associated with a haemothorax due to the tearing of pleural adhesions.

Chest radiograph shows air in the pleural cavity with a varying amount of collapse of the lung. There is rarely any evidence of lung disease.

Treatment. When a spontaneous pneumothorax is diagnosed within the first few hours after its onset, the patient is best moved to hospital if this is possible because of the slight but definite risk of a tension pneumothorax or haemopneumothorax developing. Rest at home for a short period is satisfactory if a pneumothorax has been present for a few days and is expanding satisfactorily. In the early stages some patients are shocked and in severe pain and require morphine 10–15 mg., perhaps repeated once or twice in the ensuing few hours.

No active treatment is required for a small or moderate sized pneumothorax. In all patients with a large or tension pneumothorax it is best to insert a catheter via a trochar through an intercostal space into the pleural cavity, the other end being connected to an under-water seal. The patient is instructed to cough gently and thus slowly to expel the air from the pneumothorax; expansion of the lung will then take place. In an emergency, where a patient's life is threatened by a tension pneumothorax and hospital equipment is not at hand, a needle should be pushed through a cork and into the pneumothorax; the needle can then be fixed into position with strapping and attached by a rubber tube to an under-water seal.

Occasionally the pneumothorax persists in spite of these measures in which case continuous suction can be applied to the underwater seal to encourage the visceral pleura to become adherent to the chest wall. If this fails, thoracotomy may be required. With recurrent pneumothorax pleurodesis is indicated, either by painting the pleural surfaces with a solution of silver nitrate and thus allowing the visceral and parietal pleurae to become adherent, or by thoracotomy and pleurectomy of the parietal pleura.

MEDIASTINAL CYSTS AND TUMOURS

(1) Swellings in the Mid-mediastinum

(a) *Carcinoma of the Bronchus.* This is the commonest cause of a mediastinal mass. It may be composed of the growth alone or there may be associated infiltration and enlargement of lymph-nodes.

(b) *Enlarged Lymph Nodes.* These may be due to carcinomatous infiltration (commonly from the bronchus), Hodgkin's disease, lymphosarcoma, sarcoidosis, or tuberculosis.

(2) Swellings in the Anterior Mediastinum

(a) *Retrosternal Goitre.* This is usually, but not always, associated with a goitre in the neck. It lies anteriorly behind the manubrium and may compress the trachea or other structures in the superior mediastinum.

(b) *Thymic tumours* lie in the upper anterior mediastinum. They are sometimes associated with myasthenia gravis. Some are malignant and may metastasise.

(c) *Dermoid cysts and teratomas* usually lie anterior to the upper part of the heart. Dermoids may become infected and form fistulae with surrounding structures. Both may undergo malignant change.

(d) *Pericardial Cysts (Spring-water Cysts).* These are found in the lower anterior mediastinum usually filling up the right cardiophrenic angle.

(3) Swellings in Posterior Mediastinum

Neurofibroma and Ganglioneuroma. These tumours usually lie on the paravertebral gutter. They seldom cause symptoms and are found on routine radiography, appearing as rounded opacities with clear-cut edges. Occasionally they extend into the spinal canal causing compression of the spinal cord. A neurofibroma of the first thoracic nerve often causes Horner's syndrome (p. 264).

Aortic aneurysm or aneurysmal dilatation of a pulmonary artery may appear as a mediastinal tumour.

Clinical Features. Mediastinal tumours and cysts may produce no symptoms and be found only on routine radiography. They may compress surrounding structures, causing a variety of symptoms and signs.

Investigation must always include postero-anterior and lateral radiographs of the chest. Tomography, bronchoscopy, and angiography may be required. Even with these investigations it is not always possible to make a definite diagnosis. Mediastinoscopy and thoractomy may be required both for diagnosis and for treatment.

FURTHER READING

Bates, D. V. and Christie, R. V., *Respiratory Function in Disease*, 2nd edition, W. B. Saunders Co., Philadelphia and London, 1971.

Brock, The Lord, *The Anatomy of the Bronchial Tree with Special Reference to the Surgery of Lung Abscess*, 2nd edition, Oxford University Press, London, 1954.

Crofton, J. and Douglas, A., *Respiratory Diseases*, 2nd edition, Blackwell Scientific Publications, Oxford and Edinburgh, 1975.

D'Abreu, A. L. *Practice of Cardiothoracic Surgery*, 4th revised edition, Edward Arnold, London, 1976.

Parkes, W. Raymond, *Occupational Lung Disorders*, Butterworth & Co., London, 1974.

CHAPTER SIX

THE NERVOUS SYSTEM

THE CRANIAL NERVES

THE OLFACTORY NERVE (I)

Supplies special sensation (smell) to the superior nasal concha and the opposed part of the nasal septum. Pierces the cribriform plate of the ethmoid, and enters the olfactory bulb, which lies above the medial edge of the orbital plate. It continues as the olfactory tract which passes into the indusium griseum and sweeps anteriorly and superiorly round the corpus callosum and ends in the uncus.

It serves all smell, and all of flavour except salt, sweet, bitter, and acid. These functions may be tested with non-irritant aromatic odours, such as an orange, or a bar of scented soap, and it is the ability to separate rather than to identify them which must be shown to be intact.

Function

Smell is often temporarily upset with *acute and chronic rhinitis*; derangement may remain for weeks after the other symptoms have subsided. *Permanent bilateral anosmia* may follow *head injuries*, when the olfactory bulb is sheared from the ethmoid, or may accompany *tabes dorsalis*, and some influenza-like illnesses.

Unilateral (or bilateral) anosmia may be a sign of a *meningioma* growing in the olfactory groove.

THE OPTIC NERVE (II)

Fibres of the optic nerve pass centripetally in the stratum opticum of the retina. They are separated from the vitreous humour by the hyaloid membrane, and are closely applied to the ganglionic layer of the retina. They are so arranged that those taking origin close to the optic nerve pass into it first and are situated in its periphery, whereas those from the periphery of the retina pass over the more central fibres and enter the nerve nearer its midline. Thus the most peripheral fibres are the most superficial in the retina and the most central in the nerve.

The optic nerve passes back through the optic foramen to the optic chiasma, where the fibres from the medial sides of both retinae decussate. From the chiasma the optic tracts pass back to the lateral geniculate bodies, so that the right tract carries the fibres from the right half of *both* retinae, and therefore the image of the left visual field, and *vice versa*.

The fibres relay in the lateral geniculate body; the main central connection is through the optic radiation which passes through the temporal and parietal lobes to the occipital cortex. There is also a direct pathway through the pretectal area to the Edinger-Westphal nucleus.

In the occipital cortex macular vision is represented at the occipital pole, and peripheral vision arranged above and below the calcarine fissures, which are on the medial aspects of the occipital lobes.

Visual acuity should be tested by means of test type. The *visual fields* are examined first by direct confrontation and then if a lesion is suspected with a screen. Finally the optic nerve head and retina should be inspected directly with an ophthalmoscope.

(1) Changes in *visual acuity* are commonly the result of *refractive errors* or *lens opacities*. If these are excluded then affection of the *optic nerve* should be suspected. This may be confirmed by ophthalmoscopy.

(2) Changes in visual fields are of great localising value.

(a) *Tunnel vision* results when the superficial retinal fibres are compressed by *glaucoma*, with resultant loss of peripheral field.

(b) Loss of one field, without perception of light, occurs when the optic nerve itself is diseased.

(c) Affection of the lateral part of the optic chiasma and the posterior part of the ipselateral optic nerve causes homonymous hemianopia with ipselateral central scotoma. It may occur with *chromophobe adenomas, craniopharyngiomas, anterior communicating aneurysms, meningiomas of the suprasellar region*, or *localised arachnoiditis*.

(d) Compression at the chiasma causes bitemporal hemianopia, which is the classical sign of *pituitary tumours*. It is not necessarily symmetrical, particularly in the early stages. In about half of the patients with a proven pituitary chromophobe adenoma, the initial field defect may be a central or paracentral scotoma.

(e) Lesions behind the optic chiasma cause homonymous hemianopia; their exact site must be identified by accompanying signs and symptoms. Quadrantic hemianopia is often associated with lesions of the radiation; upper quadrantic defects suggest that the temporal lobe is involved, lower quadrantic defects the parietal.

(3) The normal optic nerve head is seen as a pink disc, slightly paler in the temporal half, with clear margins, from which the retinal arterioles emerge and on which the veins converge.

Optic Neuritis and Papilloedema

The optic disc may be oedematous as in *optic neuritis* (or papillitis) and *papilloedema*: these conditions are easily separated clinically by the visual acuity. This is usually affected early and severely in papillitis, late and mildly in papilloedema.

The *common cause* of papillitis is *disseminated sclerosis*; other causes are *methyl alcohol poisoning, meningitis*, and *encephalitis*. Papilloedema is most commonly caused by *hypertension*, when the distinctive retinal changes make the diagnosis obvious. It may also result from *raised intracranial pressure*, when it is usually accompanied by headaches and vomiting. *Venous obstruction*, in the orbit or more proximally, may cause papilloedema; it may also occur in *severe anaemia* and *polycythaemia rubra*. It is commonly seen as a terminal phenomenon in *pulmonary heart disease* with marked carbon dioxide retention.

Optic Atrophy

The optic nerve head may be unduly pale, suggesting optic atrophy; this may sometimes be confirmed by showing reduced visual acuity. If optic atrophy is advanced, a dead white disc is seen. There may be no perception of light and the direct and consensual pupillary reflexes are lost; but if the absence of perception of light is unilateral the consensual pupillary reflex is retained.

Optic atrophy may result from *glaucoma*, when tunnel vision is found and the physiological cup is seen to be unduly excavated. Many other causes are recognised, and among the most important are *disseminated sclerosis, syphilis, toxins* (particularly *methyl alcohol, quinine*, and *tobacco*), as a sequel to *head injury* and as a *congenital affection*. It may also be the result of *repeated bleeding* or of long-standing *vitamin (B) deficiency*. Pressure on the nerve (from *Paget's disease of the skull, tumours* of the optic nerve or sheath, or meningiomas) obstruct its blood supply and so cause atrophy.

THE OCULOMOTOR NERVES

Oculomotor (III), Trochlear (IV), Abducent (VI)

The oculomotor nuclei lie in the midbrain (III) and pons (IV and VI). They represent the extreme cephalic extent of the somatic efferent trunk. The *oculomotor nerve* passes forward and laterally and emerges at the medial side of the cerebral peduncle. It passes through the interpeduncular fossa, and pierces the dura at the lateral side of the posterior clinoid process. It lies in the lateral wall of the cavernous sinus, and enters the orbit through the superior orbital fissure. It supplies all the eye muscles except the lateral rectus and the superior oblique. The *trochlear* nerve emerges on the posterior aspect of the pons, after decussating with the contralateral nerve. It passes round the superior cerebellar peduncle and pierces the dura just behind the posterior clinoid process, and just below the free border of the tentorium. It lies in the lateral wall of the cavernous sinus and enters the orbit through the superior orbital fissure. It supplies the superior oblique muscle. The *abducent* nerve emerges anteriorly at the inferior border of the pons. It passes forward through the cisterna pontis and pierces the dura lateral to the dorsum sellae of the sphenoid. It is sharply angulated round the petrous part of the temporal bone. It traverses the cavernous sinus closely applied to the carotid artery and enters the orbit through the superior orbital fissure. It supplies the lateral rectus muscle.

The Eye Muscles

The lateral and medial recti are simple abductors and adductors of the eyeball. When the eye is adducted the inferior and superior oblique muscles act best as simple elevators and depressors respectively. When the eye is abducted it is elevated chiefly by the superior and depressed chiefly by the inferior rectus muscles.

The superior oblique is supplied by the trochlear nerve, and the lateral rectus by the abducent. All the other muscles are supplied by the oculomotor.

Squint

Squints may be either *concomitant* or *paralytic*. Concomitant squint means congenital non-parallelism of the visual axes; it is never associated with diplopia, and both eyes have full movements if tested separately.

Paralytic squint is always acquired, and is always associated with double vision, unless the false image is suppressed, which is unusual. To discover the paralysed muscle the following points must be remembered:

(1) The false image is always the peripheral one.
(2) The false image is always seen by the affected eye.
(3) Separation of the images is always maximal in the direction of action of the affected muscle; the false image is laterally displaced with paralysis of adductors and abductors, vertically if elevators or depressors are affected.

Adductors and abductors should be tested with the gaze horizontal, elevators and depressors in full abduction or adduction.

Applied Anatomy

(1) *Lateral rectus palsy (VI)* causes a paralysis of abduction of the affected eye. If complete the gaze cannot be deviated beyond the midline in the affected eye.
(2) *Oculomotor Palsy (III)*. There is marked ptosis. When the lid is lifted the eye is seen to be abducted (and depressed) and the pupil widely dilated and non-reactive to light or other stimuli. If complete there is a complete ptosis. The eye is abducted but *not* depressed. Integrity of the *IV*th nerve is demonstrated by torsion of the eye ball on *attempted* downward gaze.
(3) *Superior Oblique Palsy (IV)*. There is paralysis of depression of the gaze when the eye is adducted.

It must be realised that these are not mutually exclusive; combinations may occur, and any or all of the lesions may be partial or complete. Bizarre combinations may be seen in *myasthenia gravis*, or when the muscles themselves are diseased, as in *malignant exophthalmos* (p. 471).

(4) *Loss of Conjugate Deviation*. Conjugate eye movement originates in the second frontal convolution; if the descending fibres are interrupted in the lower mid-brain or upper pons, conjugate deviation of the eyes is affected. This may occur temporarily following *cerebral haemorrhage* or *thrombosis*; spasmodically in *epilepsy or post-encephalitic Parkinsonism*; permanent loss occurs with destructive lesions of the upper pons, usually *vascular* or *neoplastic*. Less commonly it follows *encephalitis* or complicates *demyelinating diseases*.

The Pupils

Consist of muscle fibres arranged concentrically (sphincter pupillae) and radially (dilator pupillae). The blood supply is derived from an outer (circulus arteriosus major) and inner (circulus arteriosus minor) vascular circle, connected by radiating arterial vessels; it is supplied by the long anterior and posterior ciliary arteries. The nerve supply of the sphincter pupillae is by *parasympathetic* fibres (from the ciliary ganglion through the short ciliary nerves); the dilator pupillae by *sympathetic* fibres (from the nasociliary nerve through the long nerves).

The pupil should constrict with convergence and on exposure to light; and dilate if shaded. The path of both the light and convergence reflexes is the same as far as the lateral geniculate body. Thereafter the light reflex passes directly to the parasympathetic part of the oculomotor nucleus, whereas the convergence reflex passes back to the occipital cortex and then forward again to the oculomotor nucleus.

Applied Anatomy

(1) In *old people* and in the *presenile atheromatous conditions* vascular sclerosis and hyaline degeneration give rise to pupils which are small, unequal, irregular and relatively immobile.

(2) There is a condition known as *myotonic pupil* wherein the pupil reacts very slowly to light and convergence. It is frequently unilateral, and occurs most commonly in young women. It may be associated with absent knee and ankle jerks (*Adie's syndrome*). The aetiology is unknown, but the condition is completely benign. Neuronal degeneration has been reported in the ipsilateral ciliary ganglion.

(3) *Horner's Syndrome*. In lesions of the sympathetic nerve to the eye the pupil on the affected side is usually smaller and does not dilate to shade. There is some ptosis, and possibly enoph-

thalmos. Sweating may be reduced on the same side of the face.

Horner's syndrome is an excellent lateralising sign, but a poor localising sign; lesions are always ipselateral, but may occur anywhere on the path of the sympathetic fibres as they pass from the hypothalamus through the brain stem to the cervical cord, then emerging at the level of the first thoracic segment to join the cervical sympathetic ganglion, on to the carotid artery, with which they re-enter the skull, and finally into the globe itself. Of particular importance are lesions of the carotid artery, which may give rise to ipselateral sympathetic paralysis and contralateral hemiplegia.

(4) *Argyll-Robertson pupils* are small, unequal, eccentric, and irregular in outline. They do not react to light, but do constrict on convergence. This implies an interruption of the light reflex between the lateral geniculate body and the oculomotor nucleus; it is believed to occur in the pretectal area.

Such pupils are almost diagnostic of *syphilis*. The only other condition in which they may occur is in hypertrophic polyneuritis.

(5) Oval pupils, unequal pupils in otherwise healthy people, and pupils which show minor dilatation and contraction in time with the pulse are of no significance.

THE TRIGEMINAL NERVE (V)

The trigeminal ganglion lies in the *cavum trigeminale*, closely applied to the petrous temporal bone. Axis cylinders of the ganglion divide into peripheral and central branches; the central ones pass to the fifth nerve nuclei, extending through the pons and medulla, and lying posteriorly. The motor tract of the fifth nerve arises from the motor nucleus of V, which lies in the pons, just anterior to the middle sensory nucleus. From it all the muscles of mastication (except the buccinator) are supplied.

The peripheral axons are the sensory supply to the face and the anterior part of the scalp. They lie in three great bundles, the ophthalmic, maxillary, and mandibular nerves, each with sharply defined territory.

(1) Ophthalmic. Supplies anterior part of scalp as far back as the crown of the head, the forehead and the eye (including the cornea) and the antero-lateral part of the nose.
(2) Maxillary. Supplies the cheek, lower eyelid, side of the nose, and upper lip only.
(3) Mandibular. From the side of the head, down to the cheek, including the upper part of the ear, but missing the angle of the jaw. Also supplies the lower lip and chin.

Applied Anatomy

The nuclei may be affected in the brainstem by *syringobulbia, tumours, demyelinating* or *vascular lesions*. The ganglion may be compressed by *acoustic* or *trigeminal neuromas*, or involved in local *syphilitic meningitis*. *Trigeminal neuralgia* (p. 329) is of unknown aetiology and is not associated with signs in the nervous system.

FACIAL NERVE (VII)

The facial nucleus lies in the lower part of the pons, and fibres from it pass backwards to sweep round the sixth nerve nucleus before turning forwards to emerge from the lateral aspect of the lower border of the pons, medial to the eighth nerve from which it is separated by the *nervus intermedius*, in which secreto-motor and taste fibres travel. The three nerves then pass to the *internal auditory meatus*.

Within the temporal bone the facial nerve occupies the facial canal and bends through a right angle at the *geniculate ganglion* which receives the *nervus intermedius*. Within the facial canal the facial nerve gives off the *chorda tympani* which later joins the lingual nerve to supply taste to the anterior two thirds of the tongue.

The seventh nerve leaves the skull through the stylomastoid foramen and pierces the parotid gland, from which it emerges to supply the muscles of facial expression.

Applied Anatomy

The muscles of the forehead have bilateral cortical representation. Therefore they are relatively spared in upper motor neurone lesions affecting the face; moreover in such cases voluntary facial movements are affected more than involuntary ones, such as blinking and smiling.

In lower motor neurone lesions all the facial muscles are affected, and both voluntary and involuntary movements are paralysed. Associated lesions may contribute to better localisation.

(1) Brainstem—associated ipselateral VI nerve palsy.

(2) Cerebello-pontine angle—associated VIII and V nerve lesions.

(3) In the bony canal—associated VIII nerve lesions, sometimes hyperacusis (from paralysis of stapedius) and loss of taste over anterior two thirds of tongue.

Upper motor neurone lesions of the seventh nerve commonly occur in strokes involving the internal capsule. The nucleus may be affected in *tumours, vascular lesions*, or *poliomyelitis* affecting the brain stem. The classical lesion in the cerebello-pontine angle is the *acoustic neuroma*. The nerve is frequently affected in *acute infective polyneuritis* (p. 326).

Bell's palsy is an acute lower motor neurone palsy of the facial nerve. It is of unknown aetiology, and the exact site of the lesion is not known. The nerve is believed to become oedematous within the facial canal. Occasionally there is associated ipselateral hyperacusis or loss of taste over the anterior two thirds of the tongue on the same side. Rarely it is recurrent, sometimes bilaterally, and most rarely of all is concurrently bilateral; these latter occurrences always cast doubt on the diagnosis of simple Bell's palsy.

It is abrupt in onset, and at its worst within 48 hours. Sometimes there is a little associated pain behind the ear. If at the end of a week any movement at all is visible on the affected side an assurance of eventual complete recovery may be given; this usually takes 4 to 8 weeks, but may be as long as a year. Even if no movement is seen at the end of a week prognosis should be optimistic. Full recovery may still occur after up to three months of total paralysis. If the patient is seen in the early stages prednisolone 20 mg. four times daily for five days and then rapidly tailed off reduces the incidence of residual paralysis. If paralysis is long-standing dental splits are of value in preventing stretching of the facial muscles, and if the eye cannot be closed it must be protected, especially during sleep.

The **Ramsay-Hunt syndrome** is an acute affection of the seventh nerve by the herpes virus. It is preceded by a sore throat, and herpetic vesicles can be seen on the soft palate and external auditory meatus on the affected side. Recovery from the facial paralysis is often incomplete.

Clonic facial spasm is almost confined to elderly women. It is nearly always unilateral. Its aetiology is unknown, and it does not recover spontaneously. Its most embarrassing feature is winking, and this may be treated by surgical section of the upper fibres of facial nerve.

Habit spasm occurs in children and less commonly in young adults. It is bilateral, and can be imitated by the observer and controlled by the child voluntarily—neither of which apply to facial myoclonus. It is associated with mounting mental tension, which is in some way relieved by the grimace.

THE ACOUSTIC-VESTIBULAR NERVE (VIII)

Separate vestibular and cochlear nuclei are situated in the upper medulla and lower pons. They lie anterolaterally and are widely connected centrally.

(a) *Vestibular* nuclei to:

    (1) ipselateral cerebellar hemisphere.
    (2) medial longitudinal bundle (hence *III, IV,* and *VI*).
    (3) vestibulo-spinal tract.
    (4) ipselateral lateral lemniscus (to inf. corp. quad. and superior temporal gyrus.

(b) *Cochlear* nucleus to:

    (1) medial longitudinal bundle.
    (2) trapezoid body (to contralateral inf. corp. quad. and auditory area of temporal lobe).

great veins. The left nerve passes between the left subclavian and common carotid arteries, over the aortic arch and on to the posterior surface of the left lung. The right crosses the right subclavian artery and then passes behind the superior vena cava to the posterior surface of the right lung. It has meningeal, auricular, pharyngeal and laryngeal branches, and is the main parasympathetic supply to the thoracic and abdominal viscera.

ACCESSORY NERVE (XI)

The nucleus is in the medulla, and the nerve passes forwards and laterally through the jugular foramen, having been joined by fibres from the spinal nucleus (C1–5). These *accessory* fibres join the vagus, and pass to the larynx and pharynx. The spinal part is motor to the sternomastoid and trapezius muscles.

HYPOGLOSSAL NERVE (XII)

The nucleus lies in the medulla, and the nerve leaves the skull through the anterior condylar foramen. It passes over the hyoid bone and then turns medially to supply the muscles of the tongue.

Applied Anatomy

These last four nerves are in such close proximity that they are frequently involved together. Individual lesions do occur, however.

(a) *IX.* Loss of special and ordinary sensation to posterior third of tongue and soft palate. Test for anaesthesia in the tonsillar fossa.

(b) *X.* Paralysis of levator palati or vocal cord.

(c) *XI.* Weakness of sternomastoid, and weakness and wasting of upper fibres of trapezius.

(d) *XII.* Deviation of tongue to the affected side on protrusion.

In lower motor neurone lesions the tongue is fibrillating and wasted, in upper motor neurone lesions small and stiff.

The X, XI, and XII nuclei are involved in *bulbar* and *pseudobulbar palsies*. The *foramen magnum syndrome* results from *platybasia*; the neck is usually short, and there is a combination of upper motor neurone disease and paralysis of the lower cranial nerves; the IX, X, and XI nerves may be affected in the *jugular foramen syndrome*, from nasopharyngeal tumours or meningiomas, and the IX, X, XI, and XII nerves from *glomus jugulare tumours*, though VII and VIII are also involved frequently and at an early stage.

SPEECH

This involves the selection of words and their production. Production depends upon the integrity of the nerves and muscles concerned with articulation; their disorder is termed *dysarthria*, their complete failure *anarthria*. The selection of words depends upon the proper function of large parts of the cerebral cortex, but is possible only if the so-called speech centre is intact. This lies in the dominant hemisphere, and consists of the posterior and inferior parts of the second and third frontal gyri and the adjacent part of the temporal lobe. *Dysphasia* and *aphasia* are the terms respectively applied to difficulty in word selection or its failure. Two forms may be recognised; *expressive aphasia*, in which the word is well known to the subject, but cannot be presented for production, and *receptive aphasia*, in which the word cannot be understood. Expressive aphasia is usually associated with lesions in the anterior part of the hemisphere and receptive aphasia with more posteriorly placed lesions.

THE MOTOR SYSTEM

Anatomy

The Pyramidal Tract. It arises from the precentral gyrus. The fibres converge on the internal capsule and pass down in the cerebral peduncle. It descends through the mid-brain to the pons, where it is divided but not interrupted by the transverse pontine fibres. Some fibres cross the midline in the mid-brain and the pons and serve as upper motor neurones for the motor cranial nerve nuclei. The main bundle comes to lie anteriorly in the brain stem and finally in the pyramid which gives the tract its name. The tract crosses the midline in the lower part of the medulla, decussating with the fibres from the other side (*decussation of pyramids*). A few fibres do not cross, but pass down to the cord anteriorly and lying close to the mid-line. The main pyramidal tract eventually lies in the lateral part of the white matter of the cord and gives upper motor neurone supply to the anterior horn cells.

Stimulation of the motor area in the brain causes discrete contralateral movements, and its extirpation contralateral paralysis. Somatic representation in the cortex is very regular and remains so throughout the length of the pyramidal tract.

Applied Anatomy

Congenital abnormalities of the tract or its injury early in life may be associated with contralateral reduced growth and weakness. Vigorous movements of the unaffected limbs may cause small imitative unwanted movements on the affected side; unwanted movements may also occur at rest. *Acquired* disease of the tract causes contralateral hemiparesis. Abrupt lesions of the tract initially cause flaccid contralateral paresis. At first both plantar responses are extensor. Coma or stupor is the rule; if the dominant hemisphere is affected then aphasia is also present. After some days or a week or two the typical signs of a spastic upper motor neurone (UMN) lesion emerge.

Signs of UMN Lesion

In lesions of gradual onset these may be present from the start. The changes which may be found lie in alterations in tone, power, and the skin and tendon reflexes. Wasting is not apparent except in long-standing hemiplegia with disuse atrophy of muscles, and co-ordination is only disturbed because of weakness and stiffness of the limb.

The Face

The eyes are rarely affected. There may be weakness of the muscles of mastication, detected by deviation of the jaw on opening and weakness in keeping it open. The face is usually affected; there is spastic weakness, particularly of the lower half. The soft palate may rise asymmetrically, deviating from the affected side, and the vocal cord may be paralysed. Weakness of the trapezius is revealed on shrugging the shoulder against resistance, and of the sternomastoid by weakness in turning the head away from the affected side. Spastic weakness of the tongue causes deviation to the affected side on protrusion.

The Limbs

(a) *Spasticity.* There is increase in tone in all the muscles on the affected side but not in equal degree, being most marked in the adductors, pronators and flexors of the arm, the adductors, extensors and plantar flexors in the leg. It is such that there is initially increasing resistance to stretching, changing suddenly to rapid diminution. This action has been likened to the opening of a clasp knife. But it is this distribution of increased tone rather than its special nature which is important in the recognition of UMN disease.

(b) *Power.* All muscles are weak on the affected side, but there is uneven distribution of weakness, so that in the upper limbs flexors are stronger than extensors, and in the lower limbs extensors are stronger than flexors. In the arm the weaker muscles are the intrinsic muscles of the hand, the shoulder abductors and the extensors of the elbow, wrist and fingers. In the leg, the weaker muscles are the flexors and abductors of the hip, the flexors of the knee, and the dorsiflexors and evertors of the ankle. The hemiplegic posture results from the counterplay of the strong and weak muscles.

(c) *Skin Reflexes.* The abdominal and cremasteric reflexes are abolished or reduced on the affected side, and the plantar response is extensor. In severe hemiplegias this response may be provoked from a wide area of the affected limb. As severity decreases in degree so the sensitive area shrinks and finally only the posterior third of the lateral aspect of the sole of the foot is receptive. To be effective the stimulus may have to be noxious for example by scratching on the outer aspect of the heel with a 'Yale key'. Normally this is followed by flexion of the toes, particularly the great toe, at the metatarsophalangeal joints. To be certainly extensor, biphasic extension and flexion of the first metatarsophalangeal joint should always follow appropriate stimulation.

Signs of hemiplegia may be minimal. They are always reduced, and may be abolished, by rest in bed. In any case either weakness, hypertonia, or deranged skin reflexes may predominate. Flexor plantar responses do not exclude an upper motor neurone lesion.

THE NEUROMUSCULAR JUNCTION

Physiology

The arrival of a nerve impulse at a neuromuscular junction causes the release of acetylcholine. This stimulates a sensitive muscle area (the motor end plate) and initiates a contraction of the muscle bundle. An enzyme (cholinesterase) rapidly destroys acetylcholine, and so permits the muscle to repolarise.

Applied Physiology

Transmission may be deranged in various ways. Procaine and botulinus toxin inhibit the secretion of acetylcholine; physostigmine (eserine), neostigmine, and a number of other drugs (some now used widely as insecticides) destroy cholinesterase, and so perpetuate the actions, both central (muscarine) and peripheral (nicotine) of acetylcholine. The sensitivity of the motor end plate may be reduced either specifically, as for example by Indian arrow poison (curare), or similar substances (gallamine, mephenesin), or as part of a general muscle disorder, for example lead poisoning or potassium deficiency or excess. Disorder of conduction at the neuromuscular junction is believed to be the basis of myasthenia gravis (p. 316).

THE SENSORY SYSTEM

Anatomy

The skin is protected by a superficial and a deep network of sensory end organs. Each organ is supplied by at least two nerve fibres. Not all parts of the skin are equally sensitive. Relatively insensitive areas exist, for example over the medial and lateral condyles of the ankle, and over the elbows. Especially sensitive areas exist over the pads of the fingers and round the lips. The forehead is less sensitive than the rest of the face, and the back of the trunk less so than the front.

Non-medullated fibres conduct all modalities of sensation and pass back in bundles (sensory nerves) to the posterior horns of the spinal cord. Here they divide, and fibres carrying position sense, vibration, and light touch pass into the posterior columns without relaying; those carrying pain and temperature sensation relay in the posterior horn. The relay fibres then cross the mid-line, and pass upwards in the lateral spinothalamic tracts.

The sacral fibres enter first, and therefore occupy the most medial position in the posterior column and the most superficial in the spinothalamic tract. Conversely the cervical fibres are most lateral in the posterior columns and deepest in the spinothalamic tract.

The spinothalamic tract passes upwards through the brain stem lying superficially (lateral lemniscus) and ends in the (optic) thalamus. The posterior columns end in the gracile and cuneate nuclei in the lower medulla. Some fibres pass to the cerebellum but the main relay crosses the mid-line in the medulla, decussating with the fibres from the other side (decussation of the fillets). Having crossed the mid-line these sensory fibres lie deep to the lateral lemniscus, and pass up to the thalamus through the brain stem (medial lemniscus). In the pons they are joined by fibres from the sensory nucleus of V, bearing light touch, pressure, and postural sense from the face (quinto-thalamic tract). The trigeminal ganglion lies in the cavum trigeminale, closely related to the petrous part of the temporal bone. Its peripheral neurones conduct sensation from the face, and its central fibres pass back to three sensory nuclei in the brain stem; the lowest, receiving pain and temperature fibres from the forehead, extends as far down as the upper cervical cord (about C2). The principal nucleus lies in the pons, and it is from this that the quinto-thalamic tract takes chief origin.

Appreciation of crude sensation takes place at the level of the thalamus, but more complex sensations are relayed to the cortex. Sensation is represented in the post-central gyrus in much the same way that the motor cortex is arranged. Besides this direct representation there is an associative area (superior and inferior parietal lobules) lying behind the post-central gyrus concerned with the appreciation of spatial relationships.

Disturbance of sensation may be of two kinds. It may be reduced or absent, or abnormal sensations may be experienced. Neither decreased sensation nor any kind of added sensation alone is of localising value. It is the distribution of sensory change, and the modalities affected, together with associated signs which allow anatomical identification of lesions. Similarly, no kinds of paraesthesiae are specific, although feelings of constriction of limbs or trunk are very commonly associated with posterior column lesions.

Examination of the Sensory System

Each modality of sensation must be individually tested. First an area believed to have normal sensation must be selected, and stimuli first applied here, so that the patient is in no doubt of what he *should* feel. With each modality comparison must be made between the area being tested, the same area on the other side of the body, and the known normal area.

   (a) Pain is tested with a sharp needle or pin. Initially several
       pricks should be made rapidly over an area of about 1 sq. cm.

In this way the possibility of touching an area of apparent anaesthesia between sensory end-organs is obviated. It is important to ask the patient: 'Did it sting as a pinprick should?', not simply: 'Can you feel this?', for pin prick may be appreciated as a touch where pain sense is impaired but light touch is intact (syringomyelia, p. 312). When this has been done the pin should be firmly pressed to one point, and the patient asked to comment on the sensation. It should be felt as a pinpoint of pain. It may be that the threshold of pain is raised, but when it *is* appreciated the sensation is like a small ring of pain, often with a burning quality, rather than a pinpoint.

This is diagnostic of a partial lesion of pain pathways, but gives no information of the level at which it is affected.

(b) Temperature may be quickly tested with a cold object, such as the blade of a tuning-fork, but if impairment is discovered then careful testing with two test tubes, one filled with cold and one with hot water is necessary.

(c) Light touch can be tested by touching lightly with the finger-tip or with a piece of cotton-wool or the corner of a handkerchief. It is important to touch cleanly, and not to rub the skin; this induces tickle, which is conducted by pain pathways.

(d) Position sense should be tested by moving first small and then larger joints and asking the patient to identify the direction of movement without looking.

(e) Vibration should be tested with a tuning fork (128 c.p.s.). The handle should be firmly pressed to bony prominences, and appreciation on the two sides compared.

Abnormal sensations (paraesthesiae) are variously described as tingling, pins and needles, burning, coldness, sense of water running over the skin, formication (ants crawling on skin), gripping, and 'compression of a limb'. They imply nothing but disturbance of paths of sensation, and considered alone give no indication at what level disturbance has occurred.

Clinical Interpretation of Sensory Disturbance

(a) Peripheral Neuritis. This causes a disturbance of motor, reflex, and sensory functions, usually of about equal degree. Rarely it is almost entirely sensory, even more rarely only motor. It exists in two forms, a *polyneuritis* affecting all nerves to about equal degree, and *mono-neuritis multiplex*, in which two or more nerves are affected, others being completely spared.

(b) Posterior root lesions (*tabes dorsalis*) cause a widespread disturbance of all modalities of sensation. Degeneration occurs in the posterior columns as fibres pass into them directly; the crossing fibres are relayed, so that no degeneration occurs in the spinothalamic tracts.

(c) Lesions of the central grey matter (*syringomyelia*) catch the crossing fibres, but spare those passing directly to the posterior columns; hence pain and temperature sense are lost, but light touch preserved. Connecting neurones are also involved, so that the tendon reflexes are interrupted.

(d) Space-occupying lesions of the cord itself involve the spinothalamic tracts from within. Hence cervical and thoracic symptoms appear early, and the more superficial sacral fibres are not immediately involved (sacral sparing).

(e) Extramedullary space-occupying lesions may compress the whole cord and primarily cause upper motor neurone lesions. Later there may be root pains, involvement of long sensory tracts, and lower motor neurone signs at the level of the lesion. The circulation of cerebrospinal fluid (C.S.F.) may be obstructed (*Froin syndrome*, p. 307).

Occasionally extramedullary compression involves predominantly one half of the cord (*Brown-Séquard syndrome*), so that the posterior columns, pyramidal tracts, and spinothalamic tracts are involved on one side of the cord. This causes signs of an upper motor neurone lesion, with loss of position, vibration sense and light touch on the same side as the compression but contralateral loss of pain and temperature sensation.

(f) In the brain stem the disease can be localised by the involvement of adjacent structures. The lateral lemniscus lies superficially and the medial lemniscus deeply throughout their course. Because of this, compressing lesions tend to affect contralateral pain and temperature appreciation, whereas intrinsic lesions involve the medial meniscus and cause contralateral disturbance of position and vibration sense.

(g) Disturbances at the level of the thalamus are rare. Incomplete lesions produce contralateral sensory disturbances. Abnormal sensation, for example burning or stinging may be experienced, and the threshold to pain is increased. Once appreciated, however, there is overreaction to painful stimuli.

(h) The sensory cortex subserves all forms of discriminative sensation. Its functions have been listed as follows (modified from Gordon Holmes).

(1) It relates incoming experiences to previous sensations, and allows the recognition of similarities and differences.

(2) It allows awareness of the postural relations of separate parts of the body.

(3) It locates the sites of stimuli to the body's surface, and enables distinction to be made between one and two simultaneous contacts.

(4) It allows the recognition of the shape, size, weight, texture, and consistency of objects.

(5) It enables the attention to be focused on any given part of the body.

(6) It controls the response of subcortical centres to stimuli.

THE CEREBELLUM

Balance and Co-ordination of Movement

Co-ordination depends upon the smooth contraction of certain muscle groups (agonists) and the equally smooth relaxation of their opposers (antagonists). It is the lateral lobes of the cerebellum which are chiefly concerned in this. The function of the central lobe (vermis) of the cerebellum is to maintain balance; lesions of this lobe cause an inability to stand or to walk.

For the correct maintenance of balance, posture, and co-ordination there must be no proprioceptive defect, no weakness, and muscle tone must be normal. Only when these functions have been shown to be intact should abnormalities be certainly attributed to the cerebellum.

Disease of the lateral lobe of the cerebellum and its connections produces ipselateral derangement of movement. No abnormality is detected when the subject is completely at rest.

The inco-ordination of cerebellar disease results in a *terminal action tremor*. That is to say it occurs only with movement and is worse at the end of movement. It may be detected in various groups of muscles.

(1) The eye; it causes nystagmus on lateral and/or upward gaze.
(2) Speech becomes jerky and abnormally accentuated (scanning speech).
(3) Gait is reeling, usually towards the side of the lesion.
(4) There is loss of muscle fixation, so that if the hand and arm are held extended an abnormal posture results. Added to this there is apparent hypotonia in affected limbs. Because of this the reflexes may be reduced.

Applied Anatomy

The cerebellum is vulnerable to backward spread from infective middle ear disease, which may cause cerebellar abscess. It is very frequently affected by disseminated sclerosis, usually in the middle and superior cerebellar peduncles. Space-occupying lesions of the posterior fossa rapidly cause forward displacement of the brain stem, with obstruction of the flow of cerebrospinal fluid and internal hydrocephalus. In effect, the whole ventricular system is made to behave like a rapidly expanding cerebral tumour; consequently severe headache, papilloedema, and vomiting appear early in the course of quite small space-occupying lesions in the cerebellum.

Occasionally evidence of an upper motor neurone lesion and a cerebellar lesion occur in the same side of the body. This can be caused by one lesion in the mid-brain, catching the descending pyramidal tract before it has crossed, and the tract from the superior cerebellar peduncle to the red nucleus after it has crossed.

THE BASAL GANGLIA AND EXTRAPYRAMIDAL SYSTEM

These are a group of large nuclei situated in the white matter of the cortex just below and lateral to the anterior horns of the lateral ventricles. The corpus striatum (striped body) is divided by the descending pyramidal tract into the caudate ('tail like') and lentiform ('lens shaped') nuclei; these same fibres later separate the lentiform from the thalamic nuclei. The lentiform nucleus is seen to consist of two opposing structures, causing a medial pale and lateral darker appearance. The medial pale structure is spherical, and known as the globus pallidus (pale globe), or pallidum; the lateral darker part the putamen (shell).

In the lower vertebrates the corpus striatum is represented only by the pallidum, and for this reason is known as the palaeostriatum (old striped body); in reptiles and birds (and above) the putamen and caudate nuclei appear (neostriatum). The palaeostriatum develops from the between brain; the neostriatum develops from the same embryonic structure as the cortex. In many species the neostriatum is not separated and in man the putamen and caudate nucleus are continuous anteriorly. The structures are histologically different, in that the palaeostriatum is composed of large cells and is rich in medullated fibres, whereas the neostriatum contains smaller cells and has few nerve fibres. The red nucleus is situated high in the mid-brain. It is in two parts; a large upper two thirds containing small cells, and developing at the same time as the cerebellar hemispheres and the expansion of the cortex, and a lower third containing large cells and derived from the between brain.

The substantia nigra is a group of heavily pigmented multipolar nerve cells, situated high in the mid-brain. The subthalamic nucleus lies close to the mid-line and below the thalamus.

It appears that these nuclei are the remnants of an ancient motor system; the path of the 'palaeo' system may have been—thalamus—cortex—pallidum—lower third of red nucleus—rubrospinal tract. The path of the 'neo' system is the same, with the modifying effect of the putamen, substantia nigra, and subthalamic nuclei. Besides these pathways must be mentioned many fibres connecting the nuclei to each other, and two efferent tracts, the fasciculus lenticularis and the ansa lenticularis which pass from the globus pallidus to the medial nucleus of the thalamus, short circuiting, as it were, the cortex.

Diseases of the basal ganglia cause disorders of muscle tone and movement.

(a) There is a general increase in muscle tone. This hypertonus does not vary during flexion and extension of a joint (cf. UMN lesions), but joints in the same limb may be affected to unequal degree. Commonly the earliest and most severely affected joints are the neck, shoulder, wrist, and ankle.

The same derangement of tone may be accompanied by tremor; in contradistinction to that caused by cerebellar disease, it is present at rest and often momentarily abolished by movement. It is rhythmic, occurring 4–7 times each second. Sometimes the superimposition of tremor on rigidity causes an apparent jerkiness when the limb is passively flexed (cogwheel rigidity).

The change in tone causes great slowness of execution of voluntary movements. In addition, automatic movements such as blinking, swallowing, and arm swinging are absent or reduced and expressional facial movements much attenuated.

In acute chorea the reverse is true. There is marked hypotonia, automatic movements are increased, and facial expressions exaggerated.

(b) Unwanted movements. In some diseases unwanted movements may occur. These may be caused by the random muscular contractions seen in *chorea* (p. 137), or be of a more violent and flinging nature, as in *hemiballismus*. Slowly changing disorders of tone may cause writhing sinuous movements of limbs (*athetosis*); this may occur with chronic basal ganglia disease in young people. Unwanted movements of another kind are seen in acute chorea; additional movements may occur in either limbs, the face or trunk, when voluntary movements are being executed.

Applied Anatomy

With the exception of the nucleus subthalamicus it is usually impossible to localise disease to one or another nucleus. Commonly they are all affected to greater or lesser degree. It may be said, however, that certain diseases affect chiefly the neostriatum and others the palaeostriatum. Good examples of the former are *hepato-lenticular degeneration* (p. 465; caudate and putamen), *Huntington's chorea* (p. 315; caudate), and *chronic progressive (senile) chorea* (caudate and putamen); in contrast, the chief changes in the idiopathic form of *Parkinson's disease* (p. 313) are seen in the globus pallidus and substantia nigra.

The Cerebro-spinal Fluid

The cerebro-spinal fluid is secreted by the choroid plexuses of the ventricles. That formed in the lateral ventricles passes to the third ventricle through the foramen of Monro. Fluid in the third ventricle passes to the fourth ventricle through the aqueduct of Sylvius, and then to the subarachnoid space through two lateral apertures, the foramina of Luschka and a central foramen of Magendie. It is confined between the pia and arachnoid membranes, and bathes the surface of the brain and spinal cord. It is absorbed into the intracranial venous sinuses.

Many diseases of the nervous system are associated with changes in the pressure or composition of the cerebro-spinal fluid. Specimens for examination may be obtained by lumbar puncture. Normal values are as follows:

(i) Pressure—60–180 mm. of fluid.
(ii) Protein—200–400 mg./l.
(iii) Glucose—2·8–3·9 mmols./l.

(iv) Chloride—120–130 mmol./l.

(v) Cells—up to 3 lymphocytes/cu.mm.

Obstruction to the flow of cerebro-spinal fluid is common as a result of subtentorial space-occupying lesions, which obstruct the Sylvian aqueduct by distortion. This causes dilatation of the whole ventricular system, with very rapid rise in the cerebro-spinal fluid pressure.

A relative increase in the gamma globulin protein fraction in the C.S.F. may be found in multiple sclerosis and syphilis. This finding is particularly valuable if the total protein is not markedly raised.

The Colloidal Gold Reaction (Lange)

The protein content of the fluid consists of albumin and globulin fractions. If the globulin concentration is increased then precipitation occurs on incubation with a colloidal solution of gold. Qualitative and quantitative abnormalities may be detected by mixing CSF with serial dilutions of colloidal gold, ten in all. Characteristic patterns of precipitation are seen in a number of diseases: precipitation in the first dilutions suggests general paresis of the insane (GPI), of the middle dilutions syphilis other than GPI and in the highest dilutions some form of meningitis.

DISORDERS OF THE CENTRAL NERVOUS SYSTEM

EPILEPSY

Epilepsy, the falling sickness, has been recognised and described since earliest times. At first thought to be a general disease, it was Hippocrates who first ascribed it to a disorder of the brain. It was not until 1878 that Hughlings Jackson, as a result of clinical observations, concluded that its basis was a paroxysmal discharge in the brain. This was confirmed in 1929 by Berger who made graphic records of the brain's electrical activity, the electroencephalograph (E.E.G.), and showed that the attacks coincided with the occurrence and spread of an electrical discharge. Quite recently Lennox and Lennox have described epilepsy as 'a recurrent disturbance in the chemico-electrical activity of the brain, which manifests itself in a symptom-complex of which impairment of consciousness, perturbation of the autonomic nervous system, convulsive movements, sensory abnormalities, or psychic disturbances are the essential components'.

The aetiology is complex and obscure. Heredity is generally regarded as an important factor since a family history of epilepsy in first or second degree relatives is obtained in about 30 per cent of patients, whatever the nature of their attack. In all patients with epilepsy there are predisposing and precipitating causes, though only in some are these causes demonstrable. In addition to the constitutional factor *predisposing causes* include prenatal disorders, birth injuries and neonatal disturbances as well as the more easily recognisable traumatic, inflammatory, neoplastic, or vascular lesions of the brain; the known *precipitating causes* include exhaustion and psychological stress and, more rarely, overhydration, acute anoxia of the brain, hypoglycaemia and hypocalcaemia. In view of the possible social consequences to the patient of a diagnosis of epilepsy, there is much to be said for avoiding this label when convulsions complicate a pre-existing disorder; thus, a patient who faints from postural hypotension or cardiac arrhythmia and then has a fit as a result of cerebral ischaemia has 'syncope with convulsions' rather than epilepsy.

Clinical Features. Epileptic attacks may take the form of any type of recurrent disturbance of feeling, behaviour, or consciousness which is of primarily cerebral origin, so that their clinical varieties are legion. They may be divided into two groups, *general* epilepsy and *focal* epilepsy. All forms, however, have certain common characteristics.

(i) *They are paroxysmal,* that is to say that the attacks occur from time to time.

(ii) *They are of sudden onset,* as the word ictus, a blow, implies.

(iii) *They are of brief duration;* although attacks may be recurrent, they are individually brief, usually lasting only some minutes.

(iv) *They usually occur for no apparent reason;* although they may be associated with functional or structural changes in the brain, these changes are present and usually unchanged before and after the attack. It is usually impossible to discover exactly why any individual attack occurred.

General epilepsy may be major or minor (*grand mal* or *petit mal*). Both these forms of general epilepsy (sometimes called central epilepsy) depend in part on a disturbance in the structures of the upper brain stem which are concerned with maintaining the alert or conscious state and each has a characteristic pattern in the E.E.G.

Grand Mal. In the classical major fit there is a regular sequence of stages, though frequently one or more of these stages are absent. Sometimes the convulsion is heralded by a transient *aura,* which may take a motor, sensory, or psychic form and indicates the site of electrical discharge, but usually the first event is the *tonic stage,* at the onset of which consciousness is lost. The patient falls to the ground, and as all his muscles are in a state of rigid spasm he falls heavily and frequently injures himself. The tonic stage lasts about a minute and as respiration is in abeyance during this time the patient becomes cyanosed. After this comes the *clonic stage*: a series of convulsive movements occurs not only in the trunk and limbs but also in the jaw and tongue so that saliva may be lathered into a 'foam' or the tongue may be badly bitten. The bladder is sometimes evacuated during the clonic stage, which may last for two or three minutes. After this the patient remains in *coma,* usually for only a few minutes but sometimes for some hours; if examined at this stage he is found to have absent corneal and tendon reflexes and extensor plantar responses. On recovering consciousness he usually complains of severe *headache*. After the attack some patients pass into a state of *post-epileptic automatism*, in which they may involuntarily commit anti-social or criminal acts which bring them into the hands of the police.

Petit Mal. These attacks never arise from lesions acquired later than the neonatal period; seen therefore mainly in children, their occurrence in an adult places him in the so-called 'idiopathic' group. They consist simply of a brief interruption of consciousness, in which the patient stops what he is doing or saying for a few seconds and then carries on, or perhaps falls to the ground and immediately picks himself up again.

Focal Epilepsy. This term is used to include other ictal manifestations. The basis of such events is a *focal discharge*, and the clinical nature of the attack depends upon its site and intensity, and the patient's innate resistance to its spread, which may be of varying degree.

The attack may include movements, or any change of sensation, simple or complex. It may be so slight as almost to pass unnoticed, or so severe as to end in a general convulsion. It may be followed by a period of confusion and headache.

Brief mention may be made of *temporal lobe epilepsy* (psychomotor epilepsy), the focus of which appears to lie in the anterior part of the temporal lobe. These attacks take many forms in which organised movements, sensations, and emotions occur. Common examples are the déjà vu phenomenon, a feeling of intense familiarity, or feelings of remoteness and unreality, or of pleasure, or hallucinations of smell or taste, accompanied by pallor and sweating and often a feeling of fear. There may be convulsive movements of the limbs or smacking of the lips.

Status Epilepticus. When a series of major epileptic seizures occurs without intervening recovery of consciousness the patient is said to be in status epilepticus, a very dangerous condition which unless promptly and energetically treated may lead to death from exhaustion or hyperpyrexia. Petit mal status also occurs and gives rise to prolonged disorientation.

Diagnosis of Epilepsy. As doctors rarely have the opportunity of seeing patients in an attack, and as there are no helpful physical signs to be found between the attacks apart occasionally from scars of old injuries on the head or tongue, the diagnosis nearly always depends on a carefully taken history. Eyewitness accounts of the attacks should always be sought. On this evidence the diagnosis of grand mal and petit mal can usually be made without difficulty. Focal attacks are often more difficult to recognise as epileptic; helpful points are that they tend to recur in the same patient under the same circumstances, they have a very sudden onset and usually a brief duration.

Whatever the nature of the attack, it is important to remember that epilepsy is a symptom, and the doctor's prime duty is to discover *why* it has occurred. For this reason a careful family history, and a history of previous suspicious episodes must be sought, and a *full* clinical examination of the nervous system made including auscultation over the neck and orbits. All patients should have an E.E.G. and skull radiographs to attempt to demonstrate any focal lesion. However, electrical abnormalities are found in only a proportion of patients with epilepsy. A normal E.E.G does not exclude epilepsy. Fits may be the only manifestation of early cerebral syphilis, and so the Wasserman and Kahn tests must always be made on the blood, and if there is still reason for doubt, on the C.S.F. too.

Management of Epilepsy. When a patient presents with a recent history of epileptic fits the first question to be answered is whether he has an underlying potentially curable organic lesion. The older the patient when the seizures start the more often can an organic lesion be demonstrated; on the other hand, even in the higher age groups it is only a very small percentage of patients with epilepsy intensively investigated who are found to have a treatable organic lesion. On balance, therefore, it is wrong to perform unpleasant and occasionally harmful procedures such as air-encephalography, ventriculography, and arteriography except in patients in whom there is some special indication. In general, investigation should be limited to examination of the blood and urine, radiography of the skull and chest, which helps to exclude secondary tumours, and an E.E.G.; if the latter does not show evidence of a local spike focus or of the slow waves which suggest structural disorder of the brain, the patient should be kept under clinical observation, but not investigated further at this stage.

Even if a discoverable cause is removed the epilepsy will not necessarily by this means alone come under control. Patients with epilepsy must be allowed and encouraged to lead as normal a life as possible. Children should stay at school and adults may need help to find useful employment. The life of a patient with epilepsy should be well regulated, and hunger, fatigue, and emotional crises should be avoided as far as possible.

Anticonvulsant Drugs

The decision as to which drug should be used depends on the nature of the attack. For petit mal ethosuximide 250 mg. 4–6 times daily is the drug of choice. It is more effective and less toxic than troxidone and other drugs of the dione series.

In all other types of epilepsy treatment should be started with phenytoin sodium 100 mg. two or three times a day and this may be increased until satisfactory blood levels are achieved (therapeutic range 5–18 mg./l.). If attacks continue a second drug should be added. Those most commonly used are phenobarbitone up to 90 mg. daily, primidone up to 1·5 mg. daily, sodium valproate up to 1·2 g. daily, pheneturide up to 800 mg. daily and clonazepam up to 6 mg. daily.

Treatment should be continued until the patient has been free of attacks for at least three and preferably five years and if there are no side effects there is no reason why mild treatment should not be continued indefinitely even if the attacks are under control. Now that a patient may apply for a driving licence when free of attacks for three years, on or off drugs, there is not the same urgency to stop treatment on this account.

Surgical Treatment. In certain cases of temporal lobe epilepsy when the attacks are difficult to control, amputation of the temporal pole has brought complete relief in about 50 per cent of patients and partial relief in others. Some cases of infantile hemiplegia and of Sturge-Weber syndrome have similarly benefited from hemispherectomy.

Status Epilepticus

Urgent treatment is required, the mortality in inadequately treated patients being as high as 10 per cent. The drug of choice is diazepam 10 mg. by slow intravenous injection and this may be repeated as necessary until control is achieved. Other drugs which may be used are chlormethiazole by intravenous infusion or intramuscular paraldehyde (10 ml. in divided doses using a glass syringe). If they are ineffective intravenous short-acting anaesthetics (thiopentone and methohexitol) or the inhalation anaesthetics may be used if respiratory assistance is available. These drugs should be used in conjunction with the patient's usual anticonvulsant medication. Repeated treatments may be necessary, and careful attention to the patient's airway and if necessary treatment of secondary respiratory infection is essential.

HERPES ZOSTER (SHINGLES)

This common disease is characterised by inflammatory changes which are usually confined to one posterior root ganglion, though rarely they may involve the spinal cord. The causative virus is either identical with or closely related to the virus of chicken-pox, since it is quite common for the healthy contacts of patients with either disease to develop the other. The appearance of shingles often seems to be precipitated by injury or by some other pathological process such as spinal metastases from carcinoma or Hodgkin's disease, or other infections such as meningitis.

Clinical Features. The first symptom is usually severe pain in the distribution of the affected root or roots, often accompanied by swelling of local lymph nodes and followed a few days later by erythema and a vesicular eruption in the appropriate dermatome. At this stage there is often intense irritation as well as pain. The vesicles usually dry up into crusts in a week or so, though if the lesions become secondarily infected they may last much longer and eventually leave permanent scarring of the skin. Special mention may be made of zoster infection in the following special sites:

> (1) *Gasserian herpes* involving the first (ophthalmic) division is always serious, since it may lead to blindness either from corneal scarring following ulceration or from a panophthalmitis.

(2) *Geniculate herpes* (The Ramsay Hunt syndrome). This presents with pain in the throat or ear, followed by a vesicular eruption on the pinna, external auditory meatus or fauces and a facial palsy of lower motor neurone type. This may be accompanied by involvement of the eighth nerve, resulting in deafness or vestibular disturbance. There is reason to believe that the geniculate ganglion is not necessarily involved.

(3) *Zoster myelitis* is rare. It may present as a Brown-Séquard syndrome (pp. 276 and 306) or as a complete transverse lesion of the cord. Recovery within a few weeks is the rule.

Post-herpetic neuralgia is a very troublesome sequela which occurs particularly in elderly patients; the pain may be so severe and persistent as to induce suicidal depression.

Treatment. There is no specific treatment. To prevent secondary infection of the skin lesions they should be kept clean and dry or covered with collodion and in ophthalmic herpes atropine drops and antibiotic drops should be instilled into the eyes. Analgesics must be given to relieve the pain, but drugs of addiction should be avoided since the neuralgia may be very chronic. Post-herpetic neuralgia is sometimes improved by radiotherapy to the affected ganglia or by repeated applications of an electrical vibrator over the painful area. Accompanying depression should be treated by anti-depressants in appropriate doses.

MIGRAINE

The essential feature of migraine is a paroxysmal headache. This may be confined to one or other side of the head or may be generalised. The headache may be preceded by an 'aura' which can take the form of some visual disturbance, such as dazzles, fortification spectra or even visual loss which is usually hemianopic. There may be, separately or in addition, some numbness and tingling of face and arms, and, more rarely, dysphasia. These symptoms last for some 15–30 minutes and as they pass off the headache develops. The headache lasts on an average some 12-24 hours but may be of shorter and occasionally of longer duration, sometimes lasting several days. At its height it may be accompanied by vomiting and while the headache lasts the patient suffering a severe attack prefers to lie quietly in a darkened room, refusing all nourishment but sipping water. Its frequency is very variable but most people liable to migraine have attacks every few weeks or months.

Pathology

The patho-physiology of migraine is thought to be an initial constriction of vessels which causes the 'aura' and a later dilatation, mostly of branches of the external carotid artery, which causes the headache. The cause is unknown but there is often a family history, the attacks are often related to some emotional disturbance and are sometimes precipitated by eating certain foods, for example chocolate, citrus fruits or cheese. Most migrainous subjects are of obsessional temperament and it is typical for attacks to occur during the period of relaxation which follows a spell of intense overactivity; thus 'weekend migraine' is very common. Attacks also frequently occur premenstrually.

Migraine usually starts in the second decade and tends to diminish in frequency in later life.

In a patient liable to migraine an increase in frequency of the attacks is likely to be due to:

     (a) anxiety and overwork,
     (b) the contraceptive pill,
     (c) vascular hypertension,
     (d) the menopause,
     (e) an underlying structural lesion such as an angioma or cerebral tumour.

Treatment. This falls into three parts:

(1) The patient must be told, after appropriate steps have been taken, if necessary, that the condition, although distressing, is not medically serious.

(2) Regular sedation may be given in the form of diazepam 2 mg t.d.s. This is, in itself, sometimes enough to bring about a considerable decrease in the number of attacks and even to abolish them.

A more specific prophylactic is methysergide, a serotonin antagonist which can be given in doses of 3–6 mg. daily. Toxic effects such as skin rashes, dysequilibrium and angina are common and it may rarely give rise to retroperitoneal and other fibroses. It should be used only in intractable migraine. Clonidine hydrochloride 0·025 mg. up to six times daily is less toxic and is said to reduce attacks by some 60 per cent.

(3) Attacks are best treated by ergotamine tartrate and the important point is to introduce this substance into the body as early in an attack as possible. For this reason tablets are often disappointing in their effect and an injection of ergotamine tartrate 0·25 or 0·5 mg. may be necessary. Thus the patient should learn to inject himself, so as to avoid delay. Alternatively a suppository containing ergotamine tartrate 2 mg. may be inserted.

MIGRAINOUS NEURALGIA

This variety of paroxysmal headache differs from migraine in that the bouts are of greater frequency and shorter duration.

The headache is sharply localised to one or other supra-orbital region but may spread into the temple, eye, or cheek. Typically it wakens the patient from sleep every night an hour or two after he has gone to bed and is very intense. It lasts from 30–90 minutes and may be accompanied by

A bruit is sometimes heard for a few days after haemorrhage from an aneurysm, possibly to be attributed to vascular spasm, but this seldom persists. The commonest cause of a persistent bruit in a young person is a cerebral angioma and its discovery will thus be of significance if the symptoms are otherwise suggestive.

Investigation of Spontaneous Intracranial Haemorrhage

Whatever the clinical assessment of the likely source of haemorrhage it is desirable, in patients in whom the haemorrhage is not likely to prove rapidly fatal, to proceed to arteriography to try and visualise the source of haemorrhage and its site.

The signs will naturally determine whether the carotid tree, on one or other side, or the basilar tree is to be investigated but if there are no signs other than those of meningeal irritation or if the signs are inconclusive, carotid arteriograms should be done first. If these are normal it is important to remember that aneurysms and angiomas also occur in the posterior fossa and that a haematoma without an obvious source can be present in the cerebellum.

Treatment. If no source of the haemorrhage is discovered, treatment is traditionally by rest, good nursing, and such medical measures as will help to keep the patient alive while recovery is taking place; but even so the mortality is about 50 per cent. The possibility now arises, however, that some patients with an intracerebral haematoma may be helped by having the clot removed. This is particularly the case where there seems to be progression of signs, where coma has not been too profound or too prolonged and when the haematoma is relatively superficial.

An aneurysm may be treated surgically by direct attack, if that is possible, so that its neck may be clipped, or it may be packed around with muscle. Another method which is particularly indicated in carotid aneurysms is to tie the common carotid artery in the neck and thus reduce the thrust on the aneurysmal sac.

Some angiomas, depending on their size and situation, can be excised. This is the treatment of choice, but occasionally it may be helpful to tie off the entering arteries. Irradiation is of doubtful value.

CEREBRAL ISCHAEMIA

Apart from haemorrhage causing destruction of brain tissue directly and possibly causing more remote effects by surrounding oedema and compression, cerebral function can be disturbed by ischaemia.

The classical examples of this are where cerebral vessels are occluded by thrombosis or embolus, resulting in infarction, but more recently it has become clear that disease of the internal carotid and vertebral arteries and, indeed, of even more proximal arteries can give rise to clinical pictures indistinguishable from those which have been called cerebral thrombosis. It is no longer possible to think of cerebral ischaemia except in relation to the whole carotico-vertebral system and its cerebral branches.

The classical *source of embolus* is from the heart in the presence of either atrial fibrillation, myocardial infarction with mural thrombus, or infective endocarditis. Equally important now is atherosclerosis of the aorta and carotid or vertebral arteries from which mural thrombus, atheromatous material or platelet emboli may arise. Rarer causes of embolism are fat, tumour cells, or air.

What actually happens after occlusion by thrombosis or embolism of a cerebral vessel depends on the collateral circulation; the number of anastomotic channels available will determine the size of a given infarct or whether it will occur at all. Upon the size and situation of the infarct will depend the neurological signs.

The diagnosis between thrombosis and embolism is not so important as the diagnosis of each from haemorrhage; the onset of symptoms from embolism is the most sudden and consciousness is not usually lost.

It is now well recognised that infarction can occur without occlusion and an important advance in the understanding of atherosclerotic vascular disease is the recognition of recurrent cerebral ischaemic attacks, usually to be attributed to emboli.

Internal Carotid Artery Disease

The syndrome of the internal carotid artery with ipselateral blindness and contralateral hemiplegia has long been known but it is really carotid arteriography, by demonstrating internal carotid artery occlusion or stenosis, that has led to the recognition of these recurrent attacks. They may occur at any age from the second decade onwards but they are increasingly frequent in older people.

Clinical Features. The episodes are brief, often occurring with great frequency, usually of the same pattern and representing some focal disorder of brain function. The symptoms are characteristically transient monocular blindness with or without contralateral signs of motor or sensory disturbance and possibly dysphasia if the ischaemia is in the dominant hemisphere, occurring separately or together, possibly with confusion or other impairment of intellectual function. These symptoms may be followed in time by permanent cerebral damage, possibly extensive and of abrupt onset. In less obvious cases, in which cerebral infarction appears to be the correct clinical diagnosis, the possibility of internal carotid occlusion or stenosis deserves consideration whether the lesion is a large one causing profound hemiplegia or is causing focal symptoms only; ipselateral Horner's syndrome may be present.

Vertebro-basilar Disease

Similar brief episodes may occur when these arteries are diseased and may be distinguished by impaired vision amounting sometimes to blindness, diplopia, vertigo, dysarthria, tingling around the lips and of the tongue, ataxia, and hemiparesis or tetraparesis.

Treatment of Cerebral Ischaemia

There is no really effective treatment of an established infarct but there may be a possibility of preventing further embolic infarcts. This treatment may be *medical or surgical.*

Medical

A patient with rheumatic or arteriosclerotic heart disease may be helped by the prolonged use of anticoagulants. The same may be so if the embolus arises from the great vessels.

If, however, a cerebral vascular episode is not obviously embolic, there is no way of distinguishing with certainty between haemorrhage and thrombosis except by C.T. scanning. Unless this distinction can be made anticoagulant treatment may be unsafe.

In the recurrent cerebral ischaemia attacks, which often herald an oncoming stroke, anticoagulants may diminish the frequency of the attacks and delay or prevent the stroke.

Surgical

When the internal carotid artery in the neck is shown to be occluded, operation is rarely indicated and only if the occlusion is known to be recent. If the internal carotid artery is stenosed at its origin an endarterectomy can be performed thus increasing the total blood supply to the brain, the likelihood being that other vessels are similarly involved, and also removing a potential source of emboli. Operations on the vertebral arteries and on the vessels arising from the aortic arch are technically more difficult but are proving increasingly possible particularly in relation to the 'subclavian steal' syndrome when the subclavian artery is narrow or occluded proximal to the origin of the vertebral artery.

Diffuse Cerebral Atherosclerosis

Sometimes the effect of atheroma of the cerebral vessels is such that no obvious stroke occurs but a series of minor episodes gradually lead to a picture of intellectual impairment, into which the patient often has insight; emotional lability, bladder disturbance, and a shuffling gait—*le marche a petit pas*—are other typical features. Sometimes dysarthria and dysphagia develop and complete the picture of *pseudo-bulbar palsy*, so called because the symptoms are the same as those in progressive bulbar palsy, but are due to an upper and not a lower motor neurone lesion. Features of Parkinsonism may also appear.

VENOUS SINUS THROMBOSIS

This occurs as the result of trauma or infection. Infection from the middle ear or mastoid causes lateral sinus thrombosis and that from the face or nasal sinuses may cause cavernous sinus thrombosis or thrombosis of the superior sagittal sinus. Cerebral abscess may be a sequel.

Lateral Sinus Thrombosis

The symptoms are fever, headache and vomiting, and papilloedema may be present. Focal neurological signs are rare.

Cavernous Sinus Thrombosis

The symptoms are pain in and around the eye with proptosis and chemosis. There may be external ophthalmoplegia and papilloedema may develop.

Superior Sagittal Sinus Thrombosis

This is less common but infection may spread from the nasal sinuses and may then pass to the cortical veins giving rise to focal epilepsy and focal neurological signs.

Treatment. This is of the original infection, if present, and as a result of more effective treatment in recent years by sulphonamides and antibiotics these complications are now relatively rare and are more amenable to treatment when they occur.

INFECTIONS

Acute Pyogenic Meningitis

It results either from primary infection of the meninges and cerebro-spinal fluid (C.S.F.), or less commonly by the extension of infection from the middle ear or skull sinuses, or from a cerebral abscess.

The onset is usually acute and is characterised by fever, headache, and vomiting, with the development of a stiff neck and backache. Stupor or coma may follow. Convulsions are rare in adults. *Examination* confirms the neck stiffness and there may be a positive Kernig's sign. Other neurological signs are not found in the early stages.

The diagnosis can be confirmed by lumbar puncture, which reveals a purulent fluid containing several thousand polymorphs, increased protein, greatly decreased sugar and an organism which is likely to be meningococcus, staphylococcus, streptococcus, pneumococcus, or haemophilus influenzae. In meningococcal meningitis morbilliform rashes and petechiae often appear, but this purpuric tendency is rare in other types of meningitis.

Treatment. The principles of treatment are to try to obtain a therapeutic concentration of a suitable antibiotic in the C.S.F. as rapidly as possible. Some useful therapeutic combinations are given below.

Treatment of Bacterial Meningitis

Meningococcal Meningitis

Although sulphadiazine is effective and penetrates well into the C.S.F., resistant strains are becoming common. Treatment should therefore be started with benzylpenicillin given 4 hourly as an intravenous bolus of 3·0 mega-units, which gives an adequate concentration in the C.S.F. If the organism proves sensitive to sulphonamides, sulphadiazine 1·0 g. 4 hourly by mouth can be added to the treatment regime.

Pneumococcal Meningitis

Benzylpenicillin given as an intravenous bolus of 4·0 mega-units every 4 hours is the treatment of choice. Treatment should be continued for two weeks. In patients allergic to penicillin, erythromycin 1·0 g. I.V. 6 hourly has proved successful.

Influenzal Meningitis

Chloramphenicol in doses of 20 mg./kg. I.M. given every 6 hours is probably the preferred treatment.

Ampicillin is an alternative but dosage must be high. 50 mg./kg. given every six hours as an intravenous bolus is satisfactory.

Purulent C.S.F.—No organism seen

Benzylpenicillin 4·0 mega-units 4 hourly I.V.
Chloramphenicol 20 mg./kg. 6 hourly I.M.
as an initial treatment until the organism is identified.

Prognosis and sequelae depend upon the duration of the illness before treatment is begun, and the sensitivity of the infecting agent to the available antibiotics. Most patients do well, and death or serious sequelae occur in less than 10 per cent of cases. These include cranial nerve palsy, focal cerebral lesions, epilepsy, dementia, and hydrocephalus.

Tuberculous Meningitis

It is always secondary to tuberculosis elsewhere in the body, although this may not be manifest. It may occur at any age, most commonly in children and young adults. It is of insidious onset, and usually encephalitis is the striking early feature: this causes confusion, and ultimately stupor or coma. Epileptic fits may occur. Less commonly meningitic signs predominate. Tubercles in the choroid membrane are the only specific finding on clinical examination, but signs elsewhere may suggest tuberculosis.

Diagnosis is confirmed by examination of the C.S.F. The pressure is increased, and the fluid either clear or opalescent. There are usually 10–50 polymorphs and 50–500 lymphocytes per cu. mm., and the protein is raised. Whereas in the past expert examination would reveal the tubercle bacillus usually on direct microscopy or on animal inoculation, this is now not always so and the bacillus may only be shown, if at all, on culture.

Treatment· Streptomycin 1·0g daily I.M., isoniazid 10 mg./kg. daily and rifampicin 12 mg./kg. daily. Steroids may be given initially.

The disease was always fatal before the advent of specific chemotherapy, but with modern treatment the mortality is about 10 per cent. In general, prognosis improves with age and is most serious in infants and young people.

Viral Meningitis

Presents acutely with predominantly meningitis signs and symptoms (p. 294). Usually there is no clue to the infecting agent on clinical examination, although sometimes there may be evidence of an existing virus infection, for example the rash of herpes or the salivary gland swelling of mumps. The diagnosis again depends on examination of the C.S.F.: the pressure is raised, and the fluid is either clear or opalescent. On microscopy lymphocytes are seen, usually between 100 and 1,000 per cu. mm.

Differential diagnosis is from tuberculous meningitis: usually the abruptness of onset, the predominance of symptoms and signs of meningitis over those of encephalitis, the larger number of cells in the fluid, and absence of tubercle bacilli serve to make distinction possible.

Many viruses are capable of affecting the nervous system, but some of the commoner ones are poliomyelitis (below), herpes zoster (p. 284), and lymphocytic choriomeningitis; secondary affection may occur in herpes simplex, mumps (p. 546) and with Coxsackie and Echo viruses (p. 550).

No specific **treatment** is available for virus infections at present, but the prognosis in most cases is good. Sequelae similar to those of acute meningitis (p. 295) occasionally occur.

Poliomyelitis

This is a virus infection which is thought to gain access to the body through the nasopharynx or the alimentary tract. After an incubation period varying from 7 to 14 days, there is first a generalised bodily reaction and then invasion of the nervous system. This is confined to the grey matter, and particularly the anterior horn of the spinal cord and the motor nuclei of the brain stem.

Clinical Features. The prodromal symptoms are fever, malaise, headache, and vomiting and after three or four days, during which they sometimes remit, further symptoms referable to the central nervous system develop. These are increased headache, spinal pains, and paraesthesiae, often localised, and pains in the limbs. There is stiffness of the neck and rigidity of the whole spinal column, usually with drowsiness or irritability. In some patients recovery then occurs but in others this so-called *preparalytic stage* is followed by the appearance of *paralysis*. This usually develops rapidly but may advance for 3 to 5 days. As it develops the fever subsides. The extent and degree of the paralysis are extremely variable, but the legs are involved more often than the arms, and the arms more often than the trunk. In about 15 per cent of patients there is involvement of cranial nuclei and muscles of the face, pharynx, larynx, and tongue may be paralysed. Respiratory paralysis may result either from the involvement of the diaphragm and intercostal muscles or by involvement of the respiratory centre in the medulla. Retention of urine sometimes occurs. Reflexes may be abolished. There is no sensory loss.

The *spinal fluid* may be under increased pressure and shows pleocytosis; in the very early stages polymorphs predominate, but later lymphocytes. The protein content may be increased and this may rise further during the first month if paralysis is widespread. The sugar and chloride levels are normal.

Diagnosis. In the preparalytic stage it is from pyogenic and tuberculous meningitis and the history and spinal fluid findings are of help. The appearance of muscular fasciculation is also a sign of great value at this stage. The distinction from other forms of virus meningitis depends upon virus studies or the isolation of the poliomyelitis virus from the faeces.

In the paralytic stage, when there is a lower motor neurone paralysis with muscle tenderness, acute polyneuritis may be suspected. However, poliomyelitis is likely to be asymmetrical, and there is no sensory loss.

Prophylaxis: Poliomyelitis is now prevented by giving 3 drops of live attenuated polio virus to children at 6 months, 7 months, 8 months and $4\frac{1}{2}$ years.

Treatment. In the *preparalytic stage* rest is essential, for there is good evidence that exertion increases the likelihood of paralysis.

If *paralysis* does develop, gentle but frequent passive movements to the weak limbs are given and if pain is troublesome hot packs applied to the muscles give relief. A sedative such as amylobarbitone (15 mg. t.d.s.) is helpful.

During the acute stage of paralysis rigid splinting is to be avoided but a cradle, foot-rest and pillows should be used to prevent shortening of the paralysed muscles. Treatment is directed towards the avoidance of all unnecessary muscle activity and the prevention of painful spasm and contractures.

In the rehabilitation of the patient after the acute stage is over, early and vigorous activity is indicated.

If there are signs of *respiratory failure* the patient must be transferred to a hospital where artificial ventilation can be given.

Cases with early difficulty in swallowing and speaking due to *bulbar involvement* resemble those with respiratory paralysis and the distinction is of great importance because the treatment is different; artificial respiration may be disastrous. Those patients who are unable to prevent secretions in the pharynx from being sucked into the lungs with inspiration must be nursed semi-prone with the foot of the bed raised and must be turned from side to side every two hours.

If respiratory paralysis occurs in bulbar poliomyelitis then either postural drainage must be carried out in a respirator or a tracheostomy must be done and the patient's respiration maintained by intermittent positive pressure.

NEUROSYPHILIS

Syphilis attacks the nervous system either by a meningo-vascular process or by involving the parenchyma; the latter gives rise to tabes dorsalis or general paralysis of the insane or sometimes to a mixture of the two.

Only about 10 per cent of patients with syphilis later develop neurological manifestations, although a higher proportion have asymptomatic involvement in the early stages, characterised only by abnormalities in the C.S.F. What then happens and why only some patients develop clinical neurosyphilis are not known. Symptoms do not appear for some years after primary infection except in the rare cases of acute meningo-vascular syphilis.

Meningo-vascular Syphilis

The lesion is an endarteritis with perivascular inflammation, which is the reaction of the mesoblastic tissues to the spirochaete and its toxins. This proceeds to gumma formation, and the meningeal involvement may be focal or diffuse. The *focal form* is rare and the resulting gumma behaves like any other expanding lesion. In the *diffuse form* the symptoms are headache, often with mental confusion and possibly epilepsy, and there may be papilloedema and neck stiffness. Cranial nerve palsies may develop, the oculo-motor nerves and those in the cerebello-pontine angle being most commonly involved. Optic atrophy may also occur. In a few cases there may be hemiparesis or aphasia, usually transient.

The C.S.F. is abnormal, showing a moderate increase of protein and cells, mainly lymphocytes, and positive serological reactions for syphilis.

Treatment is by intramuscular injections of penicillin, 1 million units daily to a total of 12–15 million.

Myelitis

A spinal form of meningo-vascular syphilis may lead to a complete or partial transverse myelitis of rapid onset resulting in a variable degree of paraplegia, sensory loss, and sphincter disturbance. This occurs most commonly in the thoracic cord.

A more chronic form of meningo-myelitis usually involves the cervical portion of the cord (*cervical pachymeningitis*) and leads to wasting of the small muscles of the hand and spastic paraplegia. In this respect it resembles motor neurone disease, but the arm reflexes are usually depressed and there may be cutaneous sensory loss.

Tabes Dorsalis

This condition is not so called because the dorsal columns of the cord are involved; the name, which goes back to Hippocrates, was applied first to paraplegia associated with wasting of the back and only later, quite by coincidence, selected to describe a disease in which the posterior columns of the cord were found to be shrunken and, later, demyelinated.

Tabes tends to occur ten years or more after the primary infection and affects males more often than females. Pathologically there is thought to be a lesion of the posterior roots which starts in the lumbosacral region of the cord and may extend as far as the cervical cord. Rarely the affliction may begin in the cervical cord (cervical tabes). The effect of the lesion is to cause wasting of the posterior columns and demyelination of the fibres passing up the posterior columns; the equally severe involvement of pain fibres is not followed by demyelination because of their relay, as they enter the cord, before crossing to the opposite side.

Clinical Features. 'Lightning pains' are common and characteristic. They are irregularly occurring, sharp, momentary stabs of pain, which tend to involve one spot while the bout lasts and this spot is typically in one or other thigh, calf or ankle. It is rare for two or more spots to be involved at the same time. The pain is variously described as being like a needle or a knife plunged into the leg, but more helpful than any description is the patient's almost invariable tendency to illustrate the sudden, stabbing nature of the pain by gesture. The area where the pain has most recently struck may remain tender for a time. The bouts occur irregularly and tend to be provoked by damp weather.

Other early symptoms may be of *sphincter disturbance*, sometimes bed-wetting due to retention with overflow; *impotence*; *visual disturbances*; or *ataxia*. The unsteadiness is more noticeable in the dark when the patient is deprived of visual aid to guide his steps. Later the ataxia may become more prominent, leading to the characteristic *stamping gait*. Gastric and other *tabetic crises* may occur and *trophic lesions* such as arthropathies and perforating ulcer may develop.

On examination, the pupils are usually small, irregular in outline, fixed to light but contracting on convergence (*Argyll-Robertson pupils*). The knee and ankle jerks are absent and possibly the triceps jerks. Character-istically there is cutaneous analgesia below the knees, over the trunk to the level of T4 and down the inner arm. Deep pain in the calves and Achilles tendons is absent. There is loss of postural sense and vibration sense of variable degree in the legs. There may be ptosis and primary optic atrophy with peripheral constriction of the visual fields, though visual acuity may still be normal.

Trophic changes involve not only the hip, knee, ankle, or small joints of the feet but also the spine (*Charcot's joints*). These joints are grossly disorganised, nearly always painless and unusually mobile considering the amount of destruction present. Arthropathy of the spine may cause pain-less root lesions and in this way there may develop wasting and weakness of radicular distribution. Otherwise the power in tabes is normal, the apparent paraplegia being due to loss of position sense in the legs.

The C.S.F. in tabes may contain excess cells and protein, a positive Wassermann reaction and an abnormal Lange reaction. It is not always abnormal in all these respects and may sometimes be completely normal.

Specific treatment is by intramuscular injections of penicillin 1 million units daily to a total of 12–15 million units. This will arrest the disease but is unlikely to alter the clinical picture greatly, although lightning pains are sometimes relieved, at least temporarily. Symptomatic treatment may be required for bladder disturbance, especially if the urine is infected. Although considerable disability may result from ataxia, blindness, and arthropathies, the disease is self-limiting and death usually occurs only as a result of urinary infection. The ataxia may be improved by re-educative exercises. Arthropathies may require surgery to promote stability by arthrodesis. Perforating ulcers should have any necrotic bone removed from their base and should be treated by rest. Care should be taken to prevent further trauma.

The C.S.F. should be re-examined after six months to confirm that there is improvement, indicated by a decrease in protein and fewer cells. Although the C.S.F. is likely to become normal eventually, a persistently positive test for syphilis is not in itself an indication for further treatment.

General Paralysis of the Insane

This is a chronic spirochaetal meningo-encephalitis, the spirochaetes being in the brain; exactly how they produce the pathological changes is not yet fully understood. These changes comprise thickening of the meninges, atrophy of the convolutions, especially of the anterior two thirds of the brain, with compensatory hydrocephalus and granular ependymitis. Microscopically there is an inflammatory meningeal reaction with peri-vascular infiltration of lymphocytes and plasma cells. Nerve cells degenerate and iron pigment is deposited.

Clinical Features. The onset is usually insidious, occurring ten years or more after the primary infection. Males are more commonly affected than females.

The early symptoms are those of *dementia* and *personality change*. There may be loss of memory and of judgement, carelessness with regard to spending money and neglect of cleanliness and of general appearance. The personality change is by no means always towards ideas of grandeur and the patient may be depressed or hypochondriacal. Gradually there is complete disintegration of intellect and of personality.

Epilepsy may be an early symptom and may, indeed, be the first manifestation of the disease at a time when there is nothing to suggest its true nature.

On examination, the physical signs which accompany the dementia are a *slurring dysarthria*, often with an aphasic element so that words are not only incorrectly articulated but wrongly uttered with transposition of syllables; *tremors* of the hands, lips, and tongue; and *spastic weakness* of the legs with brisk reflexes and possibly extensor plantar responses. *Optic atrophy* and Argyll-Robertson pupils (p. 265) may also be present.

The C.S.F. is likely to show increase of protein and cells and a paretic Lange (5555544433) and tests for syphilis are always positive. It is usually also positive in the blood, but not so constantly; a negative serology cannot be taken to exclude general paralysis. If such a diagnosis seems possible the C.S.F. *must* be examined.

Treatment. Untreated general paralysis is fatal within two years or so of its onset and it was this that helped to distinguish it, at the beginning of the nineteenth century, from other forms of insanity. With the introduction of malaria therapy in the 1920's a cure was achieved in about 30 per cent of patients and arrest in a similar number. For a time this was combined with penicillin, but the latter is now generally regarded as an adequate treatment by itself. Intramuscular injections of 1 million units daily are given to a total of 12–15 million units.

If the diagnosis is made early the *prognosis* is good, with the possibility of return to normal mental function. The disease can usually be arrested and, when remission is not complete, a proportion of patients can still return to a useful life.

The C.S.F. should be re-examined after six months to ensure that there has been a satisfactory response to treatment, the important feature at this stage being a decrease of protein and cells.

Syphilitic Optic Atrophy

This may occur as an isolated manifestation of neuro-syphilis or it may accompany other clinical symptoms, either meningo-vascular or parenchymatous. The optic discs are dead white but visual acuity may be normal to a late stage, when blindness may develop quite rapidly, central vision being eventually involved in a process of gradually increasing peripheral constriction.

The C.S.F. may be abnormal, but treatment with penicillin is often ineffective in relieving the blindness or preventing its advance to involve an eye still normal at the time of treatment.

INTRACRANIAL TUMOUR

Under this heading it is convenient to include all expanding lesions inside the skull, abscesses and haematomas as well as neoplasms. Angiomas are excluded since they are congenital arteriovenous malformations and rarely behave as expanding lesions in the absence of haemorrhage.

In adults the common neoplasms are *gliomas* which are infiltrative tumours, the *meningioma*, an essentially benign tumour, and *metastatic tumours*, usually from carcinoma of the lung or breast. *Neuromas*, usually of the eighth nerve, and *pituitary tumours* are also quite common.

In children, in whom the tumours are usually found in the posterior fossa, the commonest are *medullo-blastoma* and *astrocytoma*, either of the cerebellum or the pons.

Clinical Features. Although the combination of headache, vomiting, and papilloedema is the most characteristic presentation of a cerebral tumour, it is by no means the commonest and the possibility of a tumour may arise when none of these is present. The only indication may be some progressive defect of function, either physical or mental. Thus there may be progressive deafness, visual loss, hemiplegia, and disturbance of speech or its secondary derivatives (reading, calculation, etc.); or progressive personality change or intellectual impairment.

Headache is, however, often a feature. It is usually intermittent, often localised, or lateralised, present on waking for a few hours and aggravated, or even precipitated, by coughing and straining. Although often accompanied by increased intracranial pressure it is not due to this but to a distortion or displacement of pain-sensitive structures, which are the dural sinuses, large arteries and sensory nerves. This displacement may also cause obstruction to the C.S.F. pathways and produce *papilloedema*.

Associated *vomiting* is less frequent than headache, but if present also often occurs on waking and may lead to some relief of the headache. Rarely vomiting may occur alone, usually with tumours in the posterior fossa; the probable mechanism is direct involvement of the vomiting centre.

Other symptoms which suggest the possibility of tumour are *epilepsy*, especially if of late onset, and *vertigo*, either of which may occur as an isolated symptom and precede for some time signs of an expanding lesion, in the case of epilepsy possibly for several years. If the epilepsy is focal it may localise the lesion, but if the discharge arises in the temporal lobe area it does not always lateralise it. There is, however, nothing in the pattern of the epileptic attack to indicate for certain the presence of an underlying lesion or to suggest that such a lesion is a tumour.

Mental Symptoms. These may at first consist of no more than tiredness, apathy, or lack of energy, but may proceed to personality change, intellectual impairment and gross retardation, often with incontinence.

Signs. Signs which support the suspicion of cerebral tumour are:

(1) *Papilloedema*

This occurs with obstruction of C.S.F. pathways and is more likely, therefore, with tumours involving the third ventricle, aqueduct, fourth ventricle, and its roof foramina. It is therefore more common with tumours of the posterior fossa and may not be present at all in patients with even large tumours involving the cerebral hemispheres. It must also be remembered that papilloedema occurs in other conditions, such as lateral sinus thrombosis and so-called benign intracranial hypertension; the latter occurs almost exclusively in women, sometimes in association with pregnancy, and may follow mild trauma though often the aetiology is unknown. Papilloedema must also be distinguished from retrobulbar neuritis accompanied by swelling of the disc. The distinction may not be possible simply from ophthalmoscopic appearance; but retrobulbar neuritis is associated with severe loss of visual acuity, which is not an early symptom of papilloedema.

(2) Focal Neurological Signs

If these are present, they serve to localise the tumour and may, if this localisation is characteristic, suggest its likely nature. Thus a tumour in the cerebello-pontine angles giving rise to progressive deafness, facial weakness and numbness, and ipselateral ataxia is likely to be an acoustic neuroma. A para-sagittal tumour may be a meningioma, as may be one compressing the olfactory nerve in the olfactory groove and causing anosmia. A tumour causing bitemporal field defects thereby indicates its presence in the region of the pituitary fossa and may be a pituitary adenoma, a craniopharyngioma or a meningioma. General examination of the patient, especially of the lungs or breasts, may suggest the possibility of a metastatic growth, as may the past history of a carcinoma anywhere in the body. A source of infection, either in the ear, the nasal sinuses, or the chest, suggests the possibility of abscess; and this is a common lesion too in patients with cyanotic congenital heart disease.

Special Investigations. It is always necessary to proceed to further investigation so that the presence of a tumour can be verified, its nature determined and appropriate treatment given.

(1) Radiography

Radiographs of the skull may show:

Erosion of the posterior clinoid processes, suggesting raised intracranial pressure; of the internal auditory meatus, as in acoustic neuroma; of the skull base in the region of the petrous apex and foramen ovale, as in nasopharyngeal carcinoma extending into the skull.

Expansion of the sella turcica (ballooning) as in chromophobe adenoma or its *destruction* from without as in para-sellar tumours.

Hyperostosis at the sites of election of meningioma, the vault, sphenoid wings, and olfactory grooves.

They may also show lateral *shift of a calcified pineal*, confirming the presence of an expanding lesion, or its downward shift, suggesting the presence of internal hydrocephalus, possibly secondary to tumour.

They may show *abnormal calcification*, which occurs in many tumours, but especially in slow-growing gliomas and in about half the craniopharyngiomas.

If a cerebral tumour is suspected radiographs of the chest must be always taken to exclude or reveal the presence of a bronchial carcinoma.

(2) Echo-encephalography

When X-rays of the skull are normal, when there is no abnormal calcifications and when the pineal is not calcified, echo-encephalography can be done to determine the position of the mid-line structures.

(3) Electro-encephalography (E.E.G.)

This may indicate an area of disturbed cerebral function; but a single record cannot distinguish between a vascular and a neoplastic process nor can the E.E.G. distinguish with certainty between a benign and a malignant tumour. The E.E.G. in cerebral abscess contains characteristically slow focal activity. A tumour in the posterior fossa may give rise to bilateral E.E.G. disturbances and the E.E.G. may thus help to distinguish between a posterior fossa and a cerebral hemisphere tumour.

(4) Brain Scan

This is done using Technetium 99^m, which may be taken up by various abnormal intracranial structures, including neoplasms, abscesses, haematomas, infarcts and angiomas.

(5) Computerised Transverse Axial Tomography (E.M.I. Scanner)

The development of the technique of computerised tomography of the brain has been described as the greatest advance in the use of X-rays since their discovery by Röntgen in 1895.

The brain is a soft-tissue structure with fluid-containing ventricles and subarachnoid space surrounded by bone. On plain radiography only calcium, fat and air are visible within the cranium and contrast media are necessary for demonstration of the ventricles and vasculature.

The E.M.I. scanner measures the absorption coefficient (density) of defined volumes of the brain in selected horizontal slices and presents an accurate anatomical picture in which can be identified grey and white matter and the ventricles and subarachnoid space. Lesions whose density differs from that of normal brain, e.g. tumours, abscesses, haematomas, infarcts and cerebral oedema are shown and dilatation of the ventricles due to hydrocephalus or atrophy is evident. In brain atrophy, wide cerebral sulci may also be seen. The density of tumours can be enhanced by the intravenous injection of an iodine-containing medium.

E.M.I. scanning is a rapid atraumatic method with low radiation dose. The use of the E.M.I. scanner has effected a very significant reduction in the need for other diagnostic procedures such as pneumography and angiography, which are not without danger. Lesions which are demonstrated by conventional radionucleide brain scanning are shown more clearly in E.M.I. scans.

(6) Lumbar Puncture

This may be dangerous in the presence of papilloedema and is not likely to add any information of value in cases where there is little doubt about the presence of an expanding intracranial lesion. It may, however, show increased intracranial pressure (normal is up to 180 mm. of fluid) when there is no other evidence of this and it may also show an increased protein content in the C.S.F., especially in acoustic neuroma and basal meningioma. There may be a pleocytosis, especially in cases of malignant tumours impinging on the ventricular system and it has recently been demonstrated that actual tumour cells may be identified in the C.S.F. In cerebral abscess the C.S.F. usually shows a pleocytosis, about 100 cells and mostly lymphocytic, and increased protein.

If these investigations seem to confirm the suspicion of tumour, then further neuro-radiological investigations may be done. These are:

> cerebral angiography,
> air encephalography,
> ventriculography.

Cerebral Angiography

This involves the injection of a radio-opaque dye into a carotid or vertebral artery. Injection into a carotid artery is particularly indicated if the cerebral lesion is lateralised and if there is some possibility of there being a vascular basis to the symptoms, cerebral angioma and internal carotid artery disease in particular sometimes mimicking a cerebral tumour. Angiography does not always localise an expanding lesion with certainty, especially if it is in the parietal region, but may do so accurately if there is a pathological circulation, as there not infrequently is with very malignant gliomas and metastatic growths.

Vertebral angiography is less frequently indicated but serves a similar purpose.

Air Encephalography

This is the name given to the filling of the ventricular system and the cerebral subarachnoid space with air which is injected either by lumbar or cisternal (cisterna magna) puncture.

The air in the ventricles is less opaque than the surrounding brain and the site, size, and shape of the ventricular system can thus be determined and the presence of any extracerebral, intracerebral, or intraventricular expanding-lesion can be demonstrated. Likewise it may be shown that the lesion is, in fact, one of cerebral atrophy.

Ventriculography

Air encephalography is best avoided in the presence of papilloedema or if there is no reasonable doubt about the presence of a tumour. In such cases the air can be introduced through a brain needle into the lateral ventricle through a posterior parietal burr-hole. In certain cases myodil may be introduced by this route if it is desired to demonstrate, for example, stenosis of the Sylvian aqueduct.

Treatment. At this stage the presence of a cerebral tumour may have been confirmed and if so its nature must be verified because this will determine the treatment. If investigations so far have been in favour of finding a benign rather than an infiltrating tumour, then a craniotomy should be performed. Craniotomy may also be done even if complete removal of the tumour is impossible if a substantial measure of relief can be anticipated from internal decompression, or if this is considered the safest or most effective way to verify the nature of a tumour.

If craniotomy is not done then a needle biopsy may provide the necessary verification and may confirm that the tumour is inoperable or may, on the other hand, suggest that it is operable. Exploration with a needle will also be used to find an abscess cavity, to aspirate the pus, and to instil the appropriate antibiotic.

When surgical removal of a tumour is impossible or incomplete, irradiation may be considered. If given in association with betamethasone or dexamethasone to control oedema immediate and short term results are often gratifying but the long term results are usually disappointing. This should not contra-indicate the use of radiotherapy unless the patient fails to make an initially favourable response to betamethasone or dexamethasone.

SPINAL CORD COMPRESSION

One of the most important clinical syndromes from the diagnostic point of view is that of gradual compression of the spinal cord.

Symptoms. It may occur at any age from a variety of causes and the earliest symptom may be *pain*. This pain is intermittent and precipitated or aggravated by coughing, straining, movement, jolting, and jarring. It is radicular in distribution and thus, depending on the situation of the lesion, passes down the arm or leg or is of girdle distribution round the trunk.

Following pain the next symptom from a lesion within the cervical or thoracic spine is a tendency to drag the legs on account of spasticity, especially on exertion. Progressive weakness, sensory loss, and sphincter disturbance gradually develop. A lesion within the lumbar spine causes a flaccid weakness.

Signs. The signs depend on the *level* of cord compression; it is the demonstration of a motor, sensory, or reflex *level* which leads to the diagnosis of a focal lesion of the spinal cord.

There are wasting and weakness of lower motor neurone type at the level of compression, and pyramidal weakness below it. *Reflexes* may be depressed at the level of the lesion and increased below it, with extensor plantar responses. The level of pain and temperature impairment may fall below the level of the lesion in early compression, on account of the lamination of the spinothalamic tract, but this will rise as the compression increases. The demonstration of a partial *Brown-Séquard syndrome* (i.e. pyramidal and posterior column signs more prominent on one side and pain and temperature loss more prominent on the other) confirm that the lesion is of the cord.

Compression of the conus and cauda equina cause early sphincter disturbance and impotence. A flaccid paralysis of the legs then develops, with wasting and fasciculation of the affected muscles, and sensory loss to all modalities over the lower lumbar and sacral dermatomes.

Once the suspected level of the lesion is discovered the spine must be carefully examined, especially at that level, for signs of a gibbus, other deformity, or tenderness.

Investigations

Radiological

Radiography of the spine may reveal vertebral destruction or erosion, possibly of an intervertebral foramen, or the changes of spondylosis; the latter is a particularly common cause of cord compression in the cervical region. Radiographs may also show changes of Paget's disease or of Pott's disease. A chest radiograph must be taken, since spinal metastases commonly arise from a bronchial carcinoma.

Lumbar Puncture

This is a very valuable investigation not only so that the C.S.F. may be examined but in order to do the *Queckenstedt* test to investigate the possibility of a block in the spinal subarachnoid space. This is performed by pressing on the jugular veins in the neck; if there is a free rise and fall of fluid in the manometer, there is no block. If there is no rise on jugular compression it is then necessary to press on the abdomen. If this produces a rise and fall of fluid in the manometer and further compression of the jugular veins again produces no response, then a block has been demonstrated in the spinal subarachnoid space, which confirms the suspicion of cord compression. A rise of fluid in the manometer on jugular compression, but no fall, indicates a partial block from which the same conclusion may be drawn. If there is a block the protein content of the C.S.F. is likely to be above 500 mg./100 ml. (*Froin syndrome*). If the puncture is above the level of a cauda equina compression, manometry will be normal but the protein may be increased, especially if the lesion is a neurofibroma.

Differential Diagnosis. A lesion causing focal compression of the spinal cord must be distinguished from other lesions which have a spastic paraplegia as part of the clinical picture. These are:

(1) *syringomyelia*, in which the arm reflexes are lost and there is dissociated cutaneous sensory loss,

(2) *syphilitic meningo-myelitis*, in which there may be other evidence of syphilis such as pupillary abnormalities and in which the C.S.F. shows appropriate changes.

(3) *disseminated sclerosis*, in which there is evidence of multiple lesions,

(4) *motor neurone disease*, in which there are no sensory symptoms or signs and no sphincter disturbance,

(5) *subacute combined degeneration* of the cord due to B_{12} deficiency, in which there are gastric achylia, possibly a

upper motor neurone is involved, when the expectation of life is about three years after the diagnosis has been established. With progressive bulbar palsy the outlook is similar; death results from inanition and pulmonary infection.

PERONEAL MUSCULAR ATROPHY (Charcot-Marie-Tooth)

This is a familial condition of unknown cause. There is atrophy of the anterior horn cells and posterior columns and associated interstitial neuritis of the peroneal nerves.

It presents as muscular wasting, starting in the feet and rising steadily over the years to the junction of the middle and lower thirds of the thigh. The small muscles of the hand and the distal third of the forearm may waste similarly. Despite extreme wasting power is remarkably preserved and active life for many years is the rule. All modalities of sensation are affected over the wasted muscles.

Only symptomatic treatment is possible but life expectancy is little reduced.

OCCUPATIONAL CRAMPS

This is an uncommon group of disorders affecting the muscles of the hand when engaging in vocational repetitive movements. The classical example is *writer's cramp*, but others such as seamstress's or telegraphist's cramp have been described. With increasing use of mechanical appliances they have become less common.

Characteristically the muscles are only affected when performing the particular task, for example writing. Initially there is pain in the muscles followed by cramps, eventually necessitating the cessation of the activity. No abnormality is found on examination. The only effective treatment is the complete avoidance of the painful activity for 6 to 9 months; symptomatic relief from cramp may be obtained with aspirin (300 mg.); splinting the hand and wrist is sometimes helpful.

Nothing is certainly known of the cause of the condition, but it is thought that psychological factors are important. The chief differential diagnosis is from Parkinson's disease, which may present with cramps in the hand and micrographia.

SPASMODIC TORTICOLLIS

This is an uncommon condition. It occurs only in adults, and affects the sexes equally. Outbreaks have been described following epidemics of encephalitis and rarely it is associated with Parkinson's disease. In 1959 the condition was induced in monkeys by lesions in the cephalic part of the reticular formation, the occiput turning towards the side of the lesion.

It may begin abruptly or gradually and consists of irregular spasms of the muscles supporting the head, notably of one sternomastoid. The head is irregularly displaced; usually it is rotated, occasionally flexed. It may be so slight as almost to pass unnoticed, or be so severe as to handicap the patient completely. As it persists it is associated with hypertrophy of the affected muscles and usually with derangement of the cervical spine.

Treatment consists of exercises to the neck with the object of stretching the affected muscles fully. This may be combined with amylobarbitone sodium 15 mg. t.d.s. Other drugs sometimes of use are promethazine (50 mg. t.d.s.), chlorpromazine (100 mg. t.d.s.), meprobamate (400 mg. t.d.s.) or reserpine (0·25 mg. t.d.s.). Alternatively, surgical division of the accessory nerve and upper anterior cervical roots may bring relief.

NEUROFIBROMATOSIS

This condition is usually manifest between twenty and forty and affects the sexes equally. It consists of hyperplasia of the fibrous connective tissue supporting the nerves. It occurs in a number of clinical forms.

(a) *Multiple Neurofibromata* (Von Recklinghausen's Disease)

Multiple tumours arise from cutaneous nerves, and project as lumps, some pedunculated, all over the body. There are also patches of melanotic pigmentation of the skin and often congenital spinal deformities, for example spina bifida or spondylolisthesis. There is no curative treatment, but large tumours may be excised.

(b) *Individual Neurofibromata*

These may arise from any nerve, and cause no symptoms unless the nerve passes through a constriction at the site of the tumour. Examples are:

(1) The *radial* as it pierces the lateral intermuscular septum, the *median* as it passes behind the tendonous bridge joining the origins of the flexor digitorum sublimis, and the deep branch of the *ulnar* nerve as it passes into the hand.

(2) Neurofibromata may arise on the *spinal nerve roots*, so that part of the tumour is within the spinal canal and part is in the thorax or abdomen. These so-called 'dumb-bell' tumours are occasionally discovered on chest radiography, but usually present with spinal-cord compression (p. 306).

(3) *Auditory* or (less commonly) *trigeminal nerve* tumours. They arise in the cerebello-pontine angle. They are insidious, and usually present as gradually increasing deafness and tinnitus. Vertigo may occur. This is followed by impairment of sensation of the forehead and cornea (V) sometimes complicated by corneal ulceration, and ipselateral facial weakness. Large tumours may cause ipselateral signs of cerebellar derangement (p. 277).

These tumours are all associated with raised C.S.F. protein (about 80–120 mg./100 ml.), and with expansion of the internal auditory meatus when visualised radiologically.

Treatment of all these conditions is surgical, the results depending upon the extent of the disease at the time of intervention. Rarely the tumours may undergo sarcomatous change.

(c) Rarely there is diffuse overgrowth of all the nervous supportive tissue, so as to cause hypertrophic chronic peripheral neuritis.

SYRINGOMYELIA AND SYRINGOBULBIA

Syringomyelia is a cystic degeneration of the grey matter of the spinal cord, until recently of unknown cause. There is now good evidence that in some patients, and possibly quite a large number, the primary lesion is a developmental or acquired anomaly in the region of the foramen magnum which obstructs the flow of C.S.F. from the foramina in the roof of the 4th ventricle. C.S.F. is thus forced into the central canal causing first a hydromyelia and then rupture of the ependyma permits fluid to seep into the central grey matter. Symptoms do not usually appear until early adult life or later and men are more frequently affected.

Clinical Features. The early involvement of grey matter interrupting the crossing pain and temperature fibres and the reflex arc, determines the cardinal signs of syringomyelia which are:

(1) *dissociated cutaneous sensory loss*, with loss of pain and temperature sensation and preservation of touch.
(2) *loss of reflexes.*

The process usually starts in the cervical enlargement so that the dissociated sensory loss appears over a forequarter and the arm reflexes are lost.

The *symptoms* which are likely to bring the patient under observation are:
> pain in the arm,
> wasting of small hand muscles,
> spastic weakness of the legs.

These are features which are present in a number of conditions and *on examination* the important additional diagnostic findings will be absent reflexes and dissociated cutaneous sensory loss, which may not be present over the whole forequarter and may not even be present anywhere in the arm but be confined to upper cervical dermatomes. Fasciculation, rather coarse, may be present over the arms and chest and there may be a scoliosis. Arthropathy (Charcot's joints) may be present in the cervical spine and, more rarely, in the shoulder and elbow joints.

Treatment. Radiotherapy to the affected part of the cord is thought to be helpful in some cases, especially in relieving pain. In other patients operation to restore a normal circulation of C.S.F. and decompress the expanded cord is now the treatment of choice.

Syringobulbia

Cavitation may occur in the medulla and does so usually in association with syringomyelia, but sometimes alone. The cavity has a fairly constant situation, in the postero-lateral part of the tegmentum, and involves, unilaterally or bilaterally,

(a) vestibular pathways,
(b) the descending root of the trigeminal nerve,
(c) sympathetic and taste pathways,
(d) the nucleus ambiguus,
(e) the emerging fibres of the hypoglossal nerve.

The *presenting symptoms*, which are sometimes of quite acute onset, are thus *vertigo, pain*, or *sensory loss* over the face or *hoarseness*. The *signs* are *nystagmus*, usually rotary, *dissociated sensory loss* over the face (not with a peripheral nerve distribution), *loss of taste, Horner's syndrome, vocal cord paralysis*, and a *wasted tongue*.

The condition may be slowly progressive, but may arrest and remain stationary for many years.

BASAL GANGLIA SYNDROMES

Parkinsonism

Paralysis agitans, first described by Parkinson in 1817 and later named Parkinson's disease by Charcot, is characterised by a combination in varying degree of rigidity, tremor and bradykinesia (slowness of movement) that cannot be totally accounted for by rigidity. Rigidity is the most constant feature and sometimes appears alone.

There may be a genetic factor in some 25 per cent of cases. An imbalance between the transmitter substances acetylcholine and dopamine in the striatum is now postulated and drugs which either inhibit the former (atropine and other solanaceous alkaloids) or increase the latter (levodopa) give benefit in certain cases.

Clinical Features. *Rigidity*. The effect of the rigidity is to interfere with the normal play of facial expression; with speech, so that the patient mumbles in a monotonous voice; and with posture and movement. Due to the rigidity of the neck and trunk muscles, the posture becomes stooped and there is disturbance of gait, so that starting to walk is often difficult and thereafter the patient has a tendency 'to walk at a running pace'. When walking, one or both arms may hang immobile by the side.

The patient often complains of weakness of an arm not, as he says, for picking up large things like a bucket of coal, but for picking up small things, and there is inability to perform fine finger movements. The writing becomes smaller and illegible.

Tremor. The characteristic feature of the tremor is that it is present at rest and may be momentarily inhibited by using the arm. The tremor usually starts in a hand or arm and may then involve the leg. It may remain unilateral or then involve the other side. The lower jaw may also become tremulous. Tremor stops during sleep.

In the absence of the characteristic tremor, the most important finding is *rigidity*, a resistance to passive movement at a joint throughout the full range of movement at that joint. Rigidity is found early in neck muscles, in the shoulder, wrist, and at the ankle, and may later become generalised. The small hand muscles are often *weak*, in addition to showing poverty of movement, but there is no other significant weakness and no reflex change or sensory loss. The **glabellar tap** is an interesting physical sign: blinking in response to tapping the root of the nose ceases in normal adults after a few taps, but in Parkinsonian patients it persists indefinitely.

Pathology

Paralysis agitans in the classical form is a systemic degeneration affecting a neuronal system whose nodal points seem to be the globus pallidus and substantia nigra. It usually develops in late middle age. About 100 years after Parkinson's description it became clear that a similar picture could be associated with encephalitis lethargica, coming on either at the time of the acute illness or later, the substantia nigra and its connections being the seat of an inflammatory rather than a degenerative change. More recently it has been recognised that certain features of Parkinsonism are associated with cerebral arteriosclerosis. There are, however, some distinguishing features.

Post-encephalitic Parkinsonism

In this the rigidity and tremor are identical but there may be added features which serve to distinguish it such as oculo-gyric crises, spasms of neck muscles, dribbling, a greasy skin, and behaviour disorders. The onset is nearly always before the age of forty.

Arteriosclerotic Parkinsonism

This is more easily distinguished and is commonly associated with hypertension or other evidence of vascular disorder, with dementia, pyramidal signs, sphincter disturbance, and a more shuffling gait. Tremor is less prominent than rigidity. This is a disease of old age.

Parkinsonism Due to Drugs

Parkinsonism may be a side-effect of drugs of the phenothiazine group (e.g. chlorpromazine) or of the butyrophenane group (e.g. haloperidol). These drugs can also cause oculo-gyric crises, previously seen only in post-encephalitic Parkinsonism.

Treatment

Medical. Tincture of stramonium and related drugs of the solanaceous group were for long the treatment of choice in the Parkinsonian syndrome. Then a series of synthetic drugs of the same nature was developed of which benzhexol is a useful representative. It may be given in tablets containing 2 mg. or 5 mg. up to a total of 12–18 mg. daily; it sometimes causes mental upset as a side-effect. Another useful preparation is orphenadrine 50–100 mg. t.d.s.

Following observations that dopamine was depleted in the basal ganglia of patients with Parkinsonism, dihydroxyphenylalanine (*levodopa*) (*l-dopa*) the precursor of dopamine which does not cross the blood-brain barrier, has proved effective in the treatment of about two thirds of the patients with Parkinsonism. The response is usually greater than that to the anticholinergic drugs already mentioned and bradykinesia is relieved more than rigidity and tremor. An initial dose of 250 mg. t.d.s. is gradually increased by increments of 250 mg. every three days or so and it seems that a total daily dose of between 2 g. and 8 g. will produce a satisfactory response. Side-effects are nausea, anorexia, hypotension and involuntary movements usually starting in the face. Psychiatric disturbances also occur. *Carbidopa* inhibits the extracerebral decarboxylation of levodopa and in combination with levodopa in the form of Sinemet makes more levodopa available for transport to the brain and subsequent conversion into dopamine. This permits a smaller dose of levodopa and thus lesser extracerebral side-effects, but possibly an increase in unwanted movements.

The dose is Sinemet tabs. ½ t.d.s. increasing gradually if necessary to tabs. 1 t.d.s. Alternatively Madopar may be used; this is a combination of L-Dopa and the decarboxylase inhibitor benzerizide and it is used in the same way as Sinemet.

Amantadine may also be tried in doses of 100 mg. daily for a week and 100 mg. twice daily thereafter.

If one of these L-Dopa preparations is not effective bromocriptine may be tried. This is a dopamine agonist acting directly on the dopaminergic receptors. The initial dose is 2·5 mg. daily and this may be increased by 2·5 mg. daily to 20 mg. a day and then by 5 mg. daily to 40 mg. a day.

Surgical. Recently operation has been helpful in suitable patients. The operation is a stereotactic one in which a destructive lesion is made in the globus pallidus or anterior thalamus. It is especially indicated in unilateral involvement in patients under sixty in whom there is no evidence of cerebral atherosclerosis. Tremor and rigidity are relieved more than bradykinesia and possibly operation plus levodopa will prove to be the most effective treatment.

HUNTINGTON'S CHOREA

This is an adult, hereditary, progressive chorea, with dominant inheritance, affecting the sexes equally and occurring in the third or fourth decade.

The early *symptoms* are usually involuntary movements of a fidgety and jerky character, accompanied by grimacing. As the condition progresses the arms become clumsy, the gait unsteady and signs of dementia appear, with personality change and memory and intellectual impairment.

There is no treatment and the condition usually ends in death in about fifteen years. The choreiform movements may respond to tetrabenazine 75–300 mg. daily.

FRIEDREICH'S ATAXIA

This is the commonest member of a group of heredo-familial degenerative disorders.

Pathology. Degeneration is seen in the posterior columns, less marked in the lateral columns and cerebellum, and sometimes affects the optic nerves.

Clinical Features. The onset is in the first or second decade and the first symptom is unsteadiness of the gait followed later by clumsiness of the hands. Dysarthria develops and weakness is added to the ataxia. On examination nystagmus is present, there is intention tremor of the arms, pyramidal weakness of the legs with absent knee and ankle jerks and extensor plantar responses. There is impairment of postural and vibration sense. There may be optic atrophy. Pes cavus and scoliosis are characteristic and the E.C.G. may show cardiac arrhythmia.

The condition tends to be slowly progressive and no treatment is known which will arrest its course.

MYASTHENIA GRAVIS

This is a disease characterised by abnormal fatigue of striated muscle and rapid recovery after rest. The pathology is still far from clear, but there seems to be a biochemical defect associated with abnormal behaviour of acetylcholine at the myoneural junction. The symptoms can be present in the new-born child of a mother with myasthenia gravis, and will be transient. They can come on at any age and affect the sexes about equally; the highest incidence occurs in the second and third decades and in this age group women are more commonly affected.

Clinical Features. Fatigue may occur in any muscle or muscle group but most commonly involved are those in which weakness gives rise to diplopia, dysphagia, dysarthria, and difficulty in chewing. Muscles of the trunk and limbs are involved first in about 30 per cent of the cases. Affected muscles tire quickly on exercise, for example dysarthria develops in the course of conversation or difficulty in chewing in the middle of a meal; and all symptoms tend to become worse by the end of the day and to be relieved to some extent by next morning. The disease also shows complete remissions.

Myasthenia can occur as a *symptom* in carcinomatous neuropathy and in thyrotoxicosis.

Signs. On examination there is no wasting or fasciculation and there may or may not be permanent weakness. The most important feature to demonstrate is pathological fatigue. This may be done by asking the patient to look up without blinking for a prolonged period, during which time ptosis may develop, or by asking him to raise his arm above his head thirty or forty times, a movement he may find more and more difficult to perform. In both instances power will return to normal after a few seconds' rest. There is never any reflex change or sensory loss.

Diagnosis. If the diagnosis is in doubt and weakness is present, a diagnostic test may be carried out by giving an intramuscular injection of neostigmine 2 mg. or 2·5 mg., with atropine 1·0 mg. to prevent abdominal colic. Increase in power is quite striking after 20 to 30 minutes in the patient with myasthenia gravis, but a slight improvement, particularly if only subjective, has no significance. Alternatively an intravenous injection of edrophonium 10 mg. may be given, after which the response is much more rapid, occurring in a few minutes, but possibly less prolonged.

Treatment. This is, in the first place, by tablets of neostigmine bromide (15 mg.); one or two tablets should be taken as often as is necessary to maintain normal power. Alternatively tablets of the longer-acting pyridostigmine (60 mg.) may be given in the same way.

If the weakness is severe, especially of the muscles of swallowing, an intramuscular injection of neostigmine 2 mg. may be necessary first thing in the morning and before meals.

Thymectomy is of undoubted benefit in some cases and is indicated if the response to medical treatment is unsatisfactory. It seems to be of especial benefit if the total history is short. It does not replace treatment by neostigmine, which is afterwards usually required in smaller doses.

Operation is not indicated in the first place for a thymoma, whose presence may be discovered by an abnormal mediastinal shadow on radiography; but surgery may be considered after irradiation.

DEMYELINATING DISEASES

Demyelination in the central nervous system occurs in response to various pathological processes, but under this heading will be considered only diseases in which it is possibly the primary lesion.

Multiple Sclerosis (Disseminated Sclerosis)

The commonest of these conditions is disseminated sclerosis. Patches of demyelination occur at different times and in different places throughout the central nervous system, giving rise to the 'plaques' which in their final stage form grey, translucent scars in the white matter.

The *cause* of this condition is unknown. Some still regard it as an infection, others as an allergic reaction of the nervous system or the result of a metabolic upset or deficiency disorder. The disease is more common in temperate climates and about 60 per cent of patients have their first manifestation between the ages of twenty and forty, the onset being rare below the age of fifteen or over fifty. In this country it is half as common again in women as in men. Although intercurrent infection is likely to cause at least transient deterioration, there is no clear evidence that this or trauma can precipitate the disease and the risk of operation or pregnancy in producing a relapse is no longer considered a serious one. Although there is no evidence that pregnancy influences the long-term course of disseminated sclerosis, extra care may be helpful during the puerperium.

Clinical Features. Disseminated sclerosis is essentially pleomorphic and many symptoms and signs may appear singly or together; it is the *evidence of multiple lesions* on which the diagnosis ultimately rests. Unilateral *retro-bulbar neuritis* is often an early feature, the vision in one eye becoming misty, possibly with a central scotoma, or absent. Movement of the eye may be painful and there may be swelling of the optic disc. Vision usually returns to normal, but the disc subsequently shows abnormal pallor.

There may be *weakness* of one or both legs, sometimes with a sensory level indicating a transverse lesion of the cord. Sometimes there is defect or *loss of postural sense* in one or other arm giving rise to a useless arm. There may be *numbness* or *tingling* in the hands or feet, which may also be painful. There may be *vertigo, diplopia,* sphincter disturbance, usually causing increased frequency or *urgency* but sometimes retention, or impotence. *Tremor* and *dysarthria* may develop.

In the early stages there may be complete remission of symptoms which may last for many years, but with recurrent episodes remissions are likely to be less complete and increasing permanent disability usually develops, ending in paralysis of the legs, often with painful flexor spasms, ataxia of the arms due to tremor or postural loss, and urinary infection. In many patients, however, the disorder remains fortunately mild and interferes little with ordinary life. Occasionally, and more often when the disease is of late onset, it may be steadily progressive from the first.

Diagnosis. The diagnosis depends on (1) the *demonstration* of multiple lesions, by means of symptoms and signs and (2) the *exclusion* of a focal lesion either in the brain or in the spinal cord, such as spinal tumour or cervical spondylosis, system disorders, e.g. subacute combined degeneration of the cord or Friedreich's ataxia. In doubtful cases the C.S.F. may contain changes of diagnostic help, especially a paretic Lange in the presence of normal protein, indicating a relative increase of gamma globulin. The W.R. is negative.

Treatment. There is no specific treatment which is known for certain to influence the course of the disease. Arsenic, pyrotherapy, low fat diet, intrathecal injection of P.P.D. and many others have been tried without obvious success in a disease in which spontaneous remissions make the assessment of any specific remedy difficult. Corticotrophin has, however, been shown to be helpful in the treatment of retrobulbar neuritis and in hastening recovery in other acute episodes of disseminated sclerosis; it should be given by daily injections for about a month. There are also many opportunities for symptomatic treatment which must not be ignored. A pill containing ext. belladonna sicc. 30 mg. may relieve sphincter disturbance; chlorpromazine 50 mg. t.d.s. may relieve vertigo; and patients sometimes feel the benefit of weekly, or more frequent, injections of cyanocobalamin 1,000 μg. When the patient's mobility is affected rehabilitation by physiotherapy is important. In the later stages good nursing will help the prevention of bed-sores.

Neuromyelitis Optica

This is a closely related disease in which there is demyelination in the optic nerves and in the spinal cord, where it may be limited to a few segments or be diffuse.

The cause is unknown but it may develop at an earlier age than disseminated sclerosis. The *clinical picture* is that of bilateral retro-bulbar neuritis occurring simultaneously or consecutively, followed by a transverse myelitis which causes a spastic paraplegia or quadriplegia with sensory involvement and sphincter disturbance.

Except in its most typical form the clinical picture is indistinguishable from disseminated sclerosis, unless it develops at an earlier age.

Recovery may be complete or practically so, but relapse does sometimes occur leading to symptoms and signs characteristic of disseminated sclerosis.

Treatment. Corticotrophin is given and the management is as for disseminated sclerosis.

Diffuse Sclerosis

This term includes a number of conditions whose chief feature is a widespread demyelination in the cerebral hemispheres. They usually occur early in life and both sporadic and familial types occur. They are progressive, usually rapidly, and are not necessarily symmetrical. They are characterised clinically by epilepsy, dementia, visual disturbance, and diplegia.

DISORDERS OF THE PERIPHERAL NERVOUS SYSTEM

Root Lesions

Radiculitis has been shown in recent years to be the cause of some disorders formerly referred to as neuritis (e.g. the interstitial neuritis causing sciatica); it arises usually from disorders of the spine. Of these the commonest are lesions of the intervertebral disc, which usually occur where the spine is most mobile, that is in the cervical and lumbar regions. The lesions are produced either by trauma or by degeneration and lead to a protrusion or osteophytic overgrowth (spondylosis) which may be either central or lateral. A central protrusion causes cord or cauda equina compression (p. 306); it is lateral protrusion which is considered here. A single root is usually involved, the symptoms naturally depending on the situation of the lesion.

Cervical Spondylosis

The early symptom is pain which may at first be confined to the neck but later passes down the arm. The pain is intermittent, aggravated by coughing, straining, exertion, and jarring and is distributed according to the *myotome*; that is, it appears in muscles predominantly supplied by the root involved. At the periphery tingling may occur in the fingers in accordance with the *dermatome*. The pain is often most troublesome at night.

Thus in a C6 root lesion pain passes down the outer arm and may cause tingling in the thumb and index finger; in a C7 root lesion pain passes down the posterior aspect of the arm and forearm and may cause tingling in the index and middle finger; in a C8 root lesion pain passes down the inner arm and forearm and may cause tingling of the ring and little fingers.

Signs. Neck movements are usually restricted. Weakness and fasciculation of the muscles supplied by the root involved sometimes develop. In the case of a C6 root these are predominantly biceps, brachioradialis, and the radial extensor of the wrist, and the biceps and 'supinator' jerks are depressed or absent. In the case of a C7 root the triceps, the ulnar extensor of the wrist, finger extensors, and lower pectoral muscles are affected and the triceps jerk is depressed or absent. In the case of a C8 root the finger flexors are the muscles involved and the finger jerk, if originally present, may be absent. Significant sensory loss is rarely found. Other roots are less commonly affected and involvement of more than one root at a time is unusual.

Diagnosis. The fact that cervical spondylosis is the commonest cause of a root lesion must not lead to the neglect of other possible causes, especially primary spinal tumours and metastatic deposits.

Radiographs of the cervical spine may show narrowing of the appropriate disc space and osteophytic encroachment on the intervertebral foramina.

Treatment. In the first place, if the severity of the pain warrants it, this should be rest in bed with the arm supported on pillows in the most comfortable position. Analgesics will be required for a few days and the rest should be continued for some days after the pain has subsided. Manipulation is sometimes successful but possibly dangerous. If permanent relief is not achieved in a few weeks, the wearing of a cervical spine support for 3 to 6 months is often helpful. The condition tends to recur.

Lumbar Spondylosis (Sciatica)

As in the neck, root lesions in the lumbar spine are usually attributable to spondylosis; the roots most commonly involved are L5 and S1, somewhat less commonly L4. The prominent symptom is pain which has the usual intermittent character of root pain and is precipitated by coughing, straining, jolting, and so on and is distributed in accordance with the *myotome*, with paraesthesiae at the periphery in the *dermatome*. Thus in an L4 root lesion there is pain in the anterior thigh passing down into the inner leg; in an L5 root lesion there is pain passing down the outer thigh into the outer leg; in an S1 root lesion there is pain passing down the back of the thigh into the calf. Muscle cramps, especially in the calf, sometimes develop.

Signs. With involvement of the lower lumbar and first sacral roots there is likely to be limitation of straight leg raising and there may be a scoliosis determined by spasm of the erector spinae muscles on the side of the lesion.

These may be the only abnormal signs, but weakness, wasting, and fasciculation are sometimes present; in an L4 lesion these are found in the quadriceps, and the knee jerk may be depressed or absent. In an L5 lesion the earliest and sometimes the only weakness is in the extensor hallucis longus and there is no associated reflex change. In an S1 root lesion weakness is of plantar flexion and the ankle jerk is depressed or absent. The jerks may disappear in the absence of weakness; there is seldom any significant sensory loss.

Radiographs may show appropriate changes in the lumbar spine, but they are often normal. Their main importance is in helping to rule out more serious lesions such as metastatic carcinoma.

Diagnosis. The possibility of other lesions causing radiculitis must be considered, especially primary tumours of the cauda equina and metastatic deposits. In these cases the condition is progressive, and if there is any doubt about the diagnosis lumbar puncture and myelography should be done. For lesions below the conus medullaris a radiculogram is a more appropriate investigation than a myelogram. This is performed with a dimer of methylglucamine iothalamate and/or iocarmate, the advantages being that it is water soluble and absorbed, it is less dense, the cauda equina can be seen through it and it outlines the root pouches better. If taken above the conus it will not cause any permanent damage but may produce painful muscle spasms.

Treatment. The condition varies in severity and tends to come in attacks which are sometimes fairly mild and pass off without any particular treatment. If severe, treatment in the first place should be complete rest, the patient being flat but not necessarily on the back. Bed-boards or placing the mattress on the floor, are sometimes helpful. At first analgesics may be necessary, but rest should be continued for some time after the pain has subsided and may have to be continued for 4 to 6 weeks. Thereafter gradual rehabilitation is necessary. Some advocate traction, epidural injection or manipulation and in resistant cases a plaster jacket or other lumbar support may be helpful. Operation has not proved sufficiently successful to make it the treatment of choice and should not be considered until other methods have failed to produce relief of pain. It is not likely to influence any residual weakness in the absence of pain.

The patient who has once had radiculitis from lumbar spondylosis (sciatica) should be advised against heavy lifting with the back flexed, though recurrence may take place without any apparent precipitation.

CERVICAL RIB SYNDROME

A rib arising from the seventh cervical vertebra may produce no symptoms or signs. Sometimes, however, it may produce clinical features which are likely to be predominantly either vascular or neurological.

The vascular symptoms are usually due to vascular occlusion from embolus arising from a mural thrombus which has formed in the subclavian artery distal to its narrowing as it passes over the cervical rib. The patient complains of pain in the forearm which has the character of ischaemic muscle pain, spreading sometimes to involve the whole arm. This pain develops especially with use and is relieved by rest. In addition the hand is cold and becomes blue when dependent.

The neurological symptoms are caused by involvement of the lower cord of the brachial plexus, formed by the C8 and T1 roots. There is pain down the inner arm and forearm with tingling of the ring and little fingers. This pain develops with the arm in use, especially with lifting and carrying. The patient may also complain of a weakness of the grip and of a tendency to drop things.

Signs. There is weakness and possibly wasting of the finger flexors and of the small muscles of the hand. There may be slight cutaneous sensory impairment over the inner forearm, corresponding palm, and little and ring fingers. A rib may be palpable in the supraclavicular fossa.

Radiographs may show a cervical rib and one giving rise to symptoms should be removed surgically.

NEURITIS

This is the term usually applied to disorder of a peripheral nerve from whatever cause. The cause is, however, rarely inflammatory and commonest is some form of trauma. There will be considered here the clinical features which develop when the function of certain nerves is disordered by pressure.

Radial Nerve

The radial nerve is compressed typically when the arm is hung over a chair in a drunken stupor (drunkard's palsy), but it is exposed to compression in other ways as it winds round the radial groove on the humerus.

The muscles which are thus paralysed are the brachio-radialis, the extensors of the wrist and fingers and the long abductor of the thumb. There may be a small area of cutaneous sensory loss over the first dorsal interosseous.

Ulnar Nerve

The ulnar nerve may be injured by pressure in bed, when the development of symptoms and signs is likely to be rapid; but the onset is usually more insidious and occurs in association with previous damage around the elbow in the region of the medial epicondyle, or when the ulnar groove is unusually shallow and the nerve unduly exposed, or when the nerve tends to slip out of the groove with flexion of the elbow. When there is no obvious abnormality at the elbow joint, as is sometimes the case, it has been suggested that the nerve may be compressed where it passes into the forearm between the heads of flexor carpi ulnaris.

Pain is not a feature of this compression and the earliest symptoms are numbness of the little finger and corresponding palm and inability to *adduct* the little finger so that it tends to be caught when the hand is put in a pocket or into a glove. Later, weakness progresses to involve all the interossei and wasting of these muscles appears. The numbness becomes more intense and may be found by the patient to involve the ulnar aspect of the ring finger.

Signs. There will be a variable degree of wasting and weakness of the interossei, but the bulk of the abductor pollicis brevis and its power will be normal. The function of this muscle is to abduct the thumb at right angles to the palm and the muscle bulk can be palpated alongside the first metacarpal bone. Sensory loss of variable degree will be confined to the little finger and the inner half of the ring finger. Arthritic changes may be found at the elbow, or the groove may be shallow, and the nerve tend to dislocate.

Treatment. Treatment is surgical, the nerve being transplanted from the ulnar groove, if there is evidence of disorder there, to the anterior aspect of the elbow. If the elbow seems normal the nerve may be decompressed as it passes between the heads of the flexor carpi ulnaris.

Median Nerve

Compression of the median nerve in the carpal tunnel has long been known to cause wasting of the muscles of the thenar eminence, with paralysis of abduction and opposition of the thumb, and cutaneous sensory loss over the thumb, index, middle, and radial half of the ring finger. This florid picture is, however, comparatively rare.

More recently it has been shown that milder forms of compression are responsible for acroparaesthesiae in the hand even when signs are slight or absent. This is now usually referred to as the *carpal tunnel syndrome*, which is common.

It occurs mostly in women, appearing usually for no apparent reason although, as will be seen, its development is related to use of the hands. In men there is usually a discoverable cause as, for example, arthritis of the wrist following injury, ganglion of the wrist joint, acromegaly or myxoedema. These causes do, of course, operate also in women, in whom pregnancy may be an additional precipitating factor.

The early symptoms are intermittent, usually nocturnal tingling of the fingers, usually of one hand and usually the hand the patient uses most. This tingling may spare the little finger and is sometimes most prominent in the *ring and middle* fingers. It wakens the patient, who may drop the arm out of the bed, sit up, and rub it or get up and swing it until sensation is restored.

This may happen more than once in the night. The tingling may be accompanied by pain in the hand, at the elbow or more rarely in the shoulder. The symptoms tend to be worse during a night which follows a strenuous day with the hands as, for example, doing the family washing.

As the condition progresses the patient has not only troubled nights but finds that on waking in the morning at the ordinary time the fingers feel swollen and are numb. This passes off in about twenty minutes but while present causes disability such as difficulty in doing up buttons.

Later, symptoms occur during the day. They are brought on especially by gripping, as in various forms of housework, and knitting or even holding a newspaper is sometimes enough to precipitate uncomfortable numbness so that the activity must be stopped. The tingling is sometimes painful and may be permanent.

Finally, abnormal signs may appear. They may be quite slight, and consist of weakness of the abductor pollicis brevis with cutaneous sensory impairment within the distribution of the median nerve. Sometimes there is *over-reaction* to pin-prick rather than hypoalgesia.

Diagnosis. This is rarely difficult when the history is typical and when abnormal signs, however slight, are present. Symptoms of this nature have for long been thought to arise from *cervical ribs or related anomalies*, but the neurological picture bears no resemblance to this and even if a cervical rib is discovered it can only be relevant in so far as it impedes the circulation through the subclavian artery and thus facilitates ischaemia at the wrist. *Cervical spondylosis* is also sometimes held to account for the symptoms; in this connection the not infrequent finding of tingling involving predominantly the middle and ring fingers is helpful, for this is not a radicular distribution. In general the tingling is too widespread for cervical spondylosis, which does not cause early-morning numbness.

Treatment. The early symptoms can be relieved by resting the hands and patients have often noticed this when on holiday or on coming into hospital. This is, however, rarely a practicable solution and other methods of relief must be found. Weight reduction may be of value. If the symptoms are purely nocturnal, splinting the wrist in the position of slight dorsiflexion at bed-time often ensures an untroubled night but seldom leads to permanent relief. Symptoms which are troublesome both by day and by night may be relieved by injection of hydrocortisone at the wrist, but although this can lead to permanent relief the incidence of relapse is high. With troublesome symptoms and especially when abnormal signs are present, *operation* is indicated and this is undoubtedly the most immediate and most effective method of producing lasting relief. The operation is one of decompression by division of the flexor retinaculum at the wrist. In assessing the results of this operation, which is very successful in the vast majority of patients in whom the diagnosis has been correctly made, it is important to realise that the immediate effect of the operation will be to relieve only the symptoms which are *intermittent*. Any tingling which is constant and any weakness or sensory loss may be improved immediately but, depending on its severity, will take some time to recover. If the weakness and wasting of the abductor pollicis brevis are profound then complete recovery may not take place for many months.

In myxoedema treatment of the primary condition will in most cases relieve the symptoms.

Lateral Cutaneous Nerve of Thigh

This nerve is compressed as it passes from the pelvis under the lateral aspect of the inguinal ligament where it may become involved in the origin of the sartorius muscle. This compression may give rise to numbness over the lateral aspect of the thigh and to pain. Hence the name *meralgia paraesthetica*. The pain and numbness develop usually in men in middle life and sometimes as a result of weight increase.

This pain develops typically on exertion and may be severe enough to halt the patient so that this is a cause of intermittent claudication (intermittent limping) and thus may resemble the symptoms caused by ischaemia in the leg. The pain is relieved by rest but may return with further exertion.

On examination sensory loss may be demonstrated over a somewhat variable area on the lateral aspect of the thigh corresponding to the whole or part of the distribution of the lateral cutaneous nerve.

Treatment. Weight reduction may be sufficient to relieve the symptoms but decompression of the nerve may be necessary.

Lateral Popliteal

Owing to its superficial course as it winds round the neck of the fibula, this nerve is particularly subject to pressure, for example from splints. The effect of this is to cause a flaccid foot drop with paralysis of eversion of the foot and of dorsiflexion of the foot and toes. There may be cutaneous sensory impairment over the lateral aspect of the leg and the dorsum of the foot.

Mononeuritis Multiplex

Lesions of nerves so far considered may be termed mononeuritis in the sense that only a single nerve, whether mixed or purely sensory, has been involved. In these cases the only pathological process considered has been one of compression but there are certain conditions, not due to pressure, in which there may be involvement of two or more nerves but still something less than a polyneuritis; this clinical picture is referred to as a *mononeuritis multiplex*, that is the involvement of several peripheral nerves by the same pathological process. The conditions which may give rise to this picture are:

alcoholic poisoning,
diabetes mellitus,
polyarteritis nodosa,
leprosy.

All these conditions, with the possible exception of leprosy, may at other times give rise to a true polyneuritis.

Polyneuritis

The most characteristic feature of polyneuritis is its symmetry; there is symmetrical motor, reflex, and sensory change. Tachycardia is common.

The effect of polyneuritis is usually to cause peripheral symptoms and signs, but the essential lesion may well be central. Although there are some well-recognised causes of polyneuritis, many cases remain obscure.

Symptoms. The early symptoms are usually persistent tingling and numbness of the hands and feet accompanied by peripheral weakness. They come on at varying rates and the speed of development is helpful in the diagnosis of the cause.

Signs. The signs of a polyneuritis are weakness, usually more marked peripherally, reflex loss, and cutaneous sensory disturbance, also peripheral.

Diagnosis. The clinical diagnosis of polyneuritis is not difficult but the discovery of the cause often is; and even when the cause seems established the mechanism whereby a polyneuritis occurs is difficult to understand. In some cases the vasi nervorum are affected, as for example, in *polyarteritis nodosa* and possibly *diabetes mellitus*, or as a result of some toxic effect or metabolic disturbance.

Toxic effects are produced by *heavy metals*, *chemical substances* used in industry, agriculture and the home, and *certain drugs*, for example isoniazid. Metabolic disturbances which may give rise to polyneuritis include *dietary and vitamin deficiency*, *infection*, *carcinoma*, *pernicious anaemia*, *amyloid disease*, and *porphyria*.

Acute Infective Polyneuritis

This is usually of rapid development, the onset often being associated with an upper respiratory infection and accompanied by fever. There is initially peripheral tingling, soon followed by weakness which may spread rapidly to involve *proximal muscles* and sometimes those of respiration, which is a danger to life. There is sometimes facial weakness and this is occasionally bilateral. The tendon reflexes are lost. Peripheral sensory loss may be severe but is often quite slight. The spinal fluid usually shows considerable increase in protein, up to 300 mg./100 ml. or more, but without cellular increase. This dissociation which is referred to as the *Guillain-Barré syndrome* is not, however, specific to this condition and may be found in diphtheritic, diabetic, and other forms of polyneuritis.

Treatment. Steroid therapy may be of value in the early stages but otherwise there is no specific treatment. Recovery is likely to be slow and is occasionally incomplete. The prognosis is good if death from respiratory failure can be prevented. It is therefore essential to have the patient removed to where a respirator is available if there should be any question of involvement of muscles of respiration.

Subacute and Chronic Polyneuritis

In these forms the diagnosis of polyneuritis is usually clear enough and a search must be made for the cause. Palpation of peripheral nerves may reveal hypertrophy and suggest the possibility of hypertrophic interstitial neuritis, amyloid or leprosy, but there is a tendency for nerves to hypertrophy in any long-standing chronic polyneuritis.

In *alcoholic polyneuritis* the calves are exquisitely tender and a pyruvate tolerance test shows impaired pyruvate metabolism, the cause of this neuritis probably being thiamine deficiency.

The polyneuritis may be accompanied by the syndrome of confusion, disorientation, memory loss, and a tendency to confabulation described by *Korsakoff*, or by the encephalopathy described by *Wernicke*; this is characterised by vertigo, nystagmus, ocular palsies, ataxia, and stupor. These features are likewise due to thiamine deficiency and treatment is by large doses of the vitamin intravenously.

In *lead neuritis* the extensor muscles of the wrist and fingers are almost exclusively involved and sensory symptoms and signs are rare. Other evidence of lead poisoning is not always present and a history of exposure must be sought. The diagnosis can be established by a provocative dose of calcium versenate and the demonstration of excess excretion of lead in the urine. If this is positive treatment is by means of calcium versenate.

In *diabetic polyneuritis* the symptoms are predominantly sensory and are usually confined to the legs, which may be painful. Arthropathy and perforating ulcer may develop in the feet. The diagnosis rests on the finding of diabetes mellitus which will require appropriate and energetic treatment with insulin.

In polyneuritis associated with *porphyria* (p. 462), there may be in addition abdominal pain and mental disturbance. Excess excretion of porphyrins may be found in the urine.

CARCINOMATOUS NEUROPATHY

This includes a group of neurological syndromes which appear in patients with a carcinoma, usually in the lung and far less frequently in the ovary or elsewhere. The neuropathy does not depend on the presence of metastases and the mechanism of its causation is unknown.

The neuropathy may appear before the carcinoma is discovered, may be present at the time the carcinoma is diagnosed or may appear later. Its appearance, its nature, and its extent bear no relation to the size of the carcinoma. It runs a variable course, sometimes undergoing partial spontaneous remission and is not greatly influenced by removal of the growth.

Syndromes so far recognised include polyneuritis, often predominantly sensory; neuro-myopathic pictures, with muscle wasting and weakness which is often variable and may include features of myasthenia gravis, even the response to neostigmine (p. 316); syndromes depending on cerebellar degeneration; and a clinical picture resembling subacute combined degeneration of the cord. Sometimes two or more of these clinical pictures are combined and the very fact that they are so bizarre may suggest the diagnosis.

DEFICIENCY STATES

Deficiency of thiamine causes *beriberi* which is characterised by polyneuritis sometimes with associated oedema, which may be due to associated cardiac failure. Such deficiency in temperate zones is usually due to failure of absorption associated with persistent vomiting or gastro-intestinal disease. This may be the basis of so-called alcoholic polyneuritis. Treatment is by the intravenous administration of thiamine.

Deficiency of other members of the vitamin B complex in addition to thiamine give rise to *pellagra*, which is characterised by gastro-intestinal disturbance, skin eruptions, and mental change. These features are thought to be due to a deficiency of nicotinic acid and treatment is by intravenous administration of this together with thiamine.

Deficiency of cyanocobalamin (vitamin B_{12}) may give rise to:

(1) *anaemia*,
(2) *peripheral neuritis*,
(3) *subacute combined degeneration of the cord*,
(4) *dementia*,
(5) *optic atrophy*.

The anaemia is discussed elsewhere (p. 509) and is nearly always present when the neurological symptoms develop; occasionally they occur when there is no abnormality of the circulating blood or even the bone marrow. Histamine fast achlorhydria is always present, however. In doubtful cases the diagnosis may depend on the estimation of the serum cyanocobalamin and the demonstration of its deficiency.

Subacute Combined Degeneration of the Cord

This condition, so called because of the combined involvement of the posterior and lateral columns (postero-lateral sclerosis), usually starts in the fifth or sixth decade and affects the sexes equally. The early symptoms are tingling in the hands and feet followed by increasing numbness, especially of the legs, with the development of ataxia and finally of weakness.

On examination the legs are usually flaccid and weak and the knee and ankle jerks are absent. The plantar responses are extensor and there is impairment of touch and vibration sense, often well marked in the legs and less in the arms.

The diagnosis is not difficult when there is a macrocytic anaemia and a megaloblastic bone marrow, but sometimes these are not present when gastric achlorhydria is. The diagnosis then rests between this, disseminated sclerosis of the late spinal type, and cervical spondylosis, both of which can equally give rise to a postero-lateral sclerosis. They may be distinguished by estimation of the serum vitamin B_{12} level.

Treatment. This is by injection of cyanocobalamin 1,000 μg. intramuscularly at first every second day but gradually less frequently so that eventually a maintenance dose may be given once a month; it must be continued for life.

Dementia

Mental symptoms are sometimes present in subacute combined degeneration of the cord, but may appear alone. It is important to remember the possibility of B_{12} deficiency in any case of dementia for which there is not already a satisfactory explanation, especially as it responds well to treatment with vitamin B_{12} if the diagnosis is established early.

Optic atrophy is an uncommon but very serious complication of B_{12} deficiency. It is treated in the same way as subacute combined degeneration of the spinal cord, but significant recovery is unusual.

TRIGEMINAL NEURALGIA

This is a pain in the face of unknown cause, usually severe and of a stabbing, lancinating, shooting character. The typical features are:

(1) The pain is confined to the distribution of the trigeminal nerve, involving first either the maxillary or the mandibular division and much more rarely the ophthalmic division. The pain may then spread to involve two or all divisions. It is occasionally bilateral, usually consecutively.

(2) The pain is paroxysmal, a bout of pain lasting for as little as a few seconds but not usually for more than 15 to 20 minutes.

(3) The pain is precipitated by touching the face, as in blowing the nose or in washing, or by facial movement as in talking, laughing, eating, and so on.

Such a pain usually occurs for the first time between the ages of fifty and seventy, and more often in women. Typically the first attack lasts for a few weeks and is followed by a complete remission. The pain returns after months or years and as time passes the periods of remission become shorter and the periods of pain become longer. There may, however, be no lasting remission at any time, although the pain remains paroxysmal throughout and never becomes constant.

Signs. There are no abnormal signs in the absence of any previous attempts at treatment. Patients with a similar or even indistinguishable pain who show abnormal signs may have a neoplasm, such as an acoustic neuroma, an angioma in the posterior fossa, or disseminated sclerosis. In the latter disease there is about a 2 per cent incidence of trigeminal neuralgia, but on the other hand between 5 per cent and 10 per cent of patients with trigeminal neuralgia will be suffering from disseminated sclerosis; the neuralgia in these cases being sometimes bilateral, and the treatment is the same as in the cases where no cause is discovered.

Treatment. Trigeminal neuralgia can always be relieved by numbing the face and abolishing the sensory impulses which precipitate the pain. Such numbness may, however, cause discomfort and should only be produced when the patient is likely to find it preferable to the pain. Fortunately the fact that the early attacks are likely to be brief and to remit for months or even years makes delay practicable. The early attacks are best treated with analgesics. The most effective drug is *Carbamazapine* which is really an anticonvulsant. Treatment should be started with 100 mg. t.d.s. and may be increased to 200 mg. q.i.d. Relief is obtained in about 75 per cent of patients and is usually apparent within 48 hours. Side-effects include dizziness and skin rashes. In the end more definitive treatment may be undertaken. In elderly patients in whom the pain is confined to the mandibular division this branch can be injected peripherally with alcohol. This will abolish the pain, but the nerve will regenerate and function will return. Fortunately, however, the pain does not always return with the return of function and relief may be long lasting.

If the pain is more widespread the injection must be made into the Gasserian ganglion, thus destroying the nerve cells, or an intracranial operation must be performed to divide the sensory root. Numbness after these procedures, successfully performed, is permanent and relief of pain complete. Certain dysaesthesiae sometimes develop over the face and cause some distress, but if the procedure is properly timed the vast majority of patients will be grateful for the relief of pain.

When the whole of the face is numbed patients must wear glasses with a sidepiece to protect the insensitive cornea and guard against ulceration.

GLOSSOPHARYNGEAL NEURALGIA

This is a pain similar in its characteristics to trigeminal neuralgia but in the distribution of the glossopharyngeal nerve. The pain is paroxysmal, appears in the throat and sometimes deep in the ear and is provoked by swallowing. Treatment is by the surgical division of the glossopharyngeal nerve and the two upper rootlets of the vagus nerve.

FURTHER READING

Brain's *Diseases of the Nervous System*, 8th Edition, edited by J. N. Walton, Oxford University Press, London, 1977.

Holmes, G., *Introduction to Clinical Neurology*, 3rd edition, revised by Brian Matthews, Livingstone, Edinburgh, 1969.

Merritt, H. H., *Textbook of Neurology*, 5th edition, Kimpton, London, 1973.

CHAPTER SEVEN

DISEASES OF MUSCLE

EPIDEMIC MYALGIA (Bornholm Disease)

This is an acute epidemic myalgia due to a virus of the Coxsackie group. The onset is acute and the intercostal muscles are most frequently affected. Pain is severe and respiration is shallow, rapid, and painful. A pleural rub may be heard, and affected muscles are tender. Low-grade fever is the rule, and there may be a lymphocytosis in the blood. The disease lasts 7 to 10 days and no serious complications or deaths have been reported. Treatment is symptomatic.

WASTING OF MUSCLES

Introduction. This may result as a secondary phenomenon from disuse, or because the blood or nerve supply is impaired. It may be caused by malnutrition and it occurs in old age. It may, however, present as a primary disorder of muscle or one in which muscle is chiefly involved.

Widespread weakness and wasting of muscle is an uncommon but not rare clinical phenomenon at all ages. In the past there has been much confusion in its diagnosis, and many cases still remain mysterious. Interest in recent years has served to clarify some of the clinical syndromes and use of the electromyograph (E.M.G.), measurement of serum creatine kinase (CK) levels, and histological examination of biopsy specimens has given greater precision to some diagnoses. For descriptive purposes it is convenient to separate cases of muscle wasting occurring in infancy from those first noticed in childhood or adult life. Those diseases confined to infancy will not be discussed.

THE MYOPATHIES

They are genetically determined, and are thought to represent inborn errors of muscle metabolism. Onset is usually in childhood or early adult life. Wasting is symmetrical and progress is slowly but inexorably downhill. Remissions do not occur. Similar cases frequently occur in the same family.

Clinical Features. The chief complaint is of gradually increasing weakness in the affected muscles. There are no sensory changes nor any systemic disturbance, and the only pain in the condition is from joints deprived of adequate muscular support. The disease begins proximally, and posture is usually disturbed, causing a marked lumbar lordosis. The muscles are always weak and wasted; fasciculation never occurs. Some fibres may be replaced by fat, giving the muscle an unduly bulky appearance which contrasts strangely with the weakness (*pseudohypertrophy*). Certain groups of muscles are commonly affected, and give rise to well-recognised clinical syndromes. These patterns of disease are frequently known by the names of those who first described them; it is important to realise that minor variations are the rule and that the descriptive titles given to the diseases are at best generalisations.

(1) **Pseudohypertrophic Muscular Dystrophy** (Duchenne, Erb.)
Affects principally the shoulder and hip girdles, later the calves. The muscles commonly affected by pseudohypertrophy are the deltoids, glutei, and gastrocnemius; these last cause the characteristic waddling gait. X linked.

A probable variant of the disease but one that is genetically distinct has been described by Becker. The same muscles are affected, and exhibit similar characteristics, but it is of later onset and progresses much more slowly.

Mean Age and Range in Years	Duchenne	Becker
Onset	2·8 (0–6)	11·1 (2·5–21)
Chairbound	8·6 (6–12)	27·1 (12–63+)
Death	16·0 (8–22)	42·2 (23–63+)
(Emery and Skinner 1976)		
Incidence per 100,000 population	17	1·7

(2) **Facio-scapulo-humeral Dystrophy** (Landouzy-Dejerine)
Begins in the face, and spreads centrifugally to involve the upper limb girdle and arms. No pseudohypertrophy. Autosomal dominant.

(3) **Arm and shoulder** (Erb)
Occurs between the ages of fifteen and thirty, starts in the biceps, triceps, and deltoids.

(4) **'Distal Myopathy'** (Gowers)
This is a rarity. Most cases so described are in fact suffering from cervical spondylosis (p. 320) or dystrophia myotonica (*vide infra*). A true distal myopathy starting in the hands and spreading centripetally does occur. It is not uncommon in Scandinavia, but extremely rare in this country.

(5) **Ocular myopathy** is usually confined to the ocular muscles, but sometimes affects the facial muscles, starting in the orbicularis oculi.

Diagnosis. There is usually a family history of the disease, and characteristic and symmetrical affection of muscles. The E.M.G. is characteristic, and the serum CK may be raised. Muscle biopsy may be diagnostic.

Course and Prognosis. All these conditions progress inexorably to the patient's death in 5 to 25 years. This is usually from intercurrent infection, frequently respiratory following inhalation of food or saliva. The sphincters are never affected.

No treatment influences the disease.

Benign Congenital Myopathy

Presents sporadically in childhood or early adult life with mild muscular weakness and wasting, and sometimes hypotonia. Very slowly progressive. CK levels are usually normal, but E.M.G. may show mild myopathic changes.

DYSTROPHIA MYOTONICA

Introduction

This is an hereditary disease, with onset usually in the early thirties. It is believed to represent an as yet unidentified error of metabolism.

Clinical Features. (a) *Symptoms*. Early complaints are of *weakness*, usually first manifest as difficulty in swallowing, nasal voice, and weakness of the hands. To this may be added slowness, difficulty in relinquishing grip, and stiffness, from *myotonia*.

(b) *Signs*. Weakness is manifest in the facial muscles, those of deglutition and particularly the sternomastoids, which may be greatly wasted or absent. The neck extensors, in contrast, are never affected. The hands are weak. Affected muscles may show sustained contraction on direct percussion.

Associated features are baldness, chiefly vertical, cataracts, testicular atrophy, and dementia. There is an infrequent association with diabetes mellitus. Goitres, sometimes toxic, may occur. Psychopathic behaviour is common.

Special Investigations

E.M.G. shows the typical picture of myotonia. CK levels are normal or slightly raised.

Treatment is with quinine sulphate (300 mg. t.d.s.). Prognosis is bad. The condition proceeds inexorably to death in the early forties. Anaesthetics, particularly when muscle relaxing drugs are given, are particularly hazardous.

POLYMYOSITIS

Introduction

Polymyositis is more important than the myopathies, because of its relative frequency, difficulty in diagnosis and particularly because of the prospect of effective treatment. It may be caused by a number of disease processes. It occurs equally in males and females, and although it can begin at any age it is commonest between thirty and sixty.

It may be seen in association with carcinoma of the bronchus, some collagen disorders (systemic lupus erythematosus, dermatomyositis, polyarteritis nodosa), sarcoidosis, during treatment with fluorine-containing steroids, or with Cushing's syndrome. In many cases no cause can be discovered, but when one is found it is most frequently *carcinoma of the bronchus.*

Clinical Features. It is patchy in distribution and erratic in its course. It may progress rapidly for a few months, then remit or even regress a little. It frequently affects the nuchal extensor muscles, so that the head hangs forward. No muscle is immune, including the ocular muscles, and sometimes ptosis is the first evidence of the disease. Occasionally the heart is affected. Fever, malaise, tachycardia, and pain on muscular contraction may all sometimes occur. Severe Raynaud's phenomenon is a common accompaniment.

Special Investigations. E.M.G. and muscle biopsy show typical features and enable the diagnosis to be made with certainty in a high proportion of cases. The E.S.R. may be raised, and there may be a polymorphonuclear leucocytosis in the blood. Enzymes leak from the damaged muscle into the blood in the acute stage of the disease, thus there will be elevated blood levels of CK.

Differential Diagnosis

This is chiefly from myopathy, and certain helpful features are tabulated.

	Myopathy	*Myositis*
(1) Family history	Usually present	None
(2) Age of onset	Usually before 35	Usually after 35
(3) Course	Relentless; no remissions	Erratic; remissions common
(4) Pattern of affection	Symmetrical	Patchy
(5) Extensor nuchal muscles	Spared	Affected
(6) Systemic disturbance	None	May be marked
(7) Raynaud's phenomenon	Rare	Common

Treatment is with steroids (prednisolone 5–25 mg. t.d.s.) and physiotherapy. *Prognosis* depends upon the cause, but in general the course is gradually downhill over 5 to 10 years, although long remissions are possible.

LESS COMMON CAUSES OF WEAKNESS AND WASTING OF MUSCLE

Thyrotoxic Myopathy

May occur either in association with thyrotoxicosis or myxoedema, or occasionally in euthyroid states. Eye signs of thyrotoxicosis are commonly absent. Muscular changes may precede any change of thyroid function. The effects are usually confined to the proximal muscle groups, and are worse in the legs. Hyperthyroidism may be revealed by laboratory investigation (p. 472) at this stage, and the full clinical picture is usually apparent within a few months. The muscles show typical E.M.G. changes.

Diabetic Myopathy

Occurs chiefly in middle-aged mild diabetics. It begins with pains in the thighs and legs, and goes on to moderately severe weakness and wasting of the buttocks and thighs. E.M.G. suggests denervation, but no sensory changes are found. The protein is raised in the cerebrospinal fluid and both E.M.G. and histology suggest that the disease is primarily an affection of anterior horn cells.

Lead Myopathy

Is rare in this country. It is commoner in men than women, and results most frequently from inhaling volatilised lead. It affects the arms more than the legs, and usually begins in the extensors of the fingers and wrists. Sensory changes are very rare. Frequently there is a history of industrial exposure, and often of abdominal cramps, without diarrhoea ('the dangles, with dry colic'). There may be a lead line on the gum, or a blue anal ring. Anaemia is common, and the red cells may contain punctate basiphilic granules. Collection of urine after giving chelating agents shows an excess of lead excretion.

FURTHER READING

Walton, J. N. (Editor), *Disorders of Voluntary Muscle*, 3rd edition, Churchill, Livingstone, Edinburgh, 1974.

CHAPTER EIGHT

DISEASES ASSOCIATED WITH DISORDERED IMMUNITY

Introduction

It is now realised that a number of diseases are associated with disordered immunity and in particular the mechanism of hypersensitivity and concept of auto-immune disease and immune-complex disease have gained wider recognition.

In this chapter the first part is devoted to a general summary of the immune reaction and its relationship to clinical medicine. In the rest of the chapter a description is given of certain diseases of connective tissue in which there is evidence of disordered immunity. This group includes systemic lupus erythematosus, rheumatoid arthritis, polyarteritis nodosa and dermatomyositis. Other diseases such as asthma, acute nephritis, some forms of the nephrotic syndrome, haemolytic anaemias, ulcerative colitis and a variety of skin rashes are associated with disordered immunity and are considered under the appropriate systems.

IMMUNOLOGICAL REACTIONS IN CLINICAL MEDICINE

Immunology has its roots in the observation that persons surviving certain infectious diseases seldom suffer from the same disease again. Apart from conferring specific resistance to various pathogens, it is now realised the immune system plays a fundamental role in other biological reactions of great clinical importance; the nature of these is outlined in this section.

Nature of Immune Response

The immune response is initiated by a variety of substances referred to as antigens. These are classified according to their origin as (i) hetero-antigens which originate in a foreign species, e.g. pathogenic organisms or their products, (ii) iso-antigens which originate in a genetically dissimilar member of the same species, e.g. blood group substances, (iii) auto-antigens which originate in the sensitised host, e.g. thyroglobulin. Antigenic compounds may be complex proteins or carbohydrates of large molecular size. Many antigens which initiate a specific antibody response can be observed to undergo phagocytosis by tissue macrophages (p. 338). These cells do not synthesise antibody but appear to participate in the immune response by concentrating antigen and passing it to adjacent lymphocytes. The latter cells, which are derived from precursors in bone marrow, are widely distributed in lymph nodes, spleen, marrow and lymphoid tissues of the lung and gastro-intestinal tract.

Adaptive immune responses are initiated by interaction of antigen with specific receptors on the surfaces of lymphoid cells. Two major classes of lymphocytes are recognised and these behave differently after reaction with antigen. T-lymphocytes undergo transformation and mitosis generating a population of cells specifically reactive with the inducing antigen; B-lymphocytes differentiate into plasma cells which secrete humoral antibody, but this process usually requires co-operation with T-cells. The immune reactions generated by these cellular responses therefore fall into two major categories. One is mediated by specific humoral antibody and the other by specifically sensitised T-lymphocytes (cell-mediated immunity). While it is true that antibody action may, in certain circumstances, be independent of cells, e.g. neutralisation of toxins, and that certain specific cell-mediated reactions are independent of antibody, e.g. T-cell killing of tumour cells, there remain several specific immune mechanisms which require the interaction of humoral antibody with cells such as macrophages, K-cells or mast cells. In addition, the immune response generated by the interaction of antigen with lymphocytes may locally affect other cells which do not carry the specific antigen (non-specific immunity).

(i) *Serum Immunoglobulins.* Serum antibodies are confined to the γ-globulin fraction and are referred to as immunoglobulins (Ig). They are

IMMUNE RESPONSE

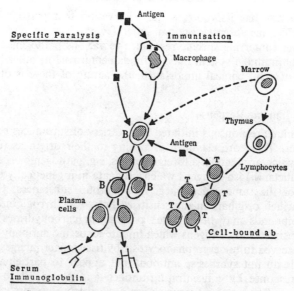

SCHEMATIC REPRESENTATION OF THE IMMUNE RESPONSE.

PROPERTIES OF HUMAN IMMUNOGLOBINS

	IgG	IgA	IgM	IgD	IgE
Structural					
Molecular weight	150,000	160,000 (serum) 370,000 (secretory)	900,000	170,000	200,000
Heavy chain classes	γ	a	μ	d	e
Light chain types	κ, λ	κ, λ	κ, λ	κ, λ	κ, λ
Carbohydrate (%)	2·9	7·5	11·8	11·3	10·7
Biological					
Serum concentration g/l.	8–17	1·5–4·5	0·5–1·5	0·003–040	0·10–1·3 μg/l
Antibody activity	+	+	+	+	+
C fixation	+	0	+	0	0
Placental transfer	+	0	0	0	0
Seromucous secretion	0	+	0		+
Tissue sensitisation	0	0	0	0	+
Combination rheumatoid factor	+	0	0		
Attachment to macrophages	+	0	+		+
B–cell receptor	0	0	+ (monomer)	+	0
Attachment to κ–cells	+	0	0	0	0

large proteins containing 2 heavy and 2 light polypeptide chains. The different classes of immunoglobulin (IgG, IgA, IgM, IgD, IgE—see below) are distinguished by the structure of their heavy chains. Each Ig chain is made up of repeating units of about 70 amino acids enclosed by a disulphide bond. This arrangement is of interest since antibodies have evolved to perform two distinct functions which are separately localised in the molecule.

(a) Each antibody combines with a specific antigen. Every individual can probably make at least 10^5 antibodies with different specificities. The portions of the molecule which interact with antigen are called combining sites and there are two on each 4 chain molecule. These sites are generated by the interaction of the N-terminal units (V_H and V_L) of heavy and light chains, which show great variability of structure and are different in antibodies of distinct specificities. The V regions are common to all classes of immunoglobulins so that antibodies of a given specificity may be distributed in all the major Ig classes.

(b) Antibodies also carry out various effector functions which are consequent upon interaction with complement or with specific cells or membranes of the body. These effector sites are in C regions of the antibody molecule and given sites are present on some immunoglobulin classes but absent from others. Only IgG and IgM have sites for complement fixation, and only IgE has a site for attachment to mast cells, which is the basis for

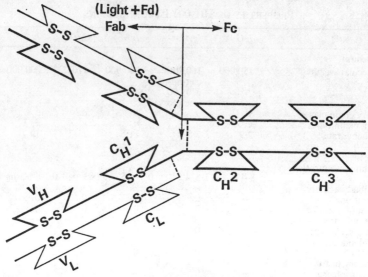

Schematic representation of the antibody molecule showing 4-chain structure, site of cleavage by the enzyme papain (arrowed) and distribution of repeating units bounded by intra-chain disulphide bonds. The units labelled V_H and V_L contain the antigen binding sites while the C_H and C_L-units carry sites for other activities such as complement fixation and membrane attachment.

sensitisation of autologous tissues. Both IgG and IgM attach to the surface of macrophages and mediate endocytosis while IgG alone attaches to K (killer) cells to initiate cell mediated antibody dependent cytotoxicity. These differences between the immunoglobulin classes account for the remarkable diversity of biological reactions mediated by serum antibody.

(ii) *Specific Cell-mediated Immunity.* In addition to the immunoglobulin response outlined above, antigenic stimulation frequently leads to the production of cells resembling small lymphocytes but carrying specific combining sites on their surface. These lymphocytes (T-cells) are derived from cells originating in bone marrow, but modified in some way by passage through the thymus gland (p. 338). Their surface receptors appear to have a structure related to that of the serum immunoglobulins, but the chemical identity of the two kinds of antibody has not been established. Cell-mediated immune responses are directed predominantly against intracellular pathogens and organised tissues. Sensitised lymphocytes after combination with antigen can exert a cytotoxic effect by producing factors which activate macrophages.

(iii) *Immunological Paralysis.* Cells of the immunological system can respond in two alternative ways to the presence of antigen. On the one hand, antigenic stimulation, as outlined above, may induce the cycle of cell proliferation and differentiation which culminates in humoral or cell-mediated immunity. On the other hand, antigen may lead to specific immunological paralysis; this is not merely a failure to produce specific antibody, but is characterised by long-lasting loss of the capacity to synthesise antibodies specific for the paralysing antigen. Injection of antigens during foetal life tends to induce specific paralysis rather than antibody production, but specific paralysis can also be induced in adults by using the appropriate antigen dose or by modifying the physical character of the antigen. The mechanisms which determine whether an antigen will induce specific paralysis rather than antibody production are not fully understood. In some instances, the removal from antigen preparations of aggregated material liable to phagocytosis converts an immunising protein antigen into one inducing specific paralysis. This suggests that, at least in these instances, the immune response is initiated by antigen which has been modified by passage through macrophages while specific paralysis follows the direct interaction of antigen with lymphocytes.

(iv) *Non-specific Cell-mediated Immunity.* Sensitised T-lymphocytes reacting with antigen undergo blast transformation and may produce cytotoxic agents capable of damaging by-stander cells. In addition, other lymphocyte products may activate macrophages which become cytotoxic for a wide range of pathogens and cells.

Disorders of Antibody Production

Clinical disorders may be associated with either diminished or increased production of antibody or lymphocytes. The most severe forms of antibody deficiency affect both cell-mediated and humoral immunity, but in other syndromes only one of these immune responses may be affected while the other remains intact.

An excessive production of Ig leading to a diffuse increase of gamma-globulin detected on electrophoresis of serum is seen in many clinical disorders (p. 342) and results from proliferation of many different clones of lymphoid cells. The proliferation of a single clone, on the other hand, leads to production of monoclonal Ig which is homogeneous on electrophoresis and belongs to a single Ig class. This occurs in multiple myelomatosis and macroglobulinaemia, in association with various lymphomata and unrelated neoplasms and also, quite commonly, as an 'idiopathic' condition without detectable underlying pathology. Clonal proliferation of lymphocytes also occurs in acute and chronic lymphatic leukaemia, but these cells rarely produce immunoglobulin.

Disorders of Antibody Production

1. **Deficient Production**
   (i) *Reduced cell-mediated and Ig responses*
   Combined Immunodeficiency
   Combined Immunodeficiency (with thymoma)
   Wiskott-Aldrich Syndrome (with thromlocytopaenia and eczema)
   (ii) *Reduced Ig response only*
   Transient hypogammaglobulinaemia of infancy
   Congenital agammaglobulinaemia
   Secondary hypogammaglobulinaemia (e.g. in Hodgkin's disease, nephrosis)

(iii) *Reduced cell-mediated response only*
Thymic aplasia (di George's syndrome)

2. Excessive Production

(i) *Diffuse hypergammaglobulinaemia*
Chronic infections
Granulomata
Hepatic disease
'Connective tissue' disease

(ii) *'Monoclonal' Ig production*
Multiple myelomatosis (IgG, IgA, IgD, or IgE)
Macroglobulinaemia (IgM)
Lymphoma
Unrelated neoplasm
Idiopathic 'gammopathy'

(iii) *Clonal Lymphocyte Proliferation*
Acute lymphatic leukaemia
Chronic lymphatic leukaemia
Burkitt's lymphoma

Reactions Mediated by Immune Responses

Humoral antibodies and cell-mediated immunity are of fundamental clinical importance, not only in regard to protective immunity, but also in a wide range of pathological states involving immediate hypersensitivity reactions, auto-antibody formation or reactions to circulating immune complexes.

(1) *Protective Immunity.* Immune reactions involve the primary interaction of antibody with the pathogen or its toxic products. Only in rare instances, however, e.g. some forms of viral immunity and toxin neutralisation, does this primary interaction constitute an effective immune response. Immunity is usually dependent on subsequent reactions of the bound antibody either with complement which leads to cell lysis, e.g. of Gram-negative bacteria, or with the surface of macrophages which promotes phagocytosis of the pathogen, e.g. pneumococci. It follows that protective immunity in systemic infections is mainly dependent upon IgG and IgM antibodies since only these can fix, complement and attach to macrophages. IgA is the predominant antibody of seromucous secretions and fulfils an important protective role at the epithelial surface of pulmonary and gastro-intestinal tracts. Although IgA does not fix complement, it can act synergistically with lysozyme, present in seromucous secretions, to cause bacterial lysis.

Whether the immune response to infection is clinically effective or not depends mainly upon the serological character of the pathogen and its distribution in the body (p. 343). Lasting immunity occurs with organisms of uniform antigenicity widely distributed in the circulation, e.g. pertussis infection. Recurrent infections may be caused by serological variants of the original infecting pathogen, e.g. pneumococcal infections, or occur after localised infections which evoke a feeble immune response, e.g. diphtheria. Immunity may be totally ineffective where the organisms persists in modified form, e.g. the herpes virus as DNA or where the lethal dose of a toxic product, e.g. tetanus toxin, is less than the immunising dose.

Patients may be susceptible to infection when specific immune responses are unimpaired, but defects occur in polymorph function or there are deficiencies of individual complement components.

(2) *Anaphylactic (Type I reactions).* These reactions which include general and localised forms of anaphylaxis depend upon an immune response fundamentally similar to that responsible for protective immunity. There has long been speculation regarding the underlying mechanism producing such dramatically divergent reactions. It is now established that immediate hypersensitivity is mediated by one class of immunoglobulin, IgE (below) and atopic individuals tend to produce this antibody in

IMMUNOPATHOLOGY—MECHANISMS AND CLINICAL ASSOCIATIONS

Mechanism	Antibody	Antigens	Clinical
Anaphylactic (Type I)	IgE	Allergens e.g. drugs, pollen	Systemic anaphylaxis Bronchial asthma, Hay fever Urticaria
Cytotoxic (Type II)	IgG or IgM	Host tissue	Hyperthyroidism, Goodpasture's syndrome, Auto-immune haemolytic anaemia.
		Viral	Post measles encephalitis
		Drugs	Haemolytic anaemia Thrombocytopaemia
Immune Complex (Type III)	IgG or IgM	DNA	Lupus erythematosus nephritis
		Serum, Drugs	Serum sickness, Arthus reaction
		Viral	Serum hepatitis (arthritis, nephritis)
		Bacterial	Glomerulonephritis Lepromatous leprosy
		Protozoal	Malarial nephrosis
		Fungal	Farmer's lung
Cell-mediated (Type IV)	Cell-mediated	Host Chemical Viral Bacterial Protozoal Helminth	Hashimoto's disease Nickel sensitivity Herpes simplex Tuberculosis Cutaneous leishmaniasis Schistosomiasis (cirrhosis)

response to antigenic stimulation. The serum concentration of IgE is very low (p. 339) and most of this antibody is attached to tissue mast cells which are then said to be sensitised. On subsequent exposure, the antigen (allergen) reacts with tissue bound IgE and as a result the sensitised mast cells undergo degranulation, liberating various pharmacologically active compounds which cause the characteristic allergic symptoms (below). Desensitisation of atopic individuals can sometimes be achieved by injecting very small doses of the allergen. This stimulates the production of IgG antibody and on subsequent, natural exposure the

IMMUNE RESPONSE TO VARIOUS INFECTIONS

Clinical Immunity	Serology	Distribution of Pathogen	INFECTIONS			
			Bacterial	Rickettsial+	Viral	Protozoal
Lasting	Uniform	Systemic or localised	Pertussis	Q-fever	Measles, Mumps, Rubella, Small-pox, Yellow-fever, Chicken-pox	Cutaneous leishmaniasic
Strain-specific	Varied	Systemic or Localised	Streptococcal, Staphylococcal, Pneumococcal	Typhus	Polio, Common-cold, Influenza	Trypanosomiasis
Poor	Uniform or Varied	Localised (or intra-cellular)	Brucella		Common-cold, Influenza, Trachoma, Gonorrhoea	Malaria
Ineffective			Tetanus		Herpes	

MECHANISM OF HYPERSENSITIVITY

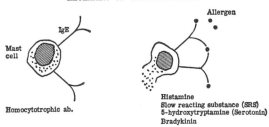

Mechanism of local and generalised anaphylaxis. Antigenic stimulation of a susceptible subject leads to synthesis of IgE antibody which becomes attached to mast cells. A subsequent exposure to the same antigen leads to its combination with cell-bound IgE and consequent degranulation of mast cells and discharge of pharmacologically active compounds which cause anaphylaxis.

allergen combines mainly with the predominant IgG (blocking) antibody so that reactions due to combination with IgE are prevented. It is apparent that the biological consequences of antibody reactions depend fundamentally upon the relative proportions of the reacting Ig classes.

(3) *Auto-antibodies (Cytotoxic Type II reaction).* The remarkable ability of the immunological system to distinguish 'self' from 'non-self' is thought to depend upon the development during foetal life of specific paralysis to auto-antigens. The appearance of auto-antibodies could, therefore, result from changes in the structure of auto-antigens (e.g. by drugs or infectious agents), entry into the circulation of antigens normally shielded from the immune system (e.g. spermatozoa, lens protein or thyroglobulin), the presence of cross-reacting heteroantigens (e.g. group A streptococci, which have antigens also present in human heart tissue) or mutation of lymphoid cells. Viral infections which cause viral antigens to be deposited on cell surfaces may also induce antibody formation against the infected tissues (e.g. as probably occurs in post-measles encephalitis).

Auto-antibodies are being found in association with an increasing num-

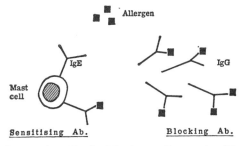

Desensitisation of an atopic subject by injecting small amounts of the allergen may induce the formation of IgG antibody. By combining with the allergen after natural exposure the IgG acts as a 'blocking' antibody and prevents combination with IgE on sensitised mast cells.

PROPERTIES OF SOME COMMON AUTOANTIBODIES

Disease	Antibody	Antigen	Test	Positive in
Rheumatoid arthritis	Rheumatoid factor (IgM)	Altered γ-globulin	Rose-Waaler / Latex-particle } agglutination	Rheumatoid arthritis 70%. S.L.E. 20%. Normal 5%. Sjøgren's syndrome 75%.
Systemic lupus erythematosus	L.E. factor (IgG, IgA or IgM)	Deoxyribonucleohistose (nuclear protein)	L.E. cell phenomenon or immunofluorescence	S.L.E. 90%. Rheumatoid arthritis 50%. Sjøgren's syndrome 75%.
Thyroiditis	IgG or IgM	Thyroglobulin / Thyroid microsomes	Precipitin reaction or Agglutination / C' fixation	Hashimoto's disease 100%. Thyrotoxicosis, Ca thyroid, non-toxic goitre 60%. Normal females 15%. Pernicious anaemia 40%.
Thyrotoxicosis	LATS (IgG)		Release of labelled hormone from thyroid	Thyrotoxicosis 60%.
Acquired haemolytic anaemia	IgG (non-agglutinating)	rH	Indirect haemagglutination (Coombs' test)	AHA 80%.
Pernicious anaemia		Intrinsic factor / Parietal cell	Binding of Radioactive Vit.^{n} B_{12} / Immunofluorescence	Pernicious anaemia 50%. Thyroiditis 30%.

ber of pathological states. In many instances these antibodies (p. 469) are directly responsible for the pathological lesions e.g. in hyperthyroidism and Goodpastures's syndrome. In other instances their presence is of diagnostic value, but several facts throw doubt upon the role of most of these antibodies in the *initiation* of pathological lesions. Many auto-antibodies occur in only a proportion of patients with the particular clinical syndrome and conversely, specific auto-antibodies are often found in the absence of the relevant disease (p. 346). In addition, their presence or level may show little correlation with the clinical state and autoimmune lesions are not usually induced by passive transfer of auto-antibodies. Long-acting thyroid stimulator (LATS) is an exception to this statement since thyrotoxicosis may occur in new-born offspring of thyrotoxic mothers who have circulating LATS. This observation strongly supports the idea that some forms of thyrotoxicosis are caused by an autoimmune reaction involving a serum IgG antibody.

(4) *Immune Complex (Type III reaction)*. Antigen-antibody complexes present in the circulation may form micro-precipitates in small blood vessels, fix complement and lead to accumulation of polymorphonuclear leucocytes, vascular occlusion and perivascular inflammation. Such lesions may occur in individuals injected with large doses of penicillin or horse serum (e.g. during passive immunisation for diphtheria or tetanus) who form antibodies which combine with the circulating antigen. The resulting syndrome, which is known as serum sickness, is characterised by glomerulonephritis, myocarditis, joint effusions, urticaria and pyrexia. Certain forms of pulmonary alveolitis which follow inhalation of fungal antigens, e.g. farmer's lung, also represent a reaction to circulating immune complexes. There is at present considerable interest in the possibility that various forms of renal disease, arthritis and periarteritis of obscure etiology are caused by a similar immune mechanism.

(5) *Cell-mediated Immunity (Type IV reaction)*. Sensitised lymphocytes of thymic origin are involved especially in immunological reactions against organised tissues carrying foreign antigens. Such antibodies are primarily responsible for rejection of foreign grafts, immunological responses to tumours and for certain forms of immunopathology, e.g. hepatic cirrhosis associated with schistosomiasis and sensitivity reactions to nickel, picryl chloride and poison ivy (p. 344). Cell-mediated immunity probably also plays an important role in specific resistance to intra-cellular infections including tuberculosis, leishmaniasis, leprosy and some viral infections, and may be responsible for many of the papular and vesicular rashes which accompany common infectious diseases. The presence of cell-mediated immunity is indicated by the delayed hypersensitivity response, i.e. an inflammatory lesion appearing 24 hours after intradermal challenge with the antigen and characterised by local infiltration of the tissue with round cells.

The importance of cell-mediated immunity in suppressing tumour growth has been demonstrated *in vitro* and is also indicated by the unusual

Large doses may be required. Occasionally *immunosuppressive drugs* (azothioprine or cyclophosphamide) may be useful but carry definite risks. *Chloroquine* in doses of 0·2–0·4 g. daily has been used but is frequently disappointing.

Prognosis. Prognosis must be guarded. There is much to commend the division of the cases into benign and malignant (Hill), in the same way as hypertension. Benign cases may progress very slowly for many years, but once the malignant phase begins, and particularly once there is marked renal involvement, the outlook is bad, patients usually only surviving a year or two.

POLYARTERITIS NODOSA (PAN)

Introduction

Polyarteritis nodosa is believed to be due to the formation of an antigen-antibody-complement complex (see p. 347). This may occur in the arterial wall causing a vasculitis, or it may be formed in the blood and deposited in the vessel wall.

The cases are best grouped into those with preceding lung involvement (30–40 per cent) and those without it (50–60 per cent). Some defy classification. In both groups there are striking constitutional effects, including loss of weight, fever, tachycardia, raised E.S.R., increased gamma-globulin levels, sometimes increased alpha 2 globulin, leucocytosis with eosinophilia (extreme if there is lung involvement), and anaemia, usually normochromic normocytic.

Clinical Features

(a) *With Lung Involvement.* The disease may start at any age, and has equal incidence in both sexes. A respiratory illness always precedes the other evidences of PAN, sometimes (25 per cent) by many years. Its features are asthma, chronic bronchitis, and recurrent pneumonia. There is no family history of asthma, and there is usually a high (albeit intermittent) eosinophilia (1,500–50,000 per cu.mm.). Radiography of the chest may show anything from transient symptomless shadows to chronic abscesses.

These symptoms are associated with a tendency to granulomatous lesions of the accessory air sinuses (Wegener's granuloma), and there may be superficial ulceration throughout the gastrointestinal tract, especially in the mouth. Other evidences of visceral granulomatoses may be found, but these are not frequent.

(b) *Without Lung Involvement.* This type occurs twice as commonly in men as in women, and increases with longevity. The incidence is maximum in the seventh decade.

(c) *Additional Features*

    (1) *Gastrointestinal involvement* occurs in 80 per cent of patients. Usual complaints are of poorly localised abdominal pain. The liver and spleen may be palpable, and shallow ulcers may occur in the gastrointestinal tract and sometimes bleed severely. About 10 per cent of cases present as an acute colitis, and may progress in a way similar to ulcerative colitis (p. 78).

    (2) *Cardiac Involvement.* The coronary vessels are involved in about half the cases, and may give rise to typical symptoms (p. 163). The heart muscle may be affected causing tachycardia and dilatation.

    (3) *Nervous Involvement.* Peripheral neuritis is common (35 per cent) and it may take the form of mononeuritis multiplex (p. 325). Focal lesions in the nervous system are less common, but do occur. They are caused by affection of cerebral vessels.

    (4) *Renal involvement* occurs in over 50 per cent of cases. It causes proteinuria with microscopic haematuria, and granular and hyaline casts. A specific glomerulitis has been described, and death from malignant hypertension or uraemia may result.

    (5) *Arthritis and Arthralgia.* A typical rheumatoid type of arthritis may occur (p. 356), less frequently there is an atypical arthralgic illness resembling rheumatic fever. Muscle pain and tenderness are common, and the pectoral muscles are frequently affected.

Special Investigations

The combination of leucocytosis, eosinophilia, and high E.S.R., should lead one to suspect the diagnosis. It may be proved by microscopy of biopsy material, either from a superficial lesion or from the pectoral muscle.

Treatment. Is general and specific, as for SLE (p. 348).

Prognosis must be guarded. Ninety per cent of patients are dead within five years of onset. Those without lung involvement survive a little longer than those with pulmonary disease.

DERMATOMYOSITIS AND SCLERODERMA

Introduction

It is probable that these two clinical syndromes represent extremes of the same pathological process. Points in favour of their unity are the identical distribution of the skin changes in both, and the presence of muscular weakness, Raynaud's phenomenon and calcinosis. They may present at any stage. Dermatomyositis occurs equally in either sex but scleroderma is commoner in women. They are much more rare than SLE or PAN, and the general manifestations of connective tissue diseases previously discussed may occur in both.

Clinical Features

(a) *Dermatomyositis.* This usually occurs between forty and sixty years. In about 20 per cent of cases an underlying neoplasm exists, but this rises to 50 per cent in new cases in men over fifty, almost all due to bronchial carcinoma. In other cases the disease often dates from an acute infection.

It may present in acute or chronic forms. The diagnostic triad is of non-suppurative polymyositis, dermatitis, and oedema. Many types of skin reaction have been recorded in the acute form but there is usually a generalised erythematous macular rash, whereas in the chronic form cutaneous telangiectases with periorbital oedema and heliotrope discoloration of the eyelids is common. All transitional forms between these rashes and the appearances of scleroderma have been recorded; calcinosis may occur. Muscular weakness is the rule, sometimes with tenderness and pain on use of muscles, including isometric contraction. Ultimately fibrosis occurs and contractures may result. The heart muscle may be affected causing a myocarditis with disproportionate tachycardia. Sometimes the oesophagus is involved, usually in the upper third, causing dysphagia.

Special Investigations. The plasma levels of creatine phosphokinase (CK) and aldolase are greatly elevated in the acute phase of the disease. Typical patterns are seen on electromyography, and muscle biopsy may be diagnostic.

Prognosis in acute dermatomyositis is bad. In about half the recorded cases death results, either from myocarditis or bronchopneumonia from involvement of the intercostal muscles. Less acute forms may merge imperceptibly into the picture of scleroderma, but the lungs and alimentary tract are usually spared.

(b) *Scleroderma.* In this condition the skin becomes hard and rigid, initially thickened from fibrosis, later atrophic and shiny, with telangiectases. It exists in two forms, local and systemic. *The local form* (morphoea) is confined to the trunk, and the lesions vary in size from a centimetre in diameter or less to great sheets encasing the whole trunk. The local form is not associated with systemic upsets, and does not usually change to the generalised form.

The commonest of the *systemic syndromes* is progressive symmetrical scleroderma with sclerodactylia (acrosclerosis). It begins insidiously with stiffness of the hand, later progressing to complete rigidity and joint fixation. The earliest sign is a disappearance of the wrinkles over the extensor surfaces of the knuckles. Later the hand seems to be encased in a hard, shiny glove, like a marble statue. Bone and joint destruction may be severe. Similarly the face may be affected, and very gradually the ability to open the mouth widely is lost and mobility of expression is impaired. The skin appears shiny, often pigmented, and with multiple telangiectases. Calcinosis in the hands is common, and severe Raynaud's phenomenon is frequent (CRST syndrome). In the *Thibierge-Weissenbach syndrome* these changes are accompanied by sclerodermatous involvement of the oesophagus and dense pulmonary infiltration. Dysphagia and dyspnoea are common complaints. Other parts of the alimentary tract and other organs, notably the heart and kidney, may be involved. Associated diseases are Sjøgren's disease and biliary cirrhosis.

Prognosis is bad, both for life and health. Death may result from intercurrent infection, cardiac failure or uraemia.

Treatment with steroids (p. 621) should be started as soon as the diagnosis is made but frequently fails to halt the progress of the disease. Penicillamine is sometimes of value.

GIANT-CELL ARTERITIS (Temporal Arteritis)

Introduction

This is not proved as a collagen disease, but is believed to represent an autoimmune reaction. It occurs in the elderly, being excessively rare before fifty-five. Commoner in women than in men, it presents local and general features.

Clinical Features

(a) *General.* Malaise, fever, weight loss, anorexia, aches and pains in muscles (see below), peripheral polyarthritis, and osteoporosis may precede local changes.

(b) *Local changes* are produced by acute inflammation of the arteries. All arteries, including the coronary vessels, may be affected, but particularly those of the scalp and brain, hence the older name of temporal arteritis.

The commonest arteries to be affected are those of the *scalp*, particularly the temporals. There is a persistent dull, throbbing headache and the skin overlying the vessels is inflamed. There is local tenderness, and arterial pulsation is absent or reduced. The temporal, occipital and facial vessels may be affected, and in severe cases there may be necrosis of the scalp. *Intracranial vessels* may be involved. Their narrowing causes turbulence in the blood flowing through them, so that loud murmurs may be heard through the skull over them. The *eye* is commonly affected, and papilloedema and blindness from retinal arterial disease is frequent. Personality changes from impairment of the blood supply to the frontal lobes are the rule, and a curious indifference to the disease marks its early stages. Later depression is common. No vessel is safe from attack and focal neurological signs may occur. The basilar artery is frequently involved leading to basilar insufficiency.

Special Investigations. The E.S.R. is always raised, and usually over 50 mm./hr. (Westergren). Leucocytosis is the rule, and the gamma-globulin levels may be raised in the plasma. Microscopy of biopsied vessels is diagnostic. They show an acute inflammatory change; the chief feature of the lesion is the presence of giant cells, though this is not a specific finding, as they may be seen in other arterial diseases. However, their profusion is such that they may reasonably give title to the disease.

Treatment is with steroids (p. 621). *Prognosis* is fairly good provided treatment is started before serious complications have occurred. The eye lesions once fully developed are little influenced by treatment, and terminal mental changes are common.

POLYMYALGIA RHEUMATICA

This is a disease of the elderly, who present with pain and stiffness of the limbs, particularly the arms, local tenderness of muscle, and malaise. Fever is usual, and the E.S.R. raised. Some patients subsequently develop an arteritis, and biopsy may demonstrate giant cells (see above). In others no arteritis occurs. The diagnosis must be made on clinical grounds; EMG and muscle biopsy are rarely useful. Treatment with small doses of steroids is usually very effective, and most patients can be weaned from the drug after a year or more.

SJØGREN'S SYNDROME

This uncommon disease is almost confined to middle-aged women. It is characterised by progressive dryness of the eyes, nose, mouth, larynx, and vagina, which is produced by atrophy of the lachrymal, salivary, and mucus glands. The patients usually present with complaints of grittiness or soreness of the eyes, sometimes with dryness of the mouth. On examination the dryness is apparent, and the lachrymal and salivary glands may be enlarged. In the later stages hyperaemia of the conjunctiva and filamentary keratitis may be seen. Polyarthritis of the rheumatoid type, and splenomegaly are occasionally found. Rheumatoid factor can be found in the serum of about 75 per cent of the patients. Treatment is unsatisfactory. Local application to the eye of methyl cellulose drops may relieve symptoms, and steroids may be tried systemically. Prognosis is generally bad.

RETROPERITONEAL FIBROSIS

A rare disorder of unknown aetiology, although in a number of patients it appears to be associated with the use of *methysergide* in treating migraine. The fibrosis extends over the posterior abdominal wall, frequently involving the ureters and producing an obstructive nephropathy. It may also obstruct the inferior vena cava or aorta. Rarely the fibrosis extends upwards into the mediastinum. It is thought to be part of a wider syndrome, which may also manifest itself as mediastinal fibrosis, ligneous thyroiditis, or localised pericaecal fibrosis.

Intravenous pyelography may show distortion of the ureters. Urine may contain leucocytes or red cells; the ESR is usually considerably raised.

Clinical features include general malaise, slight fever, low back or abdominal pain and a variety of urinary symptoms, polyuria, chronic renal failure, and sometimes anuria.

Treatment. Ureteric obstruction may be relieved surgically, and the disease thereafter treated with steroids (p. 621 or *p 645. in special Tropical Edition*).

RHEUMATOID ARTHRITIS (RA)

Introduction

Women are affected three times as frequently as men, and the usual age of onset is between twenty-five and fifty-five (mean forty years in both sexes). There is a slight (5–10 per cent) familial tendency, and the disease is essentially one of temperate climates. Dramatic remissions may be observed during pregnancy or jaundice. It affects all races.

The most obvious disorder of immunity in rheumatoid arthritis is the presence in the serum of most patients of the *rheumatoid factor*. This is an IgM globulin which will react with human IgG antigen provided that antigen is aggregated or fixed to particles (latex balls or red cells). Evidence suggests however that the rheumatoid factor does not cause rheumatoid arthritis but develops as a consequence of the disease. It seems most probable that rheumatoid arthritis is initiated by circulating immune complexes (see p. 347), but the cause is still unknown.

Clinical Features. (1) The onset is usually insidious and may be preceded by a period of general malaise with sweating and vasomotor disturbances affecting the hands. In about 15 per cent of patients the onset is acute with a widespread polyarthritis from the start.

(2) *Arthritis.* The prodromal illness is followed by the appearance of arthritis. This is essentially a peripheral polyarthritis, involving the small joints of the hands and to a less extent the feet. It usually begins in the first or second metacarpo-phalangeal joints, and rapidly involves the proximal interphalangeal joints. The distal phalangeal joints, in contradistinction to osteoarthritis, are usually spared. It spreads proximally to involve the wrists and elbows, or ankles and knees. Shoulders and hips may be affected, but this is uncommon. The cervical spine is frequently involved, with the risk of subluxation and spinal cord damage, but other parts of the spine are much less frequently affected. Occasionally one joint is affected, usually of middle size, and the disease may remain 'fixed' there for months or years.

Affected joints are tender, swollen, and hot, and movement is painful. Muscles moving the joints waste, and in advanced cases dislocation may occur. The appearance of the hands, with swollen joints, wasted muscles, sometimes dislocated fingers, and ulnar deviation is very characteristic. Radiography shows loss of joint space, soft tissue swelling, and rarefaction of bone, sometimes with small cyst formation.

(3) *Associated Features*. Commonest of these are *subcutaneous nodules*, felt most commonly over the ulnar but also found over other long surfaces or in relationship with tendons, especially around the wrist. *Chronically swollen bursae* may also appear, in particular the Baker's cyst found behind the knee-joint.

Arteritis is common but is usually symptomless. Occasionally it affects the digital vessels causing small gangrenous areas in the fingers and nail beds. Rarely it may produce a clinical picture similar to polyarteritis nodosa.

A *peripheral neuropathy* may develop, usually in the more severe cases. It varies considerably in severity. Bilateral carpal tunnel syndromes (p. 323) are common.

Anaemia is a frequent finding, and is usually normochromic and normocytic, responding poorly to iron. There may be an associated leucopenia.

Circulatory disturbances are common; the hands and feet are cold and blue, with anomalous sweating. In some cases there is generalised lymphadenopathy with splenomegaly and skin pigmentation, anaemia and leucopenia (Felty's syndrome).

Systemic involvement may also occur. *Episcleritis, iritis* and *uveitis* are seen in some cases, and in others there is *pleurisy*, with or without effusion, and progressive fibrosis of the lung. If pneumonoconiosis (p. 245) co-exists this may be extreme (Caplan's syndrome). *Pericarditis* may occur, and sometimes endocarditis causing valvular incompetence, especially mitral. Renal involvement is not uncommon, leading to progressive renal failure. It may be the result of drug treatment with penicillamine or analgesics.

Long-standing active rheumatoid arthritis may ultimately be complicated by *amyloid disease* (p. 464).

Special Investigations. There is no test specific to rheumatoid arthritis. If subcutaneous nodules are present then rheumatoid factor can be demonstrated in all the cases: if no nodules are present then this drops to 60 per cent. Unfortunately it can also be demonstrated in about 30 per cent of patients with SLE, PAN, SS and dermatomyositis. Activity of the disease may be assessed by the ESR and the ability of the serum to bind doublestrand DNA.

Treatment. This is general, local, and specific. Of the *general* measures, none is more important than rest, both physical and mental. Initially there should be a period of bed rest, and if necessary sedation. Sleep must be insured with analgesics and hypnotics. Diet should be varied and plentiful, if necessary with a vitamin supplement. Iron deficiency should be corrected if it exists; otherwise anaemia may require transfusion.

Local Treatment. In the acute phase the arthritic joints should be immobilised, preferably with light detachable plaster of Paris or plastic splints. Much relief may be found from warmth. Two perils must be avoided in this period. The first is joint fixation, to be averted by full passive movement of the affected joints at least twice daily, and the second muscle wasting. It is a counsel of perfection to aim at avoidance of wasting above and below an acutely affected joint, but it may be minimised by insisting on isometric contractions of surrounding muscles at least twelve times every hour. In the subacute phase splints may be retained for part of the day, but as soon as pain permits active voluntary movement should be encouraged. In both the acute and subacute stages much improvement may result from the local injection of 50–100 mg. of hydrocortisone into the affected joint, but repeated use may lead to a destructive arthropathy.

In the chronic phase orthopaedic and manipulative procedures including synovectomy may be of value.

Specific Measures
A. Anti-inflammatory and analgesic drugs.

(i) Salicylates remain the drugs of first choice. Soluble aspirin (4-6 g./24 hrs.) is usually satisfactory. Gastric irritation can be reduced by using enteric coated tablets. Aloxiprin (600 mg.) is a useful form of delayed release aspirin, and if given at night may reduce morning stiffness.

(ii) Indomethacin (25 mg. t.d.s.) in divided dosages is also useful. Suppositories (100 mg.) at night may also reduce morning stiffness.

(iii) Propionic acid derivatives are comparable to indomethacin in effectiveness and less toxic than phenylbutazone. They are useful in the management of acute and chronic arthritis and are analgesic and anti-inflammatory agents.

Alclofenac	1·0 g. t.d.s.
Fenoprofen	600 mg. q.d.s.
Ibuprofen	400 mg. t.d.s.
Ketoprofen	50 mg. t.d.s.
Naprosyn	250 mg. b.d.

(iv) Phenylbutazone and oxyphenbutazone are much more powerful but more toxic drugs. Gastrointestinal bleeding, skin rashes, and blood dyscarsia preclude their routine long-term administration, and important drug interactions (e.g. with anti-coagulants and hypoglycaemic agents) may occur. Nevertheless they are valuable in acute arthritis, and as short-term treatment of exacerbations of the disease.

B. Purely anti-inflammatory drugs.

(i) *Quick-acting:* steroids, corticotropin and tetracosactrin (p. 620 or p. *645 in special Tropical Edition*). These are by far the most powerful drugs currently available. There are theoretical advantages in the use of corticotropin or tetracosactrin, but a major disadvantage is that they are ineffective by mouth. In practice oral steroids are usually prescribed, and the drug of choice is prednisone (or prednisolone, therapeutically identical). Toxic side effects are common (p. 621 or *p. 645 in Special Tropical Edition*), but nevertheless they remain most effective drugs available at all stages of the disease but should only be used when it is resistant to other forms of treatment.

(ii) *Slow-acting:* gold, anti-malarials, immunosuppressives and penicillamine.

Gold. Interest has been revived in gold salts since the Empire Rheumatism Council's trial of 1961 showed benefit from a combination of IM gold injections and short courses of steroids. Toxic effects include skin rashes, blood dyscrasias and renal damage. Of these, skin rashes are by far the commonest. They can be minimised by avoiding gold in psoriatics, or other rheumatics with skin rashes. A test dose (10 mg.) should be given first, and the total dosage should not exceed 1 g., divided into 20 injections of 50 mg. each. Before each injection an inquiry for irritation at the site of the previous injection should be made, and if there was itching no more gold should be given for three months. The urine should be tested for protein before each injection, and frequent observations should be made on the haemoglobin level, and white count.

Chloroquine and its derivatives are also sometimes useful; their long-term prescription may lead to liver damage, retinal degeneration and corneal opacities. Weekly inquiry should be made for visual disturbance; the earliest sign of retinal damage is the appearance of halos round light objects. Gastro-intestinal upsets, skin rashes and depigmentation of the hair may also occur.

Penicillamine reduces the activity of the rheumatoid process. The initial dose is 250 mg. orally daily and slowly increased to a maximum of 1.5g daily. Side-effects include skin rashes, renal damage, bone marrow depression and an SLE-like syndrome.

In patients with disease resistant to all other measures either *azathioprine* or *cyclophosphamide* may be tried, but in both the risks of side effects are considerable.

Prognosis. Prognosis should be extremely guarded initially until the rate of progress of the disease has been assessed. In general it may be said that patients whose symptoms start very early or very late in life do worst, and those in middle life fare best. Some 20 per cent of patients will ultimately be seriously disabled.

Palindromic Rheumatism

Recurrent attacks of acute arthritis occur, persisting for 2–3 days and then subsiding without apparent joint damage. The hands are frequently affected. Many such cases ultimately develop into rheumatoid arthritis.

SERONEGATIVE ARTHRITIS

Arthritis which is clinically indistinguishable from rheumatoid arthritis may occur in conjunction with a number of diseases, the serum however is negative for rheumatoid factor. The tissue typing antigen HLA-B27 is common in several of the group.

Some of the more important associated disorders are:

Ankylosing spondylitis   Psoriasis
Crohn's disease   Reiter's disease
Brucellosis

PSORIATIC ARTHROPATHY

Clinical Features. The arthritis which appears similar to rheumatoid arthritis tends to attack the distal interphalangeal joints. It may be associated with considerable destruction and deformity of the fingers (arthritis mutilans). It is inclined to be less symmetrical than rheumatoid arthritis. There is usually evidence of cutaneous psoriasis together with typical pitting of the nails, though this is not inevitable.

Treatment is the same as that for rheumatoid arthritis but chloroquine may exacerbate the skin condition.

ANKYLOSING SPONDYLITIS (AS)

Introduction

This is a disease which is ten times as frequent in men as in women. It starts usually between fifteen and thirty-five years. It has a moderately strong tendency to be familial, and has been ascribed to a dominant gene with about 70 per cent penetrance in males and about 10 per cent in females. It may be significant that 90 per cent of patients have the tissue typing antigen HLA-B27. Persons poisoned with *cryolite* (sodium and aluminium fluoride) and those living in areas where there is a very high concentration of fluorine in the local water develop bone changes clinically indistinguishable from AS.

Clinical Features. (a) *Symptoms.* Clinically the commonest initial complaint is of low back pain, usually wakening the patient from his sleep in the early morning. This is associated with general stiffness of the spine. Other presenting complaints are frequent. Iritis (20 per cent) may precede all other symptoms for months or years. Non-specific urethritis occurs frequently at some time in the illness, and may present. In about 10 per cent of cases the first symptoms are from peripheral joints, usually feet, ankles, or knees. There may be tenderness of the heels, over the symphysis pubis, the greater trochanters, the ischial tuberosities, the iliac crest, or the sterno-manubrial joint. With these goes a general disturbance of health, low fever, malaise, lack of energy, and loss of weight.

(b) *Signs.* On examination the patients are usually rather tall, pale, and slender. There is a tendency to sweating, especially of the palms and soles. The normal lumbar lordosis is lost and mobility, particularly of the lumbar spine, is reduced. The respiratory excursion is poor, usually less than 2 inches. There may be pain on 'springing' the sacro-iliac joints, which may be tender on pressure. Other tender points may be found as described.

(c) *Associated Features.* The heart may be involved, and if it is the aortic valve is most commonly affected. The usual lesion found is aortic incompetence. Abdominal hernias, usually indirect inguinal, are found in up to 25 per cent of patients.

The E.S.R. is always very high in the active stage of the disease, and there may be normochromic normocytic anaemia. *Diagnosis* usually depends upon the radiographic demonstration of lesions in the sacroiliac joints. Stereoscopic views may be necessary for adequate visualisation. The earliest changes are widening of the joints with blurring of the margins; this is followed by sclerosis of the adjacent sacrum and ilium, and eventually by destruction of the joint space. The condition must be differentiated from *condensans ilii*, a benign affection of young women sparing the sacrum, and *tuberculosis*, which is usually unilateral. The spine too may be affected, and eventually all the vertebrae become joined by bridges of bone, the so-called 'bamboo' spine.

Ultimately the whole skeleton may be locked, warranting the first description (Connor, 1695) of 'An extraordinary humane skeleton, whose vertebrae, the ribs, and several bones down to the os sacrum, were all firmly united into one solid bone, without joynting or cartilage'.

Treatment. In the early stages physiotherapy may be given in an attempt to reduce ankylosis and deformity. Posture is important, and rest on a hard level bed during treatment must be insisted upon. If aspirin 0·5 g. every four or six hours fails to give adequate relief from pain, phenylbutazone 50 mg. three times daily often proves very effective but its administration must be carefully supervised (p. 537). Radiotherapy to the affected joints will sometimes arrest or retard the condition, but its use is followed by an increased incidence of leukaemia. Corticosteroids may give great symptomatic relief, but should only be given for acute exacerbations which cannot be controlled by other measures.

REITER'S SYNDROME

This is almost confined to men and may occur at any age after puberty, and consists of the association of urethritis, conjunctivitis, and arthritis, usually in that order, and sometimes accompanied by visceral manifestations. Its incidence varies between 1 and 3 per cent of all new cases of urethritis in different reported series. The aetiology of the disease is unknown but HLA-B27 is found in about 75 per cent of patients.

Clinical Features

(1) *The urethritis* follows sexual intercourse after an interval of about 1–4 weeks. It is non-bacterial, and often associated with some balanitis. It is not influenced by antibiotics. (2) *Conjunctivitis* is bilateral and follows 1–3 weeks after the urethritis. It is sometimes accompanied by uveitis,

and rarely keratitis. Usually it is mild, and lasts about a week or ten days. (3) *The arthritis* follows within a week or two of the conjunctivitis. It is usually a subacute polyarthritis of the small- and middle-sized joints; occasionally it is confined to one large joint. It is the most persistent of the triad, and may last 2 or 3 months. There may also be radiological evidence of sacro-ileitis, particularly in more chronic disease. (4) There are signs of a *general infection*, with fever, malaise, and raised E.S.R. Ulceration of the mucous membranes occurs. Plantar fasciitis is common, and may progress to the formation of a calcaneal spur. The typical associated skin lesion is *keratodermia blenorrhagica* with pustule formation on the palms and soles of the feet, but this is not common.

The disease is usually mild and self limiting, but relapses are common, and chronic affection possible, particularly if there is associated chronic prostatitis. Treatment of the urethritis is with tetracycline 25 mg. four times daily for a week, although response is variable.

Pain may be controlled by salicylates although in severe and persistent disease phenylbutazone or steroids both systemic or local may be required.

ARTHROPATHIES IN ASSOCIATION WITH SYSTEMIC DISEASE

There is a mixed group of arthropathies which complicate a number of systemic diseases. Their clinical presentation varies.

(a) **Viral infections** may cause a transient arthropathy. This occurs in rubella particularly in the adult and in viral hepatitis when it is often combined with an urticarial rash.

(b) **Bacterial infections of a joint** may be part of the clinical picture of septicaemia.

(c) **Acromegaly** is frequently associated with a polyarthritis with swelling of the joints and bony overgrowth.

GENERALISED OSTEOARTHRITIS

Although not associated with disordered immunity, this disease may conveniently be considered here. It is almost confined to post-menopausal women and there is a characteristic pattern of joint involvement, comprising the distal interphalangeal joints, the first metacarpophalangeal, the carpal joints, the intra fascicular spinal joints, especially the cervical, the tempero-mandibular and the knees. It is painful and unsightly, but rarely crippling. Treatment is symptomatic.

FURTHER READING

Copeman, W. S. C., *Textbook of the Rheumatic Diseases*, 5th edition, Livingstone, Edinburgh, 1977.

Humphreys, J. H. and White, R. G., *Immunology for Students of Medicine*, 3rd edition, Blackwell Scientific Publications, Oxford, 1970.

Samter, M., *Immunological Diseases*, 2nd edition, Little Brown & Co., Boston, 1971.

Roitt, I., *Essential Immunology*, 3rd edition, Blackwell Scientific Publications, Oxford, 1977

Dick, W. C., *An Introduction to Clinical Rheumatology*, 2nd Edition, Churchill Livingstone, Edinburgh and London, 1977.

CHAPTER NINE

DISEASES OF CALCIUM METABOLISM AND BONE

INTRODUCTION

Bone

Bone consists of connective tissue made rigid by the orderly deposition of mineral. The connective tissue of bone consists of collagen fibres lying in a polysaccharide ground substance. In this connective tissue framework are deposited crystalline bone salts which consist of calcium, phosphate and carbonate; the proportion of these ions may vary but dahlite $(CaCO_3 . 2Ca_3(PO_4)_2)$ is probably the commonest combination. In addition to calcium bone contains about one third of the total body sodium.

Calcification depends on the concentration of calcium and phosphate at the bone face and on other variables such as pH. The exact mechanism is not known but it is clear that phosphatase plays a part, perhaps by raising the local concentration of phosphate; a rise in plasma alkaline phosphatase therefore indicates an increased rate of breakdown and renewal of bone. Recently a hormone *calcitonin* has been described. It is secreted by the thyroid, parathyroid and thymus and causes deposition of calcium and phosphate in bone. Its clinical significance is not known.

After absorption vitamin D (cholecalciferol) is metabolised to more active forms. In the liver it is hydroxylated to 25 hydroxycholecalciferol. This is further modified in the kidneys to 1–25 dihydroxycholecalciferol which is very important in promoting absorption of calcium from the gut and in bone formation. When vitamin D is deficient the osteoid tissue of growing bone fails to calcify. The salts of bone are not metabolically inactive; rapid exchange can occur between the minerals in bone and those in the tissue fluids. Furthermore bone is not a static structure but is constantly being remodelled by a process of breakdown and renewal. Osteoclasts are concerned with bone resorption and osteoblasts with calcification.

Metabolism of Calcium

Calcium is absorbed from the small intestine. The average daily diet contains about 25–50 mmol. of calcium and of this about 2·5–5·0. mmol. is absorbed, the exact amount being regulated by the needs of the body. In health about 2·5–7·5 mmol. are excreted daily in the urine. Most of the body calcium is in bone. This is undergoing continuous absorption and excretion with a turnover of about 10 mmol. daily and here again calcium relase equals calcium uptake.

If the calcium in the diet is increased, balance is maintained largely by a decrease in absorption and urinary excretion rises little. Conversely, if the diet is deficient in calcium, absorption is increased and urinary excretion decreases. Vitamin D is essential for the absorption of calcium from the gut and if it is deficient calcium loss exceeds intake with subsequent decalcification of bones. Excessive urinary loss, however, is balanced by an increase in uptake and decalcification is unusual.

The plasma normally contains between 2·10–2·60 mmol. calcium/litre. A little over half of this is ionised, most of the remainder is bound to protein (chiefly albumen) and a small fraction is diffusible but un-ionised. The ionised fraction plays the most important part in the clinical states hypo- and hyper-calcaemia, although its concentration is rarely measured. Because of the binding of calcium to protein, total calcium levels are influenced by plasma protein concentration and corrections may be required. The binding of calcium and plasma albumen is also affected by pH; acidosis decreases protein-binding and thus increases the ionised fraction.

The level of plasma calcium is controlled by the *parathyroid* glands. A fall in plasma calcium increases parathormone secretion and vice versa. The actions of parathormone are:

(1) To mobilise calcium from bone and thus increase the plasma calcium concentration.

(2) To increase the renal excretion of phosphate and thus to lower plasma phosphate concentration.

(3) To stimulate production of 1–25 dihydroxycholecalciferol by the kidney (see above) and thus increase the intestinal absorption of calcium.

The non-protein-bound calcium and phosphate pass freely through the glomerulus. About 95 per cent of the filtered calcium is reabsorbed, probably by the distal tubule. The urinary excretion of calcium is only slightly dependent on dietary intake. In health it should not exceed 7·5 mmol./24 hrs. Phosphate is both reabsorbed and excreted by the renal tubules. In addition small amounts of calcium are excreted by the intestine.

HYPOCALCAEMIA
Introduction

The commonest cause of a sustained fall in plasma calcium is parathyroid hormone deficiency, for under normal circumstances any lowering of plasma calcium leads to increased secretion of parathormone with mobilisation of calcium from bone and return of the blood level to normal. Hypocalcaemia also occurs rarely in vitamin D or calcium deficiency (i.e. malabsorption, rickets or during lactation) or in renal osteodystrophy.

Long-standing hypocalcaemia produces striking structural changes in the body. Reduction in the level of ionised calcium in the blood causes increased neuromuscular excitability, and the clinical syndrome of tetany. This usually appears when the total plasma calcium level has fallen to about 1·8 mmol./litre. It is also seen in alkalosis where, although the total plasma calcium concentration is normal, the ionised fraction is reduced. It is probable too that magnesium and potassium can play a part in the genesis of tetany.

Clinical Features of Tetany

Symptoms

- (1) Paraesthesiae in lips, nose, and fingers.
- (2) Spontaneous muscle cramps.
- (3) Epileptic fits.
- (4) Laryngeal spasm in children.
- (5) Rarely arteriolar spasm, with pallor and raised blood pressure.
- (6) Psychoses may develop.

Signs

The diagnostic point is the demonstration of increased neuromuscular excitability. *Chvostek's sign* is elicited by tapping over the facial nerve as it emerges from the parotid gland beneath the zygoma. A hemi-facial twitch constitutes a positive response. Minor contractions confined to the angle of the lips should be ignored. The combination of twitching of the eyelids and the lips is usually significant but for certainty there should be movement of the whole side of the face. *Trousseau's sign* consists in the application of a sphygmomanometer cuff to the arm and raising the pressure to above the patient's systolic blood pressure for three minutes, by which time the hands should have adopted the classical 'main d'accoucheur' position—wrist and metacarpophalangeal joints flexed and fingers extended.

Signs of Long-standing Hypocalcaemia

Long-standing hypocalcaemia is associated with striking ectodermal defects. There may be coincident tetany.

- (1) Dry, scaly skin.
- (2) Loss of eyelashes, sparse eyebrows, patchy alopecia, and scanty axillary and pubic hair.
- (3) Wrinkling and brittleness of nails.
- (4) If present before they are fully formed, hypoplasia or aplasia of teeth.
- (5) Changes in nervous system; cataracts are common and so is calcification in the basal ganglia and dentate nuclei. Papilloedema occurs rarely.

Differential Diagnosis of Hypocalcaemia and Tetany

(1) **Alkalosis** usually results from hyperventilation; this is commonly hysterical but may be an epileptic phenomenon. It produces a fall in the concentration of ionised calcium in the plasma, partly by raising the pH of

the blood and partly by increasing the level of plasma citrate which combines with free calcium. Hyperventilation produces transient attacks of tetany. A history of overbreathing is diagnostic but subjects vary considerably in the amount of hyperventilation required to produce tetany. Typical findings in the blood are a reduced pCO_2, with a normal or slightly reduced bicarbonate and a normal total calcium concentration. *Treatment* consists of re-breathing from a paper bag.

Tetany may also occur with alkalosis due to acid loss from prolonged vomiting or gastric aspiration or rarely after ingestion of too much alkali.

(2) **Hypoparathyroidism** is usually the result of too radical thyroidectomy (secondary hypoparathyroidism). Transient tetany may develop soon after operation and in a few patients symptoms persist. In others the onset of symptoms may be delayed for several years. Occasionally the parathyroids are absent or non-functioning (primary hypoparathyroidism).

Clinical Features. The typical findings in parathormone deficiency are due to hypocalcaemia. They consist of tetany and sometimes epilepsy combined with widespread ectodermal defects (see above). Patients with primary hypoparathyroidism frequently develop chronic monilia infection of the skin. The plasma calcium level is low and the phosphate is high. The 24-hour urinary calcium output is usually low.

Pseudohypoparathyroidism is a rare condition in which the parathyroid functions normally but the tissues are incompletely responsive to parathormone. In addition to showing the features of hypocalcaemia these patients are short of stature and have thickset bodies, round faces, and short hands and fingers.

(3) **Osteomalacia and Rickets.** In these disorders (p. 370) there is a decrease in calcium absorption. However, a lowered plasma calcium level is unusual, presumably because the parathyroid glands maintain it at a normal level by mobilising calcium from bone, although the evidence for this is scanty. Occasionally, however, hypocalcaemia with attendant symptoms is found.

(4) The **malabsorption syndrome** may be associated with hypocalcaemia due to poor absorption of calcium and perhaps also of vitamin D.

(5) **Renal disease** can cause hypocalcaemia which may complicate chronic renal failure (see page 400). It can also result from excessive loss of calcium in the urine due to renal tubular acidosis (see page 410).

(6) Occasionally patients are seen with recurrent tetany where there is no apparent biochemical abnormality.

Treatment of Hypocalcaemia

(1) *Tetany* can be abolished by injecting calcium gluconate (10 ml. of a 10 per cent solution) slowly intravenously.

(2) The diet should be of adequate calorie value and have a high protein and calcium content. This latter is achieved by giving calcium lactate 5·0–10·0 g. daily.

(3) Patients with hypoparathyroidism are best treated with vitamin D

(50,000–200,000 units daily) by mouth. This increases calcium and phosphate absorption from the gut.

The dose must be controlled by estimation of plasma calcium and phosphate levels.

HYPERCALCAEMIA

Hypercalcaemia may result either from increased calcium absorption (vitamin D poisoning, sarcoidosis or milk poisoning) or from increased calcium mobilisation from bone as in hyperparathyroidism, or primary bone disease.

Clinical Features. Several systems are affected by hypercalcaemia.

(a) *Kidneys.* Hypercalcaemia interferes with reabsorption of water by the renal tubules producing polyuria and causing thirst. Eventually calcium may be deposited in the renal tubules producing nephrocalcinosis and renal stones.

(b) *Voluntary Muscle.* There is decreased neuromuscular excitability, which may lead to general muscular weakness.

(c) *Gastro-intestinal Tract.* Decreased excitability also affects smooth muscle causing constipation. Anorexia and vomiting are also common.

(d) Patients with hypercalcaemia may feel generally ill and depressed.

(e) *Deposits of calcium* may occur at the junction of the cornea and sclera. The deposits have a granular gritty appearance and are associated with increased vascularity.

(f) If bone is affected by the primary disease there may be pain and weakness perhaps with fractures.

(g) *Marked hypercalcaemia* produces confusion, coma, anuria and death. Such symptoms develop at a blood level between 3·5–4·0 mmol./litre.

Differential Diagnosis of Hypercalcaemia

(1) Primary Hyperparathyroidism

Usually results from one or more parathyroid adenomas; less commonly all four glands show diffuse hypertrophy. Carcinoma of the parathyroids is rare, but these tumours are always hormone-secreting. About 70 per cent of the patients are women. The disease exists in two clinical forms, with and without involvement of bone. Whether these represent two distinct fundamental disorders is not known but it seems more probable that bone changes are merely due to more severe disease, the basic cause of both types being overproduction of parathormone. Sometimes parathyroid adenomas are associated with hormone secreting adenomas in other endocrine glands, particularly the pancreas and the anterior pituitary.

HYPERCALCIURIA

Hypercalciuria is important because it may lead to nephrocalcinosis and renal stone formation. The main causes are:

(1) Hypercalcaemia (see above).
(2) Increased absorption of calcium as in vitamin D excess or sarcoidosis.
(3) Increased bone breakdown as in immobilisation and Paget's disease.
(4) Renal tubular disorders.
(5) Idiopathic hypercalciuria.

Idiopathic hypercalciuria is now thought to be a disorder of calcium absorption, although a few of these patients are believed to be suffering from mild hyperparathyroidism with a normal calcium concentration in the plasma. On a low calcium diet absorption and excretion are normal, but as the amount of calcium in the diet is increased so a larger fraction than normal is absorbed and the urinary calcium rises often to figures of 10–20 mmol./litre Ca excreted in 24 hours.

Hypercalciuria can thus be controlled by a low calcium diet but this may prove irksome. Calcium absorption can also be decreased by giving sodium cellulose phosphate (1·0 g. three times daily with meals).

RICKETS AND OSTEOMALACIA

The essential feature of both osteomalacia and rickets is a failure to calcify bone resulting in an excess of osteoid which is uncalcified bone matrix. In children the syndrome is known as rickets and in adults as osteomalacia.

Vitamin D is essential for bone calcification. It is obtained from certain foods including butter, vitaminised margarine and fish liver oils. It is also formed by the action of sunlight on the skin. Coloured people living in Britain are therefore particularly susceptible if their diet is deficient in the vitamin.

Lack of vitamin D leads to decreased absorption of calcium from the gut. This is associated with a fall in extracellular calcium concentration and it is believed (although the evidence is incomplete) that this in turn stimulates the production of parathormone. The plasma calcium is thus usually kept at normal levels, but there is an increased urinary excretion of phosphorus and the plasma phosphorus concentration is lowered. The calcification of osteoid depends in part on the solubility product of calcium and phosphorus $(Ca)^3 + (P)^2$ in the plasma and tissue fluids. When this is decreased as in vitamin D deficiency there is a failure to calcify *osteoid*. In rickets the main changes are seen where new bone is being formed from the epiphyseal cartilage. In the adult there is no new bone formation at the epiphysis but remodelling of bone continues throughout life and in osteomalacia too there is a failure to calcify new bone.

Vitamin D deficiency may be due to several causes:

(a) Dietary deficiency.

(b) Failure to absorb vitamin D—this may occur after gastrectomy or in the malabsorption syndrome.

(c) Induction of liver enzymes may lead to rapid breakdown of vitamin D; this has been reported in patients with epilepsy who have been taking phenytoin, which is a powerful enzyme-inducer, over long periods.

(d) Resistance to the action of vitamin D also occurs in chronic renal failure (see page 400) and in renal tubular disorders (see below).

Clinical Features

Rickets. The earliest clinical symptoms are tiredness and muscular weakness. There is bone pain and pain on movement. Dentition is delayed and the teeth may be deformed and quickly become carious. Swelling and tenderness of the distal ends of the radius and ulna are common, and so is the rickety rosary (costochondral swellings). Frontal and parietal bossing of the skull occurs and occipito-parietal flattening may result from the softness of the skull (craniotabes).

If the child can stand or walk, bowing of the legs may result from weight bearing, and kyphoscoliosis may appear.

Radiographs show widening and decreased density of the line of calcification next to the metaphysis, with irregularity and concavity of the metaphysis itself. In severe cases there may be rarefaction with deformities in the shaft of the bone.

Osteomalacia. Early symptoms are fatigue, stiffness and skeletal pains followed by muscular weakness and hyporeflexia. The gait is waddling and there is marked adductor spasm. Climbing up stairs may be particularly difficult. Costochondral swelling is common, and there is striking spinal curvature and the pelvic outlet is narrowed. Pathological fractures may appear in the pelvis and long bones, and may be exquisitely painful. Occasionally the plasma calcium level is low enough to produce tetany.

Radiology. Pseudo-fractures (Milkman, Looser) are the most frequent defect. These are lines of increased translucency running in from the surface of the bone, commonly found in the upper ends of the humerus and femur and in the pubic rami. They are strips of decalcification occurring in relationship to arteries or in areas of stress. In severe cases the bones show generalised decalcification with deformity and fractures.

The *biochemical* changes are similar in rickets and osteomalacia. The plasma calcium is usually a little low and occasionally considerably reduced. The plasma phosphate level is low but the alkaline phosphatase is frequently increased.

Treatment. Depends on the cause. For simple dietary deficiency, vitamin D 0·05 mg. (2,000 units) or liq calciferol (BP) 1·0 ml. (3,000 units) are sufficient. In malabsorption doses of vitamin D up to 50,000 units daily by mouth may be required, or 20,000 units can be injected weekly. Treatment should be continued until healing occurs and a watch kept for vitamin D poisoning. In coeliac disease a gluten-free diet will frequently decrease the oral vitamin D requirements.

Calcium is also required and effervescent calcium tablets (Sando-Cal) 2·0 g. daily for an adult is satisfactory.

Vitamin D Resistant Rickets. This small group have the symptoms of rickets but do not respond to small doses of vitamin D. The onset is usually late and there may be a family history. They are associated with disorders of renal tubular function.

(a) *Phosphaturic rickets* is probably due to a failure of the renal tubules to reabsorb phosphorus. The plasma calcium concentration is normal and the phosphate low. The bony lesions respond to large doses of vitamin D (50,000–500,000 units daily) and a supply of phosphorus in the form of sodium phosphates should be added to the diet.

(b) *Renal tubular acidosis* (p. 410) and *Fanconi's syndrome* (p. 410) may both be associated with rickets.

RENAL OSTEODYSTROPHY

Renal or uraemic osteodystrophy is a disease of calcium metabolism associated with chronic renal failure. The bones show a number of changes including an increase in osteoid at the metaphysis, with fibrous replacement and new bone formation elsewhere. In the blood there is a normal or lowered calcium level, a normal or raised phosphorus level and frequently evidence of acidosis. The blood urea is always raised.

There are probably several factors responsible for the clinical picture of osteodystrophy. They include:

(1) Failure to form 1–25 hydroxycholecalciferol by the diseased kidney, leading to impaired absorption of calcium.

(2) Increased parathyroid activity with enlargement of the glands and typical changes in the bones (secondary hyperparathyroidism) (see below). Rarely the parathyroids become autonomous and this leads to hypercalcaemia (tertiary hyperparathyroidism).

(3) Phosphate retention. A rise in plasma phosphate is usual in renal failure and would tend to depress plasma calcium levels.

(4) Acidosis may play a small part.

Clinical Features. In children dwarfism with bone deformities similar to those found in rickets are the most prominent features. In adults the symptoms of chronic renal failure usually overshadow the bone lesions although bone pain and fractures occasionally occur. The other feature is metastatic calcification which is occasionally palpable but is more frequently seen in radiographs. The *radiological* changes in the bones are complex and may be divided into:

(1) Changes similar to rickets (p. 371).
(2) Changes similar to hyperparathyroidism, with subperiosteal absorption of bone often most marked in the phalanges.
(3) Patchy osteosclerosis most marked in the skull. The vertebrae may show alternating bands of sclerosis and decalcification producing the 'rugger jersey' spine.
(4) Metastatic calcification may be widespread, both muscles and particularly blood vessels being affected.

Treatment. Bone symptoms can be relieved by giving vitamin D in large doses (100,000–200,000 units daily) with calcium gluconate 5·0 g. b.d. 1 alpha-hydroxycholeclaciferol may prove more useful, the initial dose being 1–2 μg. daily and reduced to 0·5–1 μg. after a few weeks. The dose of vitamin D should be controlled by blood calcium estimations.

If metastatic calcification is a problem and the blood phosphate level is raised, phosphate absorption can be decreased by giving aluminium hydroxide orally.

OSTEOPOROSIS

This may be defined as an atrophy of bone; although the volume of the bone remains the same, its content of bone tissue decreases. It affects both bone matrix and calcium and is most evident in the axial skeleton.

Aetiology

(1) *Idiopathic (senile) osteoporosis* is a common disorder. Atrophy of the skeleton is part of the general process of ageing, and starts at about the age of twenty. In certain people atrophy progresses fast enough to produce symptoms which usually appear in late life. This occurs more commonly in women than in men. There are probably several aetiological factors including androgen or oestrogen deficiency, vitamin D and calcium deficiency (particularly in the elderly), and physical and circulatory factors.

(2) In *Cushing's syndrome* and *steroid administration* a negative nitrogen balance and failure to form bone matrix are important.

(3) *Hyperthyroidism* and *acromegaly* may be complicated by osteoporosis and are associated with increase loss of calcium in the urine.

(4) *Immobilisation* leads to osteoporosis and increased excretion of calcium in the urine, sometimes complicated by stone formation.

(5) In *intestinal malabsorption* osteoporosis may co-exist with osteomalacia.

(6) *Rheumatoid arthritis* is frequently associated with osteoporosis especially in those treated with steroids.

Clinical Features. The disease may be symptomless, or there may be pains in the back, round the trunk, or down the limbs. They are made worse by jarring or flexing the spine, but rarely have the characteristics of root pain. Sudden severe back pain suggests the collapse of a vertebra. On examination, the spine is shortened so that height is lost and the distance from the ground to the iliac spine exceeds that from the iliac spine to the crown. Gross kyphosis is the rule and may decrease the vital capacity, but compression of the spinal cord is almost unknown. The consequent buckling of the trunk causes a characteristic transverse skin crease across the upper abdomen above the umbilicus. The infolded skin is keratinised, emphasising that the changes are of long standing. Radiographs show rarefaction of the spine and biconcave (cod fish) vertebrae. No typical biochemical changes are recognised.

Treatment consists of mobilising the patient and the administration of hormones and calcium. Women may be given ethinyl oestradiol 0·1 mg. daily for three weeks with a week's interval between courses. In men norandrostenolone (Durabolin) 25 mg. intramuscularly once weekly or norethandrolone (Nilevar) 10 mg. three times daily are satisfactory. A reasonably high protein diet and calcium 1·0 g. daily (calcium Sandoz three tablets daily is a useful preparation) are necessary to replace deficiencies. In older patients it is important to ensure that they are not vitamin deficient. Relief of pain often occurs within a month or so, though it is rare for radiological improvement ever to be seen.

PAGET'S DISEASE OF BONE (Osteitis Deformans)

Paget's disease usually affects a number of bones to greater or lesser degree, but some bones are completely spared. This is in distinction from osteomalacia and osteoporosis where the whole skeleton is affected, albeit unequally. Sometimes Paget's disease affects just one bone, particularly the tibia, femur, a clavicle, or a vertebra. It is rare before forty and affects men more than women in the proportion of 3 : 2. Occasionally it is familial. No disorder of metabolism has been identified, nor is there any indication that it is an inflammatory process. Two clues to its cause are the association with Hashimoto's disease and the occurrence of a similar disease in horses fed on a diet low in calcium and high in phosphorus (*big head disease*). It is said to be rare in oriental countries, where the phosphorus content of the diet is low.

The bones in order of affection are the sacrum, pelvis, spinal column (from below upwards), femur, tibia, skull, fibula, clavicle, humerus, rib. The hands and feet are almost always spared. Clearly the distribution is to some extent governed by stress and strain; the part of the skull which is particularly affected is at the sites of origin of the temporal muscles.

Clinical Features. The earliest symptom is pain, usually in the lower back, and often worse at night. Headaches are common, and there may be an unpleasant feeling of hotness from circulatory derangements. Deafness, often of nerve type, is common and the patient may have noticed increase in the size of his head. The picture may be complicated by platybasia (p. 270.) and pathological fractures are common.

Examination of advanced cases shows enlargement of the head, kyphosis, shortening of the spine and bowing of the long bones, especially in the legs. The bones are highly vascular and act as an arteriovenous shunt. This causes tachycardia, wide pulse pressure with a collapsing pulse, and dilatation of the heart. The limbs and extremities are hot, and often a murmur can be heard over affected bones. *Congestive cardiac failure* of 'high output' type may supervene. In the earliest cases these signs are absent, but there is limitation of hip movement, especially rotation, by pain.

The *serum alkaline phosphatase* level is always raised, often to great heights (350–1000 u/litre). No other biochemical abnormality is found in the blood unless the patient is immobilised, when the serum calcium level rises. The changes in the bones are essentially the result of increased resorption, and are characterised by cystic fibrosis, in this respect resembling hyperparathyroidism. Radiography shows a typical picture; there is increase in total diameter of affected bones, with thickening and broadening of the cortex, and abnormal architecture of the cortex and cancellous bone. In some cases only the proximal part of a long bone is affected, and the area immediately beyond its distal extent is rarefied (*osteoporosis circumscripta*). The disease spreads distally, progressing about 1 cm. every two years.

Complications are frequent. *Pathological fractures* are common, and generally heal well. *Deafness*, either from auditory nerve compression or otosclerosis, is ultimately the rule, and the optic nerve too may be compressed, causing *blindness*. Vertebrae may collapse and cause *spinal cord compression* and the effects of platybasia (p. 270) may be extreme. As more bone is involved so the tendency to *cardiac failure* increases. It is claimed that both hypertension and atheroma are more common than usual in Paget's disease. But the most serious (and least common) complication is the occurrence of *sarcomatous change* in the affected bone.

There are several drugs which slow down the pathological process of Paget's disease and relieve pain, but none is entirely satisfactory.

(a) Calcitonin in doses of 6–200 units daily is effective, but requires repeated injection which may be painful.

(b) Mithramycin is a cytotoxic antibiotic. The dose is 15 μg./kg. body weight given daily for five days by slow infusion.

(c) The diphosphonate, EHDP, which stabilises calcium phosphate crystals, is effective in doses of 5–20 mg./kg. daily orally. It would appear promising.

OSTEOPETROSIS (Albers-Schönberg's Disease)

The outstanding feature is a great increase in bone density so that radiographically they warrant the description of 'marble bones'. It exists in three forms foetal, juvenile and adult. The foetal form may be diagnosed radiographically *in utero*, and death always occurs shortly after birth. It is sporadic, whereas the juvenile and adult forms are familial and have Mendelian recessive characters.

Clinical Features. The *juvenile form* is severe, and death before puberty is the rule. Effects are produced by increase in size of bones, so as either to compress nerves (auditory, optic) or to encroach on the medullary cavity and to interfere with blood formation. This causes anaemia initially, later leuco-erythroblastic anaemia, ultimately marrow aplasia. Attempts at extramedullary haematopoiesis cause hepato-splenomegaly and generalised lymphadenopathy. *In adults* the disease is relatively benign. About one third of all cases sustain pathological fractures which heal badly; otherwise there are no symptoms or signs, and the diagnosis is made by chance radiography.

There is no special change in blood chemistry, but radiography shows a typically symmetrical increase in bone density. Characteristic appearances in individual bones are described, e.g. 'celery stick' in long bones, 'sandwich' vertebrae, and 'bone within bone' in the carpal and tarsal bones.

CONGENITAL ABNORMALITIES OF BONE

(a) **Osteopsathyrosis** (Osteogenesis imperfecta) exists in two forms, intrauterine and infantile. The intrauterine form causes multiple fractures *in utero* and death either before or shortly after birth. The infantile form presents as pathological bone fragility, resulting in frequent fractures. The bone changes are due to a defect in the connective tissue scaffolding of bone. Other evidence of connective tissue abnormality is found in the

TYPICAL BIOCHEMICAL CHANGES IN SOME METABOLIC BONE DISEASES

	Plasma Ca	Plasma PO_4	Plasma HCO_3	Blood Urea	Alkaline Phosphate	Urine Ca
	mmol./litre	mmol./litre	mmol./litre	mmol./litre	u./litre	mmol./24 hr.
Normal	2·10–2·60	0·80–1·50	24–28	2·5–7·1	7–105	3·0–6·0
Rickets or Osteomalacia	1·70–2·50	0·26–1·0	Normal	Normal	50–350	0·2–2·0
Osteoporosis	Normal	Normal	Normal	Normal	Normal	Normal
Primary Hyperparathyroidism	2·70–4·2*	0·26–1·3*	Normal*	Normal*	75–750	7–20
Renal Osteodystrophy (Secondary Hyperparathyroidism)	1·5–2·5	1·3–4·0	Decreased	Raised	75–750†	1·0–3·0

* If renal failure occurs figures approximate to those for renal osteodystrophy.
† Usually raised if there is bone involvement.

characteristic blue sclerotics which may however be absent in the most severe cases.

Clinically these children suffer many fractures from trivial injury. With increasing age fractures often become less frequent, probably due to greater care. Otosclerosis may develop in adult life.

(b) **Achondroplasia.** This disease appears in foetal life, and is hereditary. In most instances the pattern of occurrence is of Mendelian dominance, but sometimes recessive characters appear. There is defective ossification of bones formed in cartilage. For this reason the skull vault and spinal bones are normal, but the arms and legs are abnormally short, like those of a dachshund.

These are the typical circus dwarfs. The average height is about 4 feet; the trunk is normal but the arms and legs are short and the head misshapen. The vault appears large and the face is small with a sunken bridge to the nose. Musculature is well developed, and the hands rather small; the fingers are almost equal in length.

Many achondroplastics are stillborn, or die soon after birth. In those who survive the expectation of life is normal. No treatment is useful.

MARFAN'S SYNDROME

Marfan's syndrome is a hereditary disorder of connective tissue. There is no particular sex incidence and it can appear in incomplete forms.

The main manifestations are:

1. *Skeleton.* The bones are elongated and thin and the span exceeds the height. The palate is high arched and the hands show arachnodactyly.

2. *Cardio-vascular System.* There is necrosis of the elastic tissue of the aortic wall leading to aneurysm formation, dissecting aneurysm or aortic incompetence, sometimes with superimposed infective endocarditis.

3. *The lens of the eye* may be dislocated.

4. *The urine* may show increased excretion of hydroxyproline a constituent of collagen.

There is no treatment.

FURTHER READING

Fourman P. and Royer, P., *Calcium Metabolism and Bone*, 2nd edition, Blackwell, Oxford, 1968.

Paterson, C. R. *Metabolic Disorders of Bone*, Blackwells Scientific Publications, Oxford, 1975.

CHAPTER TEN

DISEASES OF THE KIDNEY

Introduction

The kidney has three main functions:

(1) The *excretion* of the end products of metabolism and of foreign substances and their metabolites. These include such substances as urea, uric acid and creatinine, and a large number of drugs or their breakdown products.

(2) The *maintenance* of the tissue fluids at a constant composition. The kidney is concerned not only with the concentration of various substances in the tissue fluids, but also helps to maintain the pH and volume of the latter within physiological limits.

(3) The *secretion* of hormones and hormone-like substances. These include renin erythropoietin, the active form of vitamin D (1,25-dihydroxycholecalciferol) and several prostaglandins.

There is a continual tendency for the composition of the tissue fluids to change. This results from wide variation in the intake of fluid and electrolytes and from the changes in the rate of metabolism which occur from hour to hour, resulting in uneven production of the end products of metabolism. The kidney must respond to these changes by excreting varying quantities of fluids and electrolytes; and as many of the end products of metabolism are acid it is continuously excreting hydrogen ions.

THE STRUCTURE OF THE KIDNEY

The functional unit of the kidney is the *nephron*. This consists of a glomerular tuft, situated in the cortex, and a tubule. The tuft leads into the proximal convoluted tubule which in turn leads to the loop of Henle which dips into the medulla, turns back on itself and ends in the distal convoluted tubule, which drains into a collecting tubule. There are two types of nephron: those in the outer part of the cortex which have short loops of Henle and are largely concerned with filtration and reabsorption, and those in the inner cortex which have long loops and play an important part in the countercurrent concentrating mechanism (p. 380). There are about one million nephrons in each kidney.

The *blood supply* to the glomerulus is directly from the renal artery. Efferent vessels leaving the glomerular tuft form a capillary network around the convoluted tubules, ending in a branch of the renal vein.

The cells lining the convoluted tubules and part of the ascending limb of the loop of Henle are columnar epithelium whereas those lining the rest of the loop are much flatter.

RENAL FUNCTION

THE GLOMERULUS

The glomeruli receive blood almost direct from the renal arteries at a considerable pressure. It seems probable that glomerular filtration is a passive process and that glomerular fluid is an ultrafiltrate, the formation of which depends on the balance between the capillary hydrostatic pressure forcing water and solutes through the glomerular membrane and the osmotic pressure of the plasma proteins keeping it within the vessel. Provided that the concentration of plasma proteins is constant, the rate of glomerular filtration depends therefore on the intraglomerular pressure and stresses the need for an adequate blood pressure and flow to maintain glomerular filtration.

The *glomerular filtrate* contains water with glucose, sodium, chloride, potassium, urea, uric acid, creatinine, and a number of other substances. It contains a little protein, which is reabsorbed in the proximal tubule. The volume of the glomerular filtrate is enormous, probably about 180 litres/24 hours.

The *glomerular filtration rate* (G.F.R.) can be measured. This is done by giving a substance which passes freely through the glomerular membrane and is not reabsorbed by the renal tubules. The rate of excretion of this substance is therefore the same as its rate of filtration.

TUBULAR FUNCTION

The tubules selectively reabsorb the various constituents of the glomerular filtrate so as to maintain the composition of the body fluids constant and at the same time allow the excess of electrolytes, products of metabolism, and water to pass to the collecting tubules and be excreted as urine.

The table shows the approximate composition of the glomerular filtrate and urine in 24 hours.

Substance	Amount in Glomerular Filtrate	Amount Excreted in the Urine
Sodium	600 g.	6 g.
Potassium	35 g.	2 g.
Calcium	5 g.	0·2 g.
Glucose	200 g.	—
Urea	60 g.	35 g.
Water	180 litres	1·5 l.

(After Robinson)

Reabsorption of Water

(a) *Diuresis*. About 85 per cent of the water filtered by the glomerulus is reabsorbed by the proximal tubule. It is believed that this is a passive process and follows the active reabsorption of sodium. The remaining water, greatly diminished in volume but with the concentration of sodium unaltered, then passes to the distal tubules and collecting ducts where further reabsorption occurs. This distal reabsorption is under control of the antidiuretic hormone (A.D.H.) from the posterior pituitary. Osmo-receptors in the paraventricular and supra-optic nuclei respond to changes in plasma osmolarity. Dilution of the plasma decreases the release of A.D.H. so that less water is reabsorbed in the distal tubules and collecting ducts and diuresis results.

When an osmotic diuretic is given reabsorption by the proximal tubule is decreased and the volume arriving at the distal tubule is so great that only a fraction can be reabsorbed. This is why in chronic renal failure there is a failure to concentrate urine. The increased amount of filtered urea which is not reabsorbed acts as an osmotic diuretic.

(b) *Urine Concentration*. When the osmolarity of the plasma increases, there is an increased release of A.D.H. which leads to concentration of the urine. The mechanism of this action has now been clarified. The loops of Henle as they dip into the renal medulla act as a *counter current multiplier*; sodium passes across from the ascending to the descending limbs so that as the urine descends into the loops it becomes more and more concentrated and as it ascends it becomes more dilute. The osmotic concentration which develops in the lowest part of the loops is reflected in the interstitial tissue of the medulla and renal papillae.

The action of A.D.H. is to render the cells lining the collecting ducts more permeable to water, so that when urine passes down these ducts and through the area of high osmotic concentration in the renal papillae, water is absorbed from the ducts and the urine becomes concentrated.

Reabsorption of Sodium and Excretion of Acid

One of the important functions of the kidneys is to conserve sodium, which is the chief extracellular cation, and to excrete hydrogen ions produced by the body's metabolic processes. Under normal conditions about 80 per cent of sodium reabsorption occurs in the proximal tubule, largely in association with chloride and with an osmotically equivalent volume of water. The remainder occurs in the ascending limb of the loop of Henle and in the distal tubule and is under hormonal regulation.

Sodium reabsorption is adjusted so that the total body sodium remains constant. One of the important controlling mechanisms is the hormone *aldosterone* which is secreted by the adrenal cortex. Aldosterone causes increased tubular reabsorption of sodium and excretion of potassium and is produced in response to a fall in blood volume or a decrease in renal blood flow.

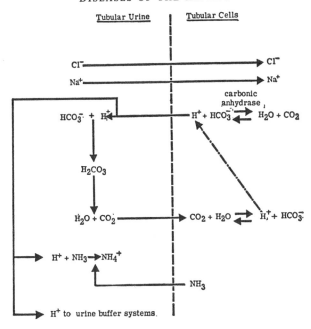

Tubular Mechanism for Excretion of Acid and Conservation of Sodium

The metabolic processes of the body lead to the production of various acids. The chief one is carbonic acid, the end result of oxidisation of food-stuffs, and this is eliminated in the form of its anhydride carbon dioxide, which is excreted through the lungs. The other important acid products of metabolism are phosphoric, sulphuric and organic acids, whose anhydrides are not volatile and must be excreted in solution through the kidneys. Although this forms only 0·2 per cent of the total H^+ production, its importance is disproportionately large. The excess hydrogen ions of these acids are absorbed by the buffer systems of the blood, mainly the sodium bicarbonate system, with the release of CO_2 which is excreted by the lungs.

The bulk of secreted hydrogen ion combines with filtered bicarbonate (see below); this normally results in removal of bicarbonate so that none is lost in the urine. Hydrogen ions are secreted in the distal tubule, and without the ability to establish a gradient of hydrogen ion from blood to tubule at this site acidosis will result. Equally, failure to reabsorb bicarbonate in the proximal tubule will overwhelm the distal H^+ excretion.

Because the kidney cannot establish a pH gradient of urine : blood greater than 4·6 : 7·3 it is necessary to reduce the number of free hydrogen ions in the urine. This is done in three ways:

(1) In an acidosis, urine hydrogen ions combine with ammonia in the tubular cell:

$$NH_3 + H^+ \rightarrow NH^+_4$$

(2) The buffer systems of the urine (largely phosphate) absorb hydrogen ions without producing too great a change in pH of the urine.

(3) Hydrogen ions combine with filtered bicarbonate (see below).

These mechanisms are important for without them the kidney could only excrete a small amount of acid (i.e. hydrogen ions).

Excretion of Bicarbonate

When hydrogen ions are excreted into the renal tubules they combine with bicarbonate:

$$H^+ + HCO_3^- \leftrightarrows H_2CO_3 \leftrightarrows H_2O + CO_2$$

The carbon dioxide thus produced diffuses back into the tubular cells to reform bicarbonate. This is one possible method of bicarbonate reabsorption, although bicarbonate ions are absorbed as such. The urine is normally bicarbonate-free on a mixed diet.

If, however, plasma bicarbonate is raised, less hydrogen ions are exchanged for sodium bicarbonate being excreted and the urine becoming alkaline. Again, if the proximal tubules are damaged or defective, bicarbonate will reach the distal tubular mechanism in excess and the urine will be alkaline with production of systemic acidosis.

Excretion of Potassium

It appears probable that all the filtered potassium is absorbed by the proximal tubules and that further potassium is excreted by the distal

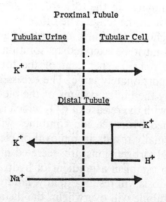

Tubular Mechanism for Excretion of Potassium

tubules. The pathway of tubular potassium excretion competes with that for hydrogen ion excretion, so that increased hydrogen ion excretion decreases potassium excretion and vice versa. Potassium is also exchanged for sodium by the renal tubules, so that if little sodium is available potassium excretion is decreased. Finally certain drugs, particularly diuretics and the adrenal steroids, increase renal excretion of potassium.

Reabsorption of Glucose and Aminoacids

This occurs in the proximal tubule. If the plasma level of glucose rises as in diabetes mellitus the reabsorbing system can no longer deal with the increased load and glucose is passed in the urine.

HORMONES PRODUCED BY THE KIDNEY

Renin is an enzyme which splits off a polypeptide *angiotensin* from plasma protein. Angiotensin is important in the control of blood pressure and blood volume. It has a direct constricting action on the arterioles and also promotes salt and water retention by stimulating the release of *aldosterone* by the adrenal cortex. Renin is released from the kidney by reduced renal circulation, usually following hypovolaemia or rarely narrowing of a renal artery or by a fall in sodium concentration in the fluid of the distal tubule.

Erythropoietin stimulates the production of erythrocytes. Overproduction may be responsible for the polycythaemia seen in some renal diseases, particularly renal tumours.

The kidney is also important in activating cholecalciferol (vitamin D) by further hydroxylating 25 hydroxycholecalciferol to *1,25 hydroxycholecalciferol* which is very active in promoting the absorption of calcium. Failure of this step in chronic renal failure may play a part in the development of renal osteodystrophy (see p. 372). The renal medulla produces several prostaglandins, one of which may be important in regulating blood pressure by lowering vascular tone.

THE URINE

Volume. The volume of urine passed in 24 hours in health usually lies between 700 and 3,000 ml. The urinary output of normal people is modified by fluid intake and by loss of fluid in sweat and the stools.

Appearance. The colour of normal urine varies from deep yellow to almost colourless. The colour is due to the presence of urochrome.

Specific Gravity. The specific gravity can be roughly estimated by a hydrometer. In health it varies between 1002 and 1032. The specific gravity of urine depends on the weight of substance in solution. Generally speaking a high specific gravity indicates that the kidney is capable of concentrating the urine. The urine SG is also high after the injection of osmotically active substances, such as glucose, mannitol, and contrast media; this occurs even when the kidney may not be capable of concentrating, because here plasma osmolarity is high.

Proteinuria. Normal adults excrete 30–100 mg. of protein in 24 hours. The amount is increased in the upright posture or after exercise. Protein is now usually detected by 'Albustix' which is a colorimetric method depending on the presence of an indicator. By this method it is possible to detect 200–300 mg. of protein per litre of urine which is at the top of the normal range. If therefore a faint trace of protein is found in the urine of an apparently normal person and if there is no suspicion of renal disease on other grounds this finding should be disregarded.

Excess protein in the urine, provided that there is no lesion of the urinary tract, indicates that protein has leaked from the blood to the urine across the glomerular membrane. Being the smallest molecule, completely retained, albumen leaks the most easily, but if the glomerular leak is severe all fractions of the plasma proteins may appear in the urine. Proteinuria is found in almost every variety of renal disease and generally speaking its presence is evidence of disease of the renal parenchyma. The amount of protein in the urine is no indication of the severity of the renal damage and it is a common experience to find only a small amount of protein in the urine of some patients with advanced renal disease (notably advanced pyelonephritis).

Symptomless Proteinuria

In patients with significant proteinuria who are otherwise symptom free it is important to avoid over-investigation, but it is necessary to exclude treatable lesions and form an idea of the seriousness of the underlying disease and of the prognosis. The first step is to decide whether the proteinuria is intermittent or persistent.

Intermittent proteinuria. In some patients proteinuria is intermittent and may be related to posture, exercise and other factors. It may occur in a wide variety of renal diseases but in young people is frequently due to **orthostatic proteinuria.** In this condition protein is found in the urine secreted when the subject is up and about, but is absent from urine secreted when he is recumbent. Urine passed on rising therefore contains no protein.

It is believed to be due to kinking of the inferior vena cava as it passes behind the liver, which occurs only in the upright posture. The rise in pressure in the inferior vena cava is transmitted to the renal veins and causes proteinuria. The condition is harmless and is unrelated to renal disease. However, before orthostatic proteinuria is diagnosed renal disease must be excluded and investigations should include renal function tests, examination of the urinary deposit and an intravenous pyelogram.

Persistent proteinuria is most commonly due to glomerulonephritis either with minimal glomerular change or to changes of the proliferative or membranous type. It may also be due to pyelonephritis or surgical renal disease. If no abnormality is found on clinical examination and renal function studies and the pyelogram are normal and the urine contains no red cells, the patient should be observed. Provided there is no deterioration in renal function over a year or two further investigation such as renal biopsy is unnecessary and the prognosis is usually good. The presence of hypertension, impaired renal function or red cells in the urine suggests progressive renal disease, may carry a worse prognosis and the diagnosis should therefore be clarified by renal biopsy.

Haematuria. Blood in the urine may arise from the kidney or from the renal tract. If it arises from the kidney it is intimately mixed with the urine; if from the lower renal tract it may appear only at certain phases of micturition. Large amounts of blood in the urine are obvious; smaller amounts give it a smoky appearance and minimal haematuria can only be detected by centrifuging the urine and examining the deposit under the microscope for red cells. Haematuria must be distinguished from haemoglobinuria and various drugs which may colour the urine red, notably phenindione.

Important causes of haematuria are:

From the Kidney	*From the Renal Tract*
Glomerulonephritis (various)	Papilloma of the urinary tract
Infarct of the kidney	Acute pyelitis or cystitis
Subacute infective endocarditis	Carcinoma of the bladder
Renal carcinoma	Prostatic infection
Overdosage with anticoagulant drugs	Tuberculosis of the renal tract
Bleeding diseases	Renal stone
Injury to the kidney	

White Cells in the Urine. White cells may be found in any inflammatory disease of the urinary tract, including glomerulonephritis, cystitis, and prostatitis. In infective conditions they may be present in such quantities as to warrant the term 'pyuria'. Pyuria may be severe enough to cloud the urine. It is important to examine a fresh sample of urine. The uncertrifuged sample should contain no more than 5 white cells/μl. in men and 10 white cells/μl. in women.

Casts in the Urine. Casts are composed of Tamm Horsfall protein, a normal constituent of urine which has solidified in the renal tubules, together with filtered plasma protein, particularly albumin. If they contain cells, either epithelial cells from the renal tubules or leucocytes or red cells, they are called *cellular casts*. If these cells have undergone cloudy swelling the casts are called *granular casts*. Casts which do not contain cells are called *hyaline casts*.

A few hyaline casts are often found in the urine of normal people and may be present in large quantities after exercise. Cellular and granular casts are found only in renal disease.

RENAL FUNCTION TESTS

Renal function resolves itself broadly speaking into filtration and reabsorption. A number of tests have been devised which assess one or other of these aspects of renal function. It must be realised that renal function tests merely indicate the degree of impairment of one aspect of renal function; they rarely indicate the nature of the underlying disease. Moreover, they are relatively insensitive and there may be considerable renal damage before these tests show evidence of impaired renal function.

The Blood Urea and Blood Creatinine

The blood urea should always be estimated in patients with suspected renal disease. Although it is a rough-and-ready test of renal function it is

USUAL URINE ABNORMALITIES IN RENAL DISEASE

Disease	Appearance	Volume	Specific Gravity	Protein	Deposit
Acute Nephritis	Smoky or red	Decreased	High	Present	Red cells, white cells and casts
Nephrotic syndrome	Normal or pale	Normal	Normal range at first, low and fixed later	Present in large amounts	Casts and sometimes red cells
Chronic renal failure	Pale	Increased	Low and fixed	Trace	Casts and few red cells
Essential Hypertension	Normal	Normal or increased	Normal range or low and fixed	0 to small amounts	Normal or excess casts
Acute renal infection	Cloudy 'fishy' odour	Often decreased	Normal range unless previous renal damage	Trace	White cells and bacteria

simple to perform and often gives as much information as more elaborate investigations.

The normal blood urea level lies between 2·5–7·1 mmol./litre. Persistent elevation indicates considerable interference with glomerular function; this may be due to primary renal disease, or be secondary to a failure of the renal circulation. Unfortunately, although the estimation of the blood urea level is easy it is not a very sensitive test of glomerular function; on a normal protein intake glomerular filtration must be reduced by about 30 per cent before there is any rise in blood urea level. The blood urea level also varies consistently with dietary protein intake and the degree of protein catabolisms, the variations becoming greater with decreasing renal function. Blood creatinine levels can be used in the same way (normal range 50–130 μmol./litre, varying with age and muscle mass) and are less susceptible to changes in diet.

TESTS OF GLOMERULAR FILTRATION RATE (G.F.R.)

The G.F.R. can be measured by giving a substance which is completely filtered by the glomerulus and is neither absorbed nor excreted by the tubules. Such a substance is the polysaccharide inulin. Under these circumstances the excretion of inulin in the urine (in mg./min.) divided by the plasma level of inulin (in mg./ml.) gives the number of ml. of plasma filtered per minute. The general calculation is given by the formula:

$$\text{G.F.R./per min.} = \frac{\text{Urine vol. per min.} \times \text{Urine concentration of inulin}}{\text{Plasma concentration of inulin}}$$

In practice inulin clearance studies are rather complicated to perform so that creatinine (a substance which occurs naturally in the blood) is often used.

Creatinine Clearance Tests

The rate of clearance of creatinine from the blood almost exactly parallels glomerular filtration although in man there is slight tubular excretion of creatinine balanced by some binding to plasma proteins. In a few patients with massive proteinuria the creatinine clearance may give an erroneously high figure for glomerular filtration. The blood creatinine levels are very constant and a 24-hour collection of urine can be used with a single plasma sample taken at some point during the collection. Generally speaking, creatinine clearance provides the most practical method of estimating G.F.R.

'Single Shot' Clearance

Substances such as ^{51}Cr EDTA or ^{125}I iothalamate which are not metabolised and are excreted only by glomerular filtration can be injected intravenously. The rate of their disappearance from the blood, which is measured by timed blood samples, is proportional to the glomerular filtration. This avoids urine collection, the least accurate step of the clearance measurement. These substances can also be used as substitutes for inulin in formal G.F.R. measurements.

TESTS OF TUBULAR FUNCTION

Urine Concentration

The kidney will fail to concentrate the urine in the face of dehydration if there is:

(1) Inadequate release of ADH.
(2) An osmotic diuresis as in diabetes mellitus or chronic renal failure.

(3) Nephrogenic diabetes insipidus—a failure of the kidney to respond to ADH.

(4) Hypercalcaemia.

Conversely poor renal perfusion prevents the kidney producing a dilute urine.

The concentration of the urine can be measured by:

(a) The specific gravity which usually varies between 1002–1032.

(b) Osmolarity which represents the total solute content of the urine and is measured by the depression of the freezing point. It varies between 100–1200 m.osmoles/litre.

The most widely used test for the concentrating ability of the kidney is:

Concentration Test

Method 1. This depends on stimulating the production of A.D.H. by dehydration. The patient is allowed to take nothing by mouth after his midday meal. He empties his bladder again next morning at 7.0 a.m., 8.0 a.m. and 9.0 a.m. (still fasting) and if renal function is normal, the specific gravity of one of these samples will be 1025 (900 m. Osm./litre). The adequacy of the dehydration is checked by weighing to ensure 3–5 per cent weight loss.

Method 2. The discomforts of dehydration can be avoided by injecting intramuscularly 5 units of pitressin tannate in oil in the morning. Urine samples are taken over the next 24 hours. The specific gravity of one specimen should exceed 1020. Excessive fluid intake should be avoided during this period.

Patients with many forms of renal disease are unable to concentrate the urine which is then found to have fixed specific gravity (about 1010).

The Ability to Produce an Acid Urine

This is an important aspect of tubular function, for if the kidney cannot secrete an acid urine it is failing in one of its most important functions, the excretion of the acid products of metabolism.

A simple test of the kidney's ability to produce an acid urine is by giving ammonium chloride by mouth in a dose of 0·1 g./kg. body weight. The urine should then become acid (pH 5·3 or less) within five hours. Failure to produce an acid urine under these circumstances indicates a derangement of tubular function.

In chronic renal failure even with a systemic acidosis, the kidney can still usually produce an acid urine but in various tubular disorders particularly renal tubular acidosis, it cannot produce a pH of less than 6·0.

ACUTE RENAL FAILURE

Acute renal failure from any cause is a serious condition with a mortality which remains about 50 per cent overall. This relates mostly to the precipitating circumstances and complications, many of them grave; no patient should die of the uraemia itself with proper management. Acute renal failure, clinically, comprises any condition in which, temporarily, the kidneys are unable to carry on their excretory and regulatory functions. There are therefore a variety of circumstances and outcomes to consider.

The *first* and most important group is reversible acute renal failure from renal hypoperfusion, usually coupled with renal intravascular coagulation (DIC), endothelial swelling within vessels and sometimes tubular necrosis. The factors which may lead to this are:

(1) Loss of circulating volume (haemorrhage, saline depletion, protein loss (e.g. burns, gut losses and massive proteinuria).

(2) Septicaemia or endotoxaemia, especially but not exclusively with gram-negative organisms.

(3) Circulating nephrotoxins. (a) exogenous, e.g. poisons and drugs especially some antibiotics. (b) endogenous, e.g. bile salts, haemoglobin from mismatched transfusions, myoglobin from crush injuries.

(4) Concealed accidental haemorrhage in toxaemia of pregnancy, probably because of DIC and renal vasoconstriction.

(5) Hypoxaemia from lung disease, heart failure, etc.

In most patients more than one factor is involved and in many most of these circumstances are present. This state of affairs may pass through three phases of increasing severity and irreversibility:

(1) A phase of *reversible renal hypoperfusion* when restoring the circulation and treatment of precipitating factors leads to immediate restoration of renal function.

(2) A phase of *established acute renal failure*, when, despite these measures, a period of days or weeks must be passed before renal function returns spontaneously. The reasons for this delay are obscure.

(3) A phase of *cortical necrosis* which may be patchy or complete; if the latter then renal function will not return.

The *second* important group is acute failure from *post renal obstruction of the urinary tract*. This may occur in the renal tubules themselves, from precipitated substances such as myeloma protein or insoluble compounds such as uric acid or sulphadiazine. More commonly, the obstruction is extra-renal from things within the ureter (e.g. stones), within the wall (e.g. tumours), or without the ureter (e.g. retroperitoneal fibrosis or tumours).

The *third* group consists of a variety of intrinsic renal diseases such as acute glomerulonephritis, severe acute pyelonephritis or amyloidosis, where filtration ceases.

The *fourth* and final group is that in which pre-existing renal damage or obstruction was present and the acute episode represents acute renal failure of any of the above varieties superimposed on this, or worsening of the primary condition.

Diagnosis of which group the patient may fall into begins alongside the management of the acute uraemia (see below). The *urine composition* is of help in distinguishing immediately reversible from established renal failure and a spot urine sample should be analysed:

Urine	Incipient Reversible	Established
Osmolarity	more than $1\cdot3 \times$ the plasma osmolarity	equal to or less than plasma
Urea concentration	above 350 mmol./litre	less than 175 mmol./litre
Specific gravity	above 1020	1010 or less
Sodium concentration	below 20 mmol./l.	30 mmol./l. or more

The next most valuable investigation is a *high dose* (2 ml./kg. of meglimine iothalamate) *pyelography* preceded by a straight X-ray of the abdomen. This will establish the presence of renal blood flow, show the size of the kidneys and demonstrate obstruction if it is present. Finally, as a diagnostic and therapeutic measure the response to a high dose (500–1000 mg.) of frusemide intravensouly over 4 hours may be tested; in a proportion of patients a brisk diuresis will be obtained. Mannitol was formerly used but the risks of pulmonary oedema and the more powerful action of frusemide have led to its being abandoned.

Clinical Features. In the first (*oliguric*) stage of acute renal failure the urinary output drops below 700 ml./24 hours (30 ml./hour). During this period urea and potassium released from cell breakdown accumulate with ever rising plasma levels. The failure to excrete hydrogen ions causes an acidosis with a fall in plasma bicarbonate. The patient becomes sleepy and stuporose, nausea and vomiting are frequent. The chief danger is cardiac arrest due to hyperkalaemia.

The *oliguric* phase usually lasts from one to twenty-one days and is followed by a *diuretic* phase. The urinary output rises sharply until the patient is passing several litres of dilute urine which is largely glomerular filtrate as the renal tubules are not yet working. The danger now is excess loss of water, sodium and potassium. Slowly the urine volume and composition return to normal as tubular function recovers.

Throughout both phases many patients have a bleeding tendency and all are highly susceptible to intercurrent infection if this has not been present from the outset.

Treatment is aimed at keeping the patient alive until spontaneous recovery of renal function occurs. The management of the precipitating circumstances may dominate the clinical picture.

Proper management requires daily measurement of the fluid and electrolyte state of the patient.

Infection should be investigated and treated promptly with the appropriate antibiotic, bearing in mind that most antibiotics are excreted in the urine. Among those which are particularly suitable are the penicillins, erythromycin and fucidin.

(a) In the *oliguric phase*, the aim is to *replace the small fluid and electrolyte losses* in urine, sweat and gastro-intestinal secretions to void overhydration and to *feed the patient a high* 3,000 Cal (12·54 mega J) diet *low in protein and electrolyte* (less than 20 mmol. of Na and of K per day). In milder forms of renal failure, where oliguria is brief and the patient not catabolic, it is possible to do this by 'conservative' management, especially if oliguria is not profound. However, better management of patients following surgery, better ante-natal care, and better management of incipient shock has resulted in many parts of the world in the virtual elimination of such cases of acute renal failure, leaving only the much more severe varieties who cannot be managed without the aid of dialysis. In managing the patient conservatively, the patient should be weighed daily, and should maintain constant weight or lose weight slowly. The fluid intake may be calculated from urinary output plus insensible loss corrected for fever (if any). Calories are best supplied as artificial carbohydrate such as Caloreen (Milner Scientific) which can be made up in a 4:1 concentration in water, or Hycal (Beecham's) which is more nauseating. Oral fat emulsions usually produces diarrhoea. Intravenous feeding is usually necessary, and a central line useful because of problems with thrombosis in peripheral veins if 50 or 33 per cent glucose is infused. Fat emulsions (Intralipid, Lipiphysan) can supply up to 2,000 Cal (8·36 mega J) l. and are invaluable and relatively free from side-effects. If protein feeding is performed I.V., a casein hydrolysate such as Aminosol may be used, but evidence suggests that mixtures of essential 1-aminoacids limit tissue breakdown still further.

With this regime some patients can be maintained until diuresis occurs. Dialysis is required if:

(a) Clinical condition deteriorates, with drowsiness, twitching, etc.
(b) Blood urea rises above 35 mmol./litre particularly if it is rising rapidly (more than 8 mmol./litre in 24 hours).
(c) Plasma potassium rises above 7·5 mmol./litre.
(d) Plasma bicarbonate falls below 15 mmol./litre.
(e) Dialysis may be required for gross overhydration.

In general patients are dialysed earlier than formerly, so that they can be maintained in better health with a more reasonable diet. In general dialysis is best performed in an experienced unit, but peritoneal dialysis can be used if the abdomen is intact to tide the patient over for transfer.

(b) In the *diuretic* phase, which may develop very quickly, the aim of treatment is to replace the large amounts of water, sodium and potassium which are lost in the urine.

Acute on Chronic Renal Failure

Patients already suffering some form of chronic renal disease are more liable to develop acute renal failure from all the causes listed above. The clinical features are similar to those in uncomplicated renal failure but the diagnosis may be suggested by finding small kidneys on the radiograph or by the presence of renal osteodystrophy.

The management is as given above but if the chronic renal disease is very advanced the patient may never recover adequate renal function and will require long-term dialysis.

NEPHRITIS

Classification

Nephritis may be defined as bilateral, non-suppurative diffuse disease of the kidneys, affecting primarily the glomerulus. There is no entirely satisfactory classification of nephritis, which can be on a basis of aetiology, pathogenesis, histology or clinical presentation. At the bedside, nephritis presents as a number of syndromes each with several causes, i.e. acute nephritis, nephrotic syndrome, recurrent haematuria. Not every patient will fit neatly into one of these groups, and it must be remembered that although certain histological changes are commonly associated with certain clinical syndromes, there is considerable overlap. Histology is more important in determining prognosis and response to treatment by steroids than it is in deciding the aetiology of the nephritis.

ACUTE NEPHRITIC SYNDROMES

The syndrome of acute nephritis usually presents as oedema which affects the face as much as the rest of the body, a decreased output of urine which contains blood and albumen, and usually some rise in blood pressure.

The syndrome of acute nephritis may occur:

(1) because of acute post-streptococcal glomerulonephritis;
(2) occasionally after other bacterial or virus infections;
(3) without any clear previous cause;
(4) As a complication of polyarteritis nodosa:
    Wegner's granuloma
    Anaphylactoid purpura
    Systemic lupus erythematosus.

Much the most common is *acute post streptococcal glomerulonephritis*, which is probably an atypical reaction to infection with β-haemolytic-streptococci of the *Lancefield Group* 12 in the throat, or types 49 or 55 in infected skin lesions. It is due to the formation of soluble antigen–antibody complexes in the blood which are trapped in the kidney and fix complement. They damage the glomerular membrane by attracting polymorphonuclear leucocytes.

ACUTE POST-STREPTOCOCCAL GLOMERULONEPHRITIS

Pathology. Macroscopically, the kidneys appear hyperaemic. On microscopy the glomeruli show inflammatory changes with increased numbers and swelling of the capsular cells, and sometimes polymorph infiltration. Electronmicroscopy shows 'humpy' deposits on the glomerular membrane which contain immunoglobins and complement. In a proportion of cases the tubular cells show some damage. Later in the evolution the glomeruli show only proliferation of the mesangial stalk.

Many of the clinical features can be explained by the morbid anatomical findings. The widespread damage to the glomeruli is responsible for blood and protein leaking into the urine. The oedema is due to a marked reabsorption of salt and water in the presence of reduced filtration by the relatively undamaged tubular cells with subsequent overloading of the circulation.

Clinical Features. Acute glomerulonephritis occurs most commonly in children and adolescents. There is usually a history of a streptococcal throat infection one to three weeks previously. The onset is fairly sudden with malaise, shivering, and fever and some patients complain of a pain in the loins or abdomen. Vomiting in children is common.

Examination shows oedema, particularly around the eyes and giving the face a characteristically puffy appearance. The blood pressure is usually moderately raised, the pressure in the neck veins is often elevated, and auscultation of the lungs often reveals fine râles from oedema. *The urine is decreased in volume during the early stages of the disease; it is of high specific gravity but low in sodium and contains protein and red cells. The amount of blood is usually sufficient to produce a smoky appearance in an acid urine.* The E.S.R. is raised. The blood urea, provided there is no previous renal damage, may be within normal limits; frequently, however, it is raised.

About 85–95 per cent of children with acute nephritis make a complete and permanent recovery. A diuresis occurs after a few days, following which the temperature settles, the oedema subsides, the blood pressure falls and the blood and protein disappear from the urine. Proteinuria, then microscopic haematuria, are generally the last of the abnormal signs to go and may take several months or even a year or more to disappear completely. In the remaining 10 per cent or so of patients the disease takes one of two courses:

(1) A few patients develop *rapidly progressive nephritis*. The symptoms and signs persist with increasing evidence of renal failure and death occurs, usually within a year, from uraemia and hypertension. In this group early epithelial crescent formation round the glomeruli is common.

(2) A further small group of patients develop complete anuria, this is a very serious complication and most of them die unless treated with dialysis.

(3) Some patients apparently make a good recovery, but continue to pass protein in the urine and although they may feel perfectly well for many months or even years they eventually develop either the nephrotic syndrome or chronic renal failure.

In adults the development of persistent renal damage is much more common, and probably no more than 50 per cent make a complete recovery, although good long-term information is lacking.

Observations. The following observations should be made on a patient with acute nephritis:

(1) Daily urine volumes.
(2) Temperature and pulse chart.
(3) Daily examination of the urine and measurement of its protein content.
(4) Daily blood pressure.
(5) Weekly E.S.R.
(6) Weekly Addis counts, if available.
(7) Renal biopsy is not required unless the disease persists or it is in some way unusual.

Treatment is designed to maintain water and electrolyte balance and to provide adequate calories until spontaneous recovery of renal function occurs. In the early stages the patient is kept in bed but is usually allowed up when his general condition improves even if there are still red cells and protein in the urine. There is no evidence that prolonged bed rest improves the prognosis.

The diet should contain at least 1,000 Calories (4·18 mega J), largely in the form of carbohydrate and fat to prevent endogenous protein breakdown, but only 20–30 g. of protein daily. It is particularly important to restrict the salt intake as the retention of salt is responsible for the oedema and raised blood pressure. Such a diet consists of bread and butter (salt free), jam, honey, cereals, and fruit. Potatoes baked in their jackets or mashed with salt-free butter are a good source of calories. The most useful fluids are barley water, fruit drinks containing glucose, or weak tea with very little milk. At the beginning of treatment fluids should be restricted to 750 ml. in 24 hours; as the urinary output increases the fluid intake is increased. The usual method of calculation is 500 ml. plus a volume equal to the amount of urine passed in the previous twenty-four hours.

On this regime a diuresis usually develops within a few days; when this occurs the patient's diet may be increased to include vegetables, milk, eggs, cheese, fish, and meat.

Procaine penicillin 600,000 units daily should be given for a few days at the beginning of treatment to clear streptococci from the throat. Otherwise there is no evidence that any drug influences the course of acute glomerular nephritis.

Complications include fits and cardiac failure. Fits can be controlled by giving diazepam 2·5–10·0 mg. intravenously. If pulmonary oedema is particularly troublesome large doses of frusemide (up to 1.0 g. daily for an adult) will induce a diuresis. An acute hypertensive crisis is best controlled by diazoxide (see p. 134).

A very small proportion of patients develop anuria which may require dialysis. This complication carries a serious prognosis and biopsy is essential at this stage.

Convalescence. As the clinical state improves the patient should make a gradual return to full activity. Proteinuria may persist for up to a year and there is nothing to be gained by prolonging convalescence until it has entirely disappeared. A gradual return to full activity should be made. On returning to normal life, chills and throat infections should be avoided as much as possible and streptococcal throat infections must be treated vigorously with antibiotics if they occur. Wholesale removal of tonsils should not be practised, but if they are grossly diseased they should be taken out at a later date.

Other Forms of Acute Nephritis

Acute nephritis due to other causes varies in its natural history. Some patients may show marked proliferative changes in the glomeruli and may ultimately develop the nephrotic syndrome (see below). A few develop proliferation of extracapillary cells with crescent formation, which is usually followed by a rapidly downhill course. The clinical course may also be influenced by any associated underlying disease.

RECURRENT HAEMATURIA

Recurrent haematuria is a syndrome in which haematuria occurs at the height of the infection and not after the lapse of some days as in patients with the more serious acute diffuse nephritis. The disorder occurs most commonly in children or young adults and most patients give a long history of repeated attacks of haematuria without oedema and without developing any evidence of impaired renal function or hypertension. Biopsy of the kidney usually shows a focal glomerular lesion or sometimes thickening of the mesangial stalk of the glomerulus. It is quite common to find IgA in the glomerulus, the reason for this is not known. Treatment should be directed to treating the infection and persuading the patient (or parents) to lead a normal life. In the majority of patients the prognosis is good, occasionally chronic renal failure develops. Warning signs are persistent proteinuria, hypertension and deteriorating renal function.

THE NEPHROTIC SYNDROME

The nephrotic syndrome is characterised by heavy proteinuria, low plasma proteins and oedema. There are a number of causes of this state:

(1) Glomerulonephritis. This accounts for 80 per cent of nephrotic syndrome in the adult. The disorder is of unknown cause. It most commonly arises *de novo*, but sometimes follows an episode of acute glomerulonephritis. It has also been called nephrotic nephritis or Type II nephritis.

(2) Diabetic nephropathy.

(3) Systemic lupus erythematosus.

(4) Amyloid disease.

(5) Anaphylactoid purpura.

(6) Thrombosis of renal veins or inferior vena cava.

(7) Poisoning by mercury, troxidone or other substances.

Pathology and Natural History of the Nephrotic Syndrome. The nephrotic syndrome is the result of excessive loss of plasma proteins in the urine. This is due to glomerular damage of differing aetiology. The smaller albumen molecules pass more easily through the damaged glomerular membrane than the larger globulin molecules and there is therefore a disproportionately large loss of albumen. With increasing glomerular disease the leak of the larger-molecular-weight proteins increases and it is possible to measure the profile of the protein leak by measuring the clearance of protein of differing molecular weights. The fall in plasma proteins, particularly albumen, leads to a low plasma osmotic pressure and diffusion of fluid into the tissue spaces, forming oedema and causing a fall in blood volume. It seems probable that the fall in blood volume stimulates the release from the adrenal cortex of excess aldosterone which in turn is responsible for the retention of more salt and water. The loss of gamma globulin which contains the circulating antibodies makes patients with this condition highly susceptible to intercurrent infections. In the early stages this protein leak may be the only disorder of renal function, but if the disease progresses there is obliteration of the nephrons and picture of chronic renal failure develops.

The nature of the glomerular lesion varies. In glomerulonephritis four types of change may be found:

(1) *Minimal Change*. In this type little abnormality can be seen in the glomerulus on light microscopy. It is believed to be due to an allergy and occasionally the allergen can be identified. It accounts for 85 per cent of childhood nephrotics and only 25 per cent in adults. Patients with minimal change usually respond well to steroids; if these are ineffective or produce excessive cushingoid changes a cytotoxic immunosuppressive agent may be tried. The ultimate prognosis is good.

(2) *Focal glomerulosclerosis* is usually associated with a slowly progressive deterioration in renal function.

(3) *Proliferative changes* are variable. The less severe lesions include subvarieties of mesangial proliferation and focal proliferation (the latter being also associated with recurrent haematuria). These changes carry a good prognosis with little if any deterioration in renal function. Severe degrees

include endo- and extra-capillary sclerosis and extra-capillary proliferation with crescent formation. Here the disease is progressive with developing hypertension, haematuria and ultimately renal failure.

(4) *Membranous Change.* The wall of the glomerular capillary is thickened by deposition of antibody and complement. The course is usually gradually downhill and it is unaffected by treatment. Membranous changes are almost confined to adults.

Both proliferative and membranous changes are associated with the deposition in the glomerulus of antigen-antibody complexes which are thought to be responsible for the damage.

The other causes of the nephrotic syndrome usually produce characteristic changes in the glomerulus (p. 414). Difficulties may arise however. Systemic lupus erythematosus may produce lesions in the glomeruli which are indistinguishable from membranous or proliferative glomerular nephritis and are due to DNA-anti DNA immune complexes. Thrombosis of the renal vein, where presumably mechanical factors are responsible for the glomerular lesion, may resemble membranous glomerular nephritis, as does mercury poisoning, which may also cause changes in the proximal renal tubules.

Clinical Features. The onset of the nephrotic syndrome is usually insidious. The appearance of oedema is preceded by a period of proteinuria; when the plasma albumen drop below a critical level (20 g./litre) oedema begins to appear. At first this may be confined to the ankles and be fleeting, but as the disease progresses it extends until finally it may affect the whole body, so that the face is pale and puffy, the legs show particularly severe distension and fluid may accumulate also in the peritoneal cavity, the pleural cavities and the pericardium. In the early stages of the disease, the blood pressure is not usually raised and the blood urea level may be normal or even low. The urine contains large amounts of protein, usually more than 5·0 g. in 24 hours; in addition it may contain red cells, the persistence of which usually indicates a severe lesion and a poor prognosis. Renal tract infection is quite a common complication and the urine may contain pus cells and organisms. The serum cholesterol level is high, the reason for this not being clear.

The *prognosis* of the disease is variable and depends on the underlying lesion. Those with minimal changes respond to treatment and those with minor proliferative lesions carry a good prognosis. In more severe lesions, whether due to glomerulonephritis, systemic lupus or amyloidosis, the ultimate prognosis is poor, about 60 per cent of patients with membranous lesions survive five years, those with severe proliferative lesions rarely survive more than two years. In such patients the oedema may persist, often fluctuating in severity. Ultimately renal failure develops. The blood pressure and blood urea levels begin to rise, the proteinuria and oedema often diminish at this stage and death ultimately ensues from renal failure. Before the introduction of antibiotics many of these patients died of intercurrent infection, but such infections can now usually be controlled.

Because of the variable nature of the glomerular lesion and its bearing on prognosis and treatment, *renal biopsy is nearly always necessary*.

Treatment. When the cause of the nephrotic syndrome has been determined it is occasionally possible to remove or treat that cause, for example drug-induced renal damage or secondary amyloid disease. In most patients, however, the only treatment possible is that of the renal disease itself.

Treatment of the nephrotic syndrome is aimed at reducing proteinuria and oedema, restoring the plasma proteins to normal and combating intercurrent infection as it arises. In the majority of adult cases all these objectives cannot be achieved, but temporary remission of symptoms is usually possible.

The main methods of treatment are:

(1) *Bed Rest*. Bed rest is inadvisable even if the patient is grossly oedamatous since it probably does not influence the course of the disease, and in the presence of the hypercoagulable state of the nephrotic syndrome, the danger of deep vein thrombosis and pulmonary emboli are increased. Wherever possible the patient should be mobilised, but if he is confined to bed he should receive 5,000 units b.d. of heparin subcutaneously.

(2) *Diet*. The chief cause of the oedema is the loss of plasma proteins and the retention of sodium. A diet with a high protein (80 g. daily), mostly as animal protein, and low salt (about 40 mEq. daily) content should be prescribed. It must be realised, however, that the speed of replacement of plasma protein is limited by the liver's ability to manufacture proteins from amino acids.

(3) *Steroid Treatment*. Nearly all patients with minimal change lesions (usually children) respond to steroids within one month of starting treatment, but the mode of action is not known. Longer treatment, or treatment of most other varieties of nephrotic syndrome, is inadvisable and may be dangerous. The nephrotic syndrome due to systemic lupus may respond but high doses of steroid are usually required.

There are many schemes of dosage and the most suitable has not yet been settled. In children aged ten years and upwards, 60 mg. of prednisolone are given daily for 14 days. The dose is then reduced by 10 mg. every five days, until a daily dose of 10 mg. is reached. If the urine is now protein-free this dose is continued for 8 weeks and then tailed off. If proteinuria persists the histology should be reconsidered and cytotoxic treatment considered. After this regime about 50 per cent of patients will have a permanent remission; the remainder will relapse, often following intercurrent infection, and will require some form of maintenance or intermittent steroid treatment.

(4) If patients fail to respond to steroids, or develop steroid toxicity, *immunosuppressive drugs* may produce a remission. *Cyclophosphamide* in doses of 3·0 mg./kg./day is the most satisfactory and is given for 8

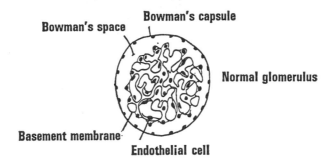

Bowman's space — Bowman's capsule

Normal glomerulus

Basement membrane — Endothelial cell

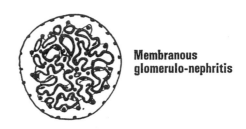

Membranous glomerulo-nephritis

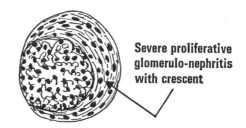

Severe proliferative glomerulo-nephritis with crescent

weeks. Weekly blood counts must be done, but leucopenia and hair loss are rare. The long-term effects of treatment on the testes or ovaries is not known, but longer courses are certainly toxic.

(5) *Diuretics* are used as symptomatic treatment for the nephrotic syndrome. Frusemide is particularly useful, especially if there is some reduction in the G.F.R. and it may be combined with spironolactone to counter the action of aldosterone and reduce potassium loss in the urine.

With large doses of diuretics the risk of hypovolaemia must be remembered, and if used intravenously the doses must always be accompanied by intravenous protein or colloid.

CHRONIC GLOMERULONEPHRITIS

Clinical Features. Chronic glomerulonephritis may follow an attack of acute glomerulonephritis or the nephrotic syndrome or it may occur without any history of renal disease. It may develop immediately after the attack of acute glomerulonephritis, or there may be a latent period of many years in which albuminuria is the only symptom of the underlying and progressive renal damage.

Sooner or later chronic renal failure develops, often complicated by severe hypertension. When this occurs the progress is usually steadily downhill and most patients are dead within two years.

CHRONIC RENAL FAILURE

Chronic renal failure may be the result of a number of pathological processes, but in the end the clinical picture is remarkably constant whatever the original cause.

The most important causes of chronic renal failure are:

Chronic glomerulonephritis	Polyarteritis nodosa
Chronic pyelonephritis	Diabetic nephropathy
Hypertension	Myelomatosis
Amyloid disease	Renal stones
Analgesic abuse	Polycystic kidneys
Systemic lupus	Renal tuberculosis

Sometimes it is difficult to decide precisely the original cause of the renal disease.

The glomerular filtration has to fall to 30 ml./minute before there is any obvious effect on renal function. As renal function deteriorates further a condition of *renal insufficiency* develops with a moderately raised blood urea but minimal symptoms. When the glomerular filtration rate reaches about 5·0 ml./minute the symptoms and signs of *terminal (end stage) renal failure* develop, and the fully developed clinical picture of uraemia emerges.

Renal Function in Chronic Renal Failure

In chronic renal failure there is a considerable decrease in the number of functioning nephrons and thus in the glomerular filtration rate. Those nephrons which remain appear to function normally so that disturbances of function are probably due to overloading of the remaining nephrons, rather than to any abnormality of the nephrons themselves. This has been called the *intact nephron hypothesis*. However, sometimes there is evidence of specific tubular defects, e.g. in pyelonephritis and polycystic kidneys there may be early and disproportionate failure to concentrate and acidify the urine. The result is a loss of flexibility of renal function *with an inability to regulate water and electrolyte balance.*

(1) **Urea and Metabolite Retention.** The excretion of urea depends on the G.F.R.; when this drops to about 30 per cent of normal, retention of urea occurs. The raised concentration of urea in the plasma increases the concentration of urea in the filtered fraction and by this means an adequate excretion is maintained. In addition to urea, sulphate and phosphate are retained together with potentially toxic substances such as phenols, guanidine compounds and aromatic amines.

(2) **Polyuria and Hyposthenuria.** The passing of large volumes of urine of a specific gravity around 1010 (300 mOsm/litre) is characteristic of chronic renal failure, this is associated with the loss of the normal diurnal rhythm of urine production so that nocturia is a common feature. This is largely an osmotic diuresis due to the increased filtered load of urea, although occasionally (particularly in pyelonephritis) damage to the tubular concentrating mechanism is contributory.

(3) **Acidosis.** Acidosis is a common feature of chronic renal failure. With the falling G.F.R., there is a decreased filtration of hydrogen ions. In addition although the kidneys are still capable of secreting an acid urine, there is a reduced production of ammonia and a reduced excretion of phosphate which are not therefore available to combine with hydrogen ions, so that total acid elimination is diminished. Also the tubules are less efficient at reabsorbing bicarbonate.

(4) **Electrolyte Disturbances.** The fall in glomerular filtration may lead to some retention of sodium and water with subsequent oedema particularly of the lungs. Hyperkalaemia may also occur and can be very dangerous. It may be due to potassium retention, but also to the acidosis in which potassium ions pass from the intra- to the extra-cellular space and are replaced by hydrogen ions. Sodium and sometimes potassium depletion may also occur, and is particularly common when there is loss of these ions from elsewhere, for instance in diarrhoea. The prolonged osmotic diuresis interferes with tubular function so that the kidney cannot respond by reducing sodium excretion.

(5) **Calcium.** The disorders of calcium metabolism are considered on p. 372.

(6) **Anaemia.** The anaemia of chronic renal failure may be due to a failure of production of *erythropoietin* by the damaged kidneys, though decreased red-cell survival is certainly present, and haemostatic disturbances may lead to increased losses.

The Early Clinical Features of Chronic Renal Failure; Renal Insufficiency

The onset of renal failure is usually insidious. Symptoms may be minimal, but may include some polyuria, nocturia, and perhaps some loss of energy. On examination the blood pressure is usually raised and the urine contains a little protein together with a few red cells and granular casts. The blood urea level is a little raised, but in the early stages of renal failure this can often be restored to normal by a diet low in protein. This stage may persist for a considerable period, sometimes years, before the classical terminal picture develops and it is in this stage that judicious management of diet, fluid intake, and electrolyte balance can keep the patient in moderately good health.

The Terminal Clinical Features of Chronic Renal Failure

For convenience these may be considered systematically:

Central Nervous System. The patient is at first *tired* and *listless* and *headaches* are common. As the disease progresses, he becomes drowsy and may finally lapse into coma. Muscular twitching and sometimes *epileptiform convulsions* may occur.

The biochemical abnormality underlying the symptoms arising in the nervous system is not clear, but it seems probable that they are due to an upset in balance of the blood electrolytes. The muscular twitching can sometimes be relieved by intravenous calcium salts.

Alimentary System. The tongue is dry and coated with a dirty brown fur, the breath has an uriniferous smell and hiccoughs, *nausea*, and *vomiting* are often distressing symptoms. Sometimes bleeding from the gastrointestinal tract occurs leading to haematemesis or bloodstained *diarrhoea*. These symptoms are caused by the excretion of urea into the gut, where it breaks down and releases ammonia. This is highly irritant.

Respiratory System and Acid Base Balance. Acidosis causes a typical gasping form of respiration known as Kussmaul breathing; Cheyne-Stokes respiration may also occur in the terminal stages.

Pulmonary oedema may occur and *dyspnoea* is a common symptom. Pulmonary infection is not uncommon and may be due to unusual bacteria such as *E. coli* or to fungi.

Cardiovascular System. *Hypertension* is frequently found in association with chronic renal failure and is probably due to several factors: increased cardiac output, sodium and water retention, and in the more severe cases, an increased production of *renin* (see p. 383). It may produce no symptoms, but more commonly the *vascular system* is severely affected. This is most easily seen in the retinae which show:

(1) Papilloedema.

(2) Soft exudates which often take the form of a star at the macula. They are caused by oedema of the retina.

(3) Haemorrhages into the retina.

(4) Thickening of the arteries with variations in calibre and tortuosity, increased light reflex, and nipping at the arteriovenous crossings.

Pericarditis frequently appears in the late stages of renal failure. It may cause chest pain and usually a loud rub. Effusions are uncommon and usually bloody. The cause is unknown.

A small proportion of patients die from heart failure or cerebrovascular accidents, although the majority die of renal failure itself.

Skin. The skin is dry and becomes yellowish or brownish in colour and since the sweat glands excrete urea or other substances normally excreted by the kidney, pruritus is common. Occasionally there is so much urea in the sweat that it crystallises on the skin to give a 'urea frost'.

Blood. Microcytic normochromic *anaemia* which is resistant to iron treatment is very common in uraemia. It is due to decreased production of red cells with some haemolysis and can only be relieved by blood transfusion.

The Skeleton. A small proportion of cases of chronic renal failure show widespread disorder of the bone which is called *renal osteodystrophy* (renal rickets, p. 372). *Pseudo-gout* due to high blood phosphate level can occur.

Endocrine System. Apart from the secondary *hyperparathyroidism* there is failure of gonadal function, *infertility*, loss of libido and *amenorrhea*, being common. Uraemia mimics *hypothyroidism* but sometimes true thyroid failure is present.

The Urine. The urine volume per 24 hours is increased and there is nocturia. It is usually of fixed specific gravity (between 1010 and 1012) and contains protein, although often in quite small amounts. Microscopy shows increased numbers of red cells and granular casts.

Treatment of Chronic Renal Failure. There is unfortunately no way of preventing the progress of renal damage in most patients with chronic renal failure. All that can be done is to help the kidney to function as well as possible under the circumstances. Patients can frequently be kept alive and in moderately good health for years. The important points in management are:

(a) *Fluid intake* should be at least 3·0 litres daily. In chronic renal failure the excretion of urea and other waste products is proportional to the urinary flow, so a high urine output is essential. It is important, however, not to overhydrate these patients since this results in oedema. They should be weighed regularly and the fluid intake adjusted to keep their weight steady. Sodium intake will have to be adjusted to the needs of the patient as sodium loss in the urine is variable. Evidence of hypernatraemia with venous congestion and rising blood pressure call for a reduced intake and frusemide in large doses (500 mg. daily) orally may be required in a crisis. Some patients lose a lot of sodium in the urine and if this is complemented by loss from vomiting or diarrhoea depletion develops with hypovolaemia and deteriorating renal function. In these circumstances sodium can be given orally in the form of sodium bicarbonate or intravenously as 0·16 M sodium lactate. Hyperkalaemia can be prevented by reducing the intake if necessary, but in the terminal stages may be impossible to control.

(b) Severe *dietary restrictions* are irksome and it is doubtful if they are useful. When the blood urea rises above 15 mmol./litre (plasma creatinine 375 μmol./litre) the daily intake of protein should be reduced to 40 g. and the diet should be largely composed of carbohydrates and fat, producing 3,000 calories. As failure becomes more severe the protein intake may be reduced to 20 g. daily, or the Giovenetti diet may be used. This diet provides the minimal necessary quantity of first class protein. This extreme type of diet requires very close supervision, since if not strictly adhered to, especially with regard to calorie intake, it results in increased catabolism weight loss and actual deterioration. For the treatment of disturbed calcium metabolism see p. 372.

(c) The *anaemia* of renal failure does not respond to haematinics. It may be treated by transfusion but the benefit is very transitory. It is fruitless to try and maintain a normal PCV by repeated transfusions and carries with it the risk of immunising the patient against transplantation antigens, or of turning the patient into a hepatitis carrier. Many of these patients get along very well with a PCV of 25 per cent or even lower.

(d) If the *hypertension* which accompanies the renal failure is very severe and in the malignant phase, it will accelerate the progression of the renal damage. It is always worth while trying to lower the blood pressure to safer levels by means of drugs (p. 131).

(e) Eventually a stage is reached at which only symptomatic treatment can be given. Chlorpromazine often prevents the nausea and vomiting and morphine may relieve discomfort and alleviate anxiety and fears.

(f) *Maintenance Haemodialysis and Renal Transplant.* When the glomerular filtration rate falls below about 3 ml./minute in patients without hypertension and 5 ml./minute in the presence of this complication terminal renal failure has been reached and the patient will die. It is now possible to maintain such patients in fair health by haemodialysis.

The patient is given a permanent external arteriovenous shunt or subcutaneous arteriovenous fistula and through this is attached to a dialysis machine for about 10 hours three times a week. The choice of patients for such treatment is not always easy, as a certain amount of mental resilience is required, and they should not be suffering from any progressive systemic disease outside the kidneys. Hypertension, however, is no bar and is usually considerably improved after dialysis has been started.

Renal transplant with either a cadaver or live donor kidney offers another method of rescuing patients with terminal renal failure, and if successful enables them to lead a more normal life than on dialysis.

URINARY TRACT INFECTION

Three clinical syndromes of urinary tract infection will be described:

(1) Acute lower urinary tract infection.
(2) Acute pyelonephritis.
(3) Chronic pyelonephritis.

The relationship between these three syndromes has long been the subject of debate. There is little doubt that lower urinary tract infection can be followed by acute pyelonephritis. The connection between acute urinary tract infection and the contracted kidneys of chronic pyelonephritis is important. In adult women, provided there is no obstruction in the urinary tract, it is very rare for acute infection to progress to chronic pyelonephritis. In adult men, where urinary infection is rare, an underlying cause should always be suspected. Children, however, are a different matter. Infection in this age group frequently means some structural abnormality of the renal tract, usually causing vesico-ureteric reflux. If the infection is not corrected there is real danger of progressive kidney damage. Finally, the clinical and pathological condition known as *chronic pyelonephritis* probably arises from several causes, of which infection is only one.

The Significance of Bacteriuria

E. coli is the common infecting organism; others include *Staphylococcus albus* or *aureus, Proteus vulgaris* (frequently associated with stones), *Pseudomonas pyocyaneus, Klebsiella* and *Steptococcus faecalis.*

The culture of a *fresh* specimen of urine (a mid-stream or catch specimen is satisfactory) is essential in the investigation of urinary tract infection. The work of Kass has shown that the urine of normal individuals does not contain more than 10,000 organisms per ml. of urine. In urinary tract infection, even if it is latent, it is usual to find more than 100,000 organisms/ml.

The clinical importance of symptomless bacteriuria depends largely on the circumstances in which it is found. In women who are not pregnant it is of little significance, it is only rarely associated with subsequent renal tract infection, and does not usually need treatment. Bacteriuria in pregnancy is discussed on p. 407. In young girls bacteriuria is more liable to be associated with structural disease of the urinary tract and requires treatment.

Acute Infections

Acute Lower Urinary Tract Infection (Urethral Syndrome)

This is a disease of women. The short female urethra allows infection to spread from the perineum to the posterior urethra and the trigone of the bladder. The urethral glands may become chronically infected and the disease become recurrent.

Clinical Features. This is a very common disease. It may be precipitated by minor trauma such as sexual intercourse (honeymoon cystitis) or complicate such conditions as prolapse. The symptoms are frequency and dysuria; general symptoms are not common. The condition frequently settles in a few days. The main dangers are:

(1) The infection may become recurrent.
(2) During the acute attack there may be reflux of urine from the bladder up the ureters causing an ascending infection and acute pyelonephritis, and in fact a proportion of patients have kidney infection although symptoms and signs suggest that infection is confined to the bladder.

Culture of the urine may show the infecting organism but is quite often sterile.

Acute Pyelonephritis

The term pyelonephritis is used to emphasise that with inflammation of the ureters and renal pelvis there is also infection of the renal parenchyma. The renal medulla is particularly involved, the high osmolality in this area interfering with the normal immune mechanism and making it especially vulnerable. It seems probable that infection reaches the kidney via the ureter, but the exact mechanism is not clear except where there is vesico-ureteric reflux.

Urinary stasis also predisposes to infection which is frequently seen therefore in *pregnancy*, in men with *bladder neck obstruction* due to prostatic enlargement and in patients with *neurological disorders* which interfere with the emptying of the bladder.

In children, outflow tract obstruction, particularly in the posterior urethra, may be combined with reflux of urine into the ureters on micturition, probably due to some congenital defect. This can be demonstrated radiologically by a *micturating cystogram*; its recognition is important since surgical correction may prevent progressive renal damage. Infection may also complicate *renal stones* and *neoplasms* with the renal tract. Finally it seems likely that other forms of parenchymal renal disease such as glomerulonephritis may predispose to bacterial infection.

In men pyelonephritis is nearly always secondary to some abnormality in the urinary tract.

Clinical Features. The onset is usually sudden, although there may be a short history of lower urinary tract infection. Symptoms include fever, shivering and rigors, general malaise, aching in one or both loins and sometimes in the suprapubic region, frequency and dysuria. On examination there is usually tenderness over one or both kidneys. There is a leucocytosis and a large number of pus cells are found in the urine.

Treatment of Acute Infection

(a) *Acute lower urinary tract infection* usually responds to a 7-day course of sulphonamide (see p. 408). Recurrent attacks may be troublesome. They require a full urological investigation to exclude a local cause and often cystoscopy and urethral dilatation may in itself lead to improvement. Simple measures including reasonable fluid intake, micturition after sexual intercourse and personal cleanliness may be helpful in preventing recurrent attacks.

(b) *Acute Pyelonephritis.* The patient is nursed in bed and given a fluid intake of at least three litres a day. A urine sample should be sent for culture and to determine sensitivity of the organism to antibiotics. Since the usual *E. coli* infection is found only in an acid urine, an alkaline mixture containing 3·0 g. each of sodium citrate and sodium bicarbonate is given two-hourly until the urine becomes alkaline and then in reduced dose to keep it alkaline. In addition, treatment is started with a sulphonamide (see p. 408). On this regime, symptoms and signs should usually subside within a few days; if they have not, a sulphonamide-resistant organism is probably responsible and the result of the initial urinary culture will reveal its nature. The sensitivity tests now show the most suitable antibiotic to use.

It is very important to eradicate infection from the kidney and the initial course of treatment which should last one week is best followed by a further one week's treatment with another antibiotic to which the infecting organism is sensitive (usually co-trimoxazole or ampicillin). The urine should be cultured one month after apparent cure to ensure that there is no persistent bacilluria.

Children, who are particularly liable to develop persistent infection with renal damage in their growing kidneys, and all patients with recurrent chronic infection require a complete urological investigation, long-term treatment with antibiotics over several months and prolonged follow-up.

Renal Infection in Pregnancy

Routine urine tests show that about 5 per cent of pregnant women have a significant bacteriuria (more than 100,000 organisms per ml.), although they may be symptomless at the time, and about 40 per cent of these bacteriuric women will develop overt urinary infection as pregnancy progresses. About 2–3 per cent of all pregnant women develop clinical renal tract infection. This is believed to be due to dilatation of the ureters and

which time the urine should become sterile and free of excess leucocytes. Thereafter the urine must be cultured at regular intervals and treatment instituted as required. In renal failure the dose of antibiotic must be halved and streptomycin should not be used. Results of treatment are often disappointing and relapses frequent.

If a patient with chronic pyelonephritis develops renal failure he should be treated as already described (p. 403). The following points, however, should be remembered:

(1) Renal failure in these patients may be precipitated by an acute exacerbation of renal infection and antibiotic treatment may induce a remission.
(2) Patients with chronic pyelonephritis are particularly prone to electrolyte disturbance, correction of which may produce considerable improvement in renal function.

DISORDERS OF TUBULAR FUNCTION

A small number of patients will be encountered who appear to have disorders of tubular function without much evidence of glomerular disease. In many of these patients the disorder is congenital but in others it is the result of various forms of renal disease, particularly chronic pyelonephritis. These disorders may be simple or multiple and may affect nearly every aspect of tubular function. Three such disorders are considered here:

Fanconi's Syndrome

Fanconi's syndrome is a proximal tubular disorder in which there is a failure of reabsorption of phosphate, amino acids, sugar, bicarbonate, and uric acid by the proximal renal tubules resulting in the appearance of these substances in the urine. It is rarely familial, without apparent cause, but more frequently is the result of endogenous or exogenous poisons acting on the tubule. Examples of the former are cystine in cystine storage disease (Fanconi–Lignac syndrome) and galactose; examples of the latter are heavy metals and antibiotics.

Clinical Features. The syndrome usually presents in childhood with polyuria, thirst, and stunting from renal rickets. Ultimately chronic renal failure develops in many cases.

Renal Tubular Acidosis

In this condition there is a failure of the tubule to produce an acid urine (below pH 6·0). This condition is often complicated by excessive calcium loss in the urine and calcification of the kidneys (nephrocalcinosis).

Two varieties are described, Type I where the defect is in the distal tubular secretion of hydrogen ion and which may be inherited or result from some types of renal disease. Type II renal tubular acidosis is due to proximal tubular defect. This may occur as an isolated phenomenon in infants when it usually recovers, or may be part of multiple proximal tubular defects as in the Fanconi syndrome described above, caused by the bicarbonate wastage.

Clinical Features. (1) *In infants* renal tubular acidosis is characterised by failure to thrive, dehydration, and vomiting. The urine is never more than slightly acid. If the child survives, renal function tends to become normal and the disease does not progress into adult life. Rickets may need treating, either with thiazides (which increase the bicarbonate reabsorption) or with carefully controlled doses of Vitamin D. If phosphate loss is also present, this should be supplemented.

(2) *In adults* the main symptoms are osteomalacia of the skeleton and calcification of the kidney which may ultimately lead to chronic renal failure. Sometimes in addition there are symptoms of potassium deficiency.

Treatment is to try and correct the acidosis by giving bicarbonate and citrates and to replace the calcium deficiency if present.

Amino-acidurias

Amino-acids are normally almost completely reabsorbed in the proximal renal tubule. They appear in the urine in two circumstances; *overflow amino-aciduria*, when because of an abnormality of amino-acid metabolism some amino-acid (or amino-acids) is produced in excess; and amino-aciduria due to *failure of reabsorption*. This occurs in the multiple proximal tubular defect referred to as the Fanconi syndrome and discussed above, when all amino-acids are present in the urine (*generalised amino-aciduria*). However, there are a number of rare conditions in which specific renal tubular transport mechanisms for amino-acids are defective. The only clinically important condition is *cystinuria*. In this disease, the defect affects a group of six dibasic amino-acids which appear in the urine in large quantities. The only important one is cystine, since it is insoluble in all but very alkaline urines and forms stones in the urinary tract. Treatment consists of high fluid intake and alkalinisation of the urine with bicarbonate, when stones may even dissolve and further formation is inhibited.

Medullary Sponge Kidney

Medullary sponge kidney (cystic disease of the renal pyramids) is not uncommon. Cysts of varying size are found in the pyramids and they communicate with the collecting tubules, which are dilated. The cysts often contain stones. The condition may be generalised, or affect one kidney, or part of one kidney. It is only found in adults and there is no preponderant sex incidence. It is not progressive and is thought to be congenital in origin. Renal function is not affected except secondarily by infection or stones.

Clinical Features. The symptoms are not specific, patients presenting with urinary infection, haematuria and stones. The diagnosis is radiological and is best shown on pyelography. The pyramids are widened, and the cysts show with the dye. The dilated collecting tubules often opacify in a fan-like fashion in the pyramids. Stones grouped like clusters of flowers are present in the medulla of the kidneys.

Management is conservative and is confined to the treatment of urinary infection or renal colic and stones. Rarely, nephrectomy for unilateral disease is indicated. When the condition is confined to one pole of one kidney partial nephrectomy can be done.

RENAL LESIONS IN SYSTEMIC DISEASE

The Kidney in Hypertension

Although hypertension causes some changes in the renal arterioles, this is not usually enough to interfere seriously with renal function and renal failure occurs very rarely in essential hypertension. In the small group of hypertensives in whom there is a very high diastolic blood pressure associated with marked arteriolar changes and papilloedema, often called *malignant or accelerated hypertension*, severe renal damage can, however, rapidly develop. Sometimes this is associated with fibrin thrombi in the arterioles and capillaries of the kidney, a fall in the platelet count, and red cell fragmentation seen in the blood film (microangiopathic anaemia). The arterioles become thickened and the afferent arterioles of the glomerulus undergo hyaline necrosis with subsequent ischaemic lesions of the glomerulus.

Clinical Features of Malignant Hypertension. In addition to the usual symptoms of severe hypertension (p. 128), the patient develops evidence of renal damage: albumen, casts, and red cells appear in the urine and the blood urea rises.

Treatment. The blood pressure must be reduced (p. 131) before severe and irreversible damage to the kidney is produced. There is some evidence that if the blood pressure is lowered early enough some of the renal changes which have already occurred may be reversible.

Unilateral Renal Disease and Hypertension

The experiments of Goldblatt showed that ischaemia of one kidney in the dog produced hypertension, and a small proportion of patients with hypertension have demonstrable unilateral renal disease. Hitherto, however, removal of the abnormal kidney, although occasionally dramatically successful, has seldom cured the hypertension.

The unilateral renal disease may be pyelonephritis, hydronephrosis, or stenosis of the renal artery. This last type exactly mimics Goldblatt's experiment and it is in this group that nephrectomy or relief of the stenosis should be successful, for it is renal ischaemia resulting in excess renin production with activation of the renin-angiotension system which is responsible for the rise in blood pressure. The problem is to separate this small group from the large number of patients with hypertension from other causes.

Clinical Features. Suspicion should be aroused if the patient is young (under 40) with severe hypertension of rapid onset and with a negative family history. Physical examination is unhelpful except that a murmur may be heard over the affected renal artery.

Pyelography may show the renal shadow to be smaller on the affected side, and the dye may be more concentrated by the ischaemic kidney and thus produce a denser shadow.

^{131}I *hippuran* is handled by the kidney in the same way as P.A.H. It can be injected intravenously and its uptake and excretion monitored by counters over the kidneys. In renal ischaemia and other forms of renal disease inequality of the traces is found. It is, therefore, a useful screening test.

If these investigations reveal unilateral renal disease which might be ischaemic the next step is to confirm the presence of stenosis by aortography which outlines the renal arterial tree. Even the presence of a stenosis, however, does not necessarily imply that the kidney is ischaemic. *Divided renal function studies*, for which under standard conditions the urine is collected from each kidney separately are rarely required.

When the kidney is ischaemic the pattern of tubular function changes. Essentially the tubules reabsorb more of the filtered load of water and proportionally even more of sodium. This means that the urine from the ischaemic kidney is:

(a) Deceased in volume.
(b) Higher in P.A.H. concentration.
(c) Lower in sodium concentration, and
(d) The inulin and P.A.H. clearances are often decreased on the ischaemic side (but this is not characteristic of ischaemia and may occur with any type of renal damage).

Treatment. The correct management is very difficult, for no test shows without doubt which patient will derive benefit from operation. Renal vein renin levels from the affected abnormal kidneys, when compared with the level in the peripheral blood, provide the best prediction of successful relief. If there is unequivocal evidence of unilateral renal artery stenosis and the other kidney is normal there is about a 50 per cent chance of relieving the hypertension by nephrectomy or by some plastic operation on the stenosed renal artery. Most patients with hypertension and renal artery stenosis can be controlled with drugs, and if possible, this course is preferable even in those patients in whom it is likely surgery will be of benefit. In general, these patients are being managed more conservatively than in the recent past.

Diabetes Mellitus

Proteinuria is common in patients with diabetes. Sometimes in addition there may be other evidence of renal involvement such as a nephrotic syndrome or chronic renal failure. It is only recently that the various renal diseases associated with diabetes have been classified. They are:

(1) *Pyelonephritis.* This is probably the commonest lesion and accounts for the majority of diabetics who develop chronic renal failure. Some diabetics have autonomic neuropathy affecting the bladder, and many are catheterised in acute episodes.

(2) *Glomerular Lesions.* There are two types:

(a) The Kimmelstiel-Wilson acellular lesion, which is characterised by nodules of eosinophilic material in the glomerular tuft and is entirely confined to diabetics.

(b) A generalised thickening with sclerosis of the basement membrane of the glomerular capillary. This change may be found in other types of renal disease.

The relationship between these changes and clinical evidence of renal disease is not clear but it would seem that the nodular lesions are not necessarily associated with clinical renal disease, which correlates much more closely with the generalised sclerosis. Glomerular lesions in diabetes are frequently associated with diabetic retinopathy.

(3) *Arterial Changes.* The smaller arteries of the kidney may show generalised sclerosis. Glomerular lesions in diabetes are frequently associated with diabetic retinopathy.

(4) *Papillary Necrosis.* In this condition the papilla may slough and it is frequently associated with acute renal infection. It may also be found in analgesic nephropathy.

Treatment is directed to controlling the diabetes as well as possible, although there is no evidence that this prevents the development of renal disease. It is very important to recognise chronic pyelonephritis, as in this group it may be possible to control the infection with antibiotics and thus halt or slow down the progress of the disease.

Subacute Infective Endocarditis

The presence of red cells in the urine is a very useful diagnostic test for subacute infective endocarditis. The kidney may show diffuse changes indistinguishable from acute glomerulonephritis or patchy lesions which affect only part of the glomerular tuft. It is believed that both these lesions are due to an allergic response. Chronic renal failure may ensue if the infection is not controlled.

Rarely larger emboli may cause frank renal infarcts.

Amyloid Disease

Amyloid disease may occur as a primary phenomenon or may complicate various systemic disorders (see p. 464). It usually produces a nephrotic syndrome and now that more accurate diagnosis is available by means of renal biopsy it does not appear to be as rare as was formerly considered.

The prognosis is variable. The primary disease is usually progressive, but if the underlying cause can be removed secondary amyloidosis can be arrested, although it is very doubtful that it will actually reverse.

Myelomatosis

Myelomatosis can damage the kidney in a number of ways. Proteinuria is common and the urine also contains immunoglobin fragments. These may gel in the renal tubules producing an obstructive nephropathy and ultimately renal failure. The rapid proliferation of cells in the bone marrow can lead to hypercalcaemia which also damages the kidney and reduces renal function.

Systemic Lupus Erythematosus

A renal lesion is an important feature of S.L.E., usually presenting as proteinuria or the nephrotic syndrome and terminating in renal failure. Rarely it presents as a progressive acute nephritis. The glomerular lesions are variable and include basement membrane thickening (wire loop appearance) and cell proliferation indistinguishable from glomerulonephritis. Due to other causes, diagnosis therefore may depend on clinical evidence of lupus elsewhere and positive tests for lupus. The disease is usually rapidly progressive in spite of treatment with steroids or cytotoxic agents, although in a few patients the downhill course is prolonged over many years.

Polyarteritis Nodosa

The arteritis frequently affects the kidney producing glomerulitis and small areas of infarction. The patient presents with acute oliguric nephritis and recurrent bouts of haematuria are a prominent feature. Occasionally the nephrotic syndrome or chronic renal failure may occur.

Anaphylactoid Purpura

A small number of patients with anaphylactoid purpura have haematuria and proteinuria or more rarely a nephrotic syndrome. Biopsy usually shows a mild proliferative lesion in the glomerulus. The prognosis is good although recovery may be slow. The course of the disease is unaffected by steroids or cytotoxic agents.

Gout

Gout may produce changes similar to those of chronic pyelonephritis. This is due to precipitation of uric acid crystals around the tubules. In severe cases it may lead to chronic renal failure. Urate stones can also cause obstructive lesions of the urinary tract. The disease is best treated with allopurinol which ultimately decreases the amount of uric acid in the kidney.

Analgesic Nephropathy

The prolonged use of analgesics is associated with the development of renal damage, the usual pathological picture being that of renal fibrosis with papillary necrosis and sometimes even detachment of the papillae. It seems that *phenacetin* is the most important analgesic involved. However, analgesics are quite often given as mixtures and it is difficult to completely exonerate other mild analgesics such as aspirin and paracetamol.

Clinical Features. The patient may present with chronic renal failure, hypertension, recurrent renal infection or haematuria. Straight X-ray may show calcification of the papillae which may outline the papilla if they are lying free in the renal pelvis. Pyelography may show small irregular kidneys similar to chronic pyelonephritis. The dye may show detachment of the papillae and may outline the spaces found by the disappearance of the pyramids.

Treatment. There is no specific treatment, but if the analgesic is stopped renal function should not deteriorate further and may actually improve. If further analgesia is required for chronic pain, the safest analgesics to give are indomethacin, ibuprofen or the fenemates, none of which have yet been shown to produce or exacerbate analgesic nephropathy.

NORMAL VALUES

Venous Plasma Concentrations

Bicarbonate	25–29 mmol./litre
Potassium	4–5·5 mmol./litre
Sodium	138–145 mmol./litre
Creatinine	50–130 μmol./l.
Urea	2·5–7·1 mmol./l.

24-hour Urine Output

Calcium	1·20–8·8 mmol.
Creatinine	9–18 mmol.
Potassium	Depends on intake
Sodium	Usually 50–200 mmol.
Urea	250–600 mmol.

Renal Function (corrected to 1·73 sq. m. surface area)

Renal plasma flow	400–750 ml./min.
Glomerular filtration rate	80–160 ml./min.
Maximum concentrating capacity—up to SG 1010–1032	800–1,200 m. osmoles/litre
Maximum acidifying capacity	pH 4·6–5·1

FURTHER READING

Wardener, H. F. de, *The Kidney*, 4th edition, J. and A. Churchill, London, 1973

Pitts, R. F., *Physiology of the Kidney and Body Fluids*, Year Book Medical Publishers Inc., Chicago, 1974.

Black, D. A. K., Edited by, *Renal Disease*, 4th edition, Blackwell Scientific Publications, Oxford, 1978.

Cameron, J. S., Russell, A. M. E. and Sale, D., *Nephrology for Nurses*, 2nd edition, William Heinemann, London, 1976.

CHAPTER ELEVEN

DISORDERS OF WATER AND ELECTROLYTE METABOLISM AND OF ACID/BASE BALANCE

Introduction

A normal man with a body weight of 70 kg. contains about 42 litres of water. The proportion of the body which is accounted for by water varies with sex and age.

Adult man: 65 per cent of weight is water.

Adult woman: 55 per cent of weight is water.

Infant: 50 per cent of weight is water.

Fat, which contains no water, also influences these figures and in very obese subjects the proportion of body weight due to water may be significantly lower.

In considering disturbances of water and electrolyte balance the body water is divided into the *intra- and extra-cellular* spaces or compartments. The intra-cellular space contains about 70 per cent and the extra-cellular space about 30 per cent of the body water.

The extra-cellular space can be further subdivided into the intravascular space and the interstitial fluid. Ions and water pass freely between these compartments and although the capillaries are largely impermeable to protein so that the concentration of protein is much higher in the plasma than in the interstitial fluid, the interstitial and plasma spaces may be regarded as a single compartment. The maintenance of an adequate volume in the intravascular compartment is however essential or circulation will fail.

The most important ions are:

		Plasma (mmol./litre)	Intracellular Fluid (mmol./litre)
Cations	Na	136–142	11
	K	4·0–5·5	164
	Ca	2·5	1·0
	Mg	1·0	1·4
Anions	Cl	95–105	0
	HCO_3	25–28	10
	HPO_4	2	110
	SO_4	1	18
	Protein	16	66
	Organic Acids	6	5

Extracellular Osmolality 285 mOsm./litre.

The intra- and extra-cellular spaces are separated by the cell membrane which is freely permeable to water but in health is largely impermeable to sodium and potassium. In health the cell water and the extra-cellular fluid are isoosmotic.

It can be seen that the main extra-cellular cation is sodium and the main intra-cellular cation is potassium. The maintenance of the high concentration gradient of these ions across the cell membrane is dependent on energy-producing metabolic activity within the cell.

Changes in the concentration of these ions in either the intra- or extracellular spaces result in the passage of water from the low concentration to the high concentration space until the osmolalities of the two spaces are again equal. The shift of water results in the shrinkage and expansion of the respective spaces.

In general, therefore, it can be stated that provided there is adequate hydration the amount of sodium in the body determines the volume of the extra-cellular fluid and the amount of potassium in the body the volume of the intra-cellular fluid.

Assessment of Volume Changes

(a) *Vascular Compartment*

A fall in the plasma volume is followed by vasoconstriction and a rise in pulse rate in an effort to maintain the circulation. This causes cold extremities, a fall in blood pressure which is more marked on standing and a fall in central venous pressure. Alternatively a rise in plasma volume is associated with a rise of blood pressure and of central venous pressure.

(b) *Tissue Fluid Compartment*

This is difficult to assess. Loss of skin elasticity when pinched is a classical but late sign of deficiency of tissue fluid. Excess will produce oedema.

(c) There is no satisfactory way of assessing the volume of intracellular water.

The sum of the anions and cations of the plasma should of necessity balance. Clinical measurements usually show a small difference between cations and anions which is called the *anion gap*. An increase in this gap may be evidence of a metabolic acidosis due to accumulation of acids such as salicylic or lactic acid.

CLINICAL DISORDERS

The diagnosis of clinical disorders of salt and water metabolism requires an awareness of the circumstances in which these disorders may occur; if these are remembered diagnosis is not usually difficult. However, it is usually much harder to assess the extent of the disorder.

The management of these conditions is made more precise by daily measurement of intake and output of water and electrolytes and estimation of plasma levels of electrolytes. The main measurements required are care-

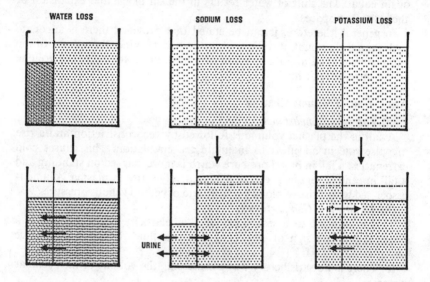

DISORDERS OF WATER AND ELECTROLYTE BALANCE.

ful records of the volume and electrolyte content of oral and intravenous fluids, the levels of sodium, potassium, bicarbonate and chloride in the plasma, and the volume of urine passed in each 24 hours. In more complicated disorders measurements of sodium and potassium concentrations in the urine may be necessary. In special cases the volume and electrolyte content of other excreta (vomit, aspirate and faeces) may be needed. Regular weighing is a most useful guide to net fluid balance.

Losses which may be expected are given below:

Aspirate ⎫ Vomit ⎭	Water, H^+ K^+ Na^+
Fistulae	Water Na^+ K^+ HCO_3^-
Diarrhoea	Water Na^+ K^+
Osmotic diuresis (as in uncontrolled diabetes)	Water Na^+ K^+

Some assessment of renal function is very useful and measurement of blood urea is usually sufficient for this purpose. Good renal function is a great help in returning the patient to normal fluid balance provided ions and water are supplied in adequate quantities. The problem is much harder when renal function is impaired.

If intake and output records are available from the start of the patient's illness the nature and degree of the disorder of electrolyte and water balance can easily be calculated. However, for most patients records are either incomplete or non-existent. Diagnosis must usually be made on clinical grounds and confirmed by plasma concentrations of electrolytes, although as will be seen below these may only give a very rough idea of the extent of the disorder. There are now methods of measuring the total body sodium and potassium, but they are not generally available for routine use and are slow and clumsy.

Finally it must be remembered that it is unusual for a single disorder to exist alone. Any change in the total body electrolytes affects the amount of water in the body, and loss of more than one electrolyte occurs frequently. Although for simplicity individual disorders are examined separately, in practice combinations are the rule.

WATER

The volume of body water depends on the amount ingested and produced by metabolic processes and the output in the urine; in addition about 500 ml./24 hrs. are lost through the lungs and skin. Diarrhoea or excessive vomiting are also factors in some patients. It is important to remember that although the volume of water in the stools is normally small (300ml./24 hrs.), a large volume passes in and out of the gut and any disturbance of this exchange can produce rapid dehydration. Healthy kidneys require to excrete at least 700 ml./24 hrs. to get rid of waste products. Many patients do not have healthy kidneys and the urine output may have to be considerably higher to prevent uraemia.

Dehydration. Isolated dehydration is not common in this country and usually results from decreased intake. Comatose or debilitated patients may not be given sufficient water. Excessive loss of water from the intestinal tract or through the kidneys is much more common, but, except in diabetes insipidus, there is a concomitant loss of electrolytes and thus a complicated picture.

In pure water deficiency shrinkage of both the intra- and extra-cellular spaces occurs (see p. 418). The main symptoms are thirst due to a rise in the osmolality of the extra-cellular fluid and in severe cases confusion or coma. Signs are not prominent except for a dry mouth. The volume of urine is low and the urine is concentrated. The plasma proteins, sodium and haemoglobin are raised. Assessment of water deficiency is not easy and will depend on the history, fluid balance charts (if available), and the clinical state of the patient. The best way to follow changes in body water is by regular weighing.

Treatment. Water should be given by mouth or intravenously as 5 per cent dextrose solution. The amount required may be difficult to assess, but the plasma sodium level or osmolality may be used as a guide.

Overhydration. This occurs when excessive water intake is combined with failure of water excretion. The common causes are acute renal failure or excessive production of antidiuretic hormone such as occurs in the first 48 hours following major surgery. Occasionally there is excessive production of an A.D.H.-like hormone, particularly in carcinoma of the bronchus. The excess water is distributed evenly through the intra- and extra-cellular spaces. Subcutaneous oedema may be present and pulmonary oedema detected by râles at the lung bases. Clinical features are confusion, convulsions and ultimately coma. The plasma electrolytes and osmolality are low although the blood urea may be raised if there is associated oliguria. The urine is of low osmolality.

Treatment. In mild cases it is sufficient to restrict water intake. If overhydration is severe it will be necessary to give hypertonic saline (2 N or 5 N) to raise the plasma sodium level (and thus osmolality) of the body water. If there is acute renal failure some form of dialysis may be needed to remove excess water.

SODIUM

The freely exchangeable sodium in the body (about 2,500 mmol.) is almost entirely confined to the extra-cellular space. There is in addition a considerable amount of sodium in bone but it is not readily available for exchange.

In health the amount of exchangeable sodium in the body depends on intake and loss in the urine. Normal kidneys are very effective in regulating excretion to keep the body sodium steady. If there is severe loss or excessive intake, particularly if renal function is temporarily or permanently disturbed, upsets in sodium balance occur.

Sodium Depletion. This can be caused by excessive loss, usually from the *gastrointestinal* tract or through the *kidneys*. Gastrointestinal loss results from vomiting, diarrhoea, and fistulae. Renal loss is usually the result of prolonged diuretic therapy, although it may also occur in uncontrolled diabetes (p. 449) or with renal tubular lesions. It is also a feature of adrenal failure.

Vomiting causes sodium deficiency, not only from loss in the vomit but also by producing an alkalosis, and thus an obligatory excretion of sodium in an alkaline urine. Decreased intake is not common in this country, but in the tropics excessive sweating plus a low salt intake can be important.

As the sodium concentration (and thus the osmolality) in the extra-cellular space falls, water is lost both in the urine and into the intra-cellular space (p. 418) so that the volume of the extra-cellular space including the blood volume decreases. Finally, this adjustment fails and the sodium concentration in the extra-cellular space falls. This means that by the time the plasma sodium is significantly reduced, considerable depletion has occurred.

Clinical Features are weakness, vomiting and cramps. The shrinkage of the extra-cellular space causes hypotension (particularly postural), lax skin and sunken facies. The plasma sodium concentration is reduced with severe depletion but owing to the fall in extra-cellular volume the plasma sodium concentration under-estimates the extent of sodium deficit. The urine volume is usually normal in the early stages with a low sodium concentration. Ultimately a fall in renal perfusion due to the low blood volume leads to a decreased urine volume and a rising blood urea.

Treatment. If charts are available, the degree of sodium depletion can be calculated, but this is unusual. There is no ideal way of establishing sodium deficiency which is suitable for routine use. A rough approximation may be obtained by multiplying the number of millequivalents the plasma sodium is below normal by the extra-cellular volume.

Deficiency in mEq. Na =

$$140 - \text{observed Na conc.} \times \frac{25}{100} \times \text{body weight in kg.}$$

This formula does not allow for the shrinkage in extra-cellular volume which occurs in sodium depletion and which tends to keep up the plasma sodium concentration. The calculated deficiency should therefore be multiplied by a factor of x2 to give a truer estimate of deficiency.

It is usual to spread the repletion of sodium over 24–48 hrs. It should also be remembered that the day to day loss of sodium may be continuing, and sodium depletion is frequently associated with water depletion so that correction of dehydration may also be required. A patient with severe sodium depletion may easily need as much as 10 litres of water and 1,000 mmol. of sodium. Sodium is usually given as N sodium chloride solution, though if the plasma sodium concentration is below 120 mmol./litre, 2 N sodium chloride should be used. If sodium depletion is associated with acidosis, due perhaps to uncontrolled diabetes or excessive intestinal loss, $\frac{1}{6}$ M sodium lactate can be infused or 100 ml. of 8·4 per cent sodium bicarbonate (1 mmol./ml.) can be added to whatever infusion fluid is used. During the repletion period, continued observation of the clinical and biochemical state of the patient is necessary.

In patients in whom it is suspected that cardiac function is impaired a careful watch must be kept on the central venous pressure and the bases of the lungs as over-rapid infusion can precipitate heart failure and pulmonary oedema.

POTASSIUM

Potassium is the major intra-cellular cation. It plays an important part in cell membrane activity and in the contraction of muscle. In health the adult male body contains about 3,000 mmol. of potassium, the amount being regulated by renal excretion, although the conservation of potassium by the kidneys is not as effective as that of sodium.

Potassium is also excreted into the gut in the bile and intestinal fluid, but is reabsorbed. If, however, there is excessive loss of intestinal fluid, depletion can occur.

The intra-cellular distribution of potassium makes the measurement of total body potassium very difficult. Unfortunately the plasma potassium concentration, though usually giving some indication of the situation, may be misleading especially as considerable depletion (up to 200 mmol. K) can occur with no fall in the plasma level and without development of symptoms. Further if potassium is passing from the cells to the circulation, plasma levels may be normal even with progressive intracellular depletion. More accurate methods of measuring total body potassium are available but are not suitable for routine use.

Potassium Depletion. Excessive loss of potassium can occur from the *gastrointestinal tract*, due to vomiting, fistulae, or prolonged diarrhoea. Prolonged use of purgatives is an occasional cause. Severe *renal loss* occurs in prolonged diuresis, usually from the use of diuretic drugs, but also in diabetes mellitus (p. 449) or the recovery phase of acute renal failure. Steroids also cause increased renal potassium loss, and it is a feature of aldosteronism (p. 481). In patients with moderate intra-cellular potassium deficiency (e.g. those receiving diuretics) surgery may cause a shift of potassium ions from the extra- to the intra-cellular space, leading to symptoms and signs of potassium deficiency.

Loss of potassium from the cell causes a fall in intra-cellular osmolality, and thus loss of water from the cell. There is some shift of hydrogen and sodium ions into the cell and thus an intra-cellular acidosis and an extracellular alkalosis. The plasma pH is therefore raised and the raised bicar-

converted to carbonic acid by the enzyme carbonic anhydrase in the red cells. This reaction is so rapid that dissolved CO_2 may be considered as an effective acid. Measurements are usually given in terms of partial pressure of carbon dioxide (pCO_2) rather than concentration of carbonic acid. Some 90 per cent of the hydrogen ions released by the dissociation of this carbonic acid combine with haemoglobin, thus preventing a large fall in blood pH. In the tissues the release of oxygen from haemoglobin allows the uptake of hydrogen ions by the imidazolyl groups on the haemoglobin molecule.

$$HbO_2 + CO_2 + H_2O \xrightarrow{\text{carbonic anhydrase}} H^+Hb + HCO_3^- + O_2$$

Oxygen in the lungs similarly causes a release of hydrogen ions which combine with bicarbonate with the formation of carbon dioxide which is excreted. In addition some carbon dioxide is carried on the amine groups of haemoglobin and plasma proteins.

$$H^+Hb + O_2 \rightarrow HbO_2 + H_2O + CO_2\uparrow$$

Maintenance of pH and Excretion of Hydrogen Ions. The stable pH of the blood is preserved by a number of buffer systems. These consist of strong bases which on the addition of hydrogen ions (acid) form weak acids. The bases and weak acids which act as buffers in this context are frequently called buffer bases and buffer acids.

The pH of the blood depends on the ratio buffer base to buffer acid. It can be derived from the equation propounded by Henderson and Hassalbalch in 1908.

$$pH = pK + \log\left(\frac{\text{buffer base}}{\text{buffer acid}}\right)$$

The buffer systems of the blood with their approximate relative buffering capacity are:

Percentage of Total Capacity		Percentage of Total Capacity	
HCO_3^-/H_2CO_3	37	Hb/HbH	34
HPO_4^{--}/H_2PO_4	5	Protein/PrH	24

If hydrogen ions are added to these buffer systems, they combine with the buffer bases to form weak buffer acids. The fall in pH resulting from the addition of acid is therefore minimised.

In the plasma the compensation is almost entirely due to HCO_3/H_2CO_3 system because CO_2 can be excreted immediately.

$$HCO_3^- + H^+ \rightarrow H_2CO_3 \rightarrow H_2O + CO_2\uparrow$$

and the ratio $\log \dfrac{HCO_3}{H_2CO_3}$ (i.e. pH) maintained at near normal levels.

Similarly if hydrogen ions are removed from the system and the pH rises, buffer acid is changed into buffer base with the release of hydrogen ions and the increase in pH is minimised.

The *total buffer base* is the sum of all the buffers (bicarbonate+protein +Hb+phosphate). If ventilation is normal then the plasma bicarbonate level reflects the total buffer base. If however there is an abnormality of ventilation then this is no longer true. This is because retention or deficit of carbon dioxide (and thus carbonic acid) will influence bicarbonate levels without altering the total buffer base, i.e.

$$\text{i.e. } H_2CO_3 \rightarrow H^+ + HCO_3^-$$
$$\downarrow$$
$$\text{Buffer base}$$

The hydrogen ion released thus reduces the buffer base, but at the same time bicarbonate is added. The net result being no change in total buffer base, but an increase in bicarbonate. The terms 'base excess' or 'base deficit' are used to indicate abnormalities of total buffer base.

The role of haemoglobin in the excretion of carbon dioxide has already been considered. In addition small amounts of hydrogen ions (about 75 mmol./24 hrs.) are produced as organic and inorganic acids (sulphuric and lactic). They are accommodated in the buffer systems of the blood and excreted in the urine. Provided the influx from the cells equals efflux through the kidneys, the pH of the blood remains constant.

Clinical Applications

Introduction. Acid/base disturbances can be divided into those which are primarily due to disorders of carbon dioxide excretion (respiratory) and those due to inequality of acid or base production or excretion (metabolic or non-respiratory). The symptoms due to acid/base disturbances are ill-defined and are often overshadowed by the primary disease. Once the possibility is recognised the diagnosis is usually not difficult.

Investigation. The bicarbonate buffer system of the blood is usually studied as it is the easiest to measure. Bicarbonate is usually estimated by the autoanalyser or the Van Slyke method using venous blood. Provided that respiratory function is normal this estimation usually gives an adequate approximation of the buffer base situation in the blood. If however there is CO_2 retention it will underestimate the deficiency in base and vice versa, so that where there is a respiratory disorder or where the situation is complicated, it is necessary to measure additionally the plasma pCO_2 or pH. The pCO_2 can be measured by the rebreathing method or by the Astrup method using capillary or arterial blood. Mixed venous blood can also be used but gives a figure about 6 mm. higher than arterial blood. If two of the three variables (pH, pCO_2 or bicarbonate) are known the third can be calculated.

Acid/base disorders are often associated with electrolyte deficiencies, so that the plasma and often urinary concentrations of sodium and potassium should be measured. Estimation of blood urea levels gives an indication of overall renal function.

Normal Values

$$\text{Plasma pH} = 7\cdot35\text{–}7\cdot45$$
$$\text{Plasma bicarbonate} = 24\text{–}28 \text{ mmol./litre}$$
$$pCO_2 = 36\text{–}42 \text{ mm.Hg.}$$

Disorders of Carbon Dioxide Excretion

1. Impaired Excretion (Respiratory Acidosis)

The carriage of carbon dioxide from the tissues to the lungs is described above. In health, ventilation is physiologically maintained so that the partial pressure of carbon dioxide in the alveoli is about 40 mm.Hg., the concentration of dissolved carbon dioxide in arterial blood being that which is in equilibrium with this partial pressure.

If there is inadequate alveolar ventilation, the partial pressure of carbon dioxide rises leading to an increase in the dissolved carbon dioxide (hypercarbia).

This causes a fall in the ratio $\dfrac{HCO_3^-}{pCO_2 \text{ (increased)}}$ and therefore a fall in pH.

The decrease is minimised by the other buffer bases combining with carbon dioxide and being converted to buffer acids with the release of bicarbonate.

$$\text{Buffer base} + CO_2 + H_2O \rightarrow \text{Buffer acid} + HCO_3^-$$

Following carbon dioxide retention the excess hydrogen ions are excreted by the kidney, producing an acid urine and reabsorption of bicarbonate by the tubules is increased.

Impaired carbon dioxide excretion occurs:

(1) Most commonly in chronic bronchitis, emphysema and asthma. It may occur acutely in bronchial obstruction with collapse.

(2) More rarely with depression of respiration in morphia or barbiturate poisoning, or from weakness of the respiratory muscles in poliomyelitis.

Clinical Features. Symptoms usually appear when the pCO_2 rises to 60 mm.Hg. The patient is dyspnoeic and cyanosed (due to the concomitant hypoxia) with a full pulse and warm extremities from peripheral vasodilation. The blood pressure is frequently raised in acute hypercapnia. Further increase in pCO_2 brings about confusion with twitching and finally coma. Papilloedema may develop due to cerebral vasodilation. The treatment is directed towards increasing alveolar ventilation and relieving hypoxia.

2. Excessive Excretion (Respiratory Alkalosis)

This is due to hyperventilation which leads to excessive loss of carbon dioxide and to a rise in the ratio $\dfrac{HCO_3^-}{pCO_2 \text{ (decreased)}}$ and a rise in plasma pH.

This is minimised by the other buffer acids converting to buffer bases with the release of hydrogen ions which combine with bicarbonate.

$$\text{Buffer acid} + HCO_3^- \rightarrow \text{Buffer base} + H_2O + CO_2$$

Renal conservation of hydrogen ions results in an alkaline urine.

Excessive excretion of carbon dioxide is often due to hysterical over-breathing and is a constant feature of salicylate poisoning; rarely it is found in subjects with alveolar block causing hypoxia but not affecting carbon dioxide excretion and it may also complicate various forms of cerebral damage.

Clinical features are increased neuromuscular excitability with twitching, paraesthiae, and tetany. The easiest treatment is to raise the pCO_2 in the alveoli by rebreathing from a bag. In those with cerebral damage careful depression of respiration with morphia is sometimes useful.

Disorders of Hydrogen Ion Excretion

1. Gain of Acid or Loss of Bicarbonate (Metabolic Acidosis)

When the rate of production of hydrogen ions exceeds the rate of excretion either because of increased ingestion of acid substances, undue metabolic production of acids or impaired excretion by the kidneys, the condition of metabolic acidosis develops.

The rise in pH is minimised by the acid combining with buffer bases,

$$\text{Buffer base} + H^+ \rightarrow \text{Buffer acid}$$

resulting in a fall in the ratio $\dfrac{\text{Buffer base}}{\text{Buffer acid}}$.

A similar state can result from the loss of bicarbonate ions.

An excessive influx of acid into the blood can arise from the following causes:

(a) Ingestion of substances which produce acid, the commonest being ammonium chloride and aspirin.

(b) Increased production of acid occurs with severe exercise, in uncontrolled diabetes mellitus and sometimes after major surgery.

(c) Tissue hypoxia as may occur in cardiac arrest leads to rapid production of lactic acid with resulting acidosis.

(d) In both acute and chronic renal failure the kidneys fail to excrete sufficient acid.

Bicarbonate deficiency follows loss of intestinal secretions due to diarrhoea or fistulae. There is frequently an associated sodium and potassium deficiency. Failure of the renal tubules to reabsorb bicarbonate with subsequent deficiency also occurs with renal tubules acidosis.

Clinical features are tiredness and weakness with increased respiration, and finally unconsciousness.

Treatment

(1) Relief of the primary cause if possible.

(2) Re-establishment of optimal renal function, i.e. correct dehydration and electrolyte deficiencies.

(3) Restoration of depleted buffer bases by the infusion of 0·16 M sodium lactate or by the addition of 8·5 per cent sodium bicarbonate (approx. 1 mmol./ml.) to whatever infusion is being used. As a rough guide the total base deficiency can be calculated:

25—Plasma bicarbonate (mmol./litre) × 0·3 body weight in Kg. This will almost certainly underestimate the deficit and further base will be required, the amount depending on the levels of plasma bicarbonate. A watch must be kept for tetany.

2. Loss of Acid or Gain of Bicarbonate (Metabolic Alkalosis)

Gain of bicarbonate is due to its excessive ingestion in the treatment of peptic ulcer. Healthy kidneys can cope with almost unlimited amounts of bicarbonate but if there is renal disease, base excess may develop. Loss of acid is usually due to vomiting or gastric aspiration. Metabolic alkalosis can also complicate potassium deficiency (p. 424).

The rise in pH results in buffer acid being changed to buffer base.

$$\text{Buffer acid} \rightarrow \text{Buffer base} + H^+$$

and a rise in the ratio $\dfrac{\text{Buffer acid}}{\text{Buffer base}}$.

The kidneys secrete an alkaline urine containing large amounts of sodium and bicarbonate.

Clinical features include clouding of consciousness and in addition there may be paraesthesiae, tetany and convulsions.

Acid loss from vomiting or aspiration is often coupled with sodium and potassium deficiency. This is due partially to loss in gastric secretion and to increased excretion in the urine.

Treatment. It is usually sufficient to correct dehydration and electrolyte deficiencies and the kidneys will excrete the excess base.

Definitions

Acid. A substance which donates hydrogen ions. Strong acids are those which are highly dissociated in solution, and weak acids are those poorly dissociated in solution.

Base. A substance which accepts hydrogen ions. A strong base accepts hydrogen ions more readily than a weak base. Important physiological bases are bicarbonate, dibasic phosphate and some amino acids.

Buffer Base. A base which takes part in the buffer systems of the body.

Acidosis and Alkalosis. These terms cannot be precisely defined. They are generally used to indicate the primary direction of the change of plasma pH, acidosis indicating a fall and alkalosis a rise in pH.

	Partial Pressure CO_2	Plasma pH	Plasma Bicarbonate
Impaired excretion CO_2 (respiratory acidosis)	Increased	Decreased	Increased
Excessive excretion CO_2 (respiratory alkalosis)	Decreased	Increased	Decreased
Retention of acid or loss of base (metabolic acidosis)	Normal or Decreased	Decreased	Decreased
Loss of acid or retention of base (metabolic alkalosis)	Normal	Increased	Increased

Plasma changes in Acid-Base Disorders.

FURTHER READING

Cameron, J. S., in *Medical Treatment* (Vol. III). Edited by K. S. Maclean and G. W. Scott, J. & A. Churchill, London, 1970.

Taylor, W. H., *Fluid Therapy and Disorders of Electrolyte Balance*, 2nd edition, Blackwell Scientific Publications, Oxford and Edinburgh, 1970.

CHAPTER TWELVE

DISEASES OF METABOLISM

DISORDERS OF CARBOHYDRATE METABOLISM

Introduction—Metabolism of Carbohydrate

Glucose is absorbed actively from the small intestine, and passes through the portal vein to the liver. Here it is phosphorylated and some is stored as glycogen, some broken down to pyruvate, and some dephosphorylated and passed into the plasma. These changes are effected by enzyme systems. Glucose passes freely through the glomerular filter, and is totally reabsorbed by the cells of the proximal tubule. If the plasma glucose level (and hence the level in the glomerular filtrate) is above about 10 mmol./litre then the tubule's power of reabsorption is exceeded, and sugar appears in the urine.

Glucose passes from the plasma into the interstitial fluid and then into the cell. Inside the cell it is again phosphorylated, and either stored as glycogen, or broken down to pyruvate and then to CO_2 and water, with consequent release of energy, or converted to fatty acids and ultimately to fat. It has been estimated from tracer studies in animals that of the total glucose which is daily metabolised 67 per cent is oxidised to CO_2 and water, 30 per cent converted to fatty acids, and only 3 per cent stored as glycogen. Sixty-five per cent of this glucose is dietary in origin, 30 per cent arises from gluconeo-genesis, and 3 per cent only from glycogen.

A number of hormones serve to regulate carbohydrate metabolism. Of these the most important is insulin, which is synthesised as a long polypeptide chain in the beta cells of the islets of Langerhans. This chain folds over on itself and through the establishment of disulphide links forms the pro-insulin molecule. Removal of the 'connecting peptide' results in the A and B chained insulin molecule, which usually polymerises in the resting state and forms the insulin granules visible by electron and light microscopy. Insulin is released and synthesised in response to a rise in plasma glucose levels and release is possibly initiated by gastrointestinal polypeptide hormones.

It circulates both in a free form and bound to the albumen and alpha-2 globulin of the plasma.

The plasma insulin level as determined by radio immune assay lies between 5–30 μU/ml. In adult diabetics normal levels are often found with a slow rise in response to glucose. Low values are found in young diabetics after prolonged insulin treatment.

The action of insulin varies in different tissues but in general it increases the uptake of glucose and suppresses the release of non-esterified fatty acids by adipose tissue.

Thyroxine is mildly hyperglycaemic in effect, but pituitary and adrenal hormones, and the secretion of the alpha cells in the islets of Langerhans, glucagon, are all hyperglycaemic. How important the hormones other than insulin are in clinical diabetes is uncertain.

DIABETES MELLITUS

Introduction

Diabetes mellitus occurs in all parts of the world. The age at which the disease is first recognised clinically ranges from early childhood to old age; over 50 per cent of patients are first diagnosed over the age of 50 years. The sex ratio was believed to show a predominance of females over males, but recent surveys suggest that it is 1:1.

It is easiest to consider it as a breakdown of the body's insulin-glucose economy. Thus, certain conditions such as steroid therapy, pregnancy, obesity, etc., may overtax the insulin resources; they may fail in idiopathic diabetes, or with primary pancreatic disease. Since the recognised disease runs in families it has been suggested that predisposition to diabetes is related to a recessive gene of low penetrance. However, there is controversy over this point, and a multifactorial aetiology and inheritance is also possible.

Prevalence

Before World War II, prevalence studies in western countries suggested a rate of 0·7 per cent. An investigation in 1946–7 based on screening by glycosuria in Oxford, Mass., indicated a prevalence of 1·99 per cent. Since then many surveys have been carried out, and it appears that the prevalence of diabetes is very low (0·1 per cent or less) in unmechanised primitive societies, rising to high levels (up to 7 per cent in some cases) in under-exercising industrial communities with extended life span. Apart from the higher proportion of more susceptible older age groups, the differences between countries can be explained largely by variations in obesity.

Pathological Chemistry

Glucose Tolerance Tests (see fig. on p. 438). After an 8–12 hr. (usually overnight) fast, the true blood sugar in arterial, capillary or venous samples ranges in most subjects from 3·0–5·5 mmol./litre per cent; these levels are regarded as normal. A fasting blood sugar over 5·5 mmol./litre is suggestive of diabetes mellitus and over 6·5 mmol./litre is now generally accepted as diagnostic. However, in many persons who sooner or later develop complications of diabetes, the fasting blood sugar, which depends on the time since the last meal, may be under 5·5 mmol./litre. A more reliable indication it obtained with tolerance tests. The oral glucose tolerance test is in widest use. After taking a fasting blood sugar sample, 50 g. (in the U.S.A. 100 g.) of glucose are given in 250 ml. water with non-caloric flavouring to prevent nausea. Further blood samples are then taken at half-hour intervals. The early form of the curve depends on the opening of the pylorus, the intestinal absorption and liver glucose uptake. Patients with rapidly emptying stomachs often show a brisk early peak (steeple or lag curve). At 2 hours, normal subjects have, according to current W.H.O. criteria, capillary auto analyser blood sugars of less than 6·0 mmol./litre per cent or venous blood sugars less than 5·8 mmol./litre.

Metabolic Consequences of Failure of Insulin Action: Diagnostic Criteria for Diabetes Mellitus

When insulin is not available, the blood glucose level rises and this leads to a high peak blood glucose and a high level after 2 hours (see the figure). On current W.H.O. recommendations diabetes is diagnosed if the capillary auto analyser blood sugar exceeds 8·0 mmol./litre at 2 hrs. in the standard glucose tolerance test. The distribution of 2 hr. capillary auto analyser blood sugars at the Bedford, 1962, survey of random subjects (see the figure on p. 437) suggests that these criteria are too strict and the more practical criterion for the diagnosis of diabetes would be a 2 hr. blood sugar of age plus 120, or even more simple, a 2 hr. capillary auto analyser blood sugar level exceeding 11·0 mmol./litre. Unfortunately, some patients with blood sugars between 8·0 and 11·0 mmol./litre have been found to develop diabetic complications.

Glycosuria. When glucose levels exceed the renal threshold glycosuria results. This may be detected in concentrations as low as 0·1 per cent by glucose-specific tests or as a reducing substance by less sensitive (0·25–2·0 per cent) means, e.g. Benedict's solution (sensitive to homogentisuric acid and other hexoses) or tablets such as those available commercially as Clinitest. Glycosuria may be due to several causes (see the figure on p. 438) and will require a glucose tolerance test to determine whether it is due to diabetes.

In all cases where diabetes is diagnosed, the renal threshold for glucose must be determined, because while glycosuria is the simplest and most widely used method for judging control, wide variations of threshold occur (see the figure on p. 439), a fact which if not recognised can result in serious errors of management. In cases where there is no fasting glycosuria, it usually develops during the rising phase of the initial glucose tolerance test, and renal threshold is easily assessed by testing half-hour urine samples with Clinitest tablets until glycosuria occurs. Such semi-quantitative methods for testing glycosuria can be used subsequently to follow control. If glycosuria is absent throughout the diagnostic glucose tolerance test, it is advisable to check the renal threshold using Clinistix or test tape with associated blood-sugar determinations on the ward, or on another test occasion using a larger glucose loading dose. If glycosuria is present in the fasting state, the renal threshold should be assessed on a separate occasion. The usual morning insulin dose, or in other cases 10–20 units of soluble insulin, is injected subcutaneously, and blood and urine samples taken every 20 minutes until glycosuria disappears—breakfast is then taken.

Besides the tendency for the renal threshold to be low in young adults, it may also fall during pregnancy and recover after parturition.

Dehydration and Shock. Intense uncontrolled glycosuria can result in an osmotic diuresis of 7–10 litres/day with resulting intense thirst. Unless adequate replacements are given, this polyuria leads to large losses of sodium and potassium.

Ketoacidosis (p. 449). Insulin failure is accompanied by ketoacidosis. This is due to:

(1) Accumulation of ketoacids.
(2) Accumulation of incompletely metabolised carbohydrate, i.e. pyruvic and lactic acid.

In the absence of insulin, adipose tissue releases large quantities of free fatty acids which circulate to the liver where they are metabolised to carbon dioxide. When this mechanism becomes overloaded, acetyl co-enzyme A accumulates in the liver and becomes condensed to aceto-acetic acid and acetone. These can be metabolised by muscle, but if produced in sufficient quantities they accumulate in the blood and appear in the urine and the breath.

The resulting acidosis causes a fall in plasma bicarbonate, and blood pH may fall to 7·0 or less.

Causes of Diabetes: Elderly, Obese, Idiopathic, Associated and Iatrogenic Types

Clearly, there are many points in the sequence of events between insulin synthesis and release, its transport clearance and action, and glucose uptake by the various organs, where abnormality or biochemical fault may upset the normal balance and produce the diabetic state.

Pancreatectomy or chronic pancreatitis removes the source of insulin production. With advancing years, protein synthesis is generally slowed down and this also applies to insulin production. It is not surprising therefore that recent studies show a high prevalence of hyperglycaemia (up to 50 per cent) among the elderly. The association recognised between obesity and diabetes reflects the relative insulin and sensitivity of tissues in overweight persons. Under-exercise and deposition of fat lead to a breakdown in the body's insulin–glucose economy despite compensatory over-production of insulin by the beta cells. In young diabetics there is an unexplained failure of the beta cells to produce insulin—virus infections are suspected of cause in some cases, in others there seems to be a genetic factor because of the tendency for diabetes to run in families. In about 80 per cent of all British and North American diabetics the disorder begins in middle or later life, usually associated with obesity. Juvenile onset cases make up most of the remainder but other causes are being recognised. Hyperglycaemia is certainly aggravated in susceptible subjects by steroid therapy, including the contraceptive pill, by pregnancy and in Cushing's disease. Changes in protein metabolism and reduced tissue sensitivity to insulin are largely responsible. The association between acromegaly and diabetes and the production of intense ketonuria when growth hormone is given to insulin-dependent diabetics indicates that this hormone, too, increases the body requirement for insulin. Other associations with diabetes, besides pregnancy, reported recently include ischaemic heart disease (45 per cent of males), ischaemic thrombotic cerebrovascular disease (over 70 per cent), and Bell's palsy (45–60 per cent). Iatrogenic causes of diabetes include bed-rest, particularly when associated with severe injuries like burns, and besides steroid treatment and the contraceptive pill, certain diuretics, e.g. thiazides, ethacrynic acid, and frusemide.

Abnormal glucose tolerance tests have also been associated with starvation and high fat diets and with Friedrickson-type IV hyperlipidaemia: the latter can be corrected by diet when the diabetes improves as well.

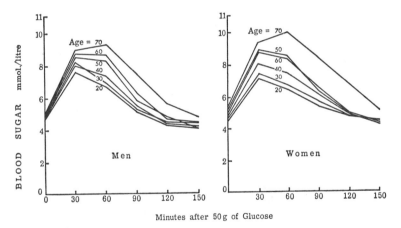

Minutes after 50 g of Glucose

THE MEAN GLUCOSE TOLERANCE CURVES IN SEX AND AGE GROUPS (40–50 SUBJECTS PER GROUP) IN APPARENTLY NORMAL PEOPLE

Symptoms and Presentation

Depending largely upon the severity and rapidity of the metabolic decompensation, hyperglycaemic patients may present in four ways, irrespective of the possible precipitating factors.

1. *Acute Onset.* The patient suffers intense polyuria, polydypsia, rapidly loses weight, becomes ketoacidotic and unless treatment is begun usually passes into coma within a few days or weeks. Less frequent symptoms include irritability, vomiting, abdominal pain, muscle cramps and

peripheral tingling. This onset is usual (but not universal) among children and adolescent diabetics, but may occur among the elderly.

2. *Gradual Onset.* There is much less intense thirst and polyuria, although nocturia may be noted. The obese may lose 0·5–1·0 kilo over a period of months, or may have gained weight lately. Pruritus vulvae or crops of boils may occur; lassitude is common, and middle-aged males may complain of loss of libido, and impotence. This onset is usual in middle life, but may be observed among younger and older patients.

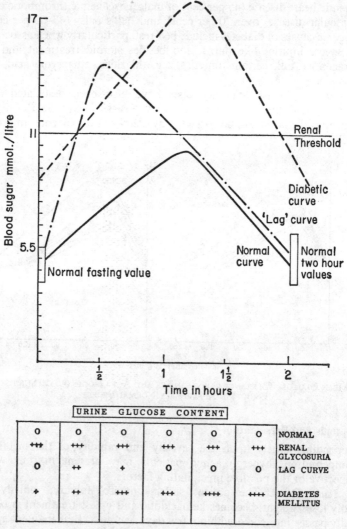

URINE GLUCOSE CONTENT						
0	0	0	0	0	0	NORMAL
+++	+++	+++	+++	+++	+++	RENAL GLYCOSURIA
0	++	+	0	0	0	LAG CURVE
+	++	+++	+++	++++	++++	DIABETES MELLITUS

GLUCOSE TOLERANCE TEST SHOWING VARIOUS TYPES OF CURVES

3. *Symptoms of Complications.* Many older diabetics present with symptoms from the complications of diabetes in the eye (cataract, retinopathy), peripheral nerves (neuropathy), kidneys (nephrotic syndrome), blood vessels (coronary artery disease, intermittent claudication, and gangrene).

4. *Asymptomatic Glycosuria.* Many adult and elderly patients are detected at the stage before symptoms (but not necessarily signs) emerge, as a result of the chance findings of glycosuria at insurance examinations

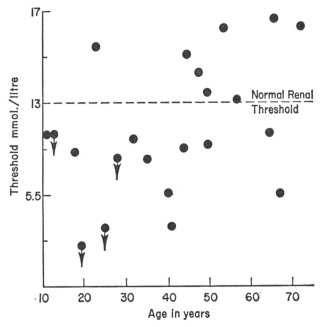

RENAL GLUCOSE THRESHOLD IN 22 DIABETIC PATIENTS.
Note the high thresholds which may be found in the older age group.

or in routine testing. This glycosuria must be distinguished from other reducing substances (with Clinistix or Testape) and from renal glycosuria by a glucose tolerance test. Because diabetics' health and subsequent enjoyment of life may be grossly impaired without the patient recognising any specific diabetic symptoms, early detection and treatment is now being widely advocated and practised.

Signs and Complications

The diabetic patient must be examined thoroughly to establish the diagnosis, to assess the severity of the metabolic decompensation and/or complications, to decide on treatment and to judge progress.

Evidence of glycosuria may be provided by penile irritation or balanitis and even glucose spots on shoes from urine splashes, and the excoriations of pruritus vulvae in women. Evidence of dehydration may be available from a dry tongue, soft eyeballs and dry skin.

   (1) *In the Eyes*

      (a) Diabetic retinopathy—ophthalmoscopic examination shows earliest a shiny 'wet' retina, then venous engorgement. Small red dots, actually capillary microaneurysms, and 'blot' haemorrhages, which may be large microaneurysms or small haemorrhages, have been detected in 95 per cent of hyperglycaemic cases after 15–25 years. Disturbances of blood

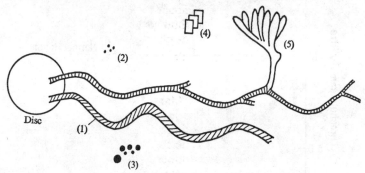

FUNDAMENTAL CHANGES IN DIABETIC RETINOPATHY.

(1) Tortuous enlarged retinal veins.
(2) Dark red 'dots'—microaneurysms (smallest not visible with clinical ophthalmoscope).
(3) Dark red 'blots'—larger microaneurysms or small haemorrhages.
(4) 'Hard exudates'—actually lipid accumulations.
(5) Skein of proliferating vessels—proliferative retinopathy (progressive loss of sight and prone to intra-ocular haemorrhage).

      lipids lead to scattered 'hard' waxy exudates. Most serious is proliferative retinopathy where delicate new vessels grow forward into the globe. These may cause haziness of the vitreous, haemorrhages, retinal detachment, fibrosis, scarring and loss of vision.

      (b) Diabetic cataracts—in older patients these are associated with generalised clouding of the lens, sometimes with (6–10) radially arranged 'faults'—sharp edged opacities like spokes in a farm wagon wheel.

      (c) Iritis rubeosa—reddening of the iris at the margin of the pupil due to microaneurysms which may lead to glaucoma.

   (2) *In the Blood Vessels*

Evidence of impaired circulation to the feet should be carefully sought (cold toes, or foot, atrophic skin, poor hair or nail growth) as gangrene here is severely incapacitating and should be prevented by foot care whenever possible. Particularly significant are small ischaemic areas which seem to be related to the obstruction of endarteries with glycoproteins.

(a) All peripheral pulses should be palpated: absent ankle pulses may occur with ageing, but are more common among diabetics.

(b) The main vessels should be auscultated for the occasional bruit, especially the abdominal aorta, renal arteries, iliac and femoral vessels. The findings should be recorded and hyperlipidaemia suspected, and if present, treated.

(c) Blood pressure should be measured lying and standing to detect sympathetic neuropathy.

(d) An electrocardiogram should be recorded.

(e) Diabetics occasionally show idiopathic ankle oedema, quite separate from the oedema of renal disease. It may occur after the start of insulin therapy: its significance is not understood.

(3) *In the Nervous System*

(a) Peripheral neuropathy. Many people over 65 years of age lose one or both ankle jerks and vibration sense over the malleoli, but these may also be signs of early diabetic peripheral neuritis. If bilateral, diabetes should be excluded. Usually confined to the lower limbs, neuropathy is associated with tingling and pain, stocking anaesthesia and, in severe cases, muscle weakness and wasting.

(b) Mononeuritis multiplex (p. 325). A peripheral nerve is suddenly affected, leading to muscle weakness and wasting and an area of anaesthesia.

(c) Radiculitis (rare). This may precede clinical recognition of diabetes. It is associated with pain, tingling or scalding sensations in the segment affected and is frequently self-limiting to about two years.

(d) Amyotrophy.

(e) Irregularity of the pupils (not uncommon) and palsies of the extra ocular muscles (rare).

(f) Damage to the autonomic nervous system causing impotence in males and loss of orgasm in females, nocturnal diarrhoea, postural hypotension and loss of sweating over the lower limbs.

(4) *In the Renal Tract* (see p. 414).

(5) *In the Skin*

(a) At blood sugar levels over 13·0 mmol./litre, glucose appears in the sweat. Skin infections, particularly boils and monilial infections of the vulva, are common in diabetics.

(b) Hypercholesterolaemia and hyperlipaemia occasionally lead to the formation of xanthomata in the skin, small hard yellowish nodules up to a few millimetres in diameter.

(c) Insulin injections may lead to changes in the skin (in 20–30 per cent of cases) either hypertrophy or atrophy (see p. 448).

(6) There is an association between tuberculosis and diabetes, and all suspected cases should have a chest radiograph.

The Classification of Diabetes

Diabetes produces a number of clinical pictures. The current W.H.O. recommendations regarding definitions and classifications are as follows:

(1) Recognised onset during growth between ages 0–14 years (*Infantile or Childhood Diabetics*). These patients usually present with severe initial symptoms and rapidly become insulin-dependent.

(2) Recognised onset between 15 and 24 years (*Young Diabetics*). These patients usually have an acute onset of symptoms and most may be expected to become insulin-dependent. However, in the tropics, cases in this age group may resemble the adult cases (see below).

(3) Recognised onset between 25 and 64 years (*Adult Diabetics*). Growth onset, insulin-dependent diabetes may occur up to the age of 22 or 23 years, but between 20 and 35 years such cases merge into the adult-onset cases who are much less insulin-dependent. These patients begin with variable symptoms and may or may not need insulin.

(4) Recognised onset over 65 years of age (*Elderly Diabetics*). These patients frequently present with symptoms of the complications of diabetes and can often be controlled without insulin.

It should be noted that all classifications refer to the age *when the diabetes was recognised, not* the current age of the patient.

In addition to these classifications by age, the W.H.O. Committee recognised certain other types of diabetes which were defined as follows:

Juvenile type diabetes. This term should refer to cases of any age group who require insulin and who are prone to attacks of ketosis.

Brittle diabetes. It was recommended that this term be used as little as possible. It refers to juvenile cases who prove difficult to stabilise swinging from heavy glycosuria and ketosis to hypoglycaemia. Erroneous urine test information due to incomplete bladder emptying, secondary to diabetic autonomic neuropathy, must be ruled out. Genuine brittle diabetics are very uncommon and the brittle state does not necessarily persist.

Insulin-resistant diabetes. This term should be reserved for patients requiring over 200 units insulin daily.

Endocrine diabetes. Cases where the disordered carbohydrate tolerance can be attributed to the endocrinological disease, e.g. Cushing's syndrome.

Treatment of Diabetes Mellitus

Introduction

In the past there have been two schools of thought, those who advocated strict control and those who felt that provided the patient was not hypoglycaemic or ketotic, little needed to be done. Longer experience suggests that only by the most careful control can complications be postponed and life prolonged. Unfortunately even the strictest control by present methods will not prevent complications developing ultimately in some cases; nevertheless the incidence of some complications—cataracts, skin infections—is less and expectation of life is far greater in those diabetics who have always been carefully controlled.

Control may be assessed by the urinary glucose provided that the renal threshold is normal and that the renal function is not impaired. It should be checked by blood-sugar estimation every three months. The patient should be 'lean and spry', neither gaining nor losing weight, eating an adequate and enjoyable diet, taking exercise reasonable for his age, free from all diabetic complications, and subject to neither hyperglycaemia nor hypoglycaemia at any time in the 24 hours. The metabolic management should be, assuming a normal renal threshold, to keep the urine as nearly sugar free as possible. Glycosuria should not exceed 5–10 g. a day, and although this is compatible with a single 2 per cent glycosuric sample, wherever possible urine samples should not contain more than $\frac{1}{2}$ per cent glucose. Obesity must be corrected.

Treatment of Adult and Elderly Diabetics

When diabetes is diagnosed in a middle-aged or elderly person, the patient should be examined carefully and any complications noted—an E.C.G. and chest X-ray should be taken and the urine tested for sugar, acetone and albumin. A midstream urine specimen should be cultured (especially in women). Any existing infection should be treated.

Obesity is often present and weight must be reduced by instituting a suitable diet, having regard to the age, occupation and exercise taken. Reduction in weight resensitizes the tissues to the endogenous insulin and many such cases can be successfully treated by diet alone providing they will cooperate. Appetite supressants such as fenfluramine or similar non-amphetamine derivatives may help in refractory obesity and are often instituted to encourage other patients to maintain weight loss after the first month of successful dieting. The doctor and patient should aim to achieve the ideal weight for the age, height, and sex, and then a diet supplying adequate but not excess calories should be prescribed, with limitation of carbohydrate. In general, patients are offered too much to eat. Only the heaviest labourers require more than 3,000 Calories (12·54 mega J) daily; most patients need between 1,800 (7·52 mega J) and 2,500 (10·45 mega J) Calories, and women rather less than men. Few patients are adequately controlled on diets containing much more than 150 g. carbohydrate in 24 hours. It is important to realise that some diabetics may take up to *four weeks* to respond fully to diet. If after 2–3 months blood sugars are not in the normal range—fasting blood glucose less than 5·5 mmol./litre or random blood sugars less than 11·0 mmol./litre—all hyperglycaemic agents should be considered.

Oral Hypoglycaemia Agents

There are many advantages in the use of oral agents for the control of diabetes mellitus. Injections are never welcome at any age, and may be impossible in the aged, handicapped or partially sighted patient. If it could be shown that these preparations were able to control (p. 439) complications as effectively as they lower the blood sugar then there would be few reservations about their use. Unfortunately, this is far from certain, indeed recently it has been suggested that the tendency to develop vascular disease may be increased in patients where hyperglycaemia is controlled by tablets and dietary restrictions neglected.

It is therefore wise to restrict the use of oral hypoglycaemia agents to those patients in whom diet manifestly fails despite conscientious effort by the patient and doctor, and whose hyperglycaemia can be controlled by tablets without recourse to insulin. Because of the ease of administration compared to rigorous dieting, oral hypoglycaemic agents are probably overprescribed.

The sulfonylureas, which stimulate the release of endogenous insulin from the remaining active beta cells, should not be used for undieted obese patients or during pregnancy. They are probably the logical therapy for nonobese elderly cases. The more useful compounds are tolbutamide, chlorpropamide and glibenclamide.

Tolbutamide and glibenclamide have short actions, and must be given two or three times daily. Clinical hypoglycaemia is rare with tolbutamide but has been observed more often with chlorpropamide, largely by neglect of the fact that the full effect of the once daily tablet develops slowly over one to two weeks. In addition doses above 250 mg. daily are rarely required and merely serve to increase the incidence of side effects without improving control of the diabetes. Acetohexamide and tolazamide are intermediate in their time of action. Hypothyroidism and jaundice from biliary stasis have been attributed to these drugs, and they occasionally cause rashes, fever, or flushing after food.

The biguanides lower the blood sugar in diabetics but parodoxically not in normal subjects. They reduce hepatic glucose release, increase peripheral insulin action, and in high doses reduce gastro-intestinal absorption.

Logically they should be tried in overweight diabetics but their general use has been hampered by the side effects, nausea, diarrhoea and vomiting. These symptoms can be reduced by starting therapy with small doses, e.g. Metformin 850 mg. b.d. with meals, increasing the dose gradually every 3–4 days. Besides the adverse side effects on the gastro-intestinal tract, biguanides should not be used in cases with hepatorenal failure. Patients taking biguanides normally show a slight rise in the concentration of lactic acid in the blood. Following excessive alcohol consumption or if they have hepatic or liver damage they may develop *acute lactic acidosis*. This presents as general malaise with clouding of consciousness and finally coma. The prognosis is poor. Treatment consists of stopping the biguanide and attempting to neutralise the acidosis by infusion of bicarbonate.

ORAL HYPOGLYCAEMIC COMPOUNDS

Approved name	Proprietary name	Average daily dose (mg.)	Strength of tablets (mg.)	Contra-indications
Sulfonylureas:				
Tolbutamide	Rastinon	1,500	500	
Chlorpropamide	Diabinase	250	100, 250	liver disease renal failure
Acetohexamide	Dimelor	1,000	500	
Tolazamide	Tolanase	250	100, 250	
Glibenclamide	Euglucon	15	5	
Glipizide	Minodiab	5		
Diguanides:				
Metformin	Glucophage	1,500	500 850	renal or liver disease

Treatment of Juvenile Diabetes

All young thin diabetics require both insulin and diet, and need to have these matched to the amount of physical exercise they take daily. Clearly a heavy worker will need more calories than a clerk. It follows that for adequate control a regular amount of activity and a regular diet are essential, and occupations which involve irregular hours, such as commercial travelling, are unsuitable careers for young diabetics to choose. Variation in diet and activity are a major problem during school years, but with patience and persistence most juvenile diabetics remain reasonably well controlled whilst being educated. In general, these children are less suitable for boarding-schools. A useful general guide is to prescribe not less than 70–80 g. protein per day, not more than 150–200 g. carbohydrate and the balance of calories needed as fat.

Insulin

Insulin is a polypeptide, and if taken by mouth is digested to its constituent amino acids. It must therefore be injected subcutaneously at least once daily. A standard insulin syringe should be used, and needles not smaller than size 19. The site of injection should be varied daily; the front of the thigh, over the deltoid muscles, and the lower abdomen are the most

EFFECTS OF SOLUBLE, PROTAMINE AND LENTE INSULIN ON BLOOD SUGAR IN THE ABSENCE OF FOOD.

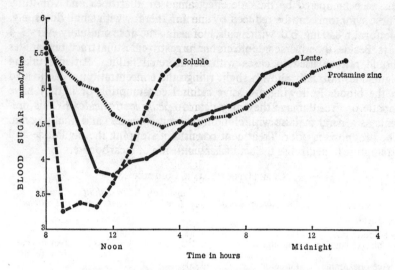

DURATION OF ACTION OF SOLUBLE, PROTAMINE ZINC and LENTE INSULIN

convenient sites for self-injection. Insulin absorption may be marginally faster in warm weather, especially in lean subjects.

Insulin is prepared from the pancreases of cattle (most British, American and Western European preparations) or pigs (Danish insulins). The species of origin is important because pig insulin is less antigenic than ox insulin and there is poor cross reactivity. Once antibodies have been established (months to years) careless conversion to a different species type has caused hypoglycaemia.

A number of highly purified insulins are now available. They have the advantage of being rarely antigenic. The main indications for their use are insulin resistance resulting from antibodies, allergy to insulin, fat atrophy and diabetes in pregnancy.

(a) *Insulin Injection BP* (*soluble insulin* S.I.) is supplied in concentrations of 20, 40, 80 or 320 units per ml. It is effective quickly but for a relatively short time.

(b) *Actrapid M.C.* Older types of insulin contain various insulin derived polypeptides and polymers. Actrapid M.C. is a highly purified monocomponent insulin and much less likely to provoke antibodies. Otherwise it is similar to Insulin Injection.

(c) *Protamine zinc insulin* (PZI) is supplied as 40 or 80 units per ml. There is usually an excess of protamine except in the isophane preparation, where this is avoided.

(d) *Insulin zinc suspension* (IZS) (Danish Insulin) is prepared either in quick-acting amorphous form (semilente) or the slow-acting crystalline form (ultralente). *Lente insulin* is a mixture of three parts of semilente and seven parts of ultralente. Mixtures of other proportions to suit individual requirements can be made. All these preparations must be shaken well before drawing up the dose.

Monocomponent insulins are now being used in insulin zinc suspensions. Monotard M.C. which is a 3:7 mixture of amorphous and crystalline monocomponent insulins has a duration of activity of about twenty hours.

(e) *Biphasic insulins* are mixtures of rapid initial acting and intermediate acting insulins; Rapitard M.C. is made up of highly purified insulins and has a duration of activity of about twenty hours.

The importance of clear prescription of insulin is stressed. The variety, strength, and dose should all be indicated, e.g. R IZS lente (40/c.c.) 20 units subcutaneously each morning. Many emergencies in practice are avoided by this simple expedient.

Many diabetics are controlled on mixtures of SI and PZI. Provided that the injection is given at once and not left to stand both may be drawn into the same syringe and injected as a mixture. Recently more use has been made of insulin zinc suspension. Most diabetics requiring less than 60 units of insulin daily can be easily controlled with lente insulin. Most patients requiring between 60 and 100 units are better managed with a mixture of SI and PZI. Those few patients requiring very large doses of insulin should receive two or more injections of soluble insulin daily.

Controlling Diabetes with Insulin

Assuming a normal renal threshold, the urine may be used as a rough index of control. The patient is taught to test the overnight urine, and then after breakfast, lunch, and tea, and immediately before bed, and to record the results. An initial dose of 20 units of SI in the morning just before or just after breakfast and 10 units just before or just after the evening meal are prescribed, and the effect on the urinary glucose observed. Changes should not be made at less than three-day intervals unless hypoglycaemia occurs. Appropriate adjustments are made until the patient is sugar free and not hypoglycaemic; this is much best done as an outpatient under normal life conditions. One caveat—all diabetics on soluble insulin in the morning must take a small mid-morning carbohydrate snack, especially if their over-night urine is sugar-free.

When control appears adequate, and more particularly in mild, easily controlled older cases, the patient may be changed to one injection daily of IZS or to a mixture of SI and PZI. It is important to remember that SI can be mixed with PZI, but not with IZS. To effect the change, the total number of units required daily is considered. If it is less than 60, then a straight change to an equivalent dose of IZS may be made (unit for unit). Some slight adjustment of this dose may subsequently be required. Between 60 and 100 units better control is achieved with mixtures of SI and PZI. Four-fifths of the total daily requirements of SI are taken, and a quarter of this given as SI, and three-quarters as PZI. Again, some slight adjustment of dose is likely to be required, always remembering that retard insulins act chiefly at night and are therefore reflected in the morning urine, and that soluble insulin acts by day. Before assuming adequate control a series of blood sugars should be estimated throughout an average day. Although sounding complicated this is a simple method of control and works well in almost all cases.

Once control is achieved the urine need be tested only once daily, but at a different time each day, so that in five days tests are made at all critical times. Hospital attendances can also become infrequent; well-controlled cases should be reviewed quarterly, when blood sugar and urine tests for sugar, ketones, and protein should be taken. Careful records of weight must be kept, and chest radiographs taken annually. Care of the feet should be emphasised, especially in the elderly, and chiropody arranged when necessary.

Complications of Insulin Treatment

(1) Repeated use of the same site for insulin injections may lead to a gross thickening of subcutaneous tissues, chiefly fat, so-called *lipohypertrophy*. It is often due to insulin being injected too deeply, directly into subcutaneous adipose tissue. In other patients the subcutaneous fat rapidly disappears at the site of injections (*lipoatrophy*). It is frequently due to insulin injections being too shallow, that is, intradermal. It usually occurs early in insulin treatment, and cannot be avoided by varying the injection site. It is usually self limiting.

(2) *Hypoglycaemia* may result from an insulin overdose; this may be caused by mis-measurement, by unwittingly using insulin of increased strength (40 or 80 instead of 20 units per ml.) or by the too-rapid action of insulin, either from increased physical activity or from failing to take an expected meal, especially the mid-morning snack, or from careless change to a preparation using insulin of a different species. Treatment, see p. 454.

Difficulties in Diabetic Control

Insulin resistance in insulin-requiring diabetics is rare. The diagnosis is usually made either when insulin is incorrectly prescribed (for 'elderly' diabetics) or incorrectly given. The common causes of failure of control if insulin is correctly prescribed and injected are:

(1) *Failure to Diet*. It is difficult to persuade patients with only minor symptoms to accept dietary restriction. Failure to comply is soon revealed by serial observation of body weight. Alcoholics, narcotic addicts, and psychopathic patients are unable to accept restrictions, and suffer accordingly.

(2) *Cryptic Infection.* Pulmonary tuberculosis is the most serious of these, chronic pyelonephritis the commonest. Septic teeth tonsils and adenoids, especially in children, may be important. Cholecystitis should be excluded.

(3) *Marked Variation in Physical Activity.* This applies particularly to schoolchildren, when great ingenuity must be used to balance diet, activity, and insulin. Some adult occupations are too irregular to be suitable.

(4) Genuine *insulin resistance* rarely exists. It occurs when there is failure of absorption of insulin from a too frequently used site at which either severe lipoatrophy or hypertrophy has occurred, when there are antibodies to insulin present in the plasma, and when there are abnormalities of intra-cellular glucose metabolism which are not wholly corrected by insulin. These cases may present as unstable, or brittle diabetics, who pass easily and rapidly from hypo- to hyperglycaemia and ketosis.

Diabetic Crisis (Ketoacidosis)

Untreated diabetes eventually leads to coma but this should not arise in cases under proper medical surveillance. However, stresses such as *intercurrent infections* frequently upset diabetic control and may create a medical emergency without coma supervening. The occurrence of glycosuria of 2 per cent or more, with ketonuria and ketonaemia, in a drowsy patient who appears ill should be regarded as a *DIABETIC CRISIS.* It must be appreciated that all degrees of crisis exist; the severity is proportional to the ketosis, not to the level of the blood sugar. In the presence of renal disease, ischaemic or other, urinary ketones are not an adequate index of ketosis. Blood ketones or plasma bicarbonate should be estimated.

While starting treatment a careful examination must be made to try to discover the initiating cause of the crisis; infection, infarction, trauma, or neglect being the commonest. But treatment is a matter of urgency, and should not be unduly delayed by prolonged search for causes. Two other words of warning. The patients should be disturbed as little as possible; routine nursing procedures may be omitted until the patient is fully conscious. Better a dirty diabetic than a clean corpse. Second, while there is ketosis there will be resistance to the action of insulin. As soon as ketosis begins to subside, sensitivity to the action of insulin increases sharply; it is possible to precipitate hypoglycaemia by too vigorous therapy. The regime detailed below is suitable for a diabetic deeply in coma. It should be discreetly interpreted for minor stages of crisis.

Treatment of Diabetic Crisis. The objects of treatment are first to treat precipitating causes, including infection; second to correct dehydration; third to replace lost electrolytes; and to re-establish the metabolism of carbohydrate.

(1) An initial blood sample should be taken for full investigations:

sugar, ketones, haematocrit. plasma bicarbonate, sodium, potassium and urea. If facilities are available, the pH of an arterial blood sample will be useful in severe acidosis. In the elderly or those with cardiac disease a central venous pressure line is useful in monitoring the rate of intravenous infusion. These results serve as an invaluable base line.

(2) *Replacement Therapy.* Intravenous replacement of lost fluid and cations is essential to prevent circulatory failure and to maintain renal function. One litre of normal saline should be given in the first half hour and a further litre in the next hour. Thereafter the infusion should be modified to the needs of the patient. If the plasma sodium rises above 150 mmol./litre, N/2 saline should be used. The plasma glucose should also be monitored and 5 per cent dextrose used if it falls below 14 mmol./litre. It is usual to avoid alkaline solutions for infusion even in face of acidosis as they can produce distortion of the acid/base balance. However if the plasma pH is very low (below pH 7·0) 100 mmol. of sodium bicarbonate should be given and the response checked by measurement of the pH of the arterial blood.

Patients in diabetic crisis are depleted of potassium and this should be given at the rate of 13 mmol./hour immediately insulin treatment is started and modified by estimation of plasma potassium concentration. When glucose passes into the cells as a result of giving insulin, potassium ions also diffuse into the cells with a resulting fall in the plasma level.

(3) *Insulin.* Soluble or Actrapid insulin should be used and can be given either by intravenous infusion which will require an infusion pump or by repeated intramuscular injections.

> (a) *Infusion.* The usual rate is 3–6 units hourly. Although the amount of insulin being given is very small and in spite of rapid clearance from the blood, a steady and adequate concentration can be maintained.
>
> (b) *Intramuscularly.* 20 units are given stat followed by 5·0 units hourly until the blood glucose level falls to 14 mmol./litre.

(4) *Antibiotics.* One million units of benzylpenicillin should be given intramuscularly at once and daily thereafter for five days.

(5) *Clinical Studies.* When appropriate insulin and antibiotic therapy has been instituted, blood may be withdrawn from the catheter inserted for intravenous therapy for chemical analysis *at two hourly intervals.* If the patient is comatose an in-dwelling catheter may be left in the bladder, and all urine withdrawn hourly and tested for ketones and sugar. An E.C.G. is useful at this stage; it may show evidence of hyper- or hypokalaemia or reveal a myocardial infarct, which may have been the initiating cause of the coma.

Subsequent Treatment. Treatment with insulin and normal saline infusion is continued until the plasma glucose level has fallen below 14 mmol./litre. Intramuscular or intravenous insulin is stopped and treatment with subcutaneous insulin resumed. 5 per cent dextrose infusion should replace normal saline but potassium replacement should continue.

Oral feeding should be resumed as soon as possible and potassium given in the form of Slow-K and potassium-rich foods such as orange juice, tomato juice or Horlicks.

Non-Keto-Acidotic (Hyper-Osmolar) Diabetic Coma

Although this condition was first described in 1886 it is only in recent years that it has been widely reported, and at the time of writing appears increasingly common. The reasons for this change are not apparent.

It occurs in elderly often obese subjects, more frequently females than males, and in the U.K. is commonest in immigrants from the West Indies. It is of insidious onset, and usually presents as disordered consciousness, ranging from mild confusion to deep coma. Focal neurological signs may develop, and epilepsy has been recorded. The outstanding features on clinical examination are deranged consciousness, dehydration (p. 422) and the absence of ketosis; the patients may be covered with a uraemic frost.

When the diagnosis is suspected it may be confirmed by measuring the blood sugar level, which is always greatly raised (above 45 mmol./litre.) The plasma bicarbonate is however normal. The plasma sodium is often above 150 mmol./litre and the blood urea above 20 mmol./litre. The plasma osmolality is raised above 380 m. Osm./litre.

Treatment consists of correcting the dehydration and hyperosmolality intravenously. The repair fluid of choice is 0·5 normal sodium chloride, supplemented by water by mouth or naso-gastric drip. Care must be taken not to provoke pulmonary oedema by too rapid intravenous therapy, and the progress of treatment can be monitored by serial haemotocrit studies. There is no indication for bicarbonate in the absence of acidosis, and hyperglycaemia is corrected with insulin.

Prognosis has been variably reported, but with earlier recognition of the condition is improving. Subsequent management of the diabetes (p. 443) is not difficult.

Hyperosmolality of comparable degree also occurs in ketotic diabetic coma, and the outstanding difference in the present group is the absence of ketotis rather than the presence of hyperosmolality. The explanation of the absence of ketosis is not at present known.

Diabetes in Special Circumstances

(a) *Pregnancy*. Diabetic women are less fertile, more prone to miscarry and to toxaemia of pregnancy and hydramnios than their healthy sisters. Their babies are more likely to die *in utero*, to be born grossly overweight, to suffer congenital malformations or to perish shortly before or after birth. Whereas the maternal mortality rate has improved markedly in the last twenty-five years, the foetal mortality in babies born to diabetic mothers remains over 10 per cent.

Diabetes almost always becomes more severe during pregnancy; indeed, it may be precipitated or unmasked by it. Insulin requirements usually increase sharply for the first trimester, remain steady for the second, and usually increase but occasionally decrease during the third. They decline very sharply after parturition and close observation is necessary to avoid hypoglycaemia. Breast feeding almost always fails, and many obstetricians artificially suppress lactation immediately after birth. Because the power of the cells in the proximal renal tubule to reabsorb glucose is impaired in pregnancy the renal threshold falls, and therefore the urinary glucose is not an adequate index of control and blood glucose levels must be estimated.

Because of the dangers of intra-uterine death, termination of pregnancy either by induction of labour or elective caesarian section is indicated at 36 weeks. Some of the fatalities in the infants can be traced to a hyaline membrane lining the alveoli, a few to hypoglycaemia, but many remain unexplained.

(b) *During Infection.* Insulin requirements increase with infection, and this is true of gastro-enteritis with vomiting and anorexia. The prescribed insulin dose should always be given, and if glycosuria or ketonuria persists it should be increased. Even minor infections in diabetes should be treated seriously.

(c) *During Surgical Operations.* Controlled diabetics undergoing short anaesthetics for elective surgery may safely forgo their treatment and food until they return to the ward. In more severe uncontrolled diabetics, or for prolonged procedures, the usual dose of insulin should be given and an intravenous infusion of 4 per cent dextrose saline set up. When the patient is unconscious estimations of the blood glucose level are made every hour. More insulin or glucose is given appropriately. When severe diabetic ketosis coexists with a surgical emergency, operation should be postponed as long as possible while the treatment for crisis is instituted. *In emergencies soluble insulin should be used as it allows more flexible control.*

DIABETES INSIPIDUS

Introduction. This is a rare disease, characterised by the excretion of a large (10–20 litres/24 hours) urinary volume and consequent great thirst. It is caused either by an absence of antidiuretic hormone from the posterior pituitary gland, or by an inability of the distal renal tubule to respond to its action. Failure of secretion may occur when disease processes affect the region of the pituitary, for example tumours (*c.* 50 per cent), inflammatory disease (*c.* 25 per cent), vascular changes (*c.* 10 per cent), trauma (10 per cent) and Hand-Schüller-Christian disease (*c.* 2–3 per cent).

Clinical Features. The effect of the diuresis is to cause intense thirst, and if fluids are withheld dehydration is rapid, and the signs and symptoms of water deficiency (p. 422), soon appear. The urinary specific gravity is always low, and the urea and chloride levels in the urine reduced. The condition should be suspected in all patients secreting over 4 litres of urine per 24 hours and drinking more than 5 litres per 24 hours. It must be differentiated from diabetes mellitus (glycosuria), terminal renal failure (proteinuria, uraemia) and hysterical over-drinking. Only the last is difficult to separate. Distinction is achieved by showing that intravenous hypertonic saline will temporarily inhibit the diuresis in hysterical patients. It has no effect in diabetes insipidus.

Symptomatic treatment is by means of pitressin, either posterior pituitary powder as snuff, or pitressin tannate (0·5–1·0 ml. daily) intramuscularly or subcutaneously (but never intravenously). A salt-free diet is also useful. Some patients are helped by thiazide diuretics and chlorpropamide is sometimes of value. Cure can only be achieved by treating the cause.

Nephrogenic diabetes insipidus is almost always congenital, very rarely the result of destruction of the distal renal tubule in pyelonephritis. The congenital form is easily recognised by the family history, its early onset, male predominance, and failure to respond to pitressin. Low sodium diets are recommended as treatment, but prognosis is poor.

Inappropriate Secretion of Anti-Diuretic Hormone

In some patients with malignant disease, almost always carcinoma of the bronchus, anti-diuretic hormone may be secreted by the tumour cells and cause water retention with progressive dilution of the plasma electrolytes and urea. This usually presents clinically as a 'low sodium syndrome' (p. 422). Treatment is by water restriction, aldosterone, and the treatment of the underlying condition.

HYPOGLYCAEMIA

Introduction. Symptoms usually appear when the blood glucose has fallen to between 2·2–2·8 mmol./litre. They seem more related to the rate of fall than to the actual level reached, and commonly occur when patients are hungry. Sometimes they can be averted by eating carbohydrate, e.g. chocolate.

Symptoms are of rapid onset and begin with slight unsteadiness, tremulousness, difficulty in concentration, and often headache. They proceed to irrational behaviour, stupor, and coma. Urine may be voided.

Signs. The patient becomes pale, sweats, and the pulse is initially rapid and jerky. When coma is complete the pulse and blood pressure are normal. Severe and prolonged hypoglycaemia may produce irreversible cerebral changes. Epileptic fits may occur and coma may proceed to death.

Causes of Hypoglycaemia

(1) *Insulin overdose*; mismeasured doses, failure to take an expected meal, over-exertion.

(2) *Reactive.*

(3) *Liver disease.* Cirrhosis, subacute necrosis.

(4) *Gastrointestinal disease*—post gastrectomy syndrome; steatorrhoea; after alcoholic excess.

(5) *Endocrine.* Hypopituitarism, hypothyroidism, adrenal insufficiency, as a premonitary occurrence in diabetes mellitus, and in insulin-secreting tumours of the pancreas.

(6) *Sarcomas, secondary carcinomatosis.*

(7) Use of *chlorpropamide*, and other *hypoglycaemic drugs*, especially in non-diabetics.

(8) Side-effects of salicylates, anti-histamines or mono-amine-oxidase inhibitors.

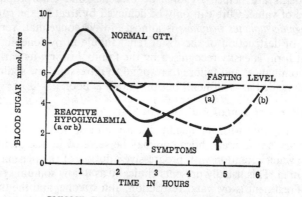

GLUCOSE TOLERANCE TESTS IN NORMAL SUBJECT
AND IN SPONTANEOUS HYPOGLYCAEMIA

Careful history and clinical examination will make nearly all these conditions sufficiently obvious. It is only when it is reactive or when it is due to an insulin secreting tumour that further investigation is usually necessary for diagnosis.

A five hour glucose tolerance test is useful in establishing a diagnosis of reactive hypoglycaemia (see figure above).

In hypoglycaemia due to an insulin producing tumour a prolonged fast (14 hours at least) will lead to a progressive fall in blood glucose (see figure on p. 455). The presence of a low plasma glucose together in an inappropriately high plasma insulin is characteristic of an insulinoma.

A number of other provocative tests are in use and may be helpful in expert hands.

Treatment. Unless von Gierke's disease is suspected, or the coma has been long-standing or very severe the patients may be revived with glucagon. A sugar-containing drink—hot sweet tea or sugar in hot water—is prepared, and an injection of glucagon 1–2 mg. intramuscularly is given. This produces a transient hyperglycaemia, with partial recovery of consciousness, during which the sweet drink can be given. Failing this, a stomach tube can be passed and the sweet drink given through this. It is better to give an intravenous injection of 20 ml. of 50 per cent glucose solution.

Subsequent treatment depends on the cause of the hypoglycaemia. If it

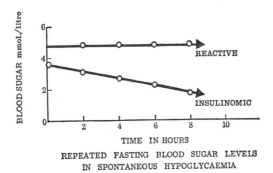

REPEATED FASTING BLOOD SUGAR LEVELS
IN SPONTANEOUS HYPOGLYCAEMIA

is due to an insulin-secreting tumour (extremely rare) this should be removed surgically. If due to 'reactive hypoglycaemia' then best results are obtained with a high-protein diet and small frequent meals.

DISORDERS OF FAT METABOLISM
OBESITY

This is a serious disease, common in prosperous communities. It results from eating more food than is required. The common cause accounting for over 90 per cent of cases of this hyperphagia is gluttony, but it may also occur in hypothalamic disorders or as a sequel to severe emotional stress. The rate of weight gain is proportional to the extent of dietary excess over requirement; once obesity is established, however, it may be maintained by quite small food intake. Fat can only be removed by eating less food than is required. Actuarial analysis shows that even minor degrees of obesity decrease the expectation of life, and gross fatness severely so. Weight is gained in myxoedema, but is not due to fat.

Obesity may occur at any age; it is most common in the prosperous years of life, and the appearance of the plump matron or city alderman is familiar. Rarely the distribution of fat is unusual. In Cushing's syndrome (p. 477) it affects the head, neck, and shoulders chiefly, and spares the legs; the reverse is true in *lipodystrophia progressiva*. This is most common in women, who show little fat above the waist, but are obese about the buttocks and legs. There is a rare association of obesity with cystic disease of the ovaries (*Stein-Leventhal syndrome*, p. 490). Many fat women have menstrual irregularities which usually remit when ideal weight is achieved.

The appearance of fat is due to hypertrophy of fat-bearing cells. If obesity appears early in life, then the actual number of fat bearing cells may be greatly increased. In some cases local hyperplasia occurs, causing painful fatty lumps in the adipose tissue (Dercum's disease). Obesity may occur in children, most frequently the young child of elderly parents. Fat accumulates generally, but is well marked in the mons pubis; this sporran of fat overhanging normal genitalia (where there is no subcutaneous fat) often leads wrongly to a diagnosis of *Frolich's syndrome*, an extremely rare condition.

The effects of obesity are widespread. Extra effort is required for all activity, and extra blood and energy for the metabolism of fat. This increases the demands on the heart and lungs, and excess obesity may itself cause heart failure from restriction of respiratory excursion. The appearance of these grotesquely bloated patients in severe congestive cardiac failure, markedly cyanosed, with polycythaemia rubra, and gross oedema (*Pickwickian syndrome*) is unforgettable. Even minor degrees of obesity may induce failure in an already diseased heart.

Direct mechanical effects of obesity too must be considered. Joints and ligaments suffer from the extra weight that they are called upon to support. Osteoarthritis is common in the knees, and skeletal pains from undue tension in ligaments are the rule. The skin creases are exaggerated, and bebecome keratinised. They are difficult to keep clean, and fungus infection and other skin sepsis is common. Because of the insulating effect of fat it is difficult for the body to lose heat. In spite of profuse sweating discomfort may be acute in hot weather. Added to these are the more mundane difficulties of obtaining appropriate clothes, rising from chairs, and entering and alighting from vehicles.

There also exists a predisposition to certain diseases. Diabetes mellitus (p. 434) is much commoner in the obese, and there is increased tendency to atheroma. Hypertensives are commonly overweight, and the risks of anaesthesia and surgery are greatly increased in the obese.

Treatment. The energy equivalent of adipose tissue is so great that exercise is of little value in treatment. It is calculated that a pound of fat would be lost for every 25 miles run! There is no benefit from hot baths, purgation, or massage. Nor is there any place for thyroid extract, which may cause irreversible exophthalmos. It may be that a few patients are helped a little by diuretics, but undoubtedly the main treatment is simply dietary restriction.

Many suitable diets for the treatment of obesity are available. Mild cases may follow a quite simple diet, merely avoiding fat and carbohydrate in normal meals. This may be reinforced by a day's starvation during the week. Drastic restriction is required in more severe degrees of obesity. The most extreme cases resemble the addiction states, and are best admitted to hospital, and supplied with only 200 calories daily; extra vitamins and iron should be given if this is undertaken. Most patients will tolerate this for 2 to 3 weeks, after which the diet may be increased to 400 calories daily. After a week or so apparent constipation occurs, from reduced faecal residue. This may be treated with methyl cellulose and liquid paraffin 15·0 ml. at night. The ultimate objects are to restore the patient to his ideal weight, to enable him to conquer his hyperphagia, and to be discharged content to eat a normal diet. These may imply a profound alteration in his way of life; simple psychotherapy and supportive interviews may be necessary for some months.

ATHEROMA AND HYPERLIPIDAEMIAS

Introduction. Arterial disease as a sequel to atheroma is a major cause of ill health. Deaths attributable to it are increasing exponentially in all civilised countries. There are many features which make it probable that it is of environmental origin. For example, man is the only mammal in which atheroma is significant; it is rarely present at birth, but increases in extent and severity throughout life. It may, however, be modified by endogenous factors. It is rarely severe in healthy women until the menopause; it is more extensive and has more complications in patients with certain maladies, for example diabetes mellitus, familial xanthomatosis, and nephrosis. It results in either abrupt or slow closure of arteries, with consequent deprivation of vital tissues of blood. It is ubiquitous and is a major cause of hospital admissions. It is the underlying cause of angina pectoris, and coronary artery disease, of cerebral vascular disease, intermittent claudication and gangrene, of much atrial fibrillation and retinal disease and most mesenteric thromboses.

	TYPE	NORMAL	I	II	III	IV	V
ELECTROPHORETIC LIPOPROTEIN PATTERNS	CHYLOMICRONS origin BETA LIPOPROTEIN PRE-BETA LIPOPROTEINS ALPHA LIPOPROTEIN						
CHOLESTEROL mmol./litre		4.7–5.7	+	+	++	NORMAL or LITTLE +	+
TRIGLYCERIDES mmol./litre		0.4–1.7	+++	NORMAL or LITTLE +	+	+	++
GLUCOSE TOLERANCE TEST		NORMAL	NORMAL	NORMAL	40% IMPAIRED	IMPAIRED	IMPAIRED
URATE mmol./litre		0.20–0.43	NORMAL	NORMAL	+	+	+

Plasma electrophoretic patterns, cholesterol, uric acid and triglyceride levels, with glucose tolerance tests in normal and hyperlipidaemic subjects. (after FREDRICKSON)

Aetiology. Of the endogenous factors, a familial history and hyperlipidaemia are the most constant associations. The technique of plasma electrophoresis has led to the easy separation of the protein fractions and subsequent staining for fat has shown where the lipids are bound to protein moieties. Plasma cholesterol and triglyceride levels have also been examined, and from these data a 'lipid profile' of the plasma has been constructed (above). The patterns of lipid carriage so derived point to at least five phenotypes (Fredrickson 1968).

Type I (Exogenous Hypertriglyceridaemia)

This is a rare disease affecting chiefly children, and inherited as an autosomal recessive. In the few adult cases recorded, no relationship with atheroma has been demonstrated. It is characterised by creamy plasma from excess of chylomicrons following about 15 hours after a fatty meal.

Type II (Hyperbeta Lipoproteinaemia)

A common disease of adult life, inherited as a Mendelian dominant character. It is strongly associated with the development of atheroma. In the heterozygotes subcutaneous xanthomata of the elbows, hands, knees and heels may occur. It may occur as a secondary phenomenon to a variety of diseases, for example, myxoedema, nephrosis, myeloma, and liver disorders.

Type III ('Broad Beta Disease')

A disease, occurring chiefly in men aged 20 to 40 years and inherited as an autosomal recessive. It is characterised by the appearance of flat linear deposits of lipids in the subcutaneous tissues, usually of the hands (planar xanthomas), and of lumpy deposits at the elbows, knees, and buttocks (tubo-eruptive zanthomas). It is strongly associated with the early appearance of atheroma.

Type IV (Endogenous Triglyceridaemia)

This is the commonest of the five groups described. It occurs in adult life, but neither its cause nor its inheritance are currently known. It is believed to reflect an imbalance between the endogenous synthesis and removal of glycerides, and is frequently unmasked by obesity. It is often seen in association with other diseases, for example, diabetes mellitus and the nephrotic syndrome. There is a strong association with early atheroma. On examination, lipaemia retinalis, eruptive xanthomata, and hepatosplenomegaly may be found.

Type V (Mixed Hyperlipidaemia)

This is an uncommon lipid pattern seen usually between 10 and 30 years. It is commonly secondary to other diseases, for example, nephrosis, diabetic acidosis, and myxoedema. Clinically it resembles type IV but recurrent bouts of abdominal pain are common. The nature of its inheritance is not yet known nor is its relationship to type IV at all clear. No certain association with early atheroma has been found.

(1) Control of Plasma Lipids

Type I   Diet with fat reduced to 50 g. daily.

Type II   Diet should be low in cholesterol and high in unsaturated fatty acids. This means a diet low in dairy produce, eggs and meat together with the use of cooking oil and margarine made from unsaturated fats.

Cholestyramine in doses 12–30 g. daily binds with cholesterol and decreases absorption and is useful when diet alone fails. Alternatively clofibrate 1·5 g. daily which also lowers serum cholesterol.

Type III   Diet should aim to lose weight and alcohol must be avoided. Clofibrate as above is a useful adjunct.

Type IV   Low carbohydrate diet.

Type V   Low carbohydrate and fat so as to produce weight loss.

(2) *Local*

In some cases parts of arteries may be resected and replaced by grafts. This is almost confined to the larger vessels, for example, the carotid and lower aorta or femoral arteries.

(3) *General*

(a) Control of predisposing factors such as heavy smoking, obesity, arterial hypertension, and lethargy.

(b) When symptoms appear, e.g. in coronary heart disease (p. 163) and arterial disease (p. 183).

GOUT

Uric Acid Metabolism

The complex compounds in the cell nucleus consist of a protein to which is joined a large polymer named nucleic acid. This is constructed of a number of nucleotides, each consisting of one molecule each of a base (purine or pyrimidine), a pentose (ribose or desoxyribose) and phosphoric acid. When nucleoprotein is broken down nucleic acid is first split off and then degraded to its constituents, ending as xanthine and finally uric acid. This diffuses from the cell into the plasma and is excreted by the kidney. The normal blood level is 0·20–0·43 mmol./litre for men and 0·14–0·33 mmol./litre for women.

It is clear that the blood uric acid may be derived from breakdown of either ingested or endogenous nucleoprotein. It may also be synthesised by the body cells from simple constituents (glycine, glutamine, and ribose phosphate) which are readily available.

Serum levels are raised in primary gout, and in conditions in which there is increased nucleoprotein turnover, for example the leukaemias (particularly myeloid), polycythaemia (primary or secondary), or chronic haemolylic anaemias. It may also be increased in renal disease associated with reduced G.F.R., or from administration of thiazide duiretics.

Introduction

Although the clinical syndrome of gout may occur in any of these conditions the relationship to the level of uric acid in the blood is by no means absolute. This and the predilection of the disease for certain specific tissues, and its precipitation and localisation by trauma, all point to there being some as yet undiscovered tissue factor concerned. The mechanism of production of hyperuricaemia in secondary gout is increased nucleoprotein turnover, or rarely renal retention. In primary gout, however, there is some evidence that increased endogenous synthesis may be the underlying cause. Relatives of patients suffering from primary gout may also develop the disease, and a proportion of them show hyperuricaemia without gout. Inheritance is determined by a single dominant gene. Primary gout does not usually develop in males under thirty and women under fifty.

Clinical Features

(1) *Arthritis.* This is usually an acute intermittent monoarthritis. The commonest joint to be affected is the first metatarso-phalangeal, but none is immune. The large joints are only occasionally affected, and a generalised polyarthritis of the rheumatoid type is a rarity. The attacks may be precipitated by overactivity, trauma, or diuresis; frequently no cause can be found. They usually begin at night, are sudden in onset, and are extremely painful. Movement is excruciatingly painful. On examination the joint is red, hot, swollen, glazed, and exquisitely tender. Left untreated the attack develops in an hour or two, and remits over six or seven days. It is frequently followed by desquamation of the overlying skin, with intense itching. The attack is accompanied by malaise and extreme irritability, with fever and leucocytosis.

(2) *Deposits* of crystals of sodium biurate occur in the subcutaneous tissues of the dorsum of the hands, the bursae, particularly the olecranon bursa, the tendons, especially in the forearm, and in the cartilage of the ears, nose, and sometimes eyelids. Typical subcutaneous deposits (tophi) vary in size from peas to pigeons' eggs. The overlying skin is thin and shiny, and the tophus may have ulcerated through and become infected. Sodium biurate is also deposited in the cartilage and juxta-articular bone of the affected joint. Most patients with chronic untreated gout show some renal damage due to deposition of sodium urate crystals. Occasionally this can cause renal failure. About 10 per cent of gouty patients develop uric acid stones.

(3) *Associated Disorders*

(a) Certain acute musculo-skeletal conditions occur more frequently than would be expected by chance in gouty subjects. These include acute tenosynovitis, acute subtendonous bursitis, and acute supraspinatous tendonitis.

(b) There is an occasional association with diabetes mellitus. The structural resemblance of the uric acid molecule to alloxan, a potent beta-cell poison will be recalled.

Diagnosis

(1) The simplest and most certain way is to puncture a tophus with a sterile needle, extract a little of the deposit on the needle point, and examine it microscopically. Typical acicular crystals are seen. Similarly sodium urate crystals can be seen in fluid, aspirated from the joint in the acute attack.

(2) Estimation of the blood uric acid level is usually valuable. It is raised to above 0·4 mmol./litre in typical cases.

Treatment

(a) *Acute Episodes*

Acute attacks of gout are best treated with phenylbutazone 200 mg. three times daily until symptoms are relieved. It is unsuitable for long-term administration and should not be used at all in patients with a history of dyspepsia. As an alternative indomethacin 50 mg. eight hourly can be used. Colchicine (0·5 mg. two-hourly) may be given, but has the disadvantage of causing nausea and diarrhoea. Prednisolone may also be used: an initial dose of 20–30 mg. should be given orally, followed by 10 mg. eight-hourly until symptoms are relieved. Once this is achieved the dose should be reduced progressively, and omitted in two to three days.

Throughout the attack the limb should be supported, and the patient remain at rest. The affected joint should be protected from the weight of bedclothes.

(b) *Management of Chronic Gout*

(1) *Diet.* The chief source of the blood uric acid is endogenous metabolism, and therefore dietary restrictions need be slight. It is wise to avoid high purine foods, and alcoholic excess, and the patient should reduce to his ideal weight. At least five pints of fluid should be drunk daily to minimise stasis and precipitation of urate in the kidney.

(2) *Excretion of uric acid.* A number of substances interfere with the reabsorption of uric acid by the renal tubule. Of these only sulphinpyrazone and probenecid need be considered. It is clear that once the diagnosis of gout is made, treatment to be wholly effective must continue for the rest of the patient's life. For this reason, toxic effects, palatability, and cost of these substances must be considered. To be effective 50–100 mg. sulphinpyrazone four times daily are required, or 0·5 g. of probenecid four times daily.

These drugs cause an increased amount of urate in the urine. If there is a history of urate stone formation or if the treatment is not effective then allopurinol may be given. This inhibits the enzyme xanthine oxidase, and so prevents the conversion of xanthine to uric acid. Initially treatment may precipitate acute attacks of gout so that it is wise to start with small doses (50 mg. three times daily) later increasing to 200–400 mg. daily in divided doses.

Whatever treatment regimen is used the aim should be to keep the blood uric acid level below 0·4 mmol./litre. If this is achieved attacks will become less frequent and eventually cease, and tophi will absorb, a process which may take a year or more.

PSEUDOGOUT

Closely resembles gout. It usually occurs in middle life, and afflicts one or more joints. It may also complicate chronic renal failure. There is a tendency for the larger joints, particularly the knee, to be affected. The attacks of acute arthritis last days, or a week or two. Occasionally 'pseudo-tophi' are seen in the ears.

Radiographs show striking calcification in cartilage, and none of the rarefied areas in bone seen in gout. Aspiration of the fluid from an acutely inflamed joint shows crystals of *calcium pyrophosphate*, as opposed to uric acid crystals in a gouty joint.

Treatment is the same as acute gout. The disease runs a prolonged course, and joints that are repeatedly affected tend to become osteo-arthritic.

PORPHYRIA

In man, porphyrins are synthesised chiefly in the liver and bone marrow, and the clinical syndromes associated with their disordered metabolism may be divided into the *hepatic* and *erythropoietic* varieties. The initial precursor is glycine, which is changed first to delta-amino-levulinic acid (ALA) and then to porphobilinogen (PBG). This is converted chiefly to uroprophyrin III with a little uroporphyrin I. The uroporphyrin III is further metabolised to protoporphyrin, and finally to haem. It is then available as a protein prosthetic group. In health up to 100 μg./24 hours of porphyrin appears in the urine, of which 60–80 per cent is coproporphyrin I; there is also some uroporphyrin present. The faecal porphyrin amounts to 200–300 μg./24 hours, chiefly coproporphyrin I.

A number of clinical syndromes are associated with disorders of porphyrin metabolism, primary or secondary. The secondary ones are asymptomatic with the exception of lead poisoning, and may occur after poisoning with a large number of substances toxic to the bone marrow. These include phosphorous, arsenic, sedormid, sulphonal, and trional. Lead is the most important, for the occurrence of abdominal colic, constipation, vomiting, and motor polyneuritis makes the differential diagnosis from acute intermittent porphyria a matter of moment. Other evidence of plumbism (*see p. 637 of special Tropical Edition only*), however, and the occurrence in the urine only of coproporphyrin III, which is colourless, and the absence of porphobilinogen, serve to distringuish it.

Of the primary porphyrias, only intermittent acute porphyria (IAP *vide infra*) is anything other than rare, and itself is uncommon. They may be divided clinically as follows:

(1) *Intermittent Acute Porphyria*

This is a dramatic disease. It appears usually in the third decade, and acute exacerbations are often precipitated by barbiturates. The sex incidence is equal, and inheritance seems governed by a dominant gene. Colic, vomiting, and constipation are reminiscent of lead poisoning. Peripheral neuritis is common, and irritability, termagantism, delirium, and hallucinations may occur. Fever, tachycardia, and moderate hypertension are common. Skin lesions, and haematologic abnormalities do not occur. Oliguria is the rule, and the urine is colourless, but as it contains large amounts of PBG and ALA it rapidly turns to the colour of port wine on standing. The diagnosis, however, depends upon chemical testing, not on any colour change.

Treatment is symptomatic. Pethidine may be used to control pain. Chloral hydrate or paraldehyde should be prescribed for sedation; barbiturates must be avoided, as they aggravate the condition and may precipitate paralysis.

(2) *Erythropoietic Photoporphyria*

It appears in childhood or adolescence, and its hallmark is dermal photo-sensitivity, presenting as solar urticaria or solar eczema. Skin reactions usually start within minutes of exposure to sunlight, and subside within 24 hours without permanent damage to the skin. The reaction has been shown to be due to a narrow band of light (400 mμ) near to the ultra-violet. This is identical with the maximum absorption band of the porphyrins.

The concentration of protoporphyrin is greatly increased in the erythrocytes and faeces. The stool may show red fluorescence with ultra-violet light.

(3) *Variegate Porphyria*

This is an hepatic type, and is common in South Africa. It is strongly familial, and its outstanding feature is skin sensitivity both to sunlight and mechanical trauma. Acute abdominal and neurological episodes may occur (*vide supra*, IAP) and the excretion of protoporphyrin and coproporphyrin in the faeces is continuously raised.

(4) *Congenital Erythropoietic Porphyria*

This is a rare inborn error of metabolism. It appears in childhood, and three-quarters of the cases are in males. It is inherited as a recessive, and a similar condition affects cattle, pigs, and possibly squirrels. Porphyrins are deposited in the bones, which are stained brown, and the teeth, which assume a lavender hue; there is a bright-red fluorescence with UVL. Porphyrins are also deposited in the skin, where they cause light sensitivity dermatitis. Histamine is released on exposure to sunlight, and a blistering eruption results. This heals with intense scarring, particularly over the nose and fingers, so that eventually scleroderma (p. 351) may be simulated. Hypertrichosis may also occur and there may be subacute haemolysis with splenomegaly. The urine is port-wine colour, and both urine and faeces contain large amounts of porphyrins, chiefly uroporphyrin I. Abdominal pains, and nervous manifestations are rare, and the patients are not sensitive to barbiturates.

Treatment is the avoidance of exposure to sunlight. Splenectomy has been performed in some cases with good effect.

CARCINOID TUMOUR

The argentaffin cells of the appendix (and elsewhere) may give rise to tumours which appear histologically to be malignant but which clinically seem relatively benign; hence the name, carcin-oid.

The tumours secrete a substance named *serotonin* (5-hydroxytryptamine, 5 H.T.) which stimulates smooth muscle. Normally it is detoxicated in the liver and probably the lungs, but if secondary hepatic carcinoid deposits have occurred, then high levels of 5 H.T. appear in the blood. This causes widespread disturbance of smooth muscle. In the bowel, watery diarrhoea is provoked. There is widespread cutaneous suffusion, most marked in the face, and punctuated by attacks of vivid flushing, lasting for a minute or two and often precipitated by alcohol. Stimulation of the smooth muscle in the bronchi may cause asthmatic spasm, with persistent wheezing. A thick white layer of fibrous tissue is deposited on the endocardium of the right side of the heart, causing pulmonary and tricuspid stenosis, and eventually leading to cardiac failure.

Some of the 5 H.T. in the body is converted into 5 hydroxy-indole acetic acid (5 H.I.A.A.), which is excreted in the urine and may be detected with Ehrlich's aldehyde reagent.

Treatment is unsatisfactory. Occasionally it is justified to remove as much of the tumour as possible as this will reduce the production of 5 H.T. blocks the action of 5 H.T. The dose is 1–2 mg. three times daily. Flushing may respond to a combination of an H_1 blocker (antihistamines) and an H_2 blocker (cimetidine). The course is variable, and patients may survive for ten years or more; the disease is always ultimately fatal.

AMYLOID DISEASE

Amyloid is an abnormal protein which may accumulate in the tissues. Some amyloid is composed of light chain residues from gamma globulins. It may be secondary to long-standing inflammation, for example, rheumatoid arthritis or tuberculosis, when it is perireticular in distribution. It may also complicate myelomatosis (p. 525). Amyloidosis can also occur as a primary condition, although a number of these cases show a slight increase in plasma cells in the bone marrow.

(1) In secondary amyloidosis infiltration occurs in the liver, spleen, kidneys, small intestines, arteries and skin. The heart is spared. More rarely endocrine glands, such as the adrenals are involved. The patient's already bad health grows worse, the skin takes on a waxy appearance, and diarrhoea and polyuria appear. Treatment is of the primary cause. There is some evidence that amyloidosis may be reversible in its early stages.

(2) When it complicates myelomatosis the kidney is specially involved, and a nephrotic syndrome may result.

(3) Primary amyloidosis affects men and women equally, and is occasionally familial. It occurs between 20 and 40, and may involve the heart, kidneys, muscles of swallowing and breathing, the peripheral nerves or the brain, the lymph nodes, liver and spleen, either singly or together. No treatment is very satisfactory but steroids (p. 620 or *see p. 645 of special Tropical Edition*) are worthy of trial.

WILSON'S DISEASE (Hepatolenticular Degeneration)

Wilson's disease is a recessive metabolic disease which is characterised by degeneration of the basal ganglia, cirrhosis of the liver, and a brownish pigmented ring at the limbus of the cornea (Kayser-Fleischer rings). The disease is due to an increased absorption and/or a decreased excretion of dietary copper which leads to a progressive increase in the total body copper with consequent damage to the tissues of the brain, liver, and renal tubules.

Clinical Features. Wilson's disease is slightly more common in males than females and usually becomes clinically recognisable between the age of fifteen and thirty years. Except in young children in whom symptoms of cirrhosis of the liver are common, neurological symptoms predominate. Tremor and rigidity of the limbs are common presenting symptoms. Dysarthria is a frequent early symptom. Rarely, symptoms of cirrhosis of the liver may predominate and the patient die of liver failure in the absence of neurological signs. The disease is usually fatal within fifteen years of onset.

Laboratory Investigation. A decreased level of serum copper and ceruloplasmin associated with an increased urinary copper excretion is diagnostic. A normal level of ceruloplasmin does not exclude the diagnosis if Kayser-Fleischer rings are present. A low serum uric acid is common. Increased aminoaciduria is usuall but not invariable.

Differential Diagnosis. The disease should be suspected in all disturbances of basal ganglion function and in all cases of juvenile cirrhosis of the liver. The presence of a Kayser-Fleischer ring is pathognomonic. Slit lamp examination is necessary in doubtful cases.

Treatment. This is directed towards removing the excess copper and decreasing dietary intake of copper. Penicillamine increases the urinary excretion of copper and is the treatment of choice (1·0–2·0 g. daily). Treatment may have to be continued indefinitely. Improvement in some patients may be striking.

FURTHER READING

Duncan, G. G., *Diseases of Metabolism*, Edited by Bondy, P. K., 7th edition Saunders, Philadelphia, 1975.

Joslin, E. P. *et al.*, *Treatment of Diabetes Mellitus*, 11th edition, Kimpton, London, 1971.

Thompson, R. H. S. and Wootton, I. D. P., *Biochemical Disorders in Human Disease*, 2nd edition, Church:ll, London, 1970.

Oakley, W. C. and others, *Diabetes and its Management*, 2nd Edition, Blackwell, Oxford, 1975.

CHAPTER THIRTEEN

ENDOCRINE DISORDERS

The system of endocrine secretions, acting in one sense as another nervous system, coordinates and controls a wide variety of functions. As in the nervous system, positive and negative feedback is crucial in its operation, and this feedback is exerted either by hormones themselves or the metabolic effects of hormones. Top level control, in the hypothalamus, integrates both these forms of feedback and the signals related to the subject's environment, such as dark or light, sleep or wakening, stress and excitement. The network of endocrine control is also held together by influences between the different hormone 'channels', both at hypothalamic-pituitary level and at the periphery where hormones act. The Table below outlines the principal control mechanisms of the pituitary gland.

ANTERIOR PITUITARY AND HYPOTHALAMIC HORMONES AND FACTORS*

Anterior Pituitary Hormone		Hypothalamic Hormone or Factor*
ACTH (adrenocorticotrophic hormone) and, as byproducts, α and β lipotrophins. (Note: MSH is *not* found in human plasma except as an artefact.)	*released by*	CRF (corticotrophin releasing factor) (The negative feedback here is through cortisol.)
FSH (follicle stimulating hormone), which in the male stimulates spermatogenesis	*released by*	LHRH (LH and FSH releasing hormone, or LRH), a decapeptide (The negative feedback here is through gonadal hormones.)
LH (luteinising hormone), which in the male stimulates interstitial cells to produce testosterone (so LH = ICSH)	*released by*	
GH (growth hormone, somatotrophin), which stimulates production of somatomedin (sulphation factor) by the liver	*released by*	GHRF (growth hormone releasing factor), the dominant control
	inhibited by	GHRIH (growth hormone release inhibitory hormone, SOMATOSTATIN) which also inhibits TSH release and several pancreatic hormones
TSH (thyroid stimulating hormone, thyrotrophin)	*released by*	TRH (thyrotrophin releasing hormone), a tripeptide, the dominant control
	inhibited by	GHRIH (and by the thyroid hormones)

(*Continued on page 468*)

(Table contd. from p. 467)
Anterior Pituitary Hormone   *Hypothalamic Hormone or Factor**

| PROLACTIN | *inhibited by* | PIF (prolactin inhibitory factor), the dominant control, thus allowing marked increase in prolactin secretion if control is 'impaired' |
| | *released by* | TRH. A prolactin releasing factor other than TRH may exist |

* The term hormone is reserved for those substances which have been well characterised and shown to have a role in human physiology.

The variety of levels at which modulation or feedback can occur deserves emphasis. Some hypothalamic factors act not only on the pituitary gland but also within the pancreas (e.g. somatostatin) or on the uterus (e.g. LHRH). Pituitary hormones may act directly on tissue receptors (e.g. prolactin on milk-producing cells), on 'non-endocrine' tissues to release secondary 'hormones' (e.g. GH on the liver to release somatomedin), or on other endocrine glands (e.g. TSH on the thyroid). The hormones secreted by target glands in their turn activate receptors which usually elicit the cellular response through a mechanism involving a second messenger, in many cases cyclic-AMP, as shown in the figure. The 'adrenergic' effects of thyroid hormones are a result of interaction at this sort of level, and it is likely that local factors such as prostaglandins also act here.

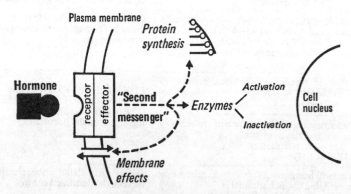

TYPICAL SCHEME OF PEPTIDE HORMONE ACTION.
Note the many points at which the effect of the hormone could be modified.

The nervous and endocrine systems, in many ways so alike, also share evolutionary origins in primitive chemical mediators, and even in man the borderline between the two systems is often academic. The 'posterior pituitary' hormones oxytocin and vasopressin (ADH, p. 380) are synthesised in the hypothalamus and secreted down axons of nerve fibres, to be released in the posterior lobe. Adrenaline at the nerve endings is a neurotransmitter; adrenaline released from the adrenal medulla is a hormone.

Hormones of the gut and pancreas, responsive particularly to stimuli from the gut and to levels of various substrates in the blood, are strongly influenced by autonomic nervous signals and themselves influence the gastrointestinal response to the vagus nerve.

GOITRE

A goitre is an enlarged thyroid gland. If it occurs in the absence of thyrotoxicosis it is a **non-toxic goitre**. The term **simple goitre** is used for the diffuse non-toxic goitre that is not uncommon in adolescent girls; it usually resolves spontaneously.

Iodine deficiency is a potent cause of goitre, and goitre is or was *endemic* in certain areas where the levels of iodine in the drinking water are low or the iodine is diverted from the thyroid gland by pollutants, fluorine or other factors. Endemic goitre has been eliminated in many areas by iodination of table salt. For reasons unknown, endemic goitre is much more frequent in women than men. The incorporation of iodine into thyroid hormone may also be blocked by anti-thyroid drugs, phenyl-butazone, sulphonylureas or PAS (which are therefore goitrogens), or by congenital deficiencies of the enzymes involved in thyroid hormone synthesis, resulting in so-called *goitrous cretinism.*

THYROTOXICOSIS

This is the clinical state associated with raised circulating levels of thyroxine (T4) *and/or* tri-iodothyronine (T3). The metabolic rate is increased, and the patient's resting state may mirror that of an athlete after a run—hot, flushed, sweaty, with a fast pulse. In adults it is due to one of two disorders: Graves' disease or toxic nodular goitre.

Clinical Features of Thyrotoxicosis

Behaviour: nervousness and irritability; inability to relax or stay still and visible hyperkinesia; shaking and fine tremor.

Hypermetabolism: weight loss with increased appetite; warm moist skin (with or without fever); diminished tolerance of warm temperatures.

Muscles: general weakness and fatigue; muscle weakness and sometimes myopathy, especially of proximal muscles.

Eyes: a staring appearance as eyelid retraction widens the palpebral fissure; when the patient looks up and then down a rim of white sclera appears over the cornea (so-called *lid-lag*).

Bowels: diarrhoea (increased frequency and/or looseness) is common.

Cardiovascular: palpitations, tachycardia persisting during sleep or occurring in paroxysms, and atrial fibrillation; angina and high-output state with flow murmurs, bounding pulse, and sometimes heart failure.

Osteoporosis or *myasthenia gravis* may occur.

Graves' Disease

This is caused by the presence of an IgG immunoglobin which stimulates the thyroid in precisely the same way as TSH, probably activating the same receptors. Pituitary TSH secretion is suppressed. This IgG may be detected by sensitive assays in which human TSH receptors are used, hence 'human thyroid stimulator' (HTS) and 'thyroid-stimulating IgG' (TSI), or by bioassay on mouse tissue; recorded as 'long acting thyroid stimuator (LATS) and LATS-protector'; patients with very human-specific IgG are positive for HTS and TSI but negative for LATS and LATS-protector. The existence of this substance, acting as it does on the whole thyroid gland and on other tissues, helps explain the various clinical features which are specific to Graves' disease and which are *not* a direct consequence of elevated levels of T4 or T3.

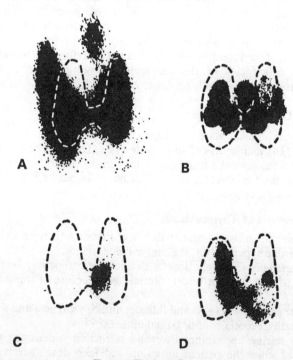

TYPICAL THYROID SCANS

The dashed line indicates the outline of a 'normal' thyroid gland, which is of course variable.

      A. Graves' disease, diffuse toxic goitre with obviously active left pyramidal lobe.

      B. Multinodular toxic goitre, with several adenomata.

      C. Autonomous toxic nodule in left lobe, suppressing the remainder of the gland.

      D. 'Cold nodule'—the white area of low uptake within the left lobe. 10 per cent are malignant, so surgery is indicated.

Specific Features of Graves' Disease

1. The disorder particularly affects women aged between twenty and forty.
2. One third of patients remit spontaneously within one to two years.
3. The thyroid is diffusely enlarged (see figure on p. 470), with a systolic bruit sometimes audible over the gland.
4. *Exophthalmos*, protrusion of the eyeball, may aggravate the staring appearance associated with both forms of thyrotoxicosis. Infiltration of the extra-ocular muscles may occur, with consequent and/or diplopia paralysis of upward gaze. In severe cases, conjunctival irritation, chemosis (inflammation of the eyelids) and even corneal ulceration may occur. *Malignant exophthalmos* is the progression of these changes to a condition of raised intraocular pressure, with pain and a risk of damage to the optic nerve. Guanethidine eye drops and systemic steroids may reduce the intraocular pressure, but if sight is seriously threatened then surgical decompression may be necessary. In *Ophthalmic Graves' Disease* the eye changes occur in the absence of thyrotoxicosis, levels of T4 and T3 being normal. About half these patients progress eventually to thyrotoxicosis.
5. *Pretibial myxoedema*, mucopolysaccharide infiltration under the skin of the shin, and *thyroid achropachy*, a form of finger clubbing which is secondary to periosteal new bone formation and soft tissue thickening, are rare but pathognomonic signs of Graves' Disease.

Toxic Nodular Goitre

A disorder which is essentially 'local' in origin, the toxic nodule is an actively secreting thyroid adenoma which has become autonomous, i.e. independent of control by the pituitary. Early in its development the levels of T4 and T3 will be normal, but attempts to restrain activity of the nodule by exogenous T3 (which reduces the circulating TSH) will fail. The patient usually presents when T4 and T3 are elevated, with features of thyrotoxicosis, and by this time the TSH levels are suppressed by the high thyroid hormone concentrations, with a consequent 'suppression' of the normal thyroid tissue around the adenoma (see page 470). On palpation, such a thyroid gland may feel lumpy, one or more nodules enlarging part or parts of the gland. Because this form of thyrotoxicosis affects an older age group than Graves' disease, and the eye signs are less noticeable, its presentation is often more subtle. Thus many older patients present with cardiac or bowel symptoms, unexplained weight loss, or myopathy, and may be lethargic or depressed rather than overactive and anxious (*apathetic thyrotoxicosis*).

Thyroid Function Tests

A selection of the most useful tests of thyroid function. Tests now superceded by improved methods, or appropriate only in very special circumstances, are omitted from this list.

Both thyroxine (T4) and tri-iodothyronine (T3) are largely in bound form in the plasma, the main carrier protein being 'thyroid binding globulin' (TBG). The *total* concentration of T4 and T3 is therefore increased when the TBG level is increased (as during pregnancy and treatment with oestrogens), and decreased when TBG is decreased. The physiologically important levels are those of the *free* unbound hormones, but these are very much more difficult to measure directly. The T3 Resin Uptake is valuable in overcoming this difficulty because the test actually 'reads' the number of binding sites on the patient's TBG which are *not* occupied by T4 or T3; the *more* such *unoccupied* sites there are, the *lower* the 'reading' of thyroid hormone concentration. With an *increase* in the number of *unoccupied* binding sites, the T3 Resin Uptake will give a falsely *low* estimate of the effective free concentration of thyroid hormones. The Free Thyroxine Index (FTI), a product of T4 × T3 Resin Uptake, combines the bias in each direction to produce a reading that is virtually independent of the TBG concentration.

Abbreviation	What Does It Measure?	Normal Range	Comment
T4	Total T4, including bound T4	70–190 nmol./l.	Increased by increased TBG (see above)
T3 resin uptake	Binding sites on TBG occupied by T3 or T4 (see above)	90–120 per cent of normal	Decreased by increased TBG (see above)
FTI	Free thyroxine as an index, 'T4 × T3 resin'	70–180 nmol./l.	Not significantly affected by TBG, correlates with free unbound T4 (see above)
ETR	Effective (i.e. free) thyroid ratio: T4 available in the presence of the patient's plasma	90–110 per cent of normal	In vitro test—gives same information as FTI but in one test
T3 (RIA)	Total tri-iodothyronine, by radio-immunoassay	1·2–3·0 nmol./l.	Particularly valuable in diagnosing thyrotoxicosis (T4 may be normal)
TSH	Hypothalamic-pituitary function, or the degree of suppression by T4 and T3 secreted autonomously	0·4–2·6 u./l. (see Figure p. 474)	Low in pituitary failure. High in 1° hypothyroidism. Response to TRH 200 ug increased in 1° hypothyroidism, suppressed in thyrotoxicosis
Scan ($_{99}$Tc or $_{131}$I)	Localisation of trapping of I (^{131}I, also, rate of total uptake)	Symmetrical, each lobe approx. 2·5 cm. × 4·0 cm. (see Figure p. 470)	May suggest size and location (e.g. retrosternal) of gland or nature of disease

Investigation and Diagnosis

Tests of thyroid function are summarised in the Table on p. 472. The serum T3 (total tri-iodothyronine, not the resin uptake) is a more reliable index than T4 in diagnosing thyrotoxicosis because the T4 is normal in some patients with thyrotoxicosis. Suppression of TSH, measured before and after injection of TRH (see graph on p. 474), is the most sensitive indicator of excessive or autonomous thyroid activity, but the test will only be necessary in borderline cases. Oversecretion of TSH by pituitary tumours is extremely rare.

Treatment

The fact that Graves' disease may remit spontaneously, and that in this condition surgical or radio-iodine therapy which restores normal thyroid function is accompanied by the later emergence of hypothyroidism in about 3 per cent of patients per year of follow-up, argues for a trial of drug therapy in such patients. In contrast, the toxic 'hot nodule' will not remit spontaneously and so merits definitive treatment. Having temporarily suppressed any iodine uptake by the normal thyroid tissue a hot nodule will take up virtually the whole of a dose of therapeutic radio-iodine, leaving the normal thyroid to resume normal function. But these comments and the following are in the nature of general guidance, the actual choice of treatment being tailored to the clinical state, age and circumstances of each patient.

Surgery (*Thyroidectomy*). This is appropriate in these situations:

(a) A significant possibility of carcinoma;
(b) Very large goitres;
(c) Pressure symptoms (whatever the apparent size of the goitre);
(d) Alternative methods of treatment refused or impossible (e.g. allergies to antithyroid drugs or radio-iodine contra-indicated).

Patients must be rendered euthyroid by carbimazole and Lugol's iodine or controlled by propanolol before operation.

Radio-iodine. In most cases this is the standard method of definitive therapy, either at the time of diagnosis or after an appropriate trial of anti-thyroid drugs. However, it is contra-indicated in patients who are or may be pregnant and those in younger age groups (although the theoretically increased risk of subsequent thyroid cancer has not been substantiated, there are additional arguments against applying radiation to fertile subjects). The full effect of the radiation will not be seen for several months, during which time anti-thyroid drugs should be prescribed.

Antithyroid Drugs. The drugs in common use are carbimazole (10 mg. qds, reducing to 5–15 mg. daily) and propylthiouracil (100 mg. qds, reducing to 50 mg. daily). Carbimazole is the less toxic but even so causes skin rashes in 5 per cent, neutropenia in 1–2 per cent, and agranulocytosis in about 0·5 per cent. of cases. Several weeks will elapse before the clinical improvement is complete. At the end of one or two years of treatment the drug may be discontinued and the TSH response to TRH measured (see graph below). If this is normal then remission has probably occurred and no further treatment is necessary, but careful and prolonged follow-up is advisable.

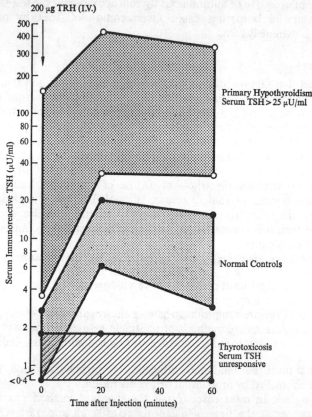

THE TRH STIMULATION TEST.

Propanolol acts peripherally to give rapid relief of many toxic symptoms and does so without influencing the levels of thyroid hormones. It may be of special value in three situations:

(1) For rapid control of cardiac effects of T4 and T3.
(2) For symptomatic relief while investigations proceed.
(3) For rapid preparation of the thyrotoxic patient and the thyrotoxic gland for thyroidectomy, as a fast acting alternative to *Lugol's iodine*.

Thyroxine 0·1–0·2 mg. daily is sometimes prescribed during or after antithyroid treatments to protect the patient from iatrogenic hypothyroidism.

Treatment of Thyrotoxicosis in Pregnancy is best managed with carbimazole, using the minimum dose which will keep the Free Thyroxine or Free Thyroxine Index (Table 2) just inside the normal range. The baby may be born with maternal HTS in the circulation, causing *neonatal thyrotoxicosis*; this needs immediate and careful control by those with special experience, so delivery should be arranged in an appropriate centre. As carbimazole is excreted in breast milk, the baby must not be breast fed.

Thyroid Crisis

Also known as thyroid 'storm' this consists of an acute exacerbation of thyrotoxicity, with especially marked hyperpyrexia and tachycardia. It can occur after thyroid surgery (or occasionally radio-iodine therapy) but is rare since patients have been rendered scrupulously euthyroid before surgery. Treatment may include physical cooling (*not* aspirin), Lugol's iodine, carbimazole, propanolol and hydrocortisone.

THYROIDITIS

Hashimoto's Disease (Autoimmune thyroiditis)

A diffuse firm goitre develops, usually insidiously but sometimes in a sub-acute manner with pain and tenderness, characteristically in a middle-aged woman. Lymphocytic infiltration of the gland, and auto-antibodies to thyroglobulin and thyroid microsomes are to be expected. Early in the disease mild thyrotoxicosis may transiently occur, but 20 per cent present with, and many more progress to, overt hypothyroidism. Other auto-immune disorders may be associated with this disease and with those cases of Graves' disease and 'primary' myxoedema who also exhibit thyroid auto-antibodies.

Subacute Thyroiditis (De Quervain's)

Although mild cases occur, the thyroid generally becomes acutely enlarged, firm, tender and painful, in a patient who is unwell and feverish. Transient hypothyroidism may be noted. There is often a history of recent respiratory infection, and the aetiology is thought to be viral. If the symptoms are not relieved by simple anti-inflammatory analgesics, prednisolone or low-dose radiotherapy may be necessary.

Riedel's Disease (Woody Thyroiditis)

The thyroid gland becomes hard as a result of intensive and locally invasive fibrosis (analogous to retroperitoneal fibrosis). It is rare, non-metastatic and can only be treated by resection.

HYPOTHYROIDISM

In the infant, thyroid deficiency produces **cretinism**, evident by slowing of growth, mental and physical retardation, a characteristic appearance and a hoarse cry. The adult form of the disease was first described by Sir William Gull in 1874; its name **myxoedema** derives from the mucoprotein thickening of subcutaneous tissue which is found in severe cases.

Clinical Features

Myxoedema: as mentioned above, a boggy non-pitting oedema which may be diffuse but is especially noticeable around the eyes and on the hands and feet.

Skin: cool, dry and coarse in texture, pale or faintly yellow in colour (aggravated by the anaemia which is often present); the hair is also dry and coarse and thin, with particular loss of the outer third of eyebrows.

Slowness: of thought, of action, of speech, of relaxation of the muscle after a reflex has been elicited (particularly at the ankle); the mental state may exhibit memory loss, dementia, neurosis or psychosis.

Hypometabolism: poor appetite yet mild weight gain; diminished tolerance of the cold; hypothermia may occur, even to the point of coma in a severe case.

Voice: may become hoarse as vocal cords thicken.

Cardiovascular: one third of patients show systolic hypertension until treated; some have angina and/or palpitations, which are not always relieved by treatment of the hypothyroidism; some are dyspnoeic on exertion.

Menorrhagia: is a common complaint.

Investigation and Diagnosis

Tests of thyroid function are summarised in the Table on p. 472. Non-specific findings may include a normochromic normocytic anaemia, raised plasma cholesterol, low voltage on the ECG, flattening of the glucose tolerance curve, and elevation of muscle enzymes. In doubtful cases an elevated TSH may provide valuable confirmation of the diagnosis (see graph on p. 474).

Hypothyroidism may be the result of the following:

Primary failure of the thyroid gland. Even in those without a convincing history of Hashimoto's disease (p. 475) there is a high frequency of thyroid auto-antibodies, suggesting an autoimmune aetiology. Defects in thyroidal enzymes occur but they are rare and are usually discovered in early childhood in the form of goitrous cretinism.

External factors affecting the thyroid. Previous treatment for thyrotoxicosis is the commonest single cause of hypothyroidism. Severe iodine deficiency within the thyroid, associated with trapping or blocking of iodine, is a rare cause, usually presenting with a goitre.

Secondary failure, due to low TSH levels. This usually occurs as part of a panhypopituitary state, which is discussed on p. 495. TRH is a very potent stimulus to TSH secretion and a TSH response to TRH may persist even in the presence of a pituitary lesion; the hypothyroidism in such cases is presumed to reflect a low average level of pituitary drive.

Treatment

Whatever the cause of the hypothyroidism, most patients need to be treated by gradual restoration of normal thyroid hormone levels using oral *L-thyroxine*, commencing with 0·05 mg. daily, increasing over three weeks to 0·02 mg. daily, at which dose level most patients are euthyroid. Any more rapid rise in thyroid hormone activity may precipitate angina or left ventricular failure, especially in the old. The adequacy and effectiveness of treatment is best assessed on clinical grounds, and confirmed by finding the dose of thyroxine at which T4 and/or TSH levels in the normal range are restored. The patient must clearly understand the life-time nature of the medication.

In external and secondary types of myxoedema the primary cause must be remedied where possible.

Myxoedema Coma

Especially in the cold of winter, the hypothyroid condition of an elderly patient may progress to such a degree that bradycardia, shallow breathing, hypoxia, carbon dioxide retention, hypoglycaemia, hyponatraemia and hypothermia all contribute to a lapse into coma. The patient is cold to the touch, with depression of central and peripheral body temperatures, often *below the range of the standard clinical thermometer*, so that the severity of the problem is not recognised. Over half the patients die, so care must be intensive but not hasty—vigorous rewarming must be avoided, the gentle action of warm blankets being safer. Rapid-acting rapidly metabolised tri-iodothyronine 20 μg. eight hourly and hydrocortisone 100 mg. eight hourly should be administered I.V., and the ECG and body functions closely monitored. As for any patient in coma and in shock, or on the brink of it, the airway, oxygenation and circulation must be maintained by appropriate means.

CUSHING'S SYNDROME

Excessive levels of glucocorticoids, if not the result of steroid treatment, arise from a disorder of the adrenal gland itself (about 20 per cent) or from an outside influence. The adrenal gland may harbour an adenoma or a carcinoma. The outside influence, which will induce adrenal hyperplasia, may take the form of an abnormally high level of ACTH from the pituitary—often driven by hypothalamic oversecretion of CRF (Table on p. 467)—or an ACTH-like peptide secreted by a non-pituitary tumour (*ectopic*). The disease that Harvey Cushing described was that in which pituitary adenomas, usually small and basophilic, over-secrete ACTH.

Many of the clinical features of the syndrome reflect impaired protein synthesis or redistribution of fat.

Clinical Features

Those Related to the Effects of Cortisol

The face is typically plethoric and mooned as the skin gets thinner and adipose tissue rounds out the chin and cheeks; the supraclavicular notch may be filled, and posteriorly fat in the upper thoracic/lower cervical area produces the 'buffalo hump'. Obesity especially affects the trunk.

Muscle. As wasting occurs the thin legs and arms contribute to the 'lemon-on-sticks' shape, and the patient suffers from fatigue and weakness, sometimes severe (steroid myopathy).

Skin. This is thin and atrophic, so that purplish striae are seen.

Vessels. Purpura, or easy bruising, is common. The blood pressure may be moderately raised. Polycythaemia may be a feature.

Nervous system. Psychoses related to the condition are relieved as steroid levels return to normal.

Bones. Osteoporosis leads to compression fractures of the vertebrae and thus spinal curvature, and pathological fractures of the ribs.

Metabolic. Glucose tolerance is often impaired. The mineralo-corticoid effects of cortisol and related compounds may result in a low serum potassium with alkalosis, but this is prominent only when very high levels of cortisol are circulating.

Androgenic Effects (*especially if an adrenal tumour is present*)

In men: impotence, increasing baldness, and acne.

In women: hirsutism (increased body and beard hair), recession of hair at the temples, menstrual irregularities or amenorrhoea, enlarged clitoris, and an increase in musculature.

Other Effects

Pituitary Tumours. Most often this is a rather small basophil adenoma, which will produce no local signs.

Adrenal Tumours. Signs related to the tumour itself are unusual but an adenocarcinoma may metastasise.

Ectopic Tumours. About 10 per cent of cases of adrenal hyperplasia are caused by secretion of an ACTH-like peptide by a cancer outside the pituitary. Typically the peptide level and therefore the adrenal output of cortisol is very high in such cases, the result being a severe Cushing's syndrome with hypokalaemic alkalosis and pigmentation. Oat-cell carcinoma of the bronchus, thymic and pancreatic islet-cell tumours are especially associated with this picture. Anaemia rather than polycythaemia may then occur.

Investigation and Diagnosis

Non-specific findings may include polycythaemia, a neutrophilia between 10,000 and 20,000, depressed lymphocyte and eosinophil counts, mild glucose intolerance with or without a raised fasting blood glucose, and hypokalaemic alkalosis.

The normal ranges are listed in the table below and specific tests are discussed below.

ADRENAL FUNCTION TESTS

PLASMA CORTISOL, nmol./l.

	09·00h	24·00h	09·00h after Dexamethasone 1 mg. at 23·00h of preceding evening
Healthy non-stressed subjects	150–700	80–220	5–150
Cushing's syndrome	400–2400	400–2400	more than 300

Response to Synacthen (tetracosactrin) 0·25 mg. IM	0 mins	30 mins	60 mins
		more than	more than
Healthy non-stressed subjects	150–700	800	800
Adrenal insufficiency	30–150	30–400	30–400
Disuse atrophy (chronically low ACTH)	30–150	30–400	30–400

Response to Insulin-induced hypoglycaemia: see Combined Pituitary Test (Table p 494)

PLASMA ACTH: normal range: 10–80 ng./l. at 09·00h; less than 10 ng./l. at 24.00h

URINARY STEROIDS: OUTPUT/24 HOURS

	Male (normal)	Female (normal)	Suppressed by Dexamethasone 2mg./day for 3–5 days
Free cortisol, nmol.	130–600	130–600	less than 100
17-Hydroxycorticoids, μmol.	11–45	11–30	less than 9
17-Oxogenic corticoids, μmol.	15–60	11–48	less than 11
17-Oxosteroids, μmol.	18–64	11–51	less than 11
Pregnanetriol μmol.	1–3	1–3	less than 0·7

The normal ranges vary slightly between laboratories. The urinary output of steroids should be interpreted in the context of the patient's weight.

Plasma Cortisol. This is often the most convenient measurement, and a low or low normal level virtually excludes Cushing's syndrome. The levels may be misleadingly high in the anxious or obese subject, or in patients with high levels of the carrier protein transcortin in the blood. A useful screening test for outpatients requires blood samples at 9.00 a.m. and 6.00 p.m. on the first day and 9.00 a.m. on the second day; dexamethasone 1 mg. is taken by mouth at 11.00 p.m. on the first day. In Cushing's syndrome the normal diurnal variation is lost and the second 9.00 a.m. cortisol is not suppressed to less than 150 nmol./litre as it would be in a normal subject. If the result of this study is not completely normal then further investigation is required.

Urinary Free Cortisol is unaffected by transcortin concentrations and accurately reflects the secretion rate of cortisol. It is diagnostically more precise than measurements of 17-hydroxycorticoids, and even more useful than plasma cortisol, provided the urine collection is accurately timed.

17-Oxogenic Corticoids include not only cortisol but several precursors and a metabolite, cortilone. While it is a more sensitive test for abnormalities of steroid synthesis such as congenital adrenal hyperplasia (adrenogenital syndrome, p. 484), it is less specific in diagnosing Cushing's syndrome because high levels occur in some hirsute patients with increased androgen production but normal cortisol levels.

17-Oxosteroids mainly reflect the androgenic steroid precursors. These are pathologically elevated in some patients with Cushing's syndrome, especially if associated with adrenal carcinoma when very high levels may occur, and in some patients with benign forms of hirsutism, including some with congenital adrenal hyperplasia (p. 484).

Dexamethasone Suppression Test. Urinary steroid excretion is suppressed in most normal or obese subjects by dexamethasone 2 mg. daily, and in most patients with adrenal hyperplasia due to pituitary ACTH by dexamethasone 8 mg. daily (but not 2 mg. daily); in most patients with adrenal tumours or an ectopic source of ACTH-like substance it cannot be suppressed even by 8 mg. daily. However, the localisation suggested by this test can be unreliable, and it is most useful in confirming the pathological nature of borderline hypercortisolism.

Responsiveness to ACTH, whether tested by injection of tetracosactrin (Synacthen) or by attempting to elevate endogenous ACTH metopirone (which blocks the final step in the synthesis of cortisol), is usually abolished in the presence of an ectopic source of ACTH-like peptide or adrenal carcinomas. About 50 per cent of benign adrenal tumours behave similarly.

Plasma ACTH levels are depressed in the presence of adrenal carcinoma or adenoma, and elevated in Cushing's syndrome of pituitary or hypothalamic origin. Most ACTH assay systems give very high readings in cases of ectopic peptide production, and some characterise the peptide in such a way as to suggest whether the origin is pituitary or ectopic. When further developed and widely available, these assays should replace several of the investigations described above.

Anatomical Localisation. Adrenal tumours may be delineated by tomography, renography, arteriography, venography, isotopic scanning with labelled cholesterol, and the E.M.I. scan (Computerised Axial Tomography). X-rays of the pituitary fossa are mandatory in every case of Cushing's, and if necessary further investigations are carried out as for a suspected chromophobe adenoma (p. 493).

Treatment

An adrenal tumour must be removed with the whole of the affected gland and the other gland must be carefully inspected. In the case of inoperable adrenal carcinoma, the excessive steroid synthesis may be controlled by the drug o-p-DDD, which is unfortunately too toxic to use in other situations. Any non-pituitary tumour secreting an ACTH-like peptide is resected.

When adrenal hyperplasia is secondary to pituitary overproduction of ACTH the choice lies between pituitary ablation (by Yttrium implant or trans-sphenoidal hypophysectomy), and bilateral adrenalectomy with pituitary irradiation when indicated. The advantages of the latter approach are the immediate reduction in cortisol levels, the temporary maintenance of pituitary function, and in particular fertility if that is appropriate, and the positive exclusion of an adrenal tumour. The disadvantage is the risk of developing *Nelson's Syndrome* (in which a ACTH-secreting tumour produces generalised pigmentation and local signs of expansion) during the period before the pituitary gland is irradiated. Maintenance therapy with corticosteroids and other hormones will be necessary following some of these forms of treatment.

ALDOSTERONISM

In its *primary* form this is related to an adenoma or hyperplasia of the adrenal cortical zona glomerulosa, producing a raised level of aldosterone in plasma and urine and—to a variable degree— hypertension, low serum potassium, metabolic alkalosis, and thus polyuria, periodic paralysis and paraesthesias. The frequency of the condition is controversial but between 1 and 10 per cent of 'essential' hypertensive patients may have the condition. About 20 per cent of hypertensive patients exhibit low plasma renin, a result of suppression by high aldosterone in some and of unknown mechanisms in others.

Aldosterone excess *secondary* to high renin and angiotensin levels is well documented in malignant hypertension (p. 130), heart failure, cirrhosis of the liver, nephrotic syndrome, salt depletion and conditions of low blood volume.

ADRENAL INSUFFICIENCY (Addison's Disease)

Atrophy of the glands in the presence of auto-antibodies to adrenal tissue is the most common cause of deficient corticosteroid production. Tuberculous infiltration was once more common, and even now this aetiology may be betrayed by adrenal calcification and an appropriate history. Rare causes include carcinoma, various infiltrations, and haemorrhage in the gland in the course of meningococcal septicaemia (Waterhouse-Friderichsen syndrome, p. 540). The circulating levels of ACTH are high in these conditions, which constitute true 'Addison's disease', but *secondary* adrenal insufficiency may occur with low ACTH levels in hypopituitary states (p. 493). In patients with diminished adrenal reserve, rifampicin may cause insufficiency by induction of liver enzymes which increase the rate of metabolism of circulating cortisol and thus shorten its half-life.

Clinical Features

Chronic Insufficiency

Pigmentation increased (an effect of ACTH), especially in skin creases, scars, and on the gums.

Weakness, fatigue, lassitude, often evident on examination.

Weight loss, anorexia, salt craving, decreased muscle mass.

Nausea, vomiting, diarrhoea, possibly dehydration.

Dizziness, perhaps related to hypotension, worse on standing.

Less frequently: hypoglycaemia, hypothermia, vitiligo, hair loss, lymphadenopathy, asthma, rhinitis, mental aberrations.

*Acute (Addisonian Crisis).*This often occurs on a background of chronic deficiency, and it may therefore include any of the features described above, particularly severe hypotension, fever, profound weakness, nausea, vomiting and diarrhoea, progressing if untreated to coma. The coma may be complicated by hypoglycaemia or hypothermia. The precipitation of the crisis in a patient with chronic insufficiency may be provoked by some major stress (e.g. an infection, an accident, an operation), or by increased salt loss (e.g. in sweat).

Investigation and Diagnosis

During the acute illness the patient is in danger of fatal collapse, so treatment should not be delayed. In the stress of any severe acute illness *other* than adrenal insufficiency the plasma corticosteroids will be elevated, so the plasma cortisol on one sample of blood taken on admission will confirm or refute the diagnosis of Addisonian crisis. The plasma ACTH, if available, indicates directly whether the condition is that of hypothalamic-pituitary failure or that of primary adrenal failure with consequent ACTH hypersecretion. The clinical clue to the level of ACTH is the degree of pigmentation.

If the situation is not acute, or if a loss of adrenal reserve rather than manifest insufficiency is suspected, the diagnostic tests fall into three groups:

(1) Baseline measurements, of plasma or urinary cortisol, or urinary 17-hydroxycorticoids or 17-oxogenic corticoids, which are persistently depressed in adrenal insufficiency (Table on p. 479).

(2) The response to ACTH, for safety and convenience in the form of the synthetic analogue tetracosactrin (Synacthen), provides a test of adrenal function which is independent of the hypothalamic-pituitary axis. A normal response in the *Synacthen test* (Table on p. 479) indicates adequate function of adrenal cortical tissue. A poor response indicates *either* adrenal gland destruction *or* a state of disuse atrophy because ACTH secretion has been chronically low (e.g. hypopituitarism, or use of oral corticosteroid drugs). If the response is poor, a three-day course of Synacthen-depot 2 mg. I.M. is followed by a second 60-minute Synacthen test. A marked improvement over the result of the first test suggests that disuse atrophy was the cause of the poor response; a persistently poor response points to primary adrenal disease.

(3) If the adrenal gland is not primarily at fault, the response of the entire system, hypothalamus-(CRF)-pituitary-(ACTH)-adrenal-cortisol, can then be tested by inducing hypoglycaemia with soluble insulin, 0·2 units/kg. body weight intravenously. Hypoglycaemia should cause sharp rises in plasma and urinary levels of corticosteroids (and ACTH, if the assay is available). The metopirone test may precipitate acute adrenal crisis as it lowers cortisol levels even lower than they already are, and this method of testing the system should be avoided in cortisol-deficient patients.

Aldosterone secretion is usually reduced, as well as cortisol, and a considerable loss of sodium and water with shifts across cell membranes produces a low plasma sodium and chloride, a raised blood urea and often a high potassium, in a hypovolaemic patient. ADH secretion may be increased and aggravate the lowering of the plasma sodium. The blood sugar may be low.

Diagnostic procedures will include, where appropriate, a search for infective and neoplastic conditions which can destroy the adrenals. Only the auto-immune type of adrenal atrophy leaves adrenal medullary secretion intact.

Treatment

The acute crisis requires immediate and generous infusion of normal saline and dextrose, to restore circulating volume and correct hypoglycaemia. Hydrocortisone hemisuccinate 100 mg.I.V. is administered stat and 6-hourly or as required. Infections must be vigorously treated. The patient's blood pressure and salt-fluid status must be carefully followed.

The long-term treatment should be based on oral hydrocortisone, between 20 and 40 mg. daily, and fluorocortisone at a dose between 0·1 and 0·2 mg. daily to supplement the mineralocorticoid effect. In establishing the proper maintenance dose, these factors should apply: the patient's subjective response, the supine and erect blood pressure, the absence of oedema, plasma cortisol levels and possibly the ACTH level. These patients are absolutely dependent on their steroid medication, which should be trebled in dose in the event of transient illness or stress and then gradually restored to normal levels. They must understand their condition and carry a card stating their situation, maintenance dose and procedure in the event of accident, and/or wear a Medic-Alert bracelet or necklace.

VIRILISATION

This is the clinical state associated with excessive androgenic effect in the female. While commonly of adrenal or ovarian origin, an abnormal end-organ sensitivity to androgens may also be important in many patients. Hirsutism (increased body and facial hair) is marked, pubic hair becomes masculine in distribution, and recession of the hairline at the temples occurs. The voice becomes deep, muscles increase in size and the clitoris enlarges. In post-pubertal women there is amenorrhoea, reduced fertility and shrinkage of the breasts. This picture may be associated with:

(1) Adrenal tumours, often with Cushinoid clinical features (p. 478) (high oxosteroids, especially with adrenal carcinoma).
(2) Congenital adrenal hyperplasia (see below).
(3) Arrhenoblastoma of the ovary (high testosterone, normal 17-oxosteroids).

Hirsutism, with no major virilisation but often with menstrual irregularities and acne, is more common. Major causes include those of virilisation and:

(4) Polycystic ovaries (see *Stein-Leventhal Syndrome*, p. 490).
(5) Mild androgen excess (compensated partial enzyme defects in the adrenal gland or ovary).
(6) Simple familial hirsutism (diagnosed by family history) or 'constitutional' hirsutism with no obvious cause.

Investigation and Diagnosis

This is especially directed at the identification of patients with tumours. Both ACTH and the gonadotrophins stimulate the adrenal glands *and* the ovary to produce androgens, and in the absence of an obvious mass on examination (which will include a full gynaecological examination) localisation of the source of the androgen can be difficult. Testosterone is the most relevant hormone in this condition, but 17-oxosteroids tend to be especially high in adrenal disorders.

Treatment

Tumours should be resected, and polycystic ovaries should be assessed by peritonoscopy. Corticosteroids and cyclical oestrogen therapy— separately or together—may be effective in reducing plasma testosterone levels and the degree of hirsutism. Courses of at least three months should be given, and management based on the clinical response and a change in testosterone levels. Long-term results are disappointing. Patients are nevertheless helped by reassurance and advice regarding cosmetic treatment.

CONGENITAL ADRENAL HYPERPLASIA (Adrenogenital Syndromes)

In these disorders there are enzyme defects along the pathway of cortisol synthesis. In the absence of a feedback system the cortisol levels would fall markedly, but plasma cortisol is protected by a very efficient homeostatic mechanism, and indeed this hormone is the only major restraint on the secretion of CRF and hence ACTH. The result of the enzyme deficiency is therefore an increased ACTH drive, which has the effect of increasing the concentration of cortisol precursors 'proximal' to the 'block', so restoring towards normal the concentrations of substances 'distal' to the block (including cortisol itself). Some of the common levels of 'block' are illustrated in the figure below. In every case the accumulating precursors or steroids have an androgenic effect overall, and in some syndromes potent mineralocorticoids are also formed in excess. While a common feature, valuable diagnostically, is the increased concentration of 17-OH-progesterone and hence urinary pregnanetriol, the actual presentation depends not only on the level of the 'block' but also its severity, and hence the age at presentation.

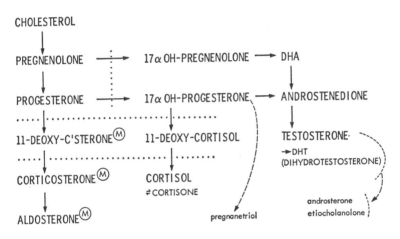

(M)-potent mineralocorticoid

OUTLINE OF ADRENAL STEROID SYNTHESIS

The dotted lines indicate levels at which enzyme deficiencies may occur, acting as a block to synthesis and so causing accumulation of precursors 'above' the block. The dashed lines indicate metabolites excreted in urine.

Typical presentations include:

(1) Perinatal and infantile. Male: phallic enlargement, 'infant Hercules' (musculature). Female: pseudohermaphroditism with genital abnormalities. Both: early fusion of epiphyses; adrenal insufficiency depends on severity of block.

(2) Delayed puberty, primary amenorrhoea.

(3) C-21 partial block: high levels of 17-OH-progesterone etc. produce virilisation, high levels of ACTH produce pigmentation.

(4) C-11 partial block: as C-21 with the addition of hypertension, produced by high levels of 11-desoxy-corticosterone (a potent mineralocorticoid).

(5) Compensated enzyme deficiencies responsible for some cases of 'idiopathic hirsutism'?

Treatment

Corticosteroids will abolish the excessive ACTH drive in these patients and restore normal androgen levels. If adrenal insufficiency is present this is treated as would be a case of Addison's disease (p. 481).

PHAEOCHROMOCYTOMA

This very rare tumour of the adrenal medulla is important as a curable cause of hypertension, and as a 'mimic' of anxiety neurosis, thyrotoxicosis and diabetes mellitus. About 10 per cent of the tumours are malignant and bilateral, and about the same proportion are associated with parathyroid adenomas or medullary carcinoma of the thyroid. The clinical features are related to the effects of excess adrenaline and/or noradrenaline.

Clinical Features

Most patients are hypertensive and complain of headaches. The hypertension is usually constant, but there occurs sometimes a characteristic picture of paroxysmal hypertension, with concurrent headaches, nose bleeds, or pulmonary oedema. Palpitations with or without tachycardia are common. Increased perspiration is a frequent complaint. Tremor, weakness, weight loss, feeling of warmth, even psychosis, with an increased metabolic rate, may at first suggest thyrotoxicosis. Anorexia and constipation are not uncommon. Although few patients complain of postural symptoms, the blood pressure may drop sharply on standing.

Investigation and Diagnosis

Tests currently in use involve measurements of excretion rates of catecholamine metabolites:

(1) As a screening test: vanillyl-mandelic acid (VMA) in urine, normally less than 25 μmol./24 hours, or 2·4 mmol./mol. creatinine excreted.
(2) As a definitive test: metadrenaline and normetadrenaline in urine. In one large series this test detected 100 per cent of patients with phaechromocytomas, whether or not their blood pressure was raised at the time, and was negative in 95 per cent of hypertensive patients without tumours.

Suppression and provocation tests are potentially dangerous and rarely indicated. Levels of blood glucose, free fatty acids and the haematocrit may be elevated. Calcium and calcitonin levels should be checked, to exclude parathyroid adenomas and medullary carcinoma of the thyroid.

Treatment

Radiological investigations and surgery should be preceded and covered by adrenergic blockade, anti-α (phenoxybenzamine) and anti-β (propanolol). During surgery both adrenal glands must be inspected.

DELAYED PUBERTY IN THE FEMALE

Regular menstruation normally commences between the ages of 10 and 16, with a mean of 12·9 years. The other major changes of puberty include breast development and nipple pigmentation, growth of pubic hair of increasingly coarse dark curled type, axillary hair growth, thickening of the vaginal epithelium and growth of the genitalia; the pelvis gradually becomes gynaecoid. Delayed puberty may be physiological and/or familial, especially in the presence of obesity. In true ovarian failure the delay in fusion of the epiphyses eventually leads to overgrowth of the long bones, such that span exceeds height, and 'bone age' on X-ray may for a time be less than actual age.

Investigation and Diagnosis

Any major disease, particularly thyroid disorders, diabetes, renal failure or chronic infection, may be contributory. As discussed on p. 484, the barrage of androgens secreted in congenital adrenal hyperplasia may impair female development. Beyond these possibilities, the main question is whether a primary ovarian defect or a failure of gonadotrophin secretion exists. If plasma and urinary FSH levels are low, the possible causes of hypopituitarism (p. 495) are pursued. Isolated gonadotrophin deficiency may be found, usually responsive to LRH, suggesting that the basic problem may be LRH failure; the line between such patients and 'late developers' is often indistinct and the initial treatment should be conservative.

High levels of FSH are consistent with:

(1) The first hint of puberty.
(2) Absence of ovaries, as in *Turner's syndrome* or *testicular feminisation.*
(3) Damage to the ovaries by cysts, tumours, trauma, surgery or irradiation.

Turner's Syndrome (Gonadal Dysgenesis)

The patients appear, act and think as women, but they are genetically male, with an OX or OX-mosaic karyotype and consequent dysgenesis of the testes. Having neither ovaries nor testes they develop—as do other mammalian male embryos when experimentally castrated in utero—into phenotypic females. Secondary sexual characteristics and the normal menstrual cycle do not appear spontaneously.

They usually present as short women or girls, under 5 feet tall, who have failed to undergo sexual maturation. Numerous other clinical features occur but are variable in their expression, as might be expected from the variety of karyotypes found in the syndrome. The features may include: webbing of the neck, a short neck, increased carrying angle at the elbow (cubitus valgus), widely separated nipples, shield-like chest, coarctation of the aorta (20 per cent), abnormalities of the urinary tract (on investigation, 60 per cent), recurrent otitis media and sometimes deafness, lymphoedema especially of the feet, hypoplastic nails and numerous pigmented naevi. Mild mental retardation with well-preserved verbal ability is not uncommon.

Treatment

Ethinyloestrodiol 0·02 mg. daily, given cyclically with norethisterone 5 mg. daily on the last ten days of the cycle, will induce menses and sexual characteristics without over-rapid fusion of the epiphyses. Higher doses of oestrogen will improve the rate of sexual development but may reduce the patient's final height.

Testicular Feminisation

Most of these patients present as females, seeking medical advice because of primary amenorrhoea or infertility. They are genetic males with a normal XY karyotype, whose testes may be located in the abdomen, inguinal canal or labia. Breasts and external genitalia are female in development with occasional slight enlargement of the clitoris, and only on investigation does it become apparent that the vagina ends blindly and there is no uterus. Testosterone production is normal in these patients, and the condition represents a diminished response to testosterone, a result of diminished conversion of testosterone to the more active dihydrotestosterone and/or a deficiency of the appropriate receptors.

INFERTILITY IN THE FEMALE

The clinical problem presents, of course, as infertility in a couple, defining 'infertility' as failure to conceive despite intent to do so over a period of more than one year, assuming normal coitus of reasonable frequency. In the majority of couples investigated there is a contributory factor in the woman. Possible factors include:

   (1) Disorders of sexual development, as discussed above.
   (2) Conditions 'hostile' to the sperm, such as genital tract abnormalities or the nature of the cervical mucus, detected by examination of post-coital semen extracted from the cervix.
   (3) Failure of implantation of the fertilised ovum.
   (4) Failure of ovulation, indicated by absence of the rises in basal temperature, or amenorrhoea. This may be secondary to major systemic disorders, including adrenal or hypo-

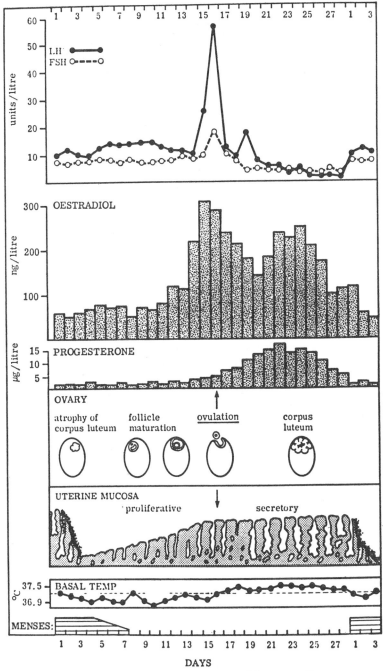

HORMONAL PATTERNS DURING A NORMAL MENSTRUAL CYCLE.

thalamic-pituitary disease, including hyperprolactinaemia, or essentially ovarian, e.g. the *Stein-Leventhal syndrome* (enlarged polycystic ovaries associated with infertility, obesity menstrual irregularities and moderate virilisation).

Treatment

Specific defects or tumours may be treated surgically. Ovulation may be induced with clomiphene, which provokes pituitary gonadotrophin release, or administered gonadotrophins. Supplementation of the hormonal milieu of the luteal phase with progestogens and oestrogens may increase the chance of implantation. Artificial insemination with the husband's sperm may overcome spermicidal barriers. Such techniques are based on the availability of hormone assays which provide precise information about the patient's cycle (see figure above).

FEMALE CLIMACTERIC (MENOPAUSE)

This can be regarded as physiological ovarian failure, leading to cessation of menstruation (menopause), sometimes preceded by menstrual irregularity. Episodes of 'hot flushes', with sweating and warmth, and symptoms of anxiety or depression may be prominent. LH and FSH levels are high. The psychological support of husband and physician is most important, with emphasis on the transient nature of the symptoms. If symptoms are severe then a combined or sequential preparation of oestrogen and a progestogen may be prescribed. Changes consequent upon the drop in anabolic oestrogen production include osteoporosis, which may become severe, a rise in risk of cardiovascular disease, reduction in vaginal secretions (occasional infections, dyspareunia), and some involution of uterus and breasts.

DELAYED PUBERTY IN THE MALE

In normal boys the earliest changes include enlargement of the testes and growth of coarse hairs in the pubic region. The scrotum develops rugal folds and darkens, the penis enlarges, axillary and then facial hair appears and the voice deepens. A mild degree of gynaecomastia is not uncommon. When the patient or his parents complain of 'delay' a family history of late puberty may be reassuring. In true gonad failure the 'bone age' by X-ray falls behind actual age and—in the absence of epiphyseal fusion—the *eunuchoid* physique emerges, span exceeding height, ground to pubis exceeding pubis to crown.

Investigation and Diagnosis

Any endocrine disorder or debilitating illness may delay puberty. When those are excluded, the diagnosis lies between a primary gonad disease, with high levels of FSH and LH (ICSH), and a hypothalamic-pituitary disorder, with low levels of gonadotrophines and bilaterally small soft testes (see hypopituitarism, p. 495).

The only cause of primary testicular failure to commonly affect puberty is **Klinefelter's Syndrome,** in which very small firm testes are associated with variable degrees of eunuchoidism, gynaecomastia, impairment of intelligence, azoospermia, sterility and typically an XXY karyotype. Very rare versions of Turner's syndrome (p. 487) also occur in the phenotypic male.

INFERTILITY IN THE MALE

In about 30 per cent of couples with clinical infertility there is a contributory factor in the husband. Only a small minority have conditions of obvious feminisation, typical Cushing's syndrome, or advanced liver disease with impaired conjugation of oestrogens. Eunuchoidism may indicate Klinefelter's syndrome. Gynaecomastia may indicate any of these conditions. In patients who are not clinically deficient in androgens, the possibilities include germinal cell aplasia, maturation (spermatogenic) arrest, a history of mumps orchitis, cryptorchidism (undescended testes) and varicocele. Semen analysis, testosterone, LH and FSH levels, and sometimes testicular biopsy are required.

Treatment

The patient with low LH or FSH levels may benefit from gonadotrophin or clomiphene treatment, while those with high levels may be prescribed an androgen such as mesterolone. Removal of even a small varicocele or correction of cryptorchidism, lowers the testicular temperature and may restore fertility.

TUMOURS OF THE TESTIS

These are rare, but occur particularly in the 20–35 age group. If the tumour is functional gonadotrophin secretion is suppressed and the other testis may be atrophied.

Type	Five-year Mortality	Special Features
Seminoma	10%	FSH frequently raised
Teratoma	30%	Spread by blood not lymph
Choriocarcinoma	100%	Raised HCG, gynaecomastia
Leydig cell (IC) tumours	± benign	Oestrogens or androgens

TUMOURS OF THE OVARY

Most cysts and neoplasms of the ovary are non-secretory, but the following tumours usually secrete hormones:

Androgens secreted	*Oestrogens secreted*
Arrhenoblastoma	Granulosa cell tumour
Hilus cell tumour	Theca cell tumour
	Luteoma (and → progesterone)
	Teratoma, chorionepithelioma (and → HCG)

PITUITARY HYPERSECRETION

For discussion of hypersecretion of these hormones refer to the appropriate page: TSH, p. 469; ACTH, p. 477; ADH, p. 453.

GIGANTISM AND ACROMEGALY

The syndromes of growth hormone (GH) excess are usually related to an *eosinophil adenoma* of the pituitary, characteristically slow in growth and insidious in clinical presentation. Only in retrospect may it be realised that the disease has been active for 20 or more years before the patient presents.

Gigantism results from excessive GH effect before the epiphyses are fused, producing the features of acromegaly but in addition long limbs and abnormal height. The all-time record for height was held by a Robert Wadlow of Illinois, who died in 1940 at an authenticated height of 8 feet 11 inches; the better known case of Goliath is not well documented. These patients especially suffer from muscular weakness and arthritis. The total effects of the tumour may include hypothalamic irritation and so hyperphagia, and compression of the remaining pituitary and so hypogonadism.

Acromegaly: Clinical Features

Headache, enlarged sella on X-ray, sometimes field defects.

Excessive tiredness, lips thick, nose bulbous, supra-orbital ridges enlarged.

Muscular aching, proximal muscle weakness.

Excessive sweating, skin thick, sebaceous, wrinkled.

Tingling in the fingers, carpal tunnel syndrome.

Progressive enlargement of hands and feet and head (perhaps noticed by change in size of gloves, shoes or hat), spadelike hands, soft and mushy grip, big feet.

Dentures stop fitting, bite over-rides, teeth become separated as the mandible enlarges.

Arthritis and backache, kyphosis, enlarged vertebrae.

Loss of secondary sexual characteristics. In women: menstrual irregularities, amenorrhoea. In men: loss of libido, impotence.

Hoarseness of voice, larynx enlarges, vocal cords thicken.

A few patients have galactorrhoea, or uncinate fits, or rhinorrhoea.

Soft tissue enlargement may include thyroid (goitre), liver and spleen.

Pigmentation is frequently present.

Investigation and Diagnosis

X-rays of the hands show increased soft-tissue thickness, tufting of the tips of the distal phalanges, increased width of phalanges and exostoses. Skull X-rays show an enlarged mandible, prominence of all the sinuses but notably the supraorbital, and in most cases enlargement of the sella. The calcaneal skin pad may exceed 30 mm. in thickness. Over 10 per cent of patients are frankly diabetic, and most have an impaired tolerance of glucose. Levels of GH in plasma are elevated even at rest and are not suppressed by oral glucose. The pituitary tumour may be investigated as one would a chromophobe adenoma (see below).

Treatment

Transphenoidal hypophysectomy, Yttrium implantation and proton beam irradiation are effective treatments. Bromocriptine, an ergotamine derivative with dopaminergic properties, will usually suppress high levels of GH, and is especially valuable for the occasional patient in whom pituitary 'ablation' fails to control the GH hypersecretion. Somatostatin (GHRIH) suppresses GH but its action is short lived, and possible side-effects on platelets prevent its general use at present.

HYPERPROLACTINAEMIA (with or without GALACTORRHOEA)

This is more common than was previously realised in patients with tumours or other lesions in the pituitary or hypothalamus, in women who are not ovulating, in hypothyroidism, and in patients receiving phenothiazines, tricyclic depressants, methyldopa, reserpine and chlordiazepoxide. If the cause cannot be removed or identified, bromocriptine restores prolactin levels to normal.

HYPOPITUITARY STATES

For purposes of discussion these can be classed as:
    (1) *Isolated hormone deficiencies*, e.g. of TSH, ACTH, FSH, and GH (producing dwarfism in an otherwise normal person).
    (2) *Pituitary chromophobe adenoma* producing varying degrees of hypopituitarism and hypothalamic disorder.
    (3) *Panhypopituitarism*, juvenile and adult.

PITUITARY CHROMOPHOBE ADENOMA

Tumours of chromophobe histology often secrete prolactin and occasionally secrete ACTH (especially following adrenalectomy, or GH, but typically act as space-occupying lesions within the sella and then the brain.

The pressure within the sella may cause a classical 'bursting' bi-temporal

The Combined Pituitary Test

This is a combination of the insulin hypoglycaemia, TRH and LHRH tests. In its complete form, the test measures the capacity of the anterior pituitary to secrete all the anterior pituitary hormones. In some patients a more selective test may be adequate.

THE FOLLOWING ARE INJECTED I.V. AT ABOUT 09·00 h:

1. *Soluble insulin*: 0·1 units/kg. body weight in suspected hypopituitarism. 0·3 units/kg. in conditions of insulin resistance. 0·2 units/kg. otherwise. (The blood glucose must fall to 2·5 mmol./l. or below for the test to be valid. It is necessary for a doctor to be present or immediately available throughout in case severe hypoglycaemia occurs and administration of glucose becomes necessary.)

2. *TRH*: 200 μg.

3. *LHRH*: 100 μg.

NORMAL ADULT LEVELS AND RESPONSES (typical ranges)

Sample	GH μg./l.	Cortisol nmol./l.	TSH u./l.	Prolactin u./l.	LH (male) u./l.	FSH (male) u./l.	LH (female) u./l.	FSH (female) u./l.
Basal	1–10	150–700	˙0–3	˙0–0·5	3–10	1–8	3–10*	3–8*
30′	peak exceeds 12	peak exceeds 800	6–20	0·3–2·0	8–35	15–11	8–25	4–11
60′			4–18	0·2–2·0	6–35	1–11	6–20	6–12
90′								
120′								

* Figures obtained in the follicular phase of the cycle. Levels are generally lower than this during the luteal phase, having risen to a peak at mid-cycle (see Figure on p. 489).

headache and radiologically visible expansion of the sella with erosion of the clinoid processes. The pressure on the optic chiasma causes loss of visual acuity, bi-temporal hemianopia, and optic atrophy. Olfactory nerves may be involved with consequent anosmia. Signs of raised intracranial pressure may appear.

Local effects on the pituitary include progressive failure of most of the hormones of the anterior and posterior lobes, and the clinical picture may gradually move towards adult panhypopituitarism

Pressure on the hypothalamus may aggravate the pituitary failure, and also provoke characteristic hypothalamic features of weight gain, somnolence and polydipsia.

Investigation and Diagnosis

For these and other tumours in the region of the sella turcica special investigations should include:

(1) A combined pituitary test (see table on p. 494)
(2) Full visual testing including perimetry for visual fields.
(3) Skull X-rays, with tomography of the sella turcica.
(4) Air encephalogram or a C.A.T. scan to detect suprasellar extension.
(5) Arteriography if an aneurysm must be excluded.

Treatment

Surgery and/or radiotherapy will be advised depending on the position and extent of the adenoma.

PANHYPOPITUITARISM

This condition may be congenital, then causing pituitary dwarfism with adult body proportions and combined failure of thyroid, adrenal and gonad function; this is rare and it is discussed fully in specialist and paediatric texts.

In the adult, panhypopituitarism (*Simmond's disease*) may be caused by infiltration of the pituitary, by neoplasms or granulomas, by trauma or by infarction. The latter is the major cause, being especially associated with major haemorrhage at the time of parturition (*Sheehan's syndrome*).

Clinical Features

History of ante- or post-partum haemorrhage. Failure of lactation and failure to resume menstruation (FSH, LH failure), uterus and vagina shrink, vaginal secretions reduced, infertility. Loss of libido, reduced pubic and axillary hair, impotence (FSH, LH and ACTH). Mild adrenal deficiency may occur (ACTH). Depigmentation and pallor (ACTH). Secondary myxoedema (TSH). Skin characteristically soft, fine and wrinkled. Hypoglycaemic episodes may occur (ACTH, GH). Mineralocorticoid function is well maintained by the renin-angiotensin system.

Investigation and Diagnosis

As discussed in each section, the several gland deficiencies should be quantitated (thyroid, p. 476, adrenal, p. 481). FSH and prolactin levels will be abnormally low, and GH will fail to respond to insulin-induced hypoglycaemia or other stimuli.

Treatment

Substitution by hydrocortisone 20 to 40 mg. daily, regular androgens, and cyclical oestrogens are advisable. Thyroxine may be added gradually, when the adrenal insufficiency has been abolished. As the best treatment for the pituitary remnant is another pregnancy, a trial of gonadotrophins may be in order. These patients should take the same precautions as those with Addison's disease (p. 481).

Hypopituitary Coma

This rare event, which should be prevented by good management, is dangerous in that it may involve the conjunction of hypoglycaemia, hypoadrenalism, hypothyroidism and hypothermia. The patient is treated specifically for these conditions and generally for shock.

HYPOTHALAMIC DEFICIENCIES

In general, the characteristics are:

(1) Diabetes insipidus may occur in association with the anterior lobe hormone deficiencies (p. 452).

(2) Visual defects tend to occur early.

(3) In a small minority only, hyperphagia, weight changes, temperature disturbance and drowsiness occur.

(4) Hyperprolactinaemia, with or without galactorrhoea.

The pathological lesions include, amongst others:

Tumours
Craniopharyngioma (calcification visible on skull X-ray; common in children)
Chromophobe adenomas (early visual changes usually occur)
Granulomas
Sarcoidosis (look for disease elsewhere)
Tuberculosis (look for disease elsewhere)
Hand-Schuller-Christian disease
Trauma of various kinds.

PLURIGLANDULAR DISORDERS

Disease states in which two or more endocrine glands are involved in the same patient:

Combined Gland Failures

(1) Hypopituitary states (p. 495)

(2) Auto-immune group (associated with HLA-B8)
Hashimoto's, Graves', myxoedema
Pernicious anaemia
Addison's disease
Insulin-dependent diabetes mellitus.

Combined Gland Hypersecretion

Multiple endocrine adenomatosis (MEA), which may occur sporadically or as a familial disorder:

MEA Type I: especially pituitary, parathyroid and pancreatic adenomas;

MEA Type II: especially parathyroid, phaeochromocytomas and medullary carcinoma of thyroid (secreting calcitonin).

OTHER ENDOCRINE FUNCTIONS

The kidney is responsible for the secretion of three substances which are hormonal in character: (a) *erythropoetin*, controlling red cell production; (b) *renin*, controlling angiotensin production (p. 383) and (c) *1-25-OH-vitamin D3*, the active form of vitamin D3 (a prohormone?). The synthesis of 1-25-OH-vitamin D3 is governed by intracellular calcium and phosphate concentration in renal tubular cells, and influenced by levels of parathyroid hormone.

The gut secretes a number of identified peptides, such as pancreozymin-cholecystokinin, gastrin, secretin, gastric inhibitory polypeptide, vaso-active inhibitory polypeptide, enteroglucagon and glucagon of pancreatic type, and many others yet to be characterised.

Prostaglandins are modified long-chain fatty acids which are synthesised close to their site of action and are then very rapidly inactivated. They have powerful modulating influences on many processes, with effects in the inflammatory reaction, in pyrexia, in spontaneous abortion, gastric secretion, control of blood pressure, platelet aggregation and smooth muscle contractions.

FURTHER READING

Williams, R. H., *Textbook of Endocrinology*, W. B. Saunders Co., London, 1974.

Hall, R., Anderson, J., Smart, G. A., and Besser, M., *Fundamentals of Clinical Endocrinology*, Pitman Medical, London, 1974.

Mazzaferri, E. L., *Endocrinology Case Studies*, ed. by T. G. Skillman, 2nd edition, Medical Examination Publishing Co., New York, 1975.

CHAPTER FOURTEEN

DISORDERS RESULTING FROM VITAMIN DEFICIENCIES

Introduction

Serious illnesses from vitamin deficiencies are rare in the Western world today. They are still sadly common in the underdeveloped countries. In this country their appearance is usually conditioned by some extra factor, neglect of an infant or elderly person, insanity, gastro-intestinal disease causing impaired absorption, alcoholism, or drug addiction. Deficiency of the accessory food factors known to be synthesised by bacteria in the gut (folic acid, nicotinic acid, riboflavin, and vitamin K) may be induced by antibiotic therapy. Certain groups of the population, for instance pregnant or lactating women, growing children, or children suffering from protracted febrile illnesses are specially at risk. Closed communities are at the mercy of cooks.

Although described separately they commonly occur together. Treatment must always include the resumption of a normal diet, and where doses of vitamins for treatment are quoted they are intended as supplements to such a diet.

VITAMIN A DEFICIENCY

Deficiency occurs endemically in the Middle East, rarely in this country, Symptoms are (1) *Night blindness* (Hemeralopia) from affection of visual purple; (2) *Xerophthalmia*, drying and thickening of the conjunctiva, progressing to (3) *Keratomalacia*, softening and inflammation of the cornea, leading to opacity and blindness; (4) *Follicular keratosis* (phrynoderma), the blocking of skin follicles with horny plugs leading to dryness and roughness of the skin surface. Similar changes are seen in myxoedema.

For details of treatment, etc., see table.

VITAMIN D DEFICIENCY

Introduction

In infants deficiency causes rickets, in adults osteomalacia. It is known that cholecalciferol (vitamin D) after absorption is hydroxylated in the liver; further hydroxylation occurs in the kidney to form 1–25 hydroxycholecalciferol which is highly active in promoting absorption of calcium from the gut.

Deficiency can therefore be caused by inadequate diet, lack of sunlight (vitamin D being formed in the skin), failure of absorption as in the malabsorption syndrome or severe renal damage (renal osteodystrophy).

Clinical Features. Osteoid is prepared at the growing ends of bones, where it heaps up and causes tender swellings which do not become calcified. This is particularly apparent in the skull (*fronto-parietal bosses*), the ribs (*rickety rosary*), and the distal ends of the long bones, particularly at the wrist. Failure of calcification also causes softening of the bones so that they bend under stress; this shows clearly as a sulcus at the line of attachment of the diaphragm (Harrison's sulcus), and in the legs (*genu valgum*, or *varum*). *Dentition* is similarly delayed and defective. The muscles are generally hypotonic; there is delay in walking and standing, with weakness, lordosis, and abdominal protuberance. If the serum calcium is low, *tetany* may result.

For details of treatment, etc., see table.

Overdosage

Symptoms are anorexia, nausea, thirst, vomiting, polyuria and drowsiness. Calcium and phosphorus levels in the serum and urine may be elevated, and tissue calcification may occur. Calcification of the kidneys may lead to hypertension and uraemia.

VITAMIN K

Deficiency causes hypoprothrombinaemia..

VITAMIN B DEFICIENCY

(a) **Thiamine deficiency** is much more likely to occur in the presence of achlorhydria and when a high proportion of the dietary calories are provided by carbohydrate.

Clinical Manifestations

(1) *Polyneuritis* (Dry beri-beri) (p. 326), less commonly myelitis. The neuritis is always associated with extreme tenderness of muscle.

(2) *Cardiac failure* with oedema, cardiac enlargement, usually regular rhythm, and circulatory hyperkinesis (high output failure). (Wet beri-beri.)

(3) *Wernicke's encephalopathy* (p. 327), in which confusion, ataxia, nystagmus, squint, and diplopia are common.

(Treatment, etc., see table.)

(b) **Riboflavine deficiency** causes widespread affection of the mucous membranes and skin, presenting as:

(1) *The tongue is sore and magenta coloured.*

(2) *Angular stomatitis*, painful red fissures at the angles of the mouth.

(3) *Cheilosis*, a stripping of the superficial epithelium at the line of closure of the lips.

(4) *Vascularisation of the cornea*, spreading in from the periphery and visible initially only on slit-lamp microscopy, later to the naked eye.

Vitamin	Solubility	Clinical Deficiency Disorder	Test for Deficiency	Prophylaxis (Daily)	Therapy (Daily)	Natural Sources
A	Fat	Xerophthalmia Keratomalacia Night blindness Follicular keratosis	Serum carotene levels	2,500–5,000 i.u.	10–25,000 i.u.	Eggs, milk, butter, vitaminised margarine, fish liver oils, coloured vegetables
D	Fat	Bone changes Hypotonia Tetany	Radiography of bones, serum alkaline phosphatase serum calcium serum phosphate	Calcium-containing foods. 400 i.u. daily, calciferol 3,000 i.u.	3–5,000 i.u.	Eggs, milk, butter, vitaminised margarine, fish liver oils
K	Fat	Hypoprothrom-binaemia	Serum prothrombin time	1–2 mg.	5–10 mg.	Spinach, cabbage, kale, cauliflower, synthesised in gut
B Thiamine (B$_1$)	Water	Beri-beri, dry or wet, Wernicke's encephalopathy (p. 327)	Pyruvate tolerance test	1–1·6 mg.	50–100 mg.	Whole grain cereals, yeast, liver
Riboflavine (B$_2$)	Water	Rubiolation of cornea, Kerato-malacia, Cheilosis Angular stomatitis Magenta tongue, Seborrhoeic dermatitis	Slit-lamp microscopy of cornea	1·4–2·5 mg.	5–15 mg.	Milk, eggs, butter, liver, yeast
Nicotinic acid (Niacin)	Water	Pellagra		10–16 mg.	100–500 mg.	Whole grain cereals, excluding maize
Pyridoxine (B$_6$)	Water	Peripheral neuritis Anaemia in infants		1–2 mg.	10–50 mg.	Whole grain cereals, yeast
Cyanocobalamin (B$_{12}$)	Water	Pernicious anaemia (p. 509)	Serum B$_{12}$	2–4 µg.	(see p. 59)	Whole grain cereals
C	Water	Scurvy	Vit. C content of white blood cells	70–150 mg.	500–1,000 mg.	Green vegetables, fresh fruit, oranges, tomatoes, black-currants

(5) Eventually *keratomalacia* with corneal opacity may develop.

(6) *Seborrhoeic dermatitis* of the naso-labial folds, ears, and chest.

(c) **Nicotinic Acid deficiency** causes the clinical syndrome of *pellagra*.

Clinical Features

(1) *Dementia*

(2) *Diarrhoea*, which is intractable and may lead to potassium deficiency.

(3) *Dermatitis*. This consists of a scaly pigmentation of the exposed skin surfaces. The tongue is affected, and has been likened to 'raw beef'. Pellagra is a disease of maize eaters. Secondary deficiency may occur in gastro-intestinal disorders and with carcinoid tumours.

(Treatment, etc., see table.)

(d) **Pyridoxin deficiency** is a rarity. Artificially fed infants given a pyridoxine deficient diet develop an anaemia with all the characteristics of iron deficiency except that it responds only to pyridoxine. They may also have convulsions. In adults, where deficiency may occur as a side-effect of *isoniazid* administration, cheilosis, glossitis, weakness, peripheral neuritis and increased susceptibility to infection may occur.

(e) **Cyanocobalamin deficiency** causes pernicious anaemia (p. 509). Peripheral neuritis, subacute combined degeneration of the cord, optic atrophy, and dementia may also occur, either in association with the anaemia or separately.

VITAMIN C DEFICIENCY

Introduction

Scurvy is seen mainly nowadays in elderly people living alone on a diet which contains no fruit or vegetables. The diet must be grossly deficient in ascorbic acid for some six months before symptoms appear.

Clinical Features. Patients feel generally ill. Signs are produced by *spontaneous haemorrhages*. These occur most frequently in the gums, which bleed at a touch, especially the interdentate papillae (*scurvy buds*). *Teeth* become loose and infected, and *foetor oris* is marked. Perifollicular haemorrhage may cause *skin purpura*, and derangement of the hairs (corkscrew hairs). Later there may be large spontaneous haemorrhages, into muscles or joints, or subcutaneous (*ecchymoses*). There is deficient haemoglobin synthesis, causing anaemia, and impaired collagen formation which gives rise to delayed wound healing.

(Treatment, etc., see table.)

CHAPTER FIFTEEN

DISORDERS OF THE BLOOD

ANATOMY AND PHYSIOLOGY

Blood contains three types of cell, red blood corpuscles (erythrocytes), white blood corpuscles (leucocytes), and platelets (thrombocytes). These cells are formed mainly in the bone marrow and normally the speed of production is regulated to ensure that just sufficient numbers of each type of cell are delivered into the peripheral blood each day to replace those which have worn out and have been removed.

Red Blood Cells

The parent cell in the bone marrow is the erythroblast, a large cell which has deeply basophilic cytoplasm, contains no haemoglobin and has one or more nucleoli in its nucleus. In the presence of adequate supplies of vitamin B_{12} and folic acid the erythroblast produces by division a smaller cell with a denser nucleus; this is the early normoblast, which still has basophilic cytoplasm. Haemoglobinisation of the cell occurs at this stage and the cytoplasm changes from the blue colour of the primitive cell through a polychromatic phase to the pink of the mature normoblast, which now has a very dense pyknotic nucleus. Disintegration of the nucleus transforms the normoblast into the young erythrocyte or reticulocyte, so-called because supra-vital staining with cresyl blue reveals a fine reticulum of polychromatic material in the cytoplasm. The fully mature erythrocyte contains no such reticulum and therefore a reticulocyte count gives a valuable indication of the rate of new red cell production. In health no nucleated red cells appear in the peripheral blood.

In the absence of adequate supplies of vitamin B_{12} or folic acid there is failure of maturation beyond the erythroblast-early normoblast phase and these large primitive cells become prematurely haemoglobinised. Anaemia characterised by large cells and a high haemoglobin content (macrocytic and hyperchromic) is the result. Iron is an essential element in the haemoglobin molecule so that iron deficiency leads to shortage of haemoglobin, but it does not interfere with the normal maturation of the red cells. Although less haemoglobin is put into each cell, the cells are smaller and thinner than normal, and the cell haemoglobin *concentration* is unaltered. The cells appear small and pale (microcytosis and hypochromia).

Small amounts of thyroid hormone, ascorbic acid, and copper are also required for efficient red cell production.

The life of each red cell in the circulation is about 120 days. At the end of that time it is broken down by cells of the reticulo-endothelial system, mainly in the bone marrow, spleen, and liver, the haemoglobin being split into two fractions. One of these contains the iron atoms and is returned to the bone marrow for re-synthesis into new red cells, forming by far the biggest source of the iron used for this purpose; the non-iron-containing fraction constitutes the bile pigment bilirubin and is transported in the blood to the liver for excretion.

White Blood Cells

(1) *The Granular Series*

The parent cell in the bone marrow is the myeloblast, a large cell with basophilic non-granular cytoplasm and a nucleus containing several nucleoli. From this is formed a smaller cell without nucleoli called the myelocyte, which acquires granules in its cytoplasm as it matures. The nucleus gradually condenses, becoming first kidney-shaped (at which stage the cell is known as a metamyelocyte) and then lobulated. The cell is now now a mature granulocyte, and is classified as neutrophil, eosinophil, or basophil according to the staining reaction of the granules in its cytoplasm. As the cell becomes older it acquires more lobes in its nucleus.

Normal blood contains $2 \cdot 0 – 7 \cdot 5 \times 10^3/\mu l$ neutrophil granulocytes, $0 – 0 \cdot 4$ eosinophils and $0 – 0 \cdot 2$ basophils $\times 10^3/\mu l$.

(2) *The Lymphocyte Series*

The parent cell is the lymphoblast, found in lymphoid tissue throughout the body as well as in the bone marrow. It looks very like a myeloblast, but can usually be distinguished by the company it keeps: i.e. it breeds lymphocytes and not granulocytes. From the lymphoblast are derived the large and small lymphocytes, cells with clear blue cytoplasm and dense nuclei; the small ones are probably the more mature cells.

The normal lymphocyte count is $1 \cdot 0 – 3 \cdot 5 \times 10^3/\mu l$.

(3) *The Monocyte Series*

The monoblast, which also closely resembles the myeloblast, is derived from reticulum cells and gives rise to the monocyte, a cell with cloudy blue cytoplasm containing a few small red granules, and a kidney-shaped nucleus.

The normal monocyte count is $0 – 0 \cdot 8 \times 10^3/\mu l$.

The Platelets

The parent cell is the megakaryocyte found in the bone marrow, a very large cell with multilobulated nucleus and granular cytoplasm. The platelets formed from it are small ($2 – 4 \mu m$.) bodies containing blue or purple granules but no nucleus.

The normal platelet count is $150 – 350 \times 10^3/\mu l$.

ANAEMIA

Definition

Anaemia is a condition of diminished oxygen-carrying capacity of the blood due to a reduction in the numbers of red cells or in their content of haemoglobin, or both.

Symptoms and Signs of Anaemia

The symptoms and signs due to the diminished oxygen-carrying capacity of the blood are common to all types of anaemia. They include general tiredness, shortness of breath on exertion, giddiness, headache, pallor (especially pallor of the mucous membranes and of the palms of the hands), palpitations, oedema of the ankles, and occasionally in older people angina pectoris (see p. 165).

Causes of Anaemia

The anaemias can be classified primarily into two groups:

(1) Those due to some failure in the quality or quantity of new red cells being produced in the marrow, and

(2) Those due to excessive loss of red cells from the circulation, either from acute or chronic haemorrhage or from abnormal haemolysis.

There is frequent overlap between these two groups since haemorrhage leads to iron deficiency, which is by far the commonest cause of the anaemias in group (1). The classification is useful for descriptive purposes, however, and can be amplified as follows:

(1) Deficient Red Cell Production

(a) Iron deficiency anaemia.
(b) Vitamin B_{12} or folic acid deficiency.
   (i) Pernicious anaemia (Addison's anaemia).
   (ii) Failure of absorption of vitamin B_{12} or folic acid due to disorders of the gastro-intestinal tract such as sprue, idiopathic steatorrhoea, and after gastro-intestinal operations.
   (iii) Tropical nutritional macrocytic anaemia.
   (iv) Macrocytic anaemia of pregnancy.
(c) The anaemia of myxoedema from lack of thyroxin.
(d) The anaemia of scurvy from lack of vitamin C.
(e) Impairment of erythroblastic activity in bone marrow:
   (i) Aplastic anaemia.
   (ii) Invasion of bone marrow in leukaemia, metastatic malignant disease, Hodgkin's disease, myelomatosis, and myelosclerosis.
   (iii) Probable toxic effect on erythroblasts in uraemia, chronic infections, malignant disease, and certain collagen diseases.

(2) Excessive Loss of Red Cells

  (a) Haemorrhage.

  (b) Abnormal haemolysis:

      (i) Due to congenital defects in the red cells, in familial acholuric jaundice, and sickle-cell anaemia.

      (ii) Due to acquired haemolysins in the blood, either of unknown cause or in incompatible blood transfusions, septicaemias, malignant disease, and erythroblastosis foetalis.

INVESTIGATION OF ANAEMIA

Haemoglobin

The average haemoglobin content of normal blood is 14·8 g. per 100 ml. (range 13·5–18·0 g. in men; 11·5–16·0 g. in women), which is consequently taken as the arbitrary 100 per cent level in most laboratories. There is still no general agreement on this point, however, and to prevent confusion the haemoglobin should always be expressed in grams per 100 ml., the percentage figure being given in addition if desired.

Red Blood Count

The red count has a wide physiological range between about $4·0–6·0 \times 10^6/\mu l$. Calculation of the haematological indices outlined below is based on the assumption that the normal red count is $5·0 \times 10^6/\mu l$ and that 100 per cent haemoglobin is 14·8 g. dl.

Haematocrit Value (or packed-cell volume)

This is the volume occupied by the red cells in 100 ml. of centrifuged blood and is normally about 45 ml. per cent.

Mean Corpuscular Haemoglobin Concentration (M.C.H.C.)

This value has been used for many years as a measure of concentration of haemoglobin within the red cells and a low value was taken as an indication of iron deficiency anaemia.

It is obtained from the formula

$$\frac{\text{Hb in grams/100 ml.}}{\text{Packed cell volume/100 ml.}} \times 100$$

The low values found in iron deficiency have however been shown to be due to the loose packing of the irregularly shaped erythrocytes when the packed cell volume is estimated by centrifugation. It is not really an estimate of cell haemoglobin concentration. If the packed cell volume is obtained from the red cell count and the mean corpuscular volume (as occurs with the Coulter 'S' Counter), a normal M.C.H.C. will be found in iron deficiency.

The haematological diagnosis of iron deficiency anaemia depends on the finding of a low M.C.V. and M.C.H. which is associated with small and irregular hypochromic erythrocytes on the stained smear (due to cells being small and thin, rather than having a low haemoglobin concentration). In addition the serum iron will be low and the bone marrow will show absence of stainable iron.

Mean Corpuscular Volume (M.C.V.)

This is the average volume of a single red cell in cubic microns and is obtained by dividing the packed-cell volume in ml. per 1,000 ml. blood by the red cells in millions per c.mm. The normal range is 78–94 fl. With the Coulter 'S' counter the M.C.V. is measured directly and is not derived from the packed cell volume obtained by centrifugation. The M.C.V. gives an indication of the size of the red cell in three dimensions.

The **Mean Corpuscular Diameter** (M.C.D.), on the other hand, being obtained by measurement of the diameter of the red cells in a stained film, gives an indication of the size of the cells in two dimensions only and takes no account of their thickness. The average normal M.C.D. is 7·2 μm., with a range of 6·7 to 7·7 μm.

Serum Iron

Normal range men 14–31 μmol./l.
women 11–29 μmol./l.

Total Iron-binding Capacity (T.I.B.C.)

Normal range 54–80 μmol./l.

Serum B$_{12}$

Normal range 150–850 pg./ml.

Serum Folate

Normal range 3–18 ng./ml.

IRON DEFICIENCY ANAEMIA

Iron Metabolism

In normal men the amount of iron excreted daily does not exceed 1–1·5 mg. Iron absorption from the upper small intestine is limited by a mucosal block mechanism, just enough being absorbed to replace the amount lost, the total body iron thus being kept fairly constant at about 4–5 g. Iron is transported in the plasma in combination with a specific fraction of the β globulin, which when fully saturated can unite with some 300–350 μg. iron per 100 ml. The normal plasma iron level, however, is only about 100 μg. iron per 100 ml., which represents approximately one-third saturation of the iron-binding capacity of the plasma. The body's reserve stores of iron, contained mainly in the liver, are about 1·5 g.; this provides enough iron for the replacement of about 3 to 4 pints of blood. Normally the iron used in haemoglobin synthesis for new red cells is nearly all provided by the catabolism of haemoglobin from old red cells and very little has to be drawn from the reserve stores.

The average daily loss of iron is at least doubled in women during the reproductive period of life by menstruation, pregnancy, and lactation. To remain in iron balance they must therefore absorb daily some 2–3 mg. instead of 1–1·5 mg. and to ensure this absorption a diet containing at least 15 mg. iron is essential. A similar iron intake is advisable for growing children, but for everyone else 5–10 mg. daily is probably adequate.

Aetiology

(a) The most important cause of iron deficiency is *haemorrhage*. If a pint of blood is withdrawn weekly from a healthy young man the blood count remains normal for about a month. By that time, however, the reserve stores of iron are exhausted and if bleeding continues at the same rate there is a shortage of iron and therefore of haemoglobin for the new red cells being poured out by the marrow. Signs of iron deficiency, therefore, rapidly appear in the blood. Clinical iron deficiency may be the result of acute haemorrhage of the same order, frequently from haematemesis or melaena, but much more often it is a consequence of chronic blood loss. Menorrhagia is by far the most important factor and its ill-effects are commonly enhanced by previous depletion of the reserve stores of iron by pregnancy and lactation. This is why iron deficiency anaemia is seen mainly in women.

(b) *Dietary deficiency of iron* occurs in those who, usually from either poverty, ignorance, or food-fad, do not eat enough of the main iron-containing foods, meat, eggs, and green vegetables. The deficiency is serious particularly in women who, as explained above, have high iron requirements.

(c) Impaired absorption of iron may be the result of achlorhydria, gastrectomy, and short-circuit operations involving the small intestine, or the malabsorption syndrome (coeliac disease, sprue, idiopathic steatorrhoea, and Crohn's disease).

Clinical Features

In addition to the usual symptoms and signs of anaemia, patients with iron deficiency often have brittle, spoon-shaped nails (*koilonychia*) and a very smooth tongue. The latter change is due to atrophy of the filiform papillae. Similar atrophic changes in the mucous membrane in the upper part of the oesophagus, and the development of a curious 'web' of delicate tissue which partially obstructs the lumen and causes dysphagia, occasionally develop and complete the picture of the *Plummer–Vinson syndrome*. The spleen is sometimes palpable.

Blood Count. Since lack of iron leads to shortage of haemoglobin but does not retard the production of red cell envelopes, less haemoglobin is put into each red cell. The red blood count is only slightly lowered, therefore, but the haemoglobin content of blood is reduced because the red cells are smaller and thus contain less haemoglobin (low M.C.H.). The haemo-globin concentration of the red cell is unaltered. In a patient with untreated iron-deficiency anaemia a reticulocyte count above 1 per cent, indicating increased turnover of red cells, suggests that haemorrhage has been an important aetiological factor. The untreated patient is also likely to have a fasting serum iron level below 50 μg. per 100 ml. and the unsaturated iron-binding capacity of the serum will be in the range of 300–400 μg. per 100 ml.

Treatment. It is important wherever possible to deal with the various factors which have led to the iron deficiency at the same time as the latter is corrected. In practice this usually means arranging appropriate treat-ment for menorrhagia or gastro-intestinal bleeding and giving advice about diet. For correcting the iron deficiency it is nearly always satisfactory to give *iron by mouth* and since ferrous sulphate is the cheapest effective preparation it is the one which should be chosen for routine use. There is some evidence that absorption of iron is better if it is not given on a full stomach, so that a good prescription is tab. ferrous sulphate 200 mg. four times daily between meals. Ascorbic acid 50 mg. twice daily, is sometimes given in the belief that it aids iron absorption; the giving of dilute hydro-chloric acid for this purpose is no longer thought to be of any value. If ferrous sulphate causes gastro-intestinal upset (nausea, diarrhoea, or con-stipation) tab. ferrous gluconate 600 mg. four times daily may be given instead.

Parenteral iron therapy is indicated:

(1) when there is a serious impairment of absorption,

(2) when severe iron deficiency has to be corrected quickly during pregnancy, and

(3) rarely when real or imagined intolerance of oral preparations makes effective treatment by mouth impracticable.

Either iron sorbitol citric acid complex (Jectofer) or iron dextran (Imferon) may be given intramuscularly and are usually effective and well tolerated. Each contains 50 mg. iron in 1 ml. The injections cause local pain and may result in staining of the skin which is transient with Jectofer but permanent with Imferon. After a test dose of 25 mg. injections of 100 mg. may be given daily or at longer intervals to a total of 1–2 g. Total dosage is calculated from the fact that about 50 mg. is required to raise the haemoglobin by 1 per cent. Toxic effects are rare if single doses do not exceed 100 mg., but Jectofer may cause fever, vomiting, disorienta-tion, temporary loss of taste, a metallic taste in the mouth and local urticaria, and Imferon fever, allergic reactions, lymph-node enlargement and arthralgia.

SIDEROBLASTIC ANAEMIAS

These are rare disorders in which varying numbers of hypochromic microcytic red cells are found in the blood and normoblasts containing an excess of iron-containing granules appear in the marrow. There are also increased iron stores in the reticulo-endothelial system and in parenchymatous organs such as the liver, pancreas and heart; the serum iron level is raised and there is complete or almost complete saturation of the iron-binding protein. Kinetic studies may show increased iron turnover but impaired iron utilisation.

Congenital Sideroblastic Anaemia

This is usually inherited as an X-linked trait and is therefore seen mainly in male patients; it sometimes responds to large doses of pyridoxine, though there is no evidence of pyridoxine deficiency.

Acquired Sideroblastic Anaemia

This may be related to underlying disease such as carcinomas, Hodgkin's disease, leukaemia or rheumatoid arthritis, or may be a side-effect of drugs such as isoniazid and cycloserine which interfere with pyridoxine metabolism.

Treatment. Pyridoxine 50–200 mg. daily should always be given for 2 months and then if there is no response steroid therapy may be tried. Since the iron overload may have serious consequences (see Haemochromotosis, p. 89) iron therapy should be avoided and blood transfusions should be given sparingly.

ANAEMIAS DUE TO VITAMIN B_{12} OR FOLIC ACID DEFICIENCY

Pernicious Anaemia (Addison's anaemia)

Aetiology. This is primarily a disease of the gastric mucosa, which in middle age or beyond fails to produce hydrochloric acid, pepsin and Castle's intrinsic factor. The cause of this failure is not known, but present evidence suggests that it is probably due to an inherited constitutional weakness; thus there is a significant familial incidence and the disease has been shown to be commoner in people of blood group A than blood group O. Gastric cytoplasmic antibodies can be demonstrated in over 80 per cent of patients, indicating a defect in the body's 'self-recognition system'. B_{12} in the diet is not absorbed in the absence of gastric intrinsic factor. The disease is very rare below the age of thirty. These patients often have prematurely grey hair.

Clinical Features. The onset is very insidious and frequently the patient does not consult his doctor until the red cell count has fallen to 1–2 million per c.mm. or even lower. This observation alone may suggest the diagnosis, since counts as low as this in the absence of severe symptoms are very rarely found in other anaemias. In addition to the symptoms common to all anaemias (p. 405), the patient may complain of recurrent soreness of the tongue and very rarely the symptoms of subacute combined degeneration of the cord (p. 328) may be the first indication of the disease. Fever is often present, but significant loss of weight is unusual. Abdominal pain and diarrhoea are common.

Examination shows pallor and in advanced cases the faint lemon-yellow colour of haemolytic jaundice due to rapid breakdown of the abnormal red cells in the circulation. About half the patients have a red raw-looking and smooth tongue. A haemic cardiac murmur, nearly always systolic in timing, can often be heard and retinal haemorrhages are sometimes present. The spleen is palpable in about 60 per cent of patients.

Investigations. *Gastric analysis* invariably reveals pentagastrin-fast achlorhydria, so that if any HCl is found in samples aspirated from the stomach after the subcutaneous injection of pentagastrin 6 μg./kg. or histamine 40 μg./kg. the diagnosis must be discarded.

Blood Picture. There is severe reduction in the red count but only moderate reduction in haemoglobin percentage, so that the M.C.H. is high, and raised M.C.D. and M.C.V. values (p. 506) show that the cells are macrocytic. Examination of the stained film shows abnormal variations in size, shape, and staining reaction and immature nucleated cells, usually normoblasts but sometimes haemoglobinised megaloblasts, may be seen. There is usually a low total white count of about 3,000–4,000 per cu.mm., the reduction affecting mainly the granulocyte cells, which also show a shift to the right (a predominance of older cells). In severe cases the platelets may also be decreased.

Bone marrow examination shows the presence of large numbers of haemoglobinised megaloblasts.

The Schilling Test. Vitamin B_{12} labelled with radioactive cobalt is given by mouth and within an hour 1,000 μg. of ordinary B_{12} is injected intramuscularly to flood the body's stores and ensure excretion by the kidneys of any of the B_{12} absorbed. The urine is collected for 48 hrs. and its content of radioactive B_{12} estimated. Normal people eliminate 15–50 per cent of the given dose in the urine, but patients with pernicious anaemia less than 10 per cent.

The serum level of Vitamin B_{12} is reduced (normal 150–850 pg./ml.).

Treatment must continue for life since the gastric atrophy is permanent. This fact should be impressed on the patient as soon as the diagnosis is made, for if the blood count is allowed to fall below normal at any time there is grave danger that irreversible changes of subacute combined degeneration of the cord will develop. Vitamin B_{12} is administered intramuscularly as cyano-cobalamin or hydroxy-cobalamin. There is a good deal of individual variation in the dosage required, but average doses are 100–1,000 μg. of vitamin B_{12} (cyano-cobalamin) every day until the blood count is normal, followed by a similar amount once every 2 to 4 weeks for maintenance. The patient's progress must of course be followed by regular blood counts. At the start of treatment there is an outpouring of new young erythrocytes into the circulation, so that the reticulocyte count rises sharply to reach a peak by about the seventh day. The degree of rise in the reticulocyte count varies with the severity of the anaemia before treatment;

when the initial red count has been very low it may reach 40 or 50 per cent. If no reticulocyte crisis occurs in response to treatment the diagnosis should be reconsidered.

Complications. *Subacute combined degeneration of the spinal cord* is by far the most important complication and is discussed on p. 328.

Carcinoma of the stomach occurs more often in patients with pernicious anaemia than in the general population and some authorities advocate annual barium meal examination or even annual gastroscopy for its early detection in such patients. It is probably an adequate precaution, however, to perform such investigations only when there is some special indication such as an unexplained rise in the sedimentation rate.

Other Macrocytic Anaemias

Macrocytic anaemia, haematologically similar to pernicious anaemia, and resulting also from lack of adequate supplies of B_{12} or folic acid in the bone marrow, may be seen under the following circumstances:

(a) Dietary deficiency, mainly of folic acid but affecting B_{12} too, occurs only in association with gross general malnutrition and has been reported mainly from India as tropical (or nutritional) macrocytic anaemia (Hindus are often strict vegetarians with very low B_{12} intake).

(b) Lesions of the gastro-intestinal tract may impair the absorption of B_{12} and folic acid. Thus macrocytic anaemia is sometimes found in patients with carcinoma of the stomach, after total gastrectomy, after operations on the small gut, particularly when multiple anastomoses or blind loops have been formed, and in patients with the malabsorption syndrome (coeliac disease, sprue, and idiopathic streatorrhoea).

(c) Alcohol is a marrow toxin and chronic alcoholism causes macrocytosis and later folate deficiency and megaloblastic anaemia.

(d) Macrocytic anaemia, which usually responds to treatment with tablets of folic acid 10 mg. daily, sometimes occurs for reasons unknown during the later months of pregnancy.

(e) Phenytoin and methotrexate sometimes causes macrocytic anaemia due to folate deficiency.

HAEMOLYTIC ANAEMIAS

Abnormally rapid breakdown of the red cells in the circulation leads to an increase in the level of bilirubin in the serum, causing latent or overt jaundice, and to an increased excretion of urobilinogen in the urine and faeces. The compensatory increase in the rate of erythropoeisis in the bone marrow causes an outpouring of new red cells into the circulation, so that a high reticulocyte count is another characteristic feature of haemolytic anaemia.

Causes. Excessive haemolysis may be due to:

(1) hereditary abnormalities in the erythrocytes, as in acholuric jaundice,

(2) haemolysins in the blood, or

(3) toxic or infective factors.

HEREDITARY ABNORMALITIES IN THE RED CELLS

(1) Acholuric Jaundice

This rare disease is usually inherited as a Mendelian dominant, being passed directly from parent to child. The sexes are affected equally. Red cells from a patient with acholuric jaundice are destroyed at a greatly increased rate when transfused into normal people, whereas normal red cells survive for the expected time when transfused into patients with acholuric jaundice. Furthermore haemolysins cannot be demonstrated in the blood. The defect therefore lies in the red cells themselves, which are smaller in diameter (about 5·6–6·2 μm.) and more spherical in shape than normal erythrocytes (*microspherocytes*) and remain in the circulation on an average for only fifteen days instead of the normal 120 days. The mean corpuscular volume and mean corpuscular haemoglobin concentration are usually normal. There is always a high reticulocyte count of 10–20 per cent, rising to 50 per cent or more during haemolytic crises. The red cells show an increased fragility in salt solutions, haemolysis starting at a salt concentration of 0·75 per cent and being complete at 0·4 per cent (normal range 0·45 to 0·3 per cent).

Clinical Features. Yellowness of the skin is usually noted during the first few years of life, but apart from this symptoms are few and slight except during the so-called haemolytic crises when the patient becomes pale, weak, and febrile. Slow spontaneous recovery usually occurs in about a month. It is now thought that some of these attacks are not episodes of increased haemolysis but of temporary marrow aplasia, since the reticulocyte count may fall and the jaundice become lighter.

The spleen is nearly always palpable and may extend to the umbilicus. About 60 per cent of patients have gallstones of 'metabolic' type, which are precipitated from the excess of bilirubin excreted in the bile; they contain pigment and calcium but no cholesterol. Cholecystectomy is, however, rarely necessary. A curious but important symptom is intractable ulceration of the legs which heals only after splenectomy.

Treatment. Splenectomy is a very satisfactory treatment which nearly always leads to permanent symptomatic cure.

(2) Sickle-cell Anaemia

This disease, which is practically confined to negroes, is inherited as a Mendelian dominant. The essential fault is an abnormal haemoglobin in the red cells which causes the latter to assume a sickle shape at the lower end of the physiological range of oxygen tension. The abnormal shape of the red cells leads to increased blood viscosity and tends to promote capillary thrombosis.

The illness presents as a chronic haemolytic anaemia, sometimes with acute crises and sometimes with thrombotic episodes, and the diagnosis is confirmed by demonstrating sickling of the red cells in a sealed preparation of blood in which the oxygen tension has been reduced. There is no effective treatment apart from transfusion for severe anaemia.

(3) **Cooley's anaemia** (thalassaemia major), due to Mendelian dominant homozygous inheritance of a metabolic fault leading to continued production of foetal haemoglobin, is found in Mediterranean peoples and usually leads to death in childhood from haemolytic anaemia. Splenectomy sometimes reduces the need for transfusion, but there is no generally effective treatment.

Thalassaemia minor, due to heterozygous inheritance of the same gene, is usually symptomless and is detected only by routine blood examination.

(4) Non-spherocytic Anaemia

In two members of this group specific enzyme defects have been demonstrated: (a) deficiency of red cell pyruvate kinase, inherited as a recessive character, and (b) deficiency of glucose-6-phosphate dehydrogenase, with sex-linked recessive inheritance.

HAEMOLYTIC ANAEMIA DUE TO CIRCULATING HAEMOLYSINS

Acquired Haemolytic Anaemia

This disease is due not to abnormalities in the red cells but to the presence of haemolysins in the blood, because:

(1) when compatible cells from patients with acquired haemolytic anaemia are transfused into normal people they survive for a normal time, whereas normal cells are quickly destroyed when transfused into patients with acquired haemolytic anaemia, and

(2) the *Coombs' test* is nearly always positive, either the direct Coombs' test demonstrating the presence of antibody adsorbed to the red cells or the indirect Coombs' test indicating a free antibody in the blood.

Acquired haemolytic anaemia, which may present in acute, subacute, or chronic clinical forms, may be seen in patients with chronic infections such as tuberculosis, syphilis, or malaria, with malignant disease, or with leukaemia or the reticuloses. Frequently, however, the underlying cause is never discovered.

Treatment. The abnormal haemolysis can usually be controlled by giving corticosteroids, which are therefore life-saving in this disease. The drug may have to be continued indefinitely, however. (See p. 621 for dangers of long-term therapy.) Dosage is very variable; the smallest daily dose which will prevent haemolysis and therefore drop in haemoglobin should be given. Splenectomy is of benefit in some patients. The abnormal haemolysis sometimes stops if the underlying cause can be treated.

TOXIC AND INFECTIVE HAEMOLYTIC ANAEMIA

Very rarely haemolytic anaemia may occur in association with severe infections, such as streptococcal or staphylococcal septicaemia or as a result of poisoning with lead or dinitro-benzene or from idiosyncrasy to drugs such as sulphonamides, amphetamine, or potassium chlorate. The presence of large numbers of Heinz bodies in red cells strongly suggests haemolytic anaemia due to chemical poisoning.

THE HAEMORRHAGIC DISEASES

A tendency to abnormal bleeding may result from:

(1) **A coagulation defect,** or lack of one of the various substances in the blood which are necessary for the formation of a firm blood-clot when blood is shed (e.g. haemophilia).

(2) **Thrombocytopenia,** which may be either idiopathic or symptomatic of some disease of the bone marrow such as leukaemia or aplastic anaemia, or

(3) Some abnormality in the **capillaries.**

Diseases in group (1) lead to persistent bleeding after injury or trauma; groups (2) and (3) constitute the *purpuras*, which are characterised by spontaneous bleeding from mucous surfaces and into the skin, causing a purpuric eruption (petechiae or ecchymoses). Purpuric spots are easily recognised since, the blood being extravascular, they do not fade on pressure.

COAGULATION DEFECTS

Physiology of Blood Coagulation

The immediate arrest of haemorrhage after injury to small blood vessels is due to vaso-constriction and plugging of the leaks by aggregations of platelets which control the bleeding until a firm blood-clot forms. Coagulation is a complex process initiated by contact of the blood with a water-wettable surface and involves the interaction of many coagulation factors; the nomenclature of these factors has now been standardised internationally, using Roman numerals:

Factor	Synonym
Factor I	Fibrinogen
Factor II	Prothrombin

(Factor III was originally tissue thromboplastin;
Factor IV calcium; and Factor VI the activated form
of Factor V; these terms are now seldom used.)

Factor	*Synonym*
Factor V	Labile factor
Factor VII	Stable factor
Factor VIII	Anti-haemophilic globulin
Factor IX	Christmas factor
Factor X	Stuart-Prower factor
Factor XI	
Factor XII	Hageman factor
Factor XIII	Fibrin stabilising factor

Contact with a water-wettable surface leads to a molecular rearrangement of factor XII which thus acquires enzymatic properties and by interaction with factors XI, IX and VIII converts factor X to its active form. Activated factor X with factor V and the platelet factor form prothrombinase, which converts prothrombin to thrombin; interaction of thrombin with fibrinogen in the presence of factor XIII leads to the formation of fibrin, which provides the framework of the blood clot. Retraction of the blood clot, which helps to draw the edges of the wound together, is due to shortening of the fibrin strands by the action of a protein liberated from the platelets.

In haemophilia and allied states the initial arrest of haemorrhage takes place normally but failure of a firm blood clot to form results in bleeding an hour or so after the injury when the vasoconstriction passes off. This also explains why in these conditions the coagulation time is prolonged, but the bleeding time is typically normal.

INVESTIGATION OF PATIENTS WITH A HAEMORRHAGIC DISEASE

Hess's Test. The sphygmomanometer cuff is placed round the upper arm and the pressure maintained halfway between the systolic and diastolic pressures for five minutes. A positive test, shown by the appearance of more than 5 purpuric spots on the arm below the level of the cuff, is found in patients with capillary defects and with severe thrombocytopenia.

Platelet Count. Purpura is usually present when the platelet count is below about 40,000 per cu.mm. Such patients also have a prolonged bleeding time and poor clot retraction.

Clot Retraction. Poor clot retraction is seen in patients with low platelet counts or more rarely when there is deficient blood fibrinogen.

Bleeding time is increased when the platelets are deficient. The lobe of the ear is pricked with a needle and the blood absorbed every 30 seconds on a piece of blotting paper which is not allowed to touch the skin. By this method the normal bleeding time is two to five minutes.

Coagulation time is increased in haemophilia and the allied coagulation-defect states. By *Lee and White's* method, using venous blood, the normal coagulation time is four to ten minutes, but a control with normal blood should always be performed as there is a wide variation in results according to the precise conditions of the test. The *partial thromboplastin time* (normal 25–55 secs) is a more sensitive test now usually preferred to the whole blood coagulation time.

Haemophilia

Deficiency of anti-haemophilic globulin in the plasma is inherited as a sex-linked recessive character, appearing only in males and transmitted to them by clinically normal female carriers. All the sons of haemophiliacs are free from the haemophiliac gene and all the daughters are carriers. When a female carrier marries a normal man half the sons are haemophiliacs and half the daughters are carriers. In practice, only two out of three haemophiliacs know of other bleeders in their families so that a typical pedigree must not be regarded as an essential diagnostic criterion. The common *symptoms* are persistent bleeding after cuts and abrasions, and after extraction of teeth (of first or second dentition), and bleeding into joints, particularly the knee joint. The severity of the haemophilic state is very variable, depending on the degree of deficiency of anti-haemophilic globulin. In severe cases major operations are very hazardous, probably carrying a mortality of about 50 per cent.

Treatment. Until the bleeding stops enough anti-haemophilic globulin (AHG) must be given I.V. daily to maintain at least 20–30 per cent of the level found in the plasma of normal people. In the past fresh plasma transfusions had to be given, since AHG rapidly disappears from stored blood or plasma; but now a cryoprecipitate of human plasma is available which can be stored frozen and enables the AHG from a pint of plasma to be given in a 20 ml. injection. This can be given to outpatients and haemophiliacs should be encouraged to attend for treatment as soon as any bleeding starts. However, they should be admitted to hospital for dental extractions and must be given AHG before operation as well as afterwards. Tooth sockets should be packed lightly with a preparation of thrombin or Russell viper venom (Stypven); this can be done most effectively with the aid of a dental splint made before the extraction.

Christmas disease has the same inheritance and clinical features as haemophilia, but the Christmas factor (which is present in normal serum) is much more stable than anti-haemophilic globulin and stored blood can be used in treatment.

Von Willebrand's disease is a rare disorder inherited as an autosomal dominant trait (and occurring therefore in both sexes) in which there is deficiency of factor VIII, but in contrast to true haemophiliacs the patients also have purpura of the skin and mucosae and a prolonged bleeding time, due to associated deficiency of the VW factor which is necessary for normal adhesion of platelets to subendothelial structures. Treatment is as for haemophilia.

Factor V deficiency is inherited in some families as a dominant trait but is extremely rare.

Factor VII deficiency is seen in patients under anticoagulant therapy and occasionally in advanced liver disease.

Prothrombin is produced in the liver from vitamin K. Vitamin K is synthesised by certain bacteria in the intestines and is also present in a number of vegetable foods; it is not absorbed properly in the absence of bile salts. Clinical prothrombin deficiency is seen in two groups of patients: newborn babies in whose intestines the vitamin-K-forming organisms have not yet become established (*haemorrhagic disease of the newborn*); and patients with *obstructive jaundice* whose intestine contains no bile salts. The former variety can be largely prevented by giving vitamin K 5 mg. intramuscularly daily to the expectant mother for a few days before delivery. Patients with obstructive jaundice should receive similar treatment, particularly if any surgical operation is contemplated, as otherwise serious haemorrhage may occur.

THE PURPURAS

Essential Thrombocytopenia (Idiopathic Thrombocytopenic Purpura)

This rare disease occurs mainly in adolescents and young adults, particularly girls, and is characterised by episodes of skin purpura and bleeding from such sites as the nose, uterus, and alimentary tract. Absence of joint pains is a useful point of distinction from anaphylactoid purpura. The platelet count is low (usually below 40,000 per cu.mm.), the bleeding time is prolonged, clot retraction is poor, but the coagulation time is normal. Hess's test is strongly positive. Gross enlargement of the spleen is uncommon, but in about one-third of the patients it becomes just palpable. As a result of haemorrhage haematological signs of iron deficiency often develop. Cerebral haemorrhage may occur.

Aetiology is obscure. There appears to be a defect in capillary endothelium. In some patients the platelet deficiency seems to be due to a splenic action, which either destroys the platelets or inhibits their release from the bone marrow; in other patients they appear to be destroyed by circulating antibodies (cf. acquired haemolytic anaemia).

Treatment. The effect of steroid therapy should first be tried, but if a complete remission does not occur or if relapse follows withdrawal of the drug splenectomy should be performed without delay. Results of operation are less satisfactory when the disease has been present for more than 12 months.

Purpura due to Capillary Damage

Purpura may be seen in any of the *acute specific fevers*, particularly meningococcal infections. It may also result from *drug sensitivity*; sedormid is the most notorious offender, but other well-known drugs which may cause it are quinine, quinidine, belladonna, phenobarbitone, thiouracil, chlorpromazine, isoniazid, sodium salicylate, carbromal, and the heavy metals. In certain drug purpuras a circulating antibody causing lysis of platelets has been demonstrated; such patients have a thrombocytopenia. Withdrawal of the drug is usually sufficient treatment, but, if not steroid therapy may be helpful. *Senile purpura* is common in elderly people, possibly as a result of degenerative changes in the capillary endothelium. The purpura of *scurvy* is due to nutritional changes in the capillary endothelium.

Anaphylactoid purpura (the Schönlein-Henoch syndrome) is characterised by purpura and allergic manifestations, namely urticaria, joint pains and swelling, and angio-neurotic oedema which affects not only the sub-cutaneous and submucous tissues but also the gut, causing intestinal colic and sometimes rectal bleeding. Classically Henoch's purpura was associated with abdominal colic and Schönlein's purpura with joint pains, but it is now recognised that the two groups often overlap.

Treatment. Subcutaneous adrenaline, 0·5 ml. of a 1/1,000 solution, and oral antihistamines should be given. If the symptoms persist corticosteroid therapy is usually effective.

APLASTIC ANAEMIA AND AGRAULOCYTOSIS

This rare disease, which usually occurs in young adults, is the result of destruction of those cells in the bone marrow which produce the red cells, the white cells, and the platelets. A similar process affecting only the granular leucocytes is termed *agranulocytosis*. Death or destruction of the parent bone-marrow cells is sometimes a toxic reaction to certain drugs, notably amidopyrin, sulphonamides, heavy metals such as gold or arsenic, thiouracil, chloramphenicol, or tridione; or to certain industrial poisons such as benzole and its derivatives. It may also result from excessive exposure to X-rays or radio-active materials. Frequently, however, the cause is unknown (idiopathic aplastic anaemia, or idiopathic agranulo-cytosis).

Clinical Features. Failure in production of red cells causes the gradual development of the symptoms and signs of anaemia; diminished or absent output of granulocytes impairs the body's defences against infection, lead-ing to painful ulceration of the throat and fever; and scarcity of platelets in the blood causes purpura and bleeding from different parts of the body.

Treatment consists in removal of the cause, if possible; fresh blood transfusion repeated as often as necessary for the correction of the anaemia; and the administration of penicillin or other suitable antibiotic to combat infection. Recovery of bone-marrow function may be assisted by androgen therapy: oxymetholone 3–5 mg./kg. by mouth should be continued for 4–6 months before being abandoned as ineffective.

Hypersplenism is a condition in which there is progressive decline in the numbers of red cells, white cells, and platelets in the peripheral blood (or any combination of the three) associated with splenomegaly of varied aetiology. The bone marrow shows not aplasia but hyperplasia. The spleen appears to be exerting some inhibitory effect on the maturation or release of cells from the bone marrow and splenectomy is frequently followed by clinical cure.

LEUKAEMIA

Leukaemia is a disease characterised by abnormal proliferation of leukopoietic tissue throughout the body. The cause is not known, but it is now generally regarded as a neoplastic process. The risk of developing it is increased by exposure to excessive radiation: there was a twentyfold increase in its incidence among survivors of the Hiroshima and Nagasaki atomic explosions; the incidence is some six times higher in patients with ankylosing spondylitis who have been treated with radio-therapy than in the general population; and radiologists have an incidence several times higher than other doctors. The risk to doctors generally, however, appears to be about twice that to the general population and in the latter the number of cases per million has doubled in the past twenty years.

Leukaemia is classified according to the type of leukocyte affected into lymphatic, myeloid, and monocytic varieties. It is also subdivided into acute and chronic types according to the speed of the clinical course.

Acute Leukaemia

Acute lymphatic, acute myeloid, and acute monocytic leukaemia present similar clinical pictures so that one description suffices for all. It may occur at any age but is most common in childhood and boys are affected more often than girls. At the start about one-third of the cases are aleukaemic (that is, have no excess of leukocytes in the peripheral blood); there may indeed be leucopenia and this with the low red cell and platelet counts may lead to a mistaken diagnosis of aplastic anaemia. Recurrent infective lesions and purpuric manifestations may occur in this phase, which may last for a few months, but when the leukaemia becomes manifest the course is usually short. More often the onset is sudden, with fever, sore throat, and bleeding from the mouth, nose, or elsewhere and it quickly becomes clear that the patient is gravely ill. Typically there is a total white count of some 20,000 to 50,000 per cu.mm. of which about 90 per cent are blast cells (lymphoblasts, myeloblasts, or monoblasts). There is always severe reduction in the red cell and platelet counts. The diagnosis can be confirmed by examination of the bone marrow. With modern treatment a remission can be induced in 50 per cent of children with acute leukaemia and the median survival in this group is now about 12 months. The incidence of remission in adults is only about 15 per cent, probably because in them the lymphoblastic type of acute leukaemia is less common.

Chronic Myeloid Leukaemia

Chronic myeloid leukaemia occurs mainly between early adult life and middle age and is rather more common in men than in women. Slowly progressive tiredness due to anaemia is usually the presenting symptom, or the patient may complain of a dragging sensation in the abdomen due to the enlarged spleen. The spleen attains a larger size in this disease than in any other seen in temperate climates and may extend into the right iliac fossa. The B.M.R. is increased and this may partly explain the nervousness, night sweats, and loss of weight which are sometimes prominent symptoms. Leukaemic infiltration of the skin sometimes occurs, and pruritus may be a troublesome symptom even when no lesions can be seen or felt. In men painful priapism, due to thrombosis in the corpora cavernosa, may be an early symptom. *Blood count* typically shows a total white count between 100,000 and 500,000, of which some 50 to 70 per cent are polymorphonuclears and 10 to 20 per cent myelocytes, and there is always moderate to severe anaemia. The *diagnosis* is usually easy in view of the enormously enlarged spleen and typical white count, but confirmation may be obtained by marrow examination. The Philadelphia chromosome is usually present, the leucocyte alkaline phosphatase is reduced or absent and the serum B12 and B12-binding proteins are greatly raised.

Myelofibrosis may be idiopathic or secondary to other conditions such as polycythaemia vera, carcinomatosis or tuberculosis. Marrow fibrosis leads to a leucoerythroblastic blood picture and haematopoesis develops in the liver, spleen and occasionally other organs. Patients are usually middle-aged or elderly and present with anaemia, weakness and splenomegaly. Bone marrow aspiration is often unproductive; trephine biopsy reveals increase in reticulin with fibrosis and new bone formation. Hyperuricaemia and clinical gout are common. The white blood count may be raised to 30–40,000 u./litre; the absence of the Philadelphia chromosome, normal leucocyte alkaline phosphatase and normal serum B12 and B12-binding proteins help to distinguish this disease from chronic myeloid leukaemia. There is no specific treatment. Increasingly frequent transfusions are usually needed and the disease runs a progressive course over 3 to 5 years.

Chronic Lymphatic Leukaemia

Chronic lymphatic leukaemia is nearly always seen in men of late middle age. The patient complains of slowly developing tiredness, due to associated anaemia, and the spleen, liver, and lymph nodes in the neck, axillae, and elsewhere are found to be enlarged. The spleen, however, does not attain the enormous size seen in chronic myeloid leukaemia. As in the latter disease the B.M.R. is raised. Priapism does not occur, but impotence is a common symptom. Infiltration of the skin may result in eruptions of various types. The blood count usually shows a total white count of up to 100,000 of which 80–90 per cent are small lymphocytes and there is always an associated anaemia.

Treatment of Leukaemia

The object of treatment is the destruction of abnormal leucocytes and the suppression of abnormal leucocyte proliferation. The drugs used fall into four groups:

(a) *Antimetabolites*, which compete directly with substances which are taken up by the cell for its metabolism. Thus, 6-mercaptopurine inhibits the uptake of purines and methotrexate the uptake of folic acid.

(b) *Alkylating agents*, which combine chemically in vivo with the chromosomes and so kill the cells or prevent their division. This group includes chlorambucil, cyclophosphamide and busulphan.

(c) *Corticosteroids*. The way in which steroid therapy exerts its beneficial effect in leukaemia is not understood.

(d) The *Plant Alkaloids* vinblastine and vincristine interfere with mitotic spindle function.

Apart from the corticosteroids all these drugs cause severe bone marrow depression and throughout the treatment frequent blood counts must be done. It has been shown that better results are obtained when combinations of drugs are given than when they are given singly or successively, presumably because the malignant cells develop drug resistance less easily (cf. anti-tuberculous chemotherapy, p. 241); and leaving intervals between courses allows the normal cells in the marrow and gastro-intestinal tract to recover and permits more of the effective agents to be given without increasing the toxic effects.

Ideally treatment should be controlled by a physician with special experience in this complex and rapidly changing subject.

Acute Lymphoblastic Leukaemia

At present the best combination for inducing remission is vincristine with prednisone; only 10 per cent of patients fail to respond and they may be tried on various combinations of 6-mercaptopurine, methotrexate, cyclophosphamide or chlorambucil.

Acute Myeloblastic Leukaemia

Treatment is much less satisfactory than for the lymphoblastic type, but has been improved by the introduction of cytosine arabinoside and daunorubicin which are given in combination with either 6-mercaptopurine or prednisone for inducing remission. Methotrexate is used for maintenance therapy.

Symptomatic Treatment. Transfusion is often required for severe anaemia in acute leukaemia and occasionally in the chronic types. Penicillin or other appropriate antibiotic should be given in large doses for infective lesions in the mouth or elsewhere. In the chronic leukaemias local lesions such as painful splenomegaly may be relieved by radiotherapy.

THE LYMPHOMAS

Hodgkin's Disease (Lymphadenoma)

The cause of Hodgkin's disease is unknown, but it is probably a malignant process. Most of the patients are young adults, though it can occur at any age, and men are affected about twice as often as women.

Clinical Features. The first symptom is usually the painless enlargement of a group of lymph-nodes, particularly in the neck but sometimes in the axillary or inguinal regions. At first the nodes feel firm, rubbery, and discrete, but later they often become matted together. In other patients mediastinal or abdominal lymph nodes enlarge before those in accessible peripheral situations and the patient may present with cough, dyspnoea, or pain in the chest or abdomen; such patients may have fever of the Pel-Ebstein type, which occurs in waves lasting a week or two separated by afebrile intervals of varying length. As the disease progresses general symptoms appear; these include itching, night sweats, fever, general malaise and anaemia. In general the development of symptoms implies a worse prognosis, but itching is an exception to this rule. Involvement of the spleen often occurs early and may be present even in the absence of splenic enlargement. Later the disease may spread to the liver; to bone, leading to severe pain in the spine, pelvis or ribs; to the nervous system, causing various symptoms including nerve palsies and cord compression; or to the lung.

Diagnosis can be established with certainty only by lymph-node biopsy.

Staging. The extent of the disease is determined by clinical examination, radiography, lymphangiography, isotope scanning, and usually by laparotomy.

Stage 1. Disease confined to one lymph-node site.

Stage 2. Disease in more than one lymph-node site, all either above or below the diaphragm.

Stage 3. Involvement of nodes on both sides of the diaphragm.

Stage 4. Sites involved outside the lymphatic system:
  A = symptom free.
  B = with symptoms.

Treatment. *Deep X-ray therapy* is the treatment of choice in Stage 1, 2, and 3A. Patients with 3B and Stage 4 disease are best treated with chemotherapy from the start. It is important that not only the affected nodes should be irradiated but all contiguous groups of lymph nodes as well. Eventually, however, the disease may recur and become widely disseminated and then some form of chemotherapy is indicated.

Cytotoxic drugs are now given in repeated courses; a number of drugs may be given together and the course of treatment repeated at intervals, even if the patient appears to be in a remission. This method seems to be giving superior results and may well be the treatment of choice. A typical course for an adult is:

Mustine 6 mg./m.^{2} I.V.	Day 1 and 8.
Vinblastine 10 mg. I.V.	Day 1 and 8.
Procarbazine 100 mg. orally.	Day 1–14 inclusive.
Prednisolone 40 mg. orally	Day 1–14 inclusive.

The courses are repeated at four to six week intervals to a total of six courses. Smaller doses are required if the white count is low.

If this combination fails to control the disease or relapse occurs other drug combinations are available. In addition symptomatic treatment may be required, such as transfusion for anaemia and analgesics for pain.

Prognosis. The prognosis depends on the extent of the disease at diagnosis, on the presence or absence of symptoms, and on the histology. Patients whose biopsy shows a lymphocyte-predominant picture have the best prognosis and those with lymphocyte depletion the worst; the other types come between these two.

Of patients whose disease is localised and who are therefore treated with radiotherapy about 80 per cent survive 5 years and about 50 per cent 10 years or longer. Of those who require treatment with cytotoxic drugs about 50 per cent survive 5 years.

Non-Hodgkin Lymphomas

These consist of lymphomas derived from the lymphatic system (lymphosarcomas) or from histiocytes. They can be classified as:

Lymphocytic lymphoma ⎫	
Lymphoblastic lymphoma ⎬ Lymphosarcomas	
Histiocytic lymphoma ⎭ Reticulum cell sarcoma	

The histological appearance gives an important guide to the prognosis. Patients in whom the lymphocytic cells are arranged in a nodular pattern have the best outlook and often survive for many years particularly if the disease is localised. Those in whom the normal pattern is replaced by a diffuse sheet of lymphoblasts or malignant histiocytes have the worst prognosis; the disease is often generalised from the start and few patients survive more than two years, although vigorous cytotoxic treatment may perhaps improve this outlook.

Clinical Features. These are very like those of Hodgkin's disease and range from an isolated enlarged lymph node to generalised lymphadenopathy in a very ill patient. Involvement outside the lymphatic system may occur early, particularly in the liver and bone marrow but often affecting other organs. Sometimes malignant lymphocytes appear in the peripheral blood in quite large numbers and this may make the distinction from chronic lymphatic leukaemia difficult.

Treatment depends on the histology and the extent of the disease.

Localised disease with well-differentiated lymphocytes, particularly in the elderly, responds well to radiotherapy and this may be all that is needed. If the disease is localised but the malignant cells are lymphoblasts or malignant histiocytes the radiotherapy may be followed by a course of chemotherapy. Generalised disease requires chemotherapy and several regimes are available. COP is widely used and consists of:

Cyclophosphamide 600 mg./m^2 i.v. on day 1 and 8
Vincristine (Oncovin) 1·5 mg. i.v. on day 1 and 8
Prednisolone 40 mg. daily for 1 week

After two weeks without drugs the course is given again and this pattern is repeated for up to 1 year providing the blood count is satisfactory. Adriamycin may be added to the regime.

In the elderly, particularly if the lymphocytes are well differentiated, long-term treatment with chlorambucil 2·0–5·0 mg. daily, perhaps combined with intermittent prednisolone, can also be very effective. With vigorous treatment it is possible to increase the 2-year survival to about 50 per cent, but side-effects can be troublesome. In the very old and frail when the disease is asymptomatic it is often best to withhold treatment.

Follicular Lymphoma

Histologically the lymphocytes are arranged in a characteristic follicular pattern and this disease may be regarded as a nodular lymphocytic lymphoma.

Clinical Features. The disease may be localised or generalised from the beginning. It usually produces few or no symptoms for several years, but may enter a more malignant phase when it can be difficult to treat.

Treatment. Radiotherapy may eradicate disease which is localised. Generalised disease requires cytotoxic drugs, either low dosage chlorambucil or COP (see above).

POLYCYTHAEMIA RUBRA VERA (Erythraemia)

This is a disease of middle age and is commoner in men. It is characterised by hyperplasia of the erythroblastic, leucoblastic, and megakaryocytic tissue of the bone marrow; and although the clinical picture is dominated by the greatly increased number of red cells in the peripheral circulation, there may eventually be exhaustion of the marrow cells, leading to aplastic anaemia, or the leucoblastic tissue may continue to proliferate as the erythroblasts die out, so that the final picture may be that of frank leukaemia.

It is now recognised that in a small proportion of patients with polycythaemia (about 9 per cent) there is an underlying renal lesion, neoplasm-cyst or hydronephrosis. In such patients there is presumably increased production of erythropoeitin by the kidney. Nephrectomy may cure the polycythaemia.

Clinical Features. The patient usually complains of headache, dizziness, and tiredness and has a very plethoric cyanosed appearance. The spleen is nearly always palpable. Congestion of the capillary bed leads to haemorrhage from various sites (for example, after dental extraction), while arterial thromboses in the brain, limbs, and elsewhere are also common, no doubt as a result of the increased blood viscosity. There is also an increased incidence of peptic ulcer and of gout.

The *red count* may be up to 10,000,000 per cu.mm. or even higher with an equivalent increase in the haemoglobin level. The white count is usually raised to about 20,000 per cu.mm. and the platelet count to 500,000 per cu.mm. or more.

Treatment. The treatment of choice is an intravenous injection of radioactive phosphorus (^{32}P) in a dosage of 5–7 millicuries. This is usually followed by very satisfactory clinical remission, but the patient must be carefully followed up as further treatment is often necessary after about three years. Alternatively, the patient may be kept symptom-free by regular venesection of a pint or so of blood every three or four weeks.

MYELOMATOSIS

This is a neoplastic proliferation of plasma cells in the bone marrow and rarely in other organs such as the liver, spleen, and lymph-nodes, occurring mainly in late middle-age. It is more common in men than in women.

Clinical Features. The commonest initial symptom is bone pain, often in a rib or vertebra, but sometimes the first indication is an unexplained anaemia or fever or rarely a bleeding tendency due to thrombocytopenia. There are seldom any abnormal physical signs; splenomegaly and enlarged lymph-nodes are very rare. Radiographs of the skeleton may show generalised demineralisation or characteristic punched-out osteolytic lesions particularly affecting the skull, ribs and vertebral column. Pathological fractures and collapse of vertebrae may occur. Anaemia from impaired erythropoeisis is usual and haemolytic anaemia may develop; ultimately thrombocytopenia is the rule. Plasma cells rarely appear in the peripheral blood.

The plasma cells produce an abnormal protein which on electrophoresis is found to move with the beta or gamma globulins. This protein is responsible for the very high sedimentation rate which is frequently found and in about one-third of the patients is associated with Bence-Jones protein in the urine; this precipitates when the urine is heated to about 70° C., but re-dissolves before boiling point is reached. Myeloma proteins are mono-clonal: i.e. in any individual patient they belong to a single immunoglobulin class (see Table, p. 339). The IgM proteins are referred to as macroglobulins. Bence-Jones proteins are made up of the light polypeptide chains of immunoglobulins. Proteinuria often occurs in myelomatosis even in the absence of Bence-Jones protein. Progressive renal failure may ensure, apparently due to plugging of the renal tubules by casts; such obstruction may be precipitated by intravenous pyelography, which should therefore be avoided. A few patients also have renal amyloidosis, while in others hypercalcaemia may lead to further damage to the kidneys.

The diagnosis can usually be established by marrow examination. The prognosis is very variable, but most patients die within two years.

Treatment is unsatisfactory. The best drug is probably *melphalan*. The dose is 10 mg. daily for seven days, and the course may be repeated at monthly intervals. It can be combined with steroids. A close watch must be kept for leucopenia or thrombocytopenia. As an alternative cyclophosphamide combined with steroids may be useful. The pain from local involvement of bone can be relieved by radiotherapy, and transfusion may be required to correct anaemia.

FURTHER READING

Wintrobe, M. M., *Clinical Haematology*, 7th edition, Kimpton, London, 1975.

CHAPTER SIXTEEN

INFECTIOUS DISEASES

DEFINITION

Although the term 'infectious disease' might logically be applied to any illness which results from invasion of the body by a micro-organism, its use is customarily restricted to those diseases which spread by direct contact from patient to patient. This chapter therefore deals mainly with those diseases for which isolation or 'barrier nursing' is required to prevent spread of infection.

INFECTION AND IMMUNITY

The result of any infection depends partly on the virulence and numbers of the invading organisms and partly on the state of the patient's defences against them. The state of his defences depends partly on his *natural immunity*, which may be good or bad according to his race and heredity and may have been reduced by such factors as malnutrition, worry, and overwork, and partly on *acquired immunity* resulting from previous infection or prophylactic inoculation with this particular organism. Such inoculations given to stimulate the formation of antibodies constitute *active immunisation*, and are widely used in the prevention of such diseases as smallpox, diphtheria, tetanus, enteric fever, and poliomyelitis. *Passive immunisation* means conferring temporary protection against a disease by injecting serum containing the specific antibodies; such serum is obtained from humans who have recovered from the disease or from horses actively immunised for this purpose.

Carriers. Some people after recovering from an infectious disease continue to harbour the specific organisms and may transmit them from time to time to susceptible persons, either by direct contact or by infecting food or water. This carrier state is particularly important in the spread of enteric fever.

Routes of Infection. The invading organism usually gains access to the patient either in inspired air ('droplet infection') or in contaminated food or drink.

Incubation Period. This is the time which elapses between the access of organisms to the tissues of a susceptible individual and the onset of the first clinical symptoms. Its duration varies widely in the different infectious diseases, but remains fairly constant in each of them. The approximate length of the incubation period of the common specific fevers is:

Less than 7 days	Cerebrospinal meningitis
	Diphtheria
	Scarlet fever
10 to 14 days	Measles
	Whooping cough
	Smallpox
	Enteric fever
14 to 21 days	Chicken-pox
(usually nearer *21*)	German measles
	Mumps

The incubation period is occasionally helpful in diagnosis if the date of exposure to a particular infection is known. The period of *quarantine* or isolation of contacts, used in serious diseases such as smallpox and where there is some special risk, is obtained by adding a few days (to be on the safe side) to the known incubation period.

Stage of Invasion. At the end of the incubation period the infecting organism or its toxic products become distributed throughout the body and give rise to the symptoms and signs of the disease. Common to all infectious diseases are fever, headache, general malaise, loss of appetite, dry furred tongue, hot dry skin, and scanty highly coloured urine; but in addition each has special features, which in many include a typical rash, which enable diagnosis to be made.

Barrier Nursing

To prevent direct transmission of organisms from patients with proven or suspected disease to other patients the technique known as 'barrier nursing' is employed. Preferably the patient is isolated in a separate room; if he must remain in a general ward the space between the adjoining beds is increased and a screen placed at the foot of the bed serves as a reminder that barrier precautions are being observed. Gowns are provided for all medical and nursing staff attending the patient; these may be hung within the 'barrier' with the 'dirty' side outermost or outside the barrier with the 'dirty' side turned inwards. The hands must be washed before removing the gown and again after leaving the barrier. For diseases spread by droplet infection masks should also be worn. To prevent indirect transmission of infection the patient's cutlery, crockery, and linen are kept separate, everything that has been near him being considered a possible source of infection.

Scheme of Prophylactic Inoculations for Children

Age	Vaccine	Interval	Notes
During first year of life	Diph/Tet/Pert and first dose of oral Polio vaccine		The first dose should not be given before 3 months; a better immunological

Age	Vaccine	Interval	Notes
	Diph/Tet/Pert and second dose of oral Polio vaccine	Preferably after an interval of 6–8 weeks.	response is obtained if it is not given until 6 months of age.
	Diph/Tet/Pert and third dose of oral Polio vaccine.	Preferably after an interval of 6 months	
During second year of life	Measles vaccine	After an interval of not less than 3–4 weeks.	
At 5 years old or school entry	Diph/Tet and oral Polio vaccine		These may be given at 3 years to children at nursery school, day nurseries or homes.
Between 10–13 years of age	B.C.G. vaccine		For tuberculin negative children.
At 15–19 years or on leaving school	Polio vaccine Tetanus toxoid		

Antigens for primary immunisation are now given later, at an age when antibody responses are no longer depressed by the presence of maternal antibody and the child is able to make antibody more efficiently.

Precautions. Routine vaccination of children against smallpox is no longer recommended in the U.K. since the risk of contracting the disease is now less than the risk of developing a serious complication of vaccination. *Encephalopathy* is a rare complication of whooping-cough vaccination and it is more likely to occur in infants with a history of convulsions; such children should be given combined diphtheria and tetanus vaccine instead of triple vaccine. Children with a history of asthma, hay fever, or eczema have a high incidence of *allergic reactions* after injections; they must be kept under observation for an hour after inoculation, therefore, and adrenaline must be immediately available for injection if needed. When a severe local reaction occurs after the first injection of triple vaccine it is probably the whooping-cough component which is responsible and for the subsequent injections it may be advisable to use only the combined diphtheria and tetanus vaccine.

When does the Rash come Out?

It is important to remember the day of the disease on which the specific eruption usually appears in the exanthemata. The following is a useful mnemonic:

	Disease	*Rash appears on*
Really	**Rubella**	1st day
Sick	**Scarlet Fever**	2nd day
People	**Small Pox**	3rd day
Must	**Measles**	4th day
Take	**Typhus**	5th day
No	**Nil**	—
Exercise	**Enteric**	7th day

BACTERIAL INFECTIONS

DIPHTHERIA

Diphtheria is an infection of the throat, nose or larynx (or occasionally the skin) and although the organism, *C. diphtheriae*, remains localised to this site, it produces a powerful exotoxin which becomes widely distributed and may cause serious or fatal effects on other parts of the body. The amount of exotoxin produced by different strains of the organism varies a good deal and that is one reason why some patients are much more severely ill than others. Another reason for the variation in clinical severity is the state of the patient's immunity at the time of infection.

Immunity. Immunity to diphtheria may be acquired in three ways:

(1) After recovery from an attack of the disease.
(2) After repeated subclinical infection, that is, as a result of coming into contact from time to time with organisms insufficient in either numbers or virulence to cause a full-scale attack of diphtheria.
(3) As a result of active immunisation by inoculation. It is because of the widespread inoculation of children that this killing disease is much less common than it used to be; if immunisation were universally practised, as it should be, there would be no cases.

The Schick Test is used to detect whether an individual has immunity against diphtheria. Diphtheria toxin 0·2 ml. is injected into the skin of the left forearm and 0·2 ml. of the same toxin which has been heated to 70° C. to destroy its potency is injected into the skin of the right forearm as a control. The result is read in 5 to 7 days, as follows:

Positive. An area of redness and swelling at the site of injection on the left arm, with no reaction on the right (control) arm. This indicates that the person tested has no antitoxin with which to neutralise the toxin injected; in other words, he is *susceptible* to diphtheria.

Negative. No reaction in either arm. The injected toxin has been neutralised by anti-toxin and the subject is therefore *immune* to diphtheria.

Positive plus 'Pseudo Reaction'. There is redness and swelling on both arms, but more on the left (test) arm than on the right (control) arm. The reaction on the right arm and part of the reaction on the left are due to some factor in the injection other than the actual toxin; the extra reaction on the left must be due to unneutralised toxin and the subject is therefore *susceptible* to diphtheria.

Negative plus 'Pseudo Reaction'. There is equal redness and swelling on both arms; the subject is *immune* to diphtheria.

Active Immunisation

All children should be immunised against diphtheria. The Schick test is used on adults who are exposed to special risk of infection, for example nurses and medical students, and those shown to be susceptible are immunised.

Immunisation of children may be effected by three injections of alum-precipitated toxoid (A.P.T.), but it is better to give a combined triple vaccine against diphtheria, whooping cough, and tetanus. The first dose of 0·3–0·5 ml. of A.P.T. is given between three and nine months, the second of 0·5 ml. is given four weeks later and the final boosting dose of 0·2 ml. at the age of four. Adults are immunised in the same way, but if the preliminary Schick tests show a 'positive plus pseudo' result unpleasant reactions may follow the use of A.P.T. and it is better to use toxoid-antitoxin floccules (T.A.F.). This is given in three doses of 1 ml. each at intervals of two weeks and rarely causes any side effects.

Clinical Features of Diphtheria

Diphtheria is classified clinically according to the exact site of infection. The commonest variety is *faucial* diphtheria, in which the characteristic membrane of the disease forms in the throat. There is a short incubation period of only three or four days from exposure to infection. Points which help to distinguish diphtheria from streptococcal tonsillitis are:

(1) The throat is not so sore and the temperature usually not so high, but the general exhaustion and toxaemia are much greater.

(2) The lymph-nodes in the neck are usually enlarged to a greater extent, in severe cases causing a collar of swelling sometimes referred to as the 'bull-neck'.

(3) The exudate in the throat is not confined to yellowish spots on the tonsils, but forms a continuous greyish sheet of membrane which often extends forwards over the soft palate and

backwards on to the pharyngeal wall and is so firmly adherent that any attempt to wipe it off leaves a bleeding surface.

Less common and more difficult to diagnose are *nasal diphtheria*, in which the membrane is confined to the nose, where it may lead to a blood-stained nasal discharge; and *laryngeal diphtheria*, a very dangerous form in which the membrane on the larynx may obstruct breathing and necessitate emergency tracheotomy. *Cutaneous diphtheria* is very rare in this country, but in troops serving in the East during the war it was a common cause of so-called 'jungle-sores' or 'desert-sores', the true nature of which was often not appreciated until the development of post-diphtheritic paralysis.

Complications

The complications of diphtheria are due to the effects on the heart and nervous system of the exotoxin absorbed from the lesions in the upper respiratory tract or skin.

Carditis may occur during the second week and is characterised by vomiting, a greyish pallor, a weak rapid pulse, low blood pressure, diminished urinary output, usually with some albuminuria, and sometimes pain over the heart. Conduction defects such as heart block may be found. Sudden death is not uncommon in these cases, but no permanent cardiac lesion results in patients who recover.

Paralysis. Paralysis of the palate is the commonest type and causes a nasal voice and regurgitation of food through the nose. It usually appears in the second or third weeks and may extend to the pharyngeal muscles, causing difficulty in swallowing, or rarely to the intercostal muscles or diaphragm, causing weakness in breathing and necessitating treatment with a mechanical respirator. There is sometimes paralysis of the ciliary muscle, causing difficulty in reading, and lateral rectus (sixth nerve) palsy is not uncommon. Towards the fifth or sixth weeks peripheral neuritis may occur, causing weakness in the limbs of varying degree. Complete recovery from all types of diphtheritic weakness occurs, but may take as long as six months.

Treatment

Antitoxin and Antibiotics

Although a throat or nasal swab should always be taken whenever diphtheria is suspected, the disease is so dangerous that treatment must invariably be started at once without waiting for the result of the culture. The most important measure is the immediate administration of antitoxin. The dose varies from about 8,000–100,000 units, according to the severity of the infection and it is usual to give half the total dose intramuscularly and then if there has been no serum reaction within 15 to 30 minutes to give the remainder, warmed to body temperature, by slow intravenous injection. The latter route should be avoided, however, in patients giving a history of allergic phenomena, owing to the serious risk of fatal anaphylaxis; and any patient who develops vomiting, wheezing, urticaria, or collapse must be given 0·5 ml. of 1:1,000 adrenaline subcutaneously without delay and an antihistamine, for example promethazine 25 mg., by slow intramuscular injection. It is usual also to give intramuscular benzyl penicillin, 100,000 to 500,000 units every four hours with erythromycin 250 mg. four-hourly, but it should be stressed that these are less important than the antitoxin.

Nursing

The patient is nursed flat in bed with only one pillow and as complete rest is essential everything, including feeding, must be done for him. In patients with acute carditis these conditions may have to be maintained for some two or three months. Local treatment of the throat probably does more harm than good, but ordinary cleanliness of the mouth is important. If palatal and pharyngeal paresis occur tube-feeding may become necessary.

Control of Outbreaks

When a case of diphtheria occurs in a closed community such as a school or a hospital ward the parents and medical officer of health are notified and the patient is transferred to an infectious diseases hospital. The parents of contacts are also notified and combined active and passive immunisation of the latter is carried out. Antitoxin 1,000 units is given into the deltoid of one arm and the first 0·5 ml. of A.P.T. into the other. Four weeks later the second injection of 0·5 ml. of A.P.T. completes the procedure.

Sometimes an outbreak of diphtheria can be traced to a healthy *carrier* and it is important that his infection be eradicated to prevent further spread of the disease. This can sometimes be achieved by giving large doses of penicillin, 2–4 million units daily, combined with sulphadimidine 4–6 g. daily for up to a week. If the infection persists tonsillectomy may be indicated.

WHOOPING COUGH (Pertussis)

Whooping cough is an infection of the respiratory tract by either *Bordetella pertussis* or a virus. In this country at present it is the most serious of the acute specific fevers of childhood, not only causing many deaths in young children, particularly under the age of twelve months, but also occasionally leading to serious damage to the bronchi and lungs (see bronchiectasis, p. 214). Asthma in childhood also sometimes dates from an attack of whooping cough. Infants receive no passive immunity from the mother and are therefore susceptible to the infection from birth.

Clinical Features. After an incubation period of about 7 to 14 days the child develops what is thought at first to be an ordinary cold on the chest, but within a week of onset the paroxysms of coughing have usually become so severe and typical that the diagnosis is obvious. A characteristic paroxysm consists of a deep inspiration followed by a rapid series of explosive coughs during expiration. The tongue protrudes, the face and lips become deeply cyanosed and the attack may end with the inspiration of air through a partially closed glottis, producing the classical whoop. Paroxysm may follow paroxysm until a little sticky mucus is expectorated or until the child vomits and sinks back exhausted. During the spasms of coughing the tongue may be abraded against the lower incisors, causing a traumatic ulcer on the fraenum; rectal prolapse, hernia, and haemorrhage, particularly under the conjunctiva, may also be induced.

In young infants, however, cough is often not such a prominent symptom. Instead, procedures such as feeding or changing may induce cyanotic attacks, in which the child becomes flaccid, blue, and alarmingly lifeless. There may also be frequent vomiting. Furthermore, immunised subjects may have a mild form of the disease without the typical paroxysmal cough or whoop. The diagnosis may remain very obscure until the appearance of a few feeble whoops at the end of attacks. The preliminary catarrhal stage is short in duration but highly infectious; the paroxysmal stage and whooping may continue for many weeks but the infectivity is now very slight.

Diagnosis. The paroxysmal coughing is virtually diagnostic, but bacteriological confirmation may be obtained by isolation of *B. pertussis* on 'cough plates' (a Petri dish held in front of the patient's mouth) or better, by taking a post-nasal swab. *B. pertussis* does not grow readily, however, and special culture media are essential. It is now thought that patients with negative cultures have virus infection. The blood count shows a lymphocytosis, but young children have a high lymphocyte count in health so that no significance should be attached to a count of less than 70 per cent of 20,000.

Complications. Acute bronchitis and *broncho-pneumonia* are the most serious complications and account for most of the deaths which occur in infancy and in old age. *Collapse* of broncho-pulmonary segments, or less often of lobes of the lung, from plugging of bronchioles or bronchi by sticky mucus may lead to bronchiectasis if allowed to persist. A radiograph should be taken, therefore, and appropriate physiotherapy instituted if necessary. *Otitis media* is the other common infective complication. *Convulsions* occur more often in whooping cough than in any of the other specific fevers. *Spontaneous pneumothorax* may occur.

Treatment. Erythromycin 12·5 mg./kg. body weight orally four times daily in the first week of infection may attenuate the symptoms and should be given to infants under one year old. Feeding is often a problem; the diet is most likely to be retained if given after an episode of vomiting. Cyanotic attacks in infants should be treated by freeing the airway and re-establishing breathing by gentle pressure on the chest. It may also be advisable to nurse such a child in an oxygen tent. Phenobarbitone 8–32 mg. has a calming effect and may reduce the number of paroxysms and ephedrine 16–32 mg. relieves or prevents bronchial spasm.

Prophylactic Inoculation. Suspended whooping cough vaccine may be given subcutaneously or intramuscularly. It is best given as a combined triple vaccine against diphtheria, whooping cough, and tetanus (p. 528).

SCARLET FEVER

When seen in historical perspective many infective diseases go through periods of increased or decreased severity, and scarlet fever at the present time is a much less serious illness than it was in the first two decades of this century. It is a haemolytic streptococcal infection which is distinguished from other diseases due to the same organism by its typical rash; this rash indicates that the streptococcus concerned is of a strain which produces a special erythrogenic toxin and that the patient is susceptible to its action.

The **Dick test** is performed by injecting 0·2 ml. of erythrogenic toxin into the skin of the forearm, no control injection in the other arm being necessary. A red swollen area at the site of injection in twenty-four hours shows that the person tested is *susceptible* to the toxin (Dick positive); no reaction shows that he is *immune* (Dick negative). The test is little used at the present time.

Clinical Features. After a short incubation period of less than a week the illness starts abruptly with sore throat, fever, shivering, and often vomiting. Small children may not complain of sore throat, but examination shows that the tonsils and fauces are very red and swollen and the tonsils may be covered with patches of soft, yellowish exudate. At first the tongue is covered with a white fur, which peels off from the edges during the next two or three days, leaving a clean surface with enlarged red papillae—the 'strawberry' or 'raspberry' tongue.

The *rash* appears on the second day and is described as a punctate erythema; the skin is a bright scarlet colour and on close inspection is seen to be covered with minute red spots. It appears first behind the ears and on the side of the neck and spreads rapidly over the whole body, but avoiding the area round the mouth (giving the so-called 'circum-oral pallor') and tending to be particularly heavy in flexures such as the axillae, cubital fossae, and groins. After about a week 'pin-hole desquamation' of the skin starts: little round pieces of dead skin flake off, temporarily leaving small holes in the superficial layers of the epidermis.

Septic Scarlet Fever, in which there is suppuration of cervical lymphnodes as well as extensive septic infection in the throat, and **Toxic Scarlet Fever,** in which there is overwhelming toxaemia characterised by circulatory failure, delirium and stupor with minimal faucial reaction and rash, are severe and often fatal forms of the disease fortunately rare at the present time.

Complications. Local spread of infection may cause peritonsillar abscess (quinsy), retropharyngeal abscess, sinusitis, and cervical adenitis while aspiration may cause bronchitis and pneumonia, but none of these is common nowadays.

Late complications, occurring some three weeks after the original illness, are those which may follow any streptococcal tonsillitis, namely acute nephritis, rheumatic fever and anaphylactoid purpura.

Treatment. For the mildest form of the disease oral penicillin (phenoxymethyl penicillin) 250 mg. four times daily or phenethicillin 125 mg. four times daily is satisfactory. For more severe infections benzyl penicillin 250,000 to 1,000,000 units should be given 6-hourly I.M. for the first two days, followed by oral penicillin. To ensure eradication of haemolytic streptococci and minimise the risk of acute nephritis and rheumatic fever it is wise to continue penicillin therapy for ten days. Patients allergic to penicillin may be given erythromycin 250–500 mg. orally every 6 hours for 10 days.

ENTERIC FEVER

Enteric is the name applied to a group of diseases which consists of *typhoid fever* and *paratyphoid A, B, and C*. They are due to closely related salmonella organisms, short thick motile gram-negative bacilli which can be distinguished from most of the non-pathogenic organisms of the coli-typhoid group by their inability to ferment lactose. Typhoid and paratyphoid B occur all over the world, the latter being the most common of the enteric fevers in this country; paratyphoid A is found mainly in the East; paratyphoid C is rare.

Method of Spread. Enteric fever is spread by contamination of food or water by excreta from carriers or from patients with the disease. It is therefore prevalent in countries whose standards of sanitation are low and armies on active service in the tropics are at special risk. The sharp reduction in the incidence of the disease which occurred in this country at the end of the nineteenth century was due to the introduction of methods of sewage disposal which prevent access to the water supplies. In countries with good sanitation outbreaks can usually be traced to unsuspecting carriers of the disease who are engaged in the handling of foodstuffs.

Clinical Features. After an incubation period of about a fortnight there is usually a gradual onset of *headache, aching* in the limbs, *tiredness, cough*, and *fever*, which typically rises in 'step-ladder' fashion by about half a degree (C.) daily to reach a height of perhaps 39–40° C. towards the end of the first week. For the next week, or sometimes much longer, the temperature continues at this high level, showing very little variation throughout the twenty-four hours. The pulse usually does not show the increase in rate which accompanies most febrile illnesses, a *relative bradycardia* of less than 100 per minute being frequently maintained through the whole course of the illness. *Cough* and signs of bronchitis or even broncho-pneumonia are common in the first few days and may dominate the clinical picture at this stage.

In suspected cases watch must be kept about the end of the first week for the appearance of the characteristic *rash*. In typhoid this consists of a few 'rose-spots', which can easily be overlooked but which nevertheless are very typical of the disease. They occur particularly on the abdomen or chest and appear for a few days in a succession of crops of tiny pink spots, each not more than 1–2 mm. in diameter and each one lasting for only 24 hours or so. It is useful, therefore, to make a ring with a skin pencil round each spot seen so that the next day if any new ones have appeared it is clear at a glance that they are a new crop. In paratyphoid the rash is often much more profuse and may be composed of much larger less clearly defined elements which tend to coalesce with each other, producing an eruption rather like that of measles. The spleen often becomes palpable at about the same time as the rash appears.

Most patients are constipated during the first few days, but towards the end of the second week the abdomen becomes distended and *diarrhoea* sets in. By this time if the attack is a severe one the patient is very gravely ill and may pass into the 'typhoid state', in which he remains throughout the 24 hours in what has been called a 'coma-vigil', drowsy and confused but continually muttering to himself, plucking at the bedclothes, and groping for non-existent objects. The faeces are now fluid and light yellow in colour ('pea-soup stools') and up to twenty may be passed in 24 hours.

Gradual improvement usually occurs during the third and fourth weeks; the temperature settles by lysis, the diarrhoea stops, the mind becomes clearer and the other symptoms also slowly disappear. Very occasionally relapse occurs in convalescence: the writer has seen one patient before the antibiotic era who went through the whole course of typhoid fever three times within six months before making a complete recovery.

Diagnosis

Blood culture is by far the best way of establishing the diagnosis, and as the organisms circulate in the blood only during the first week it is extremely important that blood should be taken for culture as early as possible, preferably during the first three days.

Blood count typically shows a leucopenia, but this is not a constant finding, particularly in paratyphoid, and in the presence of bronchitis or other complication there may even be a slight leucocytosis.

Agglutinations (Widal test). As a rise in the agglutinin titre during the illness is the most important evidence of active infection, blood should be taken for this estimation at the same time as the initial blood culture during the first few days, and again during the second week. Quite high titres of 'H' (flagellar) agglutinin may be found in the blood of healthy people who have been inoculated with T.A.B., but a rising titre of 'O' (somatic) agglutinins is usually indicative of enteric infection. A high titre of 'Vi' (virulence) agglutinin is also usually significant.

Complications. The two most serious complications of typhoid are liable to occur during the third week of illness, when sloughs separate from the Peyer's patches in the ileum leaving deep ulcers which may *perforate* or cause serious *haemorrhage*. Such *perforations* are easily overlooked clinically. By the time they occur the patient is in such a weak state that very little peritoneal reaction takes place and nothing approaching the dramatic pain and tenderness of the patient with a perforated peptic ulcer is to be expected; the only clue may be a sudden worsening of the general clinical condition, with a fall in the temperature and a rise in the pulse and respiration rates and the appearance of minimal abdominal tenderness. Before the days of antibiotics surgical closure of the perforation gave the only hope of recovery, but patients receiving chloramphenicol can usually be treated conservatively. *Haemorrhage* is more common than perforation; it is suggested by sudden faintness, pallor, and sweating, and diagnosed by the appearance of bright-red blood in the next stool passed. Transfusion is occasionally necessary but surgery never.

Venous thrombosis, particularly in the femoral vein, is common.

Parotitis is a dangerous complication which should be prevented by careful attention to the hygiene of the mouth.

Cholecystitis, with the subsequent formation of gall-stones containing *Salmonella typhi*, and *acute arthritis*, are rare complications.

Typhoid abscesses in bone and periostitis causing the stiff and painful *typhoid spine* are very rare sequelae which may appear years after the original infection.

Treatment. The prognosis of typhoid has been greatly improved since the introduction of chloramphenicol, which is usually very effective. A satisfactory scheme of dosage for an adult is 1·5 g. twice daily for the first five days, then 0·75 g. twice daily for a week, and finally 1 g. daily for a few more days. Agglutination titres are lower and relapses more common than in untreated patients but the relapses usually respond satisfactorily to further courses of chloramphenicol. Subsequent development of the carrier state is no commoner in treated than in untreated patients, but chloramphenicol usually fails to eradicate the organisms from carriers and for this purpose cholecystectomy remains the most useful measure.

Ampicillin, in doses of 8 g. daily, is also effective but rather slower in producing a response than chloramphenicol.

Patients with typhoid must of course be nursed with strict barrier precautions. They should be given a high-calorie low-roughage diet.

Prophylactic immunisation against the enteric fevers is achieved by giving T.A.B.C. vaccine intramuscularly, 0·5 ml., followed a week later by a second inoculation of 1 ml. Those living in endemic areas should receive 'booster' doses of 0·5 ml. annually.

STAPHYLOCOCCAL FEVER

Staphylococci may invade the bloodstream from abscesses in any part of the body, the most common primary lesions being skin boils and carbuncles, lung abscess, osteomyelitis, and renal carbuncle. Factors tending to promote bloodstream invasion are the early incision of abscesses and attempts to evacuate pus by squeezing, and general debility due to chronic fatigue, malnutrition, or serious underlying disease such as diabetes or leukaemia.

Outbreaks of antibiotic-resistant staphylococcal infection have become a serious menace in hospital wards in recent years, the organism being disseminated by contact with such articles as blankets and bed-curtains, and by healthy carriers.

Clinical Features. The initial staphylococcal lesion may be an apparently trivial one, unsuspected by the patient as the source of his subsequent severe illness. The onset of septicaemia is heralded by *rigors* and *fever* which is usually high and remittent or intermittent in type. Profuse *sweats* are common and sometimes there is a relative bradycardia. Metastatic *abscesses* develop in various sites, notably the lungs, joints, muscles, and skin, and purpura is also common. Bacterial endocarditis should be suspected when there are changing cardiac murmurs and when septicaemia persists in the absence of obvious staphylococcal lesions elsewhere. Some anaemia and leucocytosis are usual and the diagnosis is clinched by a positive *blood culture*.

Treatment. In spite of modern antibiotic therapy the mortality rate is still high. When staphylococcal septicaemia is suspected clinically, blood should be taken for culture and treatment started with benzylpenicillin 10 mega units daily together with flucloxacillin 2·0 g. daily. Treatment should be continued for at least two weeks (six weeks if endocarditis is suspected). If a satisfactory response is not obtained, sodium fusidate 500 mg. thrice daily can be added to the treatment. If blood culture reveals other organisms antibiotic treatment should be adjusted accordingly.

CEREBROSPINAL FEVER (Meningococcal Meningitis)

This disease is endemic throughout the world and in this country it is seen mainly during the winter months. From time to time epidemics occur, usually localised ones in residential institutions such as military barracks. Sporadic cases are commonest in infancy, while outbreaks affect adolescents and young adults.

Transmission is by droplet infection from patients and carriers and in susceptible contacts the meningococcus enters the bloodstream from the nasopharynx, causing a septicaemia. Usually, but not always, the infection then becomes localised to the meninges.

Clinical Features

(1) **Usual Meningitic Form.** After an incubation period of two or three days the illness starts rather suddenly, often with a shivering attack or rigor, followed by fever, severe headache, and vomiting. Convulsions are common in children. Within a few days signs of acute meningeal irritation develop: these are *neck rigidity* and a positive *Kernig's sign*. About 30 per cent of patients have a macular rash which rapidly becomes purpuric and is of great help in clinical diagnosis. Although the eruption may be profuse,

there are frequently only a few lesions which are easily overlooked unless a careful search is made for them.

Diagnosis is established by lumbar puncture, which reveals turbid fluid under increased pressure. The fluid contains large numbers of polymorphs, and meningococci can be demonstrated either by microscopy of a stained film or on culture.

(2) **Fulminating Meningococcal Meningitis.** This rapidly fatal but fortunately rare form starts very abruptly with high fever and within a few hours the patient is in coma with signs of acute meningitis and a profuse petechial rash. In spite of treatment death usually occurs within 24 to 48 hours.

(3) **Waterhouse-Friderichsen Syndrome.** Also fortunately rare, this syndrome is the result of bilateral adrenal haemorrhages accompanying the purpura of acute meningococcal (and other) septicaemias and is usually seen in children. Acute adrenal insufficiency leads to vomiting, collapse, and low blood pressure. Cortisone 200–300 mg. daily must be given in addition to antibiotic therapy but rarely averts the fatal outcome.

(4) **Chronic Meningococcal Septicaemia.** This curious, recurrent, and often puzzling disease, which has become much rarer since the introduction of the sulphonamides and antibiotics, causes little constitutional upset but presents with bouts of low fever, accompanied by headache, joint pains, and a maculo-papular rash on the trunk and limbs. On the legs the eruption may mimic erythema nodosum and sometimes, though not always, it contains purpuric elements. Such attacks may recur at varying intervals over a period of many months. The diagnosis is confirmed by isolation of the meningococcus on blood culture.

Treatment. The meningococcus is sensitive to both the sulphonamides and pencillin. Suitable dosage of sulphadiazine for an adult is 1·5 g. four-hourly for two days, then 1 g. four-hourly for two days, and finally 1 g. six-hourly for three or four days. During this time it is particularly important to maintain an adequate fluid intake. Patients who are gravely ill or vomiting should be given 1 g. by slow intravenous injection every four hours and in addition should receive benzylpenicillin 3·0 mega units intramuscularly every four hours. Penicillin alone must be used systemically in large doses, in view of its poor penetration of the blood-brain barrier.

VIRUS INFECTIONS

SMALLPOX (Variola)

There are three varieties of the smallpox virus. The first causes true Asiatic smallpox (*variola major*), which has a high mortality rate; the second causes a much milder disease (alastrim or *variola minor*); and the third is the one used for vaccination, which, though it retains the power to stimulate immunity against smallpox, can no longer itself cause a serious disease.

Routine vaccination of children is no longer recommended in the U.K. since the risk of contracting smallpox is now less than the risk of a serious complication of vaccination, which is given therefore only to people at special risk, such as doctors and nurses, and those travelling to endemic areas.

Clinical Features. After an incubation period of about a fortnight (exactly 12 days in most patients) there is sudden onset of headache, fever, shivering, severe pain in the back, and generalised aching in the limbs. In the most severe cases a prodromal purpuric rash may be seen almost from the start, but the true eruption of smallpox does not appear until the third day. Mucosal lesions are often the first to appear and may be very extensive in the mouth and throat. When the disease is very severe the skin of the whole body may be covered by the rash (confluent smallpox), but usually it can be seen that the peripheral parts of the limbs are more thickly covered with spots than the proximal limb segments and the trunk. Each spot starts as a red discoloration (a *macule*), but within about 24 hours it becomes thick and raised so that it can be felt with the finger (a *papule*). About three days later the centre of the papule becomes soft and filled with clear serous fluid, so that it is now a *vesicle*; and secondary infection of the fluid with pyogenic bacteria changes it in a few days into pus, so that the lesion now becomes a *pustule*. All the spots go through this series of changes at approximately the same time. A day or two after the appearance of the rash the patient's temperature may come down and his general condition improve, but a few days later, when the lesions have become pustular, the fever returns and he again becomes gravely ill. Most of the deaths (up to 25 per cent of the patients in some epidemics of variola major; 16 out of 64 patients in one outbreak dealt with by the writer) occur during the pustular stage, though in the most severe but fortunately rare form of the disease (*haemorrhagic smallpox*) death occurs within 48 hours of the onset with signs of bleeding into internal organs and from various mucosal surfaces. In patients who recover, the temperature slowly settles over a period of a week or so as the pustules gradually dry off into crusts and scabs. Since the crusts contain living virus, the patient has to be kept in isolation until they have all come away: this may take several weeks, the last to separate being the deep-seated scabs in the palms of the hands and soles of the feet.

Modified Variola Major and Variola Minor. Variola major modified by partial immunity from past vaccination and variola minor are relatively trivial illnesses with only slight constitutional upset and a rash which may be very difficult to distinguish from that of chicken-pox.

Diagnosis. In distinguishing mild smallpox from chicken-pox the following points are helpful:

(1) The lesions of chicken-pox are set more superficially in the skin and tend to be smaller.

(2) In chicken-pox the lesions are more profuse on the trunk than on the extremities; the reverse is true of smallpox,

(3) In chicken-pox the eruption appears in a series of crops, so that at any one time lesions at different stages of maturity can be found; in smallpox the lesions are all at the same stage.

(4) Recent successful vaccination excludes smallpox.

(5) The diagnosis of smallpox can be confirmed within a few hours by electronmicroscopy of scrapings from the base of a lesion.

(6) Virus culture on the chorio-allantoic membrane of a chick embryo is the only positive proof of smallpox, but takes 72 hrs.

Complications include broncho-pneumonia, otitis media, conjunctivitis, corneal ulceration and resultant opacity, cardiac failure, and encephalitis.

Treatment. There is no specific therapy against the virus of smallpox, but the stage of secondary pyogenic infection can be cut short by the administration of a suitable antibiotic. Penicillin by injection or one of the tetracyclines by mouth may be given for this purpose and if necessary changed later when the *in vitro* sensitivities of the organism isolated from the lesions have been established. Skilled nursing is of great importance, particular attention being paid to the care of the mouth, eyes, and skin.

Action to be taken when Smallpox is suspected

(1) The Area Medical Officer must be notified immediately.

(2) If the diagnosis is confirmed the patient is transferred at once to a special smallpox hospital.

(3) All members of the hospital staff and all who have been in contact with the patient must be vaccinated or revaccinated. N-methylisatinthio-semicarbazone ('Marboran') given by mouth to contacts within the incubation period has been reported as giving remarkable protection and may replace vaccination for this purpose. The dose is 1·5–3 g. twice daily for four days.

In addition the Area Medical Officer will take further action to trace the source of infection and to prevent further spread; this will include disinfection of the patient's house and keeping his family and other contacts under supervision for at least 16 days.

Prevention by Vaccination

Edward Jenner introduced vaccination at the end of the eighteenth century after noting that milkers who had had cowpox (vaccinia) appeared to be immune to smallpox. This is because the virus of smallpox is attenuated by passage through the cow, though it retains its antigenic properties.

Technique of Vaccination. Fresh glycerinated calf lymph is obtained from the public health laboratory service and stored in a refrigerator. Secondary infection is least common when the vaccination is performed over the deltoid area. The skin at the chosen site is cleaned with soap and water and dried with a sterile towel; alternatively ether or acetone may be used, but spirit and iodine should be avoided as they may kill the virus and so prevent the vaccination taking. Using a rubber bulb a drop of lymph is ejected from the capillary tube on to the prepared area of skin and a sterile Hagedorn needle, held parallel to the skin, is moved rapidly up and down through the lymph, just sufficient pressure being applied to penetrate the epidermis at the point of the needle. This is the *multiple pressure technique*, which is superior to the old scratch method as it limits the depth of penetration of the virus into the skin and reduces the incidence of complications. About 10 pressures are recommended for primary vaccination and 30 pressures for revaccination. After a few minutes (during which time the area should not be exposed to direct sunlight) excess lymph is dabbed off and a dry sterile dressing is applied.

Results of Vaccination. Successful vaccination may be indicated by three types of reaction:

(1) The *primary reaction* (obtained in people who have not been vaccinated before) is the appearance by the third or fourth day of a papule which develops through a vesicular stage to become a pustule by the seventh day (when the result is read). During this week there may be fever, malaise, and axillary adenitis. A scab forms in the second week and separates in the third week, leaving a permanent pitted scar.

(2) The *accelerated reaction* is seen in people with partial immunity. The lesion goes through its stages more quickly and may never become pustular.

(3) The *immune reaction*, seen in people with a higher degree of immunity, consists simply of a small itchy papule on the second or third day which disappears without becoming vesicular.

Contra-indications to vaccination. Vaccination should be avoided in infants with eczema since it may cause a generalised pustular rash which may be fatal (eczema vaccinatum); it should be postponed if possible in patients with septic skin lesions; and it should be avoided if possible in people with conditions predisposing to generalised vaccinia (hypogammaglobulinaemia, long-term steroid therapy and blood dyscrasias such as leukaemia).

Complications of Vaccination are very rare and particularly so in infancy.

Encephalitis (see p. 551) is much the most serious and has a mortality of about 50 per cent. Its incidence is about 1 in 100,000 vaccinations.

Generalised vaccinia, in which lesions occur on the skin all over the body from widespread dissemination of the virus, is also very rare except in people with eczema, who should not be vaccinated unless exposed to special risk.

Secondary infection of the vaccination site and *accidental inoculation* of other areas of skin by scratching are commoner and less serious complications.

Foetal mortality is high in women vaccinated during the first three months of pregnancy and this time should consequently be avoided for vaccination whenever possible.

CHICKEN-POX (Varicella)

The virus of chicken-pox is identical or closely allied to the virus of herpes zoster (shingles); susceptible children who come into contact with shingles frequently develop chicken-pox, while less often adult contacts of the latter disease may develop shingles.

Clinical Features. After an incubation period of up to three weeks the illness may start with a day of vague malaise, headache, fever, and a transient prodromal rash, before the specific eruption appears, but more often the rash is the first sign of the disease. Vesicles appear first in the mouth and throat and soon rupture, leaving ulcers which may cause a good deal of pain and difficulty in swallowing. The skin rash, unlike that of smallpox, is most profuse on the trunk and sparsest at the periphery of the limbs; and instead of all the lesions going through their various stages together, the spots appear in a succession of crops over several days, so that at any one time papules, vesicles, pustules and crusts can be seen together. The papules develop within a few hours into small round vesicles containing clear fluid set in the superficial layers of the skin. Within two or three days they become pustules and then dry up into crusts.

Constitutional upset is usually slight, though the enanthem (mucosal lesions) may cause much discomfort and the exanthem (skin rash) much itching. The disease is more severe in adults, who may develop patchy consolidation in the lungs and may subsequently be found to have scattered calcified opacities on chest X-ray.

Complications are unusual. Secondary infection may lead to boils, impetigo, cellulitis, or conjunctivitis. More serious but very rare are polyneuritis, tranverse myelitis, and encephalitis.

Diagnosis from smallpox; see p. 540.

Treatment is purely symptomatic. Irritation of the skin can be relieved by the application of calamine lotion containing 1–2 per cent phenol, or by warm boracic baths, and anti-histamine tablets may be helpful.

MEASLES (Morbilli)

Next to whooping cough this is the most serious of the infectious fevers of childhood at the present time. Passive immunity from the mother prevents infection in the first three months of life, but thereafter the child becomes highly susceptible.

Clinical Features. About ten to fourteen days after exposure to infection there develops what appears to be a common cold, with fever, running nose and eyes, sneezing, and cough. Examination of the mouth, however, reveals an eruption of tiny white spots like grains of salt set on a slightly reddened base, usually best seen on the mucous membrane inside the cheeks opposite the molar teeth. These are *Koplik's spots* and they are diagnostic of measles. If thcy are overlooked the erroneous impression that the child simply has a cold may appear to be confirmed on the third day, when the temperature may come down to normal, but this opinion is finally refuted on the fourth day, when the rash appears on the skin.

Transient prodromal rashes are sometimes seen during the first three days, but the true *morbilliform eruption* appears on the fourth day as pink macules, about 3–5 mm. in diameter, which first appear behind the ears and quickly spread over the face, trunk, and limbs. Within a day or two the lesions enlarge and become papular, many of them coalesce into large, irregular, blotchy areas, and their colour gradually changes to a darker red. The temperature rises again with the appearance of the rash and continues for several days before finally subsiding as the lesions fade.

Complications are mainly due to secondary bacterial infection of the respiratory tract. *Broncho-pneumonia* is the most serious of them, particularly in very young children, and should always be suspected in a severely ill child with a persistent cough. *Otitis media* is fairly common. *Corneal ulceration* and potential blindness should be prevented by careful treatment of any conjunctival inflammation which occurs.

Treatment. The virus of measles is not susceptible to any form of specific treatment, but antibiotics are of value for the prevention and cure of secondary bacterial complications. Save in the mildest cases it is probably wise to give a course of penicillin, starting with the appearance of the rash and continuing for up to a week. Procaine penicillin 300,000 units twice daily may be given intramuscularly, but phenoxymethyl penicillin 250 mg. six-hourly, is almost as satisfactory and avoids the necessity of injections.

Prevention. Effective measles vaccines are now available and the best course for inducing *active immunity* is probably to give 0·5 ml. killed vaccine intramuscularly followed by 0·5 ml. of live vaccine one month later. A rise in temperature may occur after live vaccine and it should not be given to children under 9 months, to pregnant women or to patients with infective or neoplastic disease. Rapid *passive immunisation* lasting two or three weeks can be achieved by the intramuscular injection of gamma globulin, from 150 to 900 mg. during the first five days after exposure to infection. Large doses prevent the attack of measles; smaller doses have the advantage that, although an attack of measles may occur, it will be a mild one and recovery from it will leave lifelong immunity.

Subacute Sclerosing Panencephalitis (SSPE)

This is a very rare disease of children and young adults due to latent infection of the nervous system with Measles virus; it is one of the so-called 'slow' virus infections characterised by very long incubation periods (2 years or more). The clinical features are progressive dementia, fits, myoclonic movements and various focal neurological signs and most patients die within two years of the onset. The C.S.F. shows a paretic Lange and the EEG reveals characteristic periodic complexes.

GERMAN MEASLES (Rubella)

This is a less infectious disease than true measles and even in towns many people reach adult life without acquiring it. It causes little constitutional upset and is never fatal, but when acquired by women in the first four months of pregnancy it may lead to development defects in the foetus. Cataract, glaucoma, disorders of retinal pigmentation, deaf mutism, and congenital heart disease are the lesions commonly caused. There is also an increased incidence of abortion, miscarriage, and stillbirth, but fetal injury is not inevitable and a proportion of women who have had rubella early in pregnancy do produce healthy live babies. It is now recommended that girls who have not had rubella should be given a single dose of live attenuated rubella virus, Cendehill strain, between the ages 11–14. No other vaccine should be given within 3–4 weeks. This vaccine must not be given to pregnant women because of the risk of foetal damage, or to patients with Hodgkin's disease or leukaemia or to those on immuno-suppressive therapy.

Clinical Features. After an incubation period of two to three weeks the rash is usually the first indication of the disease, and takes the form of small pink macules and papules which remain distinct units and do not run together as in true measles. There are no Koplik's spots in the mouth. The only other notable feature is generalised lymph-node enlargement, affecting particularly the nodes at the back of the neck. There are rarely any general symptoms of illness and the rash usually fades in two or three days. In adults a transient mild arthritis is common.

No **treatment** is needed. The disease may be prevented in women in early pregnancy who have been exposed to infection by giving high-titre im-munoglobulin if available; protection lasts for three weeks. Ordinary gamma globulin is of little value.

MUMPS (Epidemic parotitis)

Mumps is a relatively trivial illness in young children, but if contracted after puberty it may have serious complications. There are undoubted advantages, therefore, in 'getting it over' early in life, and only if a child is in a weak state of health from some other illness should any steps be taken to isolate him from this infection.

Clinical Features. After an incubation period of three weeks or a little longer the patient develops fever, malaise, and stiffness in the jaw, and examination reveals swelling of one or more of the salivary glands. Usually the parotid glands are affected and fill out the hollow between the angle of the jaw and the mastoid process. Sometimes the submandibular glands are affected too, or occasionally they are involved alone. There is no rash and usually the fever and glandular swellings subside within a few days.

The *diagnosis* is usually easy, but if there is doubt it can be confirmed by isolation of the virus from saliva, or by demonstrating a rising antibody titre in two specimens of serum taken at the onset of illness and a fortnight later.

Complications are almost confined to adolescent and adult patients and usually arise a few days after the swelling of the salivary glands.

Orchitis is the commonest complication, being seen in about 25 per cent of patients. It is usually unilateral and causes severe pain and swelling of the testicle. Very rarely it may be bilateral and result in sterility.

Oophoritis is less common and causes severe lower abdominal pain and vomiting.

Prostatitis should be suspected in patients with unexplained fever and perhaps some frequency of micturition.

Mastitis, causing pain and swelling of the breast, may be seen in either sex.

Pancreatitis is characterised by severe upper abdominal pain, fever and vomiting.

Meningitis. Routine lumbar puncture in patients with mumps usually reveals a pleocytosis in the C.S.F., so that invasion of the nervous system by the virus is common, but in only about 10 per cent of cases is there clinical evidence of meningitis (headache, fever, vomiting, and neck rigidity). These symptoms usually subside within two or three days and the prognosis is excellent.

Encephalitis, characterised by severe headache, fever, vomiting, perhaps cranial nerve palsies, drowsiness, and coma, is much more serious and carries a mortality of about 50 per cent.

Treatment. There is no specific treatment and no method of inducing either active or passive immunity has yet been shown to be effective. However, patients with orchitis gain relief from systemic steroids.

ORNITHOSIS (Psittacosis)

This virus is acquired by contact with infected birds, who do not themselves necessarily appear ill. Originally described in parrots, it can, however, be transmitted by other birds, including canaries and budgerigars.

Clinical Features. After an incubation period of one to two weeks there is gradual onset with cough, fever, headache, backache, and general malaise. The pulse usually remains low in relation to the temperature, but in fulminating cases with high fever and delirium rising pulse and respiratory rates indicate a poor prognosis. Though clinical signs of pulmonary consolidation are often absent, radiographs usually show evidence of pneumonia spreading out from the hilum of the lung. The white blood count is low or normal.

The disease acquired from parrots is often more severe than that spread by other birds. Convalescence is usually slow and prolonged.

Diagnosis may be confirmed by a complement fixation test using psittacosis antigen.

Treatment. Tetracycline is the drug of choice and should be given in doses of 0·5 g. four-hourly for a week. In view of the possibility of case to case transmission by droplet infection the patient should be nursed on barrier precautions.

ACUTE INFECTIOUS MONONUCLEOSIS (Glandular Fever)

An infective agent which fulfils Koch's postulates has not yet been found, but there is strong evidence linking the disease with the Epstein-Barr (E.B.) virus, which is also associated with Burkitt's lymphoma and acute leukaemia. Rarely, an attack of infectious mononucleosis is followed by Hodgkin's disease.

It is a common disease, seen mainly in young adults, but its infectivity is low, though small outbreaks occur quite often in hostels and similar institutions. There is evidence that the virus is transmitted in saliva, either by kissing, or sharing of drinking vessels.

Clinical Features. The main symptoms are fever, which is usually low and long-continued, lassitude, general malaise, and sometimes sore throat, but the severity and course of the disease are very variable. Some patients simply feel a little tired for a week or two, while others are gravely ill with high fever, headache, and severe sore throat; and although this acute stage does not usually last for more than a week or so, general debility and depression may persist for up to six months. The prognosis, however, is excellent; the disease is never fatal and all patients makes a complete recovery. Examination usually reveals enlarged lymph nodes in the neck and elsewhere and the spleen can often be felt. Many patients have a transient macular rash and palatal petechiae are common.

Subclinical hepatitis is very common but actual jaundice infrequent. E.C.G. evidence of myocarditis has been reported in 16 per cent of patients. Acute abdominal pain simulating appendicitis, benign lymphocytic meningitis, transient thrombocytopenic purpura and rupture of the spleen are rare manifestations.

Diagnosis depends on:

(1) The *white blood count* which after an initial leucopenia is usually raised with an excess of monocytes and lymphocytes, many of which are seen in the stained film to have a characteristic abnormal appearance ('glandular fever cells').

(2) The *Paul-Bunnell* test is positive in about 90 per cent of cases. It depends on the fact that in glandular fever the serum contains an unknown factor which agglutinates sheep's red cells. Occasional false positive results occur, but a titre of 1:64 or

higher, and particularly a rising titre during the illness, may be taken as significant. If the Paul-Bunnell test is negative, the possibility of toxoplasmosis or cytomegalovirus infection should be considered.

(3) Antibodies against the E.B. virus found in the IgM fraction of the plasma proteins are evidence of recent infection by the virus and are found in a high proportion of cases.

Treatment. The duration of fever and debility may be reduced by a week's course of prednisolone, starting with 40 mg. daily, but this should be reserved for severely ill patients. There is no specific treatment, and prolonged convalescence is often necessary.

CYTOMEGALOVIRUS INFECTION

Intra-uterine infection with this virus causes severe generalised disease at birth or severe brain damage some months later; infection later in childhood or in adult life is common but usually remains subclinical. Sometimes, however, it causes fever and lymphocytosis with many atypical lymphocytes, but the Paul-Bunnell test and tests for Epstein-Barr virus antibody (both positive in infectious mononucleosis) are negative. The diagnosis may be confirmed by isolation of the virus, usually from the urine, or by demonstrating antibody to cytomegalovirus by complement-fixation and indirect haemagglutination tests.

INFLUENZA

Of the three strains of influenza virus, A is more common than B and C is rare. There is no correlation between the clinical severity of the illness and the strain of virus and no cross-immunity between the strains. Variation in the antigenic structure of the virus occurs from time to time and limits the effectiveness of vaccines. Epidemics of influenza A tend to occur every two to three years and influenza B every four to five years. Factors leading to occasional pandemics, as in 1918 and 1957 (the 'Asian flu') are unknown. Between epidemics the virus is probably kept going in a chain of sporadic infections in man; some of these may be subclinical. Transmission is by droplet infection.

Clinical Features. After an incubation period of one to two days there is sudden onset with fever, shivering, headache, profound malaise, and severe aching in the back and limbs. Cough, sneezing, and upper respiratory catarrh are usually relatively slight. Remittent fever and general prostration continue for up to a week and the temperature settles by lysis. In some patients convalescence is very slow and post-influenzal debility and depression may persist for months.

Influenzal pneumonia. Particularly in the 1918 pandemic pneumonia was a common complication and a common cause of death, but in recent years it has been comparatively rare. It is due to secondary bacterial infection with *H. influenzae*, staphylococci, streptococci, or pneumococci.

Treatment. There is no specific treatment, though the appropriate chemotherapy should of course be given for any bacterial complication. Aspirin 0·6 g. four-hourly helps to relieve symptoms during the febrile stage.

Prophylaxis. Vaccines containing inactivated strains of A and B virus give partial immunity for about six months and are of limited value if given just before an epidemic.

EPIDEMIC VOMITING

This very common virus infection typically causes small outbreaks of several cases in a family.

Clinical Features. Onset is abrupt with nausea and vomiting and sometimes there is mild fever and diarrhoea as well. Constitutional upset is very mild and complete recovery usually occurs within two days.

Diagnosis is usually obvious from the occurrence of multiple cases and the short duration of symptoms and no *treatment* is necessary.

OTHER VIRUS CONDITIONS

In addition to the well-recognised virus diseases, it is now realised that there are several groups of viruses which may cause a variety of clinical syndromes. Among the most common are:

COXSACKIE AND ECHO VIRUS GROUP

These viruses may cause:

(a) **Meningitis** (Benign lymphocytic)

This presents with fever, headache, nausea and a stiff neck. The cerebrospinal fluid contains a hundred or so cells per c.mm. which are predominantly lymphocytes.

(b) **Epidemic Myalgia** (Bornholm disease) (p. 332).

ADENOVIRUS GROUP

An acute upper respiratory tract infection which is sometimes no more than a common cold, but it may be a more severe influenza-like illness with fever, sore throat, cough, and sometimes painful enlargement of the lymphatic glands. Areas of pneumonic consolidation and concomitant conjunctivitis have been reported.

HAND, FOOT AND MOUTH DISEASE

This infection with Coxsackie A viruses is distinct from foot and mouth disease of animals, which is caused by another picornavirus. It is seen mainly in young children, but adults in the family are often affected too. It occurs mainly in summer and autumn.

Clinical Features. After an incubation period of 3–6 days there is a mild febrile illness lasting only a few days. On the second or third days a maculopapular rash, later becoming vesicular, appears on the fingers, toes and lateral borders of the feet and painful ulcers develop in the mouth. These lesions heal within about a week.

Diagnosis. The clinical picture is quite characteristic but if necessary the diagnosis can be confirmed by virus studies. The virus may be present in the faeces for several weeks after infection.

POST-INFECTIOUS ENCEPHALITIS AND ENCEPHALOMYELITIS

This condition is a very rare sequel to acute specific fevers such as whooping cough, measles, and mumps and less often to others such as chicken-pox, German measles, scarlet fever, and glandular fever; it is no commoner after severe than mild attacks. It also sometimes follows vaccination and other immunising procedures. It has been suggested that the underlying cause may be an antigen-antibody reaction and sometimes improvement does seem to follow treatment with ACTH or cortisone.

Clinical Features. Symptoms appear within a week or two of the onset of the original infection or vaccination. Headache, malaise, vomiting, irritability, drowsiness, or coma are common; other patients present with fits or sudden paresis mimicking a cerebral vascular accident; while in others the clinical picture is dominated by signs of meningitis, cranial nerve palsies, and transient lower motor neurone weakness in the limbs. Mortality is highest, about 50 per cent, in encephalitis following smallpox or vaccination, but even in the other groups it does not fall below 10 per cent and is often higher. Moreover, many of those who recover are left with a disability such as hemiplegia, cranial nerve palsies, mental defect, or a Parkinsonian syndrome.

INFECTIVE DISEASES for which barrier nursing is unnecessary.

WEIL'S DISEASE (Epidemic Spirochaetal Jaundice)

The causal organism, *Leptospira icterohaemorrhagiae*, is excreted in the urine of infected rats. Man acquires the infection either by ingesting food or drink contaminated by rat urine or by immersion in contaminated water, since the spirochaete is able to gain entry through the nasal mucosa or through minor skin abrasions. In this country leptospirosis is therefore mainly seen as an occupational disease of people working in damp rat-infested places, notably sewer workers, miners, canal and dock-workers, farm-hands and fish-cleaners.

Clinical Features. After an incubation period of between one and two weeks there is rapid onset of fever, headache, pains in the back and limbs. Injection of the conjunctivae is often a very striking feature. The name 'icterohaemorrhagiae' implies jaundice and purpura, but clinical jaundice is seen in only about 75 per cent of patients; it appears during the first week. Features which help in distinguishing the disease from infective hepatitis are the profound prostration, heavy albuminuria, purpuric rash, and sometimes haemoptysis, haematemesis, melaena, or bleeding from the gums. There is usually a leucocytosis. Some patients develop signs of meningeal irritation and some proceed from oliguria to anuria and uraemia; the mortality rate is about 15 per cent.

Diagnosis is established by identifying the spirochaete by dark-ground illumination of specimens of blood taken during the first few days or urine during the third week. The organism can also be isolated by intraperitoneal inoculation of guinea-pigs with blood or urine. A rising titre of serum agglutinins also occurs but does not give diagnostic information until the clinical illness is more or less over.

Treatment. To be effective penicillin must be given early in the illness, in large doses such as 3 million units six-hourly. If there is no improvement after three days oxytetracycline 1·5 g. six-hourly may be given a trial. Antileptospiral serum is also effective if given during the first few days; it is injected either intravenously or intramuscularly in doses of 20–40 ml.

BRUCELLOSIS (Undulant Fever; Malta Fever)

The causative organism is a gram-negative cocco-bacillus which is transmitted to man in infected milk. In this country the usual infecting organism is *Brucella abortus*, which is prevalent throughout the world and is transmitted in cow's milk. *Brucella melitensis* is transmitted in goat's milk and is found particularly in the Mediterranean area, where it causes Malta fever. *Brucella suis* infects pigs and is rarely transmitted to man.

The disease is an occupational hazard of farm workers and slaughtermen since infection can be acquired through the skin and mucosae, but others may be infected by drinking unpasteurised milk. There is reason to think it may be more common in this country than is generally realised.

Clinical Features. Typical undulant fever has an incubation period of between one and three weeks, followed by headache, malaise, anorexia, constipation, and a bout of fever which usually settles by lysis after about ten days. Cough and profuse sweating are common and the spleen is usually palpable. After the temperature has been normal for a few days another bout of fever begins and these febrile episodes may continue recurring at short intervals for many months. During the course of the illness arthritis is common. One joint is usually affected at a time, the pain and swelling subsiding after a few days and then appearing elsewhere. The joints most often affected are the hip, knee, shoulder, ankle, and wrist, but occasionally the small joints of the fingers and toes or of the spine may be involved. Peripheral neuritis, orchitis, and albuminuria are less common complications.

Abortus fever as seen in this country is on the whole clinically milder and sometimes takes such a prolonged and insidious course that the more appropriate label *chronic brucellosis* is often used. Recurrent bouts of drenching night sweats without serious general ill-health should always suggest this diagnosis and the other clinical features mentioned above may also be seen.

Diagnosis. *Blood culture* is the most satisfactory way of establishing the diagnosis, but the organism is difficult to isolate (even under increased CO_2 tension) so that sterile cultures do not rule out this disease. *Urine culture* is occasionally positive. A rising *agglutinin titre* during the illness is helpful; dilutions up to 1:5,000 should be tested, since agglutination may be found in the higher dilutions but absent in the lower ones. The brucellin skin test is of doubtful value. The *blood count* usually shows a leucopenia and perhaps mild anaemia.

Treatment. Tetracycline 0·75 g. six-hourly and intramuscular streptomycin 0·75 g. twice daily, with a vitamin B preparation such as becosym forte two tablets three times daily, should be given for two weeks. A second course of treatment may be necessary for patients with chronic brucellosis.

Prevention of infection may be achieved by attention to personal hygiene by those handling cattle, pigs, and goats; pasteurisation of milk; a clean water supply; and disinfection of excreta, particularly urine, from patients with the disease.

TETANUS

It is estimated that in Britain each year this preventible disease is contracted by 200–300 people and kills half of them. *Clostridium tetani* is a normal inhabitant of the alimentary tract of horses and sheep, so that its spores are particularly prevalent on cultivated land, and as it is a strict anaerobe it thrives especially in deep penetrating wounds contaminated with soil or road dust. The wound, however, may be a trivial one which heals before the tetanic symptoms appear. These are due to a powerful exotoxin which is absorbed by muscle end-plates at the site of infection and travels along motor nerves to the central nervous system.

Clinical Features. The incubation period is very variable and is important in prognosis: tetanus appearing within a few days of a wound is usually fatal, while if symptoms are delayed for two or more weeks the disease is likely to be mild. Local muscular weakness near the site of infection, attributable to the action of the toxin on the motor end-plates, may precede the generalised spasms. These are usually heralded by trismus (hence the term lockjaw), which may be accompanied by spasm of the facial musculature causing the classical '*risus sardonicus*'. Tonic spasm spreads to the trunk, causing opisthotonus and board-like rigidity of the abdomen. Fever is commonly present.

The *paroxysmal stage* starts in severe cases within two days of the appearance of trismus; the longer it is delayed the better the prognosis. Paroxysms are precipitated by stimuli such as feeding and other nursing attentions, clinical examination or even simply external noises. The whole body is thrown into painful spasm, with arching of the back, extension of the limbs and clenching of the teeth; this may subside after a few seconds or persist for several minutes. In severe cases the paroxysms recur with increasing frequency until death occurs from exhaustion.

Treatment. Specially staffed and equipped tetanus units have been established in Britain and strenuous efforts should be made to have the patient transferred without delay to the nearest of these. The patient should be nursed in a quiet room with shaded light.

(a) Human antitetanus immunoglobulin (Humotet, Wellcome) is the antitoxin of choice since it avoids the serious allergic reactions which may follow horse serum antitoxin; the dose is 30–300 IU/kg. body weight, given intramuscularly. Even though the neurotoxin is fixed to the nervous tissue by the time clinical signs of tetanus appear, it is important to give antitoxin to deal with toxin still circulating in the blood or being produced at the wound site.

(b) *Wound Toilet.* An hour after the antitoxin has been given, surgical debridement of the wound should be carried out under light general anaesthesia.

(c) *Antibiotic Therapy.* As a prophylaxis against broncho-pneumonia procaine penicillin 450,000 units and benzyl penicillin 500,000 units should be given twice daily.

(d) *Control of Muscular Spasms.* For successful management of severe cases continuous skilled medical supervision throughout the 24 hours is necessary. Intravenous succinylcholine 0·2 per cent at a rate of 1–1·5 ml. (2–3 mg.) per minute controls most of the spasms, but occasionally much faster administration is needed for a few seconds and at these times respiration ceases and the lungs must be inflated with oxygen delivered through an anaesthetic machine. For the latter purpose tracheal intubation should be carried out as soon as satisfactory relaxation has been obtained and later a tracheotomy may be done. The foot of the bed should be blocked to prevent accumulation of secretions in the air passages, which are cleared every hour by a sucker attached to a catheter which is passed through the tracheotomy tube. From time to time the patient is allowed to come round so that an attempt may be made to feed him, but in the early stages this must be done through an intragastric tube. Intravenous therapy to maintain fluid and electrolyte balance is also essential.

Prophylaxis. *Active immunisation* if generally adopted could wipe out this disease. Tetanus toxoid should be given to all children in the combined triple vaccine with diphtheria and pertussis (see p. 528). Alternatively tetanus toxoid alone may be given in three doses of 1 ml., the second six to twelve weeks after the first and the third six to twelve months after the second. If an individual actively immunised in this way receives a wound he should be given a further dose of toxoid instead of antitetanic serum.

Passive immunisation. All non-immunised patients with tetanus-prone wounds should be given antitoxin. Human antitetanus immunoglobulin

(Humotet, Wellcome) should be used, since it provides better protection and has none of the disadvantages of horse serum antitoxin; the dose is 250–500 IU intramuscularly. At the same time the first immunising dose of absorbed toxoid should be given.

TOXOPLASMOSIS

Infection with the protozoon *toxoplasma gondii* is common, but only rarely causes clinical disease; it is mainly acquired by eating undercooked meat from infected animals.

Congenital toxoplasmosis may lead to choroido-retinitis, or less often to lesions in the brain which may calcify and may cause hydrocephalus.

Acquired toxoplasmosis causes lymphadenopathy and may mimic infectious mononucleosis, or Hodgkin's disease. The *diagnosis* may be suspected from the histology of a node removed by biopsy and the toxoplasma may be isolated by mouse inoculation. Antibody tests, particularly the dye test, and a skin test may also help: intradermal inoculation of toxoplasma antigen causes a reaction which is maximal in 24–48 hrs.

Treatment. Spiramycin (50–75 mg./kg. daily) may give good results in children with ocular infections, but has little effect on lymphadenopathic toxoplasmosis.

CAT-SCRATCH FEVER

This disease, whose causative organism has not yet been isolated, is transmitted by the scratch of apparently healthy cats.

Clinical Features. A few days after the scratch a small indolent ulcer or sore may appear at the site of inoculation and a week or two later the regional lymph nodes become very enlarged. There may be some fever at this stage but constitutional upset is slight. The affected lymph nodes sometimes suppurate, but recovery without serious complications or sequelae is the rule though adenitis may persist for some months. The white blood count is normal and aspirated pus is sterile.

Treatment. A course of tetracycline, 250 mg. six-hourly for five days, may prevent suppuration.

ACTINOMYCOSIS

The organism *Actinomyces bovis* occurs in pus as 'sulphur granules' of up to 1 mm. in diameter and is anaerobic. The disease is much more common in men than in women.

Clinical Features. There are three clinical varieties:

(1) *Actinomycosis of the jaw* is the commonest type. Infection through the mucous membrane of the gum leads gradually to woody induration of all the tissues of the jaw and overlying skin, through which multiple

sinuses eventually discharge. There is little pain or constitutional upset and the regional lymph nodes are not usually involved.

(2) *Ileocaecal actinomycosis* causes a hard irregular mass in the right iliac fossa and in time fixation to the overlying skin and sinus formation occurs. The disease may spread to the liver, spleen, and other organs and is frequently fatal.

(3) *Actinomycosis of the lung* is the least common type. Cough, dyspnoea, fever, and pain in the chest occur and in the later stages induration and sinuses appear in the chest wall.

Diagnosis depends on identification of the 'sulphur granules' in the pus.

Treatment consists of the administration of penicillin in high dosage for a prolonged period and surgical eradication of the disease wherever possible.

FURTHER READING

Cruickshank, R., *Medical Microbiology,* 12th edition, Churchill Livingstone, Edinburgh and London, 1973.

Lawson, J. H., *A Synopsis of Fevers and their Treatment*, 12th Edition, Lloyd-Luke, London, 1977.

CHAPTER SEVENTEEN

TROPICAL DISEASES

MALARIA

Malaria is by far the commonest and most important of the tropical diseases and is responsible for some millions of deaths each year. It is prevalent in areas where there are both anophelene mosquitoes and enough warmth and humidity to allow the parasite to develop in them. There are four varieties of human malaria, due to infection respectively with *Plasmodium vivax* (benign tertian malaria). *Plasmodium falciparum* (malignant tertian malaria), *Plasmodium malariae* (quartan malaria), and *Plasmodium ovale* (benign tertian malaria). *P. vivax* is responsible for most of the malaria seen in India and South-east Asia; *P. falciparum* is the common malarial parasite in Africa; *P. malariae* and *P. ovale* are both comparatively rare.

Life-cycle of the Malarial Parasite. Sexual forms of the plasmodium (*gametocytes*) circulate in the blood at a certain stage of malaria and when they are ingested into the stomach of an anophelene mosquito the male and female gametocytes unite, penetrate the stomach wall and form an oocyst. After some one to three weeks (the time varying with the temperature) *sporozoites* are liberated from the oocyst, find their way to the salivary glands and so back to the bloodstream of man. They quickly disappear from the blood to enter liver cells, where the pre-erythrocytic stage of development takes place. After $8\frac{1}{2}$ days (*P. vivax*) or $6\frac{1}{2}$ days (*P. falciparum*) numerous *merozoites* are liberated and enter circulating red blood corpuscles, or, in the case of *P. vivax*, *P. malariae*, and *P. ovale* infections—but not *P. falciparum*—they may enter new liver cells. In the latter site they may lie dormant for many months and are probably responsible for the relapses which are common in these three infections but do not occur in *P. falciparum* (malignant tertian) malaria. In the red cell the merozoite develops first into a ring form, then by asexual reproduction into a *schizont* from which a new batch of merozoites (the number varying with the species) are liberated into the blood on rupture of the red cell. This asexual reproduction takes some 48 hours in the tertian malarias and 72 hours in quartan malaria, the characteristically spaced rigors and fever occurring when the new shower of merozoites enters the blood. Each merozoite enters a new red cell and several cycles of schizogony usually occur before some merozoites invading red cells develop not into schizonts but into male or female gametocytes. The cycle is then complete.

Clinical Features. For the first few days there is usually either continuous or remittent fever with general malaise, headache, and vomiting, but by the end of a week the typical periodicity, with rigors on every alternate or every third day, is often becoming apparent. In relapses it may be a striking feature from the beginning. In some patients, however, no regular pattern ever emerges, probably because they harbour two or more 'families' of parasites at different stages of development. The typical attack of malaria starts with a cold stage with shivering or *rigors*, lasting from a few minutes to a couple of hours, followed by a *hot stage* in which the patient has a severe headache, vomiting, a hot dry skin, and high fever, and finally profuse *sweating* for an hour or two brings down the temperature and the patient feels better. He may then remain well, with a normal temperature, until the next attack two or occasionally three days later. By the time the patient has had two or three rigors his spleen has often become palpable. Some patients develop a crop of herpes febrilis on the lip or face with each relapse of malaria.

Diagnosis depends on finding the malarial parasite in a thick blood smear and then identifying the species in a thin blood film. Recognition of the plasmodium can be learnt only by practical study, however, and no description of its various forms will be given here.

Complications of Malignant Tertian (Subtertian) Malaria

These occur only in people with little or no acquired immunity to malaria; they are therefore seen particularly in visitors to malarious areas who have not taken a prophylactic antimalarial drug and in people living in areas where there is good malaria control who nevertheless acquire the infection.

(1) *Cerebral malaria.* Red cells containing *P. falciparum* sometimes adhere to capillary walls in sufficient numbers to impair blood flow and cause disturbances in cerebral function from anoxia. *Clinically* cerebral malaria usually presents with high fever and drowsiness, often rapidly proceeding to coma, or there may be epileptiform fits and hemiplegia or other evidence of focal cerebral lesions. There is a high mortality and treatment must be started at the earliest possible moment, even while awaiting confirmation of the diagnosis from the blood film examination.

(2) *Blackwater fever* is a variety of acute haemolytic anaemia with haemoglobinuria seen in patients with malignant tertian (falciparum) malaria who have been treated, often rather irregularly and inadequately, with quinine. It has therefore become extremely rare now that quinine has been largely superseded by the newer antimalarial drugs. The patient complains of headache, fever, rigors, and vomiting; he may become jaundiced within 24 hours or so; and he passes dark urine containing oxyhaemoglobin or methaemoglobin. In severe cases oliguria or anuria may occur and haemodialysis may be life-saving.

Relapses

Relapses of *P. vivax* and *P. ovale* infection commonly recur for two years after the patient leaves a malarious area, but are rare thereafter; *P.*

malariae (quartan) infection may recur for five years or longer. Falciparum malaria does not relapse.

Treatment

(1) *Acute Attacks of Malaria.* The drug of choice is chloroquine, which is put up in 250 mg. tablets containing 150 mg. base. The initial dose is four tablets, followed by two tablets in six hours and two tablets on each of the next two days. Patients who are gravely ill or vomiting should be given intravenous chloroquine sulphate 200 mg. (base) in 5 ml. distilled water and this dose may be repeated in eight hours if necessary.

In falciparum infections occurring in an area where resistant strains are common, a short course of quinine sulphate 650 mg. three times daily for two days followed by a single dose of Fansidaz (pyrimethamine 75 mg. and sulphadoxine 1·5 g.) is very effective.

If the patient is gravely ill quinine can be given by infusion over four hours in doses of *10 mg./kg. twice daily. With liver or kidney damage the dose should be halved. When the patient responds the dose can be increased to 20 mg./kg.

(2) *Prevention of Relapses.* The most effective drug for eradicating pre-erythrocytic forms of *P. vivax* and *P. malariae* from the liver is primaquine diphosphate 7·5 mg. of base (1 tablet) two or three times daily for two weeks. This course may be started at the same time as the chloroquine course described above.

(3) *Suppressive Therapy.* The following are recommended for suppressing malaria during residence in an endemic area. Administration should start as soon as the area is entered and continue for four weeks after it has been left. Clinical malaria may, of course, appear thereafter.

> (a) Pyrimethamine 1 tablet (25 mg.) weekly—suitable for most areas except those with resistant strains.
> (b) Proguanil monohydrochloride 100 mg. daily—suitable for India.
> (c) Maloprim (pyrimethamine and dapsone) 1 tablet weekly should be used in S.E. Asia owing to the high incidence of resistant strains of *P. falciparum*.

Malaria prevention may be achieved by:

(1) Measures to prevent the breeding of anophelene mosquitoes.
(2) Protecting humans from mosquito bites by:

> (a) Mosquito-proofing of houses and other buildings by fitting wire-meshing to windows and doors and regular spraying with D.D.T.
> (b) Sleeping under mosquito nets.
> (c) Wearing protective clothing and applying a repellent lotion to exposed parts, particularly when going out at night.

* As quinine base.

AMOEBIASIS

Although infection with the protozoon *Entamoeba histolytica* is not confined to hot climates, clinical amoebiasis is very much more common in tropical countries where relatively low standards of hygiene permit faecal contamination of food.

Entamoeba histolytica is found in man in a vegetative form, which exhibits active amoeboid movements, and a non-motile cystic form. The vegetative forms invade the wall of the colon producing ulcers with undermined edges separated from each other by areas of healthy mucosa. From the colon amoebae may be carried in the portal bloodstream to the liver to cause amoebic hepatitis or so-called amoebic abscesses. In the lumen of the gut the amoebae encyst and develop a tough outer envelope; it is these cysts passing out in the faeces which are infective to other humans. If amoebae are swallowed they are destroyed by the digestive juices of the upper alimentary tract, but the cysts are able to survive until they reach the large bowel, where they develop into the mature vegetative form.

Clinical Features

Clinically amoebiasis may present in several different ways:

(1) **Acute Amoebic Dysentery.** This is usually more insidious in its onset than bacillary dysentery and there is less fever and constitutional upset. The patient complains of lower abdominal colic and has frequent loose motions containing blood and mucus. Diagnosis is readily established by microscopic examination of a specimen of mucus from a freshly passed stool, which reveals active vegetative forms of *Entamoeba histolytica* (see below).

(2) **Chronic Amoebic Colitis.** Many patients never develop acute dysenteric symptoms, but pass rather gradually into a state of vague ill-health; they lose weight, complain of general tiredness and irritability and suffer recurrent exacerbations at varying intervals in which they pass a number of loose motions, usually in the morning, with a good deal of colic and flatulence. The stools usually contain mucus but no blood. Examination often reveals thickening and tenderness of the caecum, and during exacerbations appendicitis may be closely mimicked.

Diagnosis remains in doubt until the organisms have been identified and they may be much more elusive than in the acute dysenteric form of the disease. As the cysts are much more difficult to identify than the active amoebae, and as the latter rapidly lose their motility when the stool becomes cool, arrangements should be made for the patient to pass the specimen near the laboratory where it is to be examined. A small portion of mucus is selected, mixed with a little saline on a slide, covered with a cover slip, and quickly searched with the 2/3 microscope objective. A higher power is used for final identification of the *Entamoeba histolytica* which, in contrast to the non-pathogenic *Entamoeba coli*, shows very active amoeboid movements and contains ingested red blood cells in its cytoplasm. Cysts of *Entamoeba histolytica* are pearly white in appearance, and contain four nuclei and a greenish refractile chromatoid bar; they can be identified with certainty only by pathologists with wide experience of this type of work.

Sigmoidoscopy may reveal deceptively small-looking ulcers (they are flask-shaped in section and may extend quite widely into the submucosa) separated by areas of normal mucous membrane. This is in contrast to bacillary dysentery and ulcerative colitis, both of which show a generally inflamed mucosa. In the more chronic cases, however, the lesions are often confined to the caecum and ascending colon, so that the rectum and pelvic colon appear normal, but even in these patients sigmoidoscopy may be very helpful in diagnosis by providing a fresh specimen of mucus for microscopy.

(3) **Hepatic Amoebiasis.** Though usually a complication of acute amoebic dysentery, amoebic hepatitis is sometimes seen in endemic areas in people who give a history of only slight recurrent looseness of the stools. The patient presents with fever and pain in the right upper quadrant of the abdomen. Examination reveals an enlarged and tender liver, and there is often impaired resonance at the right base and a high immobile diaphragm on radiological screening. There is usually a leucocytosis but jaundice is very rare. Cloroquine provides a therapeutic test of the diagnosis; the inflammation rapidly resolves when it is given and the temperature should be normal after two or three days. If not, either the diagnosis is wrong or there is an associated amoebic abscess in the liver.

(4) **Amoebic Abscess in the Liver.** Pathologically the difference between amoebic hepatitis and amoebic abscess in the liver is probably simply a matter of degree; the 'abscess' contains the debris of necrotic liver tissue, but no pus cells. Such an abscess may develop many months or even years after the original infection. It may also be clinically silent until a late stage, as in a patient of the writer's, an army sergeant in a combatant unit who remained symptom-free and on active service until admitted to hospital following the rupture of a large liver abscess into the peritoneal cavity. This latter event is very unusual; more commonly the abscess points upwards and may rupture into the pleura, or into the lung and bronchus with subsequent expectoration of sputum aptly likened to anchovy sauce.

Treatment. Metronidazole is a safe and effective amoebicide which has replaced emetine as the drug of first choice in this disease. It is given by mouth in doses of 400–800 mg. t.d.s. for 10 days. Older regimes of treatment such as the following are still occasionally used:

Days 1–3 : Emetine hydrochloride 60 mg. intramuscularly daily.
Days 1–5 : Oxytetracycline 250 mg. six-hourly.
Days 6–16: Emetine bismuth iodide 0·2 g. daily by mouth.
Days 14–35: Diodoquin tablets 0·6 g. three times daily.

Emetine by injection may have toxic effects on the myocardium, so that patients must be kept in bed while it is being given and the treatment should be stopped if tachycardia, fall in blood pressure or flat T waves in the electrocardiogram appear. To minimise the vomiting caused by E.B.I. the drug should be given in gelatin capsules (which prevent gastric irritation) and preferably last thing at night combined with an anti-histamine such as promethazine 25 mg. and a sedative such as amylobarbitone 200 mg. in the hope that the patient may 'sleep through his nausea' and so retain the drug.

Treatment of Hepatic Amoebiasis. Amoebic hepatitis usually responds quickly to emetine by injection, but chloroquine is the drug of choice for this condition since it is less toxic and even more effective. Chloroquine is a relatively feeble amoebacide, of no value in intestinal amoebiasis; it is effective in hepatitis because it is concentrated some thirty times in the liver. An adult should be given 600 mg. of base (4 tablets), followed by 2 tablets six hours later and then 2 tablets daily for two to three weeks. Failure of the temperature to settle a few days on this treatment suggests that there is a large abscess in the liver which requires aspiration.

VISCERAL LEISHMANIASIS (Kala-azar)

This disease is endemic in the Far East, India, East Pakistan, the Middle East, the Sudan, Kenya, the Mediterranean seaboard and parts of South America. The causative organism is the protozoon *Leishmania donovani*, which is transmitted from man to man by sandflies of the genus *Phlebotomus* and parasites reticulo-endothelial cells in the liver, spleen, bone marrow and occasionally lymph nodes.

Clinical Features. After an incubation period which is usually several months but may be as long as three years, the illness usually starts insidiously and runs a long chronic or relapsing course. There are bouts of fever lasting from a few days to a few weeks; these are accompanied by night sweats and separated by apyrexial phases of variable length. Meanwhile the spleen slowly and progressively enlarges until eventually it may extend into the right iliac fossa. Hepatomegaly of lesser degree is common and occasionally there may be enlarged lymph nodes too. The blood count reveals anaemia and leucopenia. In the later stages the patient may become grossly wasted.

Diagnosis is established by identifying the parasites. These are rarely found in peripheral blood films, but more often in smears of bone marrow or splenic pulp obtained by percutaneous aspiration. The formol-gel and Chopra tests are useful ancillary investigations, but are not specific since they are positive in all conditions characterised by a raised serum globulin level.

    (1) *Formol-gel test.* Add one drop of commercial formalin to 1 ml. of serum. The test is positive if the serum becomes opaque in 10–30 minutes.

    (2) *Chopra test.* Add a few drops of 4-per-cent solution of a pentavalent antimony preparation to a 10-per-cent solution

of serum in distilled water. The test is positive if the mixture becomes opaque within a few minutes.

Treatment

Pentavalent antimony compounds have replaced trivalent preparations since they are much less toxic. *Sodium antimony gluconate* is given intravenously, 0·3–0·6 g. daily dissolved in 6–10 ml. of sterile distilled water, for three to ten days. Alternatively the aromatic diamidine *pentamidine isethionate* is another effective drug which may be given if the patient fails to respond to the antimony preparation, or relapses. The dose is 2–4 mg. per kg. body weight dissolved in 5–10 ml. sterile distilled water and given by daily intravenous injection for ten to fourteen days.

Cutaneous Leishmaniasis

Within two years of receiving treatment for kala-azar some patients develop depigmented patches, usually on the face, shoulders and upper part of the chest, and later papular lesions may appear on these areas. The condition usually responds to a further course of treatment.

TRYPANOSOMIASIS (SLEEPING-SICKNESS)

This disease, which is endemic in tropical Africa, is due to infection with the flagellated protozoa *Trypanosoma gambiense* or *T. rhodesiense*. The organisms are spread from man to man by the tsetse fly, in which part of their life cycle occurs, and wild game also probably provide a reservoir of infection.

Clinical Features. The early symptoms are fever, anaemia, enlarged and tender lymph nodes in the neck and elsewhere, splenomegaly, and pleomorphic skin rashes, but eventually the central nervous system is invaded and lassitude and somnolence, often with dysarthria, tremors, and fits, now dominate the clinical picture. Patients who develop these neurological symptoms run a slowly downhill course over a period of months or years and invariably die if untreated.

Diagnosis is established by identifying the trypanosome in smears of blood, bone marrow, or material obtained by lymph-node puncture.

Treatment. (1) Cases without C.N.S. involvement. If the C.S.F. shows no increase in globulin or lymphocytes the relatively toxic drug tryparsamide need not be used. Instead a course of eleven weekly intravenous injections of *suramin* is given, starting with a test dose of 200 mg. and if there is no reaction giving 1 g. at each subsequent injection. This drug may cause renal damage, so that the urine should be tested for albumen before each injection. Vomiting and skin rashes are other side-effects. If suramin has to be abandoned on account of toxicity or failure to cure a course of *pentamidine isethionate* should be given as for kala-azar.

(2) **Cases with C.N.S. involvement,** as shown by neurological signs or C.S.F. changes. Melarsoprol (Mel.B), a trivalent arsenical which cross the blood-brain barrier, has largely replaced tryparsamide because of the

latter's toxicity and the increasing emergence of trypanosomes resistant to it. Three I.V. injections of Mel.B are given on days 1, 3 and 5, each containing 3·6 mg./kg. body weight (maximum dose 200 mg.), and the course may be repeated after 3 weeks if the nervous system is severely affected. Toxic effects include vomiting, rashes and rarely hepatitis or encephalopathy.

Prophylaxis. Control of the tsetse fly is the most important measure in prevention. Those exposed to infection should be given pentamidine isethionate 3 mg. per kg. body weight in 3 ml. sterile distilled water by intramuscular injection every six months.

BACTERIAL INFECTIONS

LEPROSY (Hansen's Disease)

This is a disease of low infectivity which is endemic in many parts of Asia, Central Africa, and South America. Infection with the acid-fast causative organism, *Mycobacterium leprae*, is acquired only by close contact over a prolonged period and the incubation period is therefore difficult to determine, though it may be several years.

Clinical Features. (1) **Tuberculoid Leprosy.** This is the benign variety of the disease in which small numbers of organisms stimulate a vigorous response by the tissues. The main reaction occurs in peripheral nerves: the patient complains of numbness, tingling, and loss of pain and temperature sense in the distal parts of the limbs and the affected nerves can be felt as hard thick cords. The great auricular nerve is very commonly affected. In addition, round, depigmented and anaesthetic areas appear on the skin. The disease usually runs a self-limiting course and the patient is non-infectious.

(2) **Lepromatous Leprosy.** This is the malignant variety of the disease: the patient's resistance to infection is low and granulomatous lesions teeming with *M. leprae* spread over the skin, particularly on the face and ears. As in the tuberculoid variety the earliest lesions are probably in the nerve fibrils, from which extension occurs into the skin and up the nerve trunks, but as there is very little inflammatory response nerve function is not disturbed until much later in the course of the disease. After a number of years of progressive ill-health death usually results from intercurrent infection.

Diagnosis is established by identifying the characteristic acid-fast bacilli in scrapings from skin lesions but as bacilli are very scanty in the tuberculoid type, radial nerve biopsy may be necessary.

Treatment. The sulphones are specific therapy for leprosy, the active substance being 4–4' diaminodiphenylsulphone (D.D.S.). This is given by mouth on two days each week, starting with 100 mg. each dose for the first month, 200 mg. the second month, 300 mg. the third month, and then continuing with 400 mg. per dose indefinitely. During sulphone therapy ferrous sulphate 200 mg. three times daily, intramuscular vitamin B_{12} 100 microgrammes twice weekly, with added yeast and Marmite, should be given to counteract the tendency to anaemia. Patients who develop severe toxic reactions to dapsone, such as hepatitis or haemolytic anaemia, or in whom the organisms become dapsone-resistant, may now be treated effectively with clofazimine (Lamprene) 100–200 mg. three times weekly.

Notification. Leprosy is a notifiable disease in Great Britain.

BACILLARY DYSENTERY

This is the result of infection with gram-negative bacilli of the genus *Shigella*, which cause acute inflammation and ulceration of the colon. The common pathogenic varieties of *Shigella* are *Sh. dysenteriae* (Shiga bacillus), *Sh. flexneri* and *Sh. sonnei*. The disease is spread by contamination of water with faeces from patients and carriers and although it is widespread throughout the world it is much more common in the tropics than elsewhere. Food may be infected by flies or by unsuspected carriers engaged in the transport or preparation of salads and other cold dishes. Severe bacillary dysentery in the tropics is usually due to *Sh. dysenteriae* or *Sh. flexneri*; in this country the milder disease due to *Sh. sonnei* is usually seen, mainly as small recurring outbreaks in residential institutions.

Clinical Features. The incubation period is up to one week. The disease starts abruptly and in its severest form (usually due to *Sh. dysenteriae shiga*) causes high fever, vomiting, and profuse diarrhoea with blood and mucus in the stools. There is rapid dehydration and the patient may collapse and die within a few hours. At the other end of the scale sonnei dysentery as seen in this country causes slight fever, colicky abdominal pains, vomiting, and diarrhoea, often without blood or mucus in the stools and with minimal constitutional upset. Complete recovery takes place within a week or so. In cases of intermediate severity symptoms may last for two or three weeks, but unlike amoebiasis this disease seldom if ever becomes chronic.

Acute *arthritis*, usually limited to one of the large joints of the limbs, sometimes develops within six months of infection with *Sh. dysenteriae* or *Sh. flexneri*. The joint pain and swelling may persist for some months.

Diagnosis. Microscopic examination of a specimen of mucus from the stool, mixed with a little saline on a slide and covered with a cover slip, shows an exudate with pus cells, red blood cells and macrophages, and the organism may be isolated by culture on McConkey's medium.

Treatment. Mild dysentery is best treated symptomatically as there is no evidence that antibiotics speed recovery. Antibiotics are used in severe infections but it is important to choose the correct drug as determined by sensitivity tests as resistant strains are common. Among the antibiotics used are tetracycline 500 mg. 6 hourly, oral streptomycin 0·5 g. 6 hourly or ampicillin 500 mg. 6 hourly.

For severely ill patients complete rest and good nursing are of great importance and intravenous saline may be needed to combat dehydration and sodium depletion. For the first day or so only bland fluids should be given by mouth, in sufficient quantities to ensure a urinary output of at least 1 litre in 24 hours.

CHOLERA

This disease is due to infection with the 'comma vibrio' and is found particularly in India and the Far East. Epidemics occur from contamination of food or water supplies with faeces from patients or convalescent carriers; there are no chronic carriers. The severity varies very widely in different epidemics; in some the disease is relatively mild, while in others mortality rates of 75 per cent have been reported.

Clinical Features. After an incubation period of two to six days sudden diarrhoea begins and within an hour or so mucus-flecked fluid uncoloured by faecal material may be pouring from the patient, who is also vomiting, complaining of cramps and in acute circulatory collapse. Oliguria or anuria inevitably follow and death may occur within 48 hours. In milder cases complete recovery occurs within two or three weeks.

Diagnosis is established by culturing the vibrio from the stools.

Treatment. The most urgent measure is fluid and electrolyte replacement. In view of the circulatory collapse it is usually necessary to cut down on a vein to set up an intravenous infusion and two pints of normal glucose saline should be run in quickly, followed by a pint of alkaline hypotonic saline (6·0 g. sodium chloride and 18·0 g. sodium bicarbonate per litre) within the first two hours. But if there are severe cramps, little thirst and a good urinary output (indicating a predominant salt deficiency) the first pint should be hypertonic saline (16 g. sodium chloride per litre). It may be necessary to continue intravenous therapy for 48 hours. The amount of fluid given in all must obviously depend on the clinical state of the patient, but at least one third of it should be alkaline hypotonic saline. In view of the risk of pulmonary oedema the patient must be carefully watched for warning symptoms and signs such as cough, dyspnoea, basal râles, or rising jugular venous pressure.

A course of tetracycline, furazolidine or chloramphenicol, which inhibit most strains of the vibrio, should also be given.

Prophylaxis. Vaccination is effective for up to six months. Two doses of 0·5 ml. and 1 ml. are given at an interval of one week. Further booster doses of 1 ml. are necessary every six months for those who remain in endemic areas.

PLAGUE

Plague is endemic in the Far East, India, Central Africa, and parts of South America. The causative gram-negative bacillus, *Pasteurella pestis*, is transmitted by fleas from rats and other rodents to man.

Clinical Features. (1) **Bubonic plague** is by far the most common type. After an incubation period of two to four days there is sudden fever and grave constitutional upset, often with delirium. Enlarged and tender lymph nodes (buboes) appear after two or three days, usually in the groins but occasionally in the neck or axillae.

(2) **Septicaemic** and (3) **Pneumonic** plague are both rare; they are characterised by fever and profound toxaemia, with cough and signs of broncho-pneumonia in the latter variety, but buboes do not form. The mortality rate varies in different epidemics and may be as high as 80 per cent. Recovery from septicaemic or pneumonic plague is rare.

Diagnosis is established by isolating the organism from the blood or from material aspirated from a bubo.

Treatment. Combined therapy with the following drugs probably gives the best results, though even in treated cases the mortality rate may not fall below 20 per cent:

(1) Streptomycin 0·5 g. intramuscularly every four hours until the temperature is normal, and then 1 g. daily until a total of 15 g. has been given, and

(2) Chloramphenicol *or* tetracycline 0·5 g. every six hours for a week or 10 days.

Control of Outbreaks. Patients must be strictly isolated, all excreta being disinfected with care and fomites burnt. Attendants should wear protective overalls, rubber gloves, and plastic face-masks and their clothes should be treated with malathion. Contacts must be vaccinated, either with Haffkine's heat-killed vaccine two 3 ml. doses at an internal of 10 days, or a single dose of the more efficient living avirulent vaccine. This gives protection for six months. In addition, contacts should take sulphadiazine 1 g. three times daily until a week after the last exposure and must be instructed to drink plenty of fluids during this time. Equally important is the energetic prosecution of campaigns against the rat and flea population of the district.

RELAPSING FEVER (Famine Fever)

The causative organisms, spirochaetes of the genus *Borrelia*, are transmitted by lice and ticks. The disease is found in southern Europe, South America, the Middle East, Africa, and India.

Clinical Features. The incubation period is usually about a week, but varies from a day or so to a fortnight. The onset is remarkably sudden, with giddiness, headache, fever and rigor, pains in the back and limbs and sometimes vomiting. There is continuous high fever for several days and the patient soon becomes gravely ill, restless, and often delirious, with enlargement of the liver and spleen, sometimes purpura, and occasionally in severe cases, jaundice. On the fifth or sixth day the temperature drops to normal and there is a sudden dramatic clinical improvement, but after a week or so the first of a small series of relapses occurs, each febrile bout tending fortunately to be less severe than the last. The mortality rate is very variable in different epidemics, but may be as high as 30 per cent.

Diagnosis is established by identifying the spirochaete in the blood during the bouts of fever.

Treatment. Either tetracycline by mouth, 0·5 g. six-hourly, or benzyl penicillin by injection, 500,000 units six-hourly, should be given for four days. In addition, if the patient is not jaundiced he should be given a single intravenous injection of neoarsphenamine 0·45 g.

YAWS

This disease, due to the *Treponema pertenue*, is non-venereal but is spread by direct contact from patient to patient. The highest incidence is among children over the age of eighteen months.

Clinical Features. The first sign is a papular skin rash, which eventually ulcerates. Hyperkeratosis of the soles of the feet is common and there may be lymphadenopathy and lesions in the bones and periosteum. The disease usually runs a very chronic course over many years.

Diagnosis is established by identifying the *Treponema pertenue*. The Wassermann reaction is also positive.

Treatment. Oxytetracycline 0·5 g. six-hourly for five days is usually very effective. A second course should be given if the W.R. is still positive after three or six months.

SCHISTOSOMIASIS (Bilharzia)

This disease is due to infestation with trematodes (flukes) of the genus *Schistosoma*. Three species of *Schistosoma* are pathogenic to man: *S. haematobium* is found in Central and North Africa, especially in Egypt; *S. mansoni* is fairly widespread throughout Africa, in the West Indies and along the east coast of South America; *S. japonicum* is found in the Far East. The habitat of the adult worm is the vascular system, *S. haematobium* being found in the portal vein and its branches and in the vesical, uterine, and haemorrhoidal veins, while *S. mansoni* inhabits chiefly the portal and mesenteric veins. *S. haematobium* produces terminally spined eggs, which are found mainly in the urine; *S. mansoni* produces laterally spined eggs found mainly in the faeces. The irritation caused by these spined eggs is the initial cause of the symptoms.

Life Cycle. If the egg reaches water it hatches into a free-swimming larva which enters the intermediate host, a fresh-water snail. In the snail the larva forms into a sporocyst, which gives off a number of daughter cysts and these in turn produce enormous numbers of bifid-tailed cercariae which escape into the surrounding water. These cercariae have an independent life of about 48 hours, during which time they may gain access to human host by penetrating the unbroken skin or buccal mucosa. They pass via the bloodstream and lungs to the liver, where they develop within about two months into adult male and female worms. Thereafter the females start producing the spined eggs.

Clinical Features. After an incubation period of about three months. *S.*

haematobium infestation causes haematuria, frequency, and dysuria, and though the illness is usually mild the symptoms are intractable. *S. mansoni* infestation has a shorter incubation period of about two months, followed by cough, headache, malaise, fever and rigors, abdominal pain, and enlargement of the liver and spleen. The general symptoms are usually followed by diarrhoea, with blood and mucus in the stools, due to the ulcerative and polypoid lesions in the colon. Urticarial and other skin rashes are often found and eosinophilia is common. Cirrhosis of the liver with ascites is a late complication of this variety of the disease. *S. japonicum* causes lesions very similar to those of *S. mansoni*, but there is frequently involvement of the central nervous system, causing cranial nerve palsies, hemiplegia, fits, or coma.

Diagnosis is established by identifying the eggs in the urine or faeces.

Treatment. Patients with no neurological symptoms should be given oral niradazole (Ambilhar) 25 mg./kg. body weight in divided doses daily for 7–10 days. It may cause E.C.G. changes or hallucinations, tremor and convulsions and may colour the urine red. Patients with cerebral symptoms and those who fail to respond to niradazole should be given intravenous sodium antimony tartrate, which is a more effective but also a more toxic drug. Injections are given on alternate days, starting with 30 mg., 60 mg., 90 mg. and then 120 mg. for nine injections. Great care must be taken to ensure that none of this preparation is injected outside the vein, as it is intensely irritant, and the injection should be given very slowly to the fasting patient. As it is a cardiac depressant it may cause hypotension and the patient should lie down for an hour after each injection.

RABIES

This viral infection is acquired from the bite of a rabid animal; it causes an encephalitis which is invariably fatal after a few days of increasing restlessness, mental excitement, hyperaesthesia, hydrophobia and convulsions. Combined active and passive immunisation started soon after the bite prevents the development of the disease in a high proportion of cases.

The U.K. has been free of rabies for many decades, but since the second World War it has been increasingly prevalent among susceptible wild carnivores on the continent of Europe, notably the red fox. Strict application of animal importation regulations is essential if the disease is to be kept out of Britain.

The Incubation Period is usually 20–50 days, but may be over a year.

Prophylaxis. When a human being is bitten by a domestic animal in an area in which rabies is endemic the animal should be kept under observation by a veterinary surgeon. If the animal remains well after 10 days no further action need be taken; but if the animal becomes sick during this period, the human patient must be given anti-rabies treatment. Humans bitten by wild animals, or by domestic animals who run away, must also be treated. Rabies is not likely to be contracted unless the skin has been penetrated with introduction of saliva into the wound.

Post-Exposure Treatment. The wound should be washed immediately with soap and water and iodine or 40–70% alcohol applied. In the Accident and Emergency department the wound is washed again and surgical treatment given if necessary. If it is decided to give anti-rabies treatment (see above) half the dose of rabies antiserum or human anti-rabies immunoglobulin (HRIG) is given into the wound area and the other half intramuscularly.

The total dose of rabies anti-serum is 40 i.u./kg and of HRIG 20 i.u./kg. The former causes serum sickness in about 40 per cent of adults and before it is given the patient should be tested for sensitivity to avoid anaphylaxis; HRIG is therefore to be preferred but is at present in short supply and very expensive. In addition to this passive immunisation a course of vaccine to produce active immunisation is started. Human diploid cell (HDC) vaccine is the best; 1 ml. is given intramuscularly on days 0, 3, 7, 14, 30 and 90.

TYPHUS FEVER

There are several varieties of typhus due to closely related rickettsiae. The most important is epidemic or louse-borne typhus, due to *R. prowazeki*. Other varieties are murine typhus, which is transmitted chiefly by fleas; Rocky Mountain fever, 'fievre boutonneuse' (prevalent along the Mediterranean coast), and Queensland or 'Q' fever, transmitted chiefly by ticks; and tsutsugamushi fever and scrub typhus, transmitted chiefly by mites.

Epidemic Louse-borne Typhus has been one of the scourges of armies since prehistoric times and an aftermath of civil disasters which lead to overcrowding and destitution. Lice become infected by sucking blood from a patient with typhus and transmit the rickettsiae to other people in their faeces, which are rubbed into scratches and other lesions in the skin.

Clinical Features. The incubation is usually twelve days, with a range of five to fourteen days. There is usually a gradual onset with headache, shivering, backache, general malaise, and tenderness of the eyeballs, but by about the third day the patient is more seriously ill and has a flushed face, injection of the conjunctivae and tachycardia out of proportion to the fever. Epistaxis is common. About this time the temperature gradually rises towards its maximum (which is usually between 102–105° F.) and remains at this level with only slight morning remissions throughout the rest of the illness. The rash appears on the abdomen on the fifth day and spreads to the chest and shoulders; the limbs are sometimes involved too, but never the face. It takes many forms, but there are usually macules of varying sizes, a subcuticular mottling and sometimes petechial elements. As the rash develops the patient sinks into a stuporose and often delirious state from which he is difficult to rouse. By the second week the spleen is often palpable and the urine is scanty and contains albumen and casts. In patients who recover the temperature settles by lysis during the third week. The clinical severity and mortality rate of typhus vary widely in different epidemics, but in general most patients do recover.

Diagnosis is confirmed by the *Weil-Felix reaction*, which demonstrates a high agglutinin titre in the serum against B. proteus OX 19.

Murine Typhus (and the other varieties of endemic rickettsial infection mentioned above) differ from epidemic louse-borne typhus in being primarily diseases of rodents and other small animals, from which infection is transmitted to man by fleas, ticks, and mites. The clinical illness is very similar to that of the epidemic disease, though usually much milder.

Diagnosis. The Weil-Felix reaction demonstrates agglutinins against B. proteus OX 19 in flea-borne murine typhus (as in epidemic typhus); against B. proteus OXK and only slightly OX 19 in mite-borne typhus; and against OXK, OX 19, and OX 2 in varying degrees in tick-borne typhus.

Treatment. Tetracycline 0·75 g. should be given six-hourly for forty-eight hours and then 0·5 g. six-hourly until the temperature has been normal for two days. Intravenous glucose-saline may be required to combat dehydration; intramuscular chlorpromazine 50–100 mg. or morphine 15 mg. may be needed to control delirium.

Control of Outbreaks. The important measures are (1) Delousing of patients on admission with D.D.T., their clothes being disinfested or burned. (2) Delousing of the population. This may be done by spraying dicophane dusting powder (which contains 10 per cent D.D.T.) into all apertures in the clothing, which must not be changed for 10 days thereafter. (3) Vaccination of doctors, nurses, and others specially exposed to infection with the Cox type yolk-sac vaccine, two doses of 1 ml. being given at an interval of two weeks followed by booster doses of 1 ml. every four months. Protective clothing must be worn while dealing with infested patients.

LASSA FEVER

This is an acute viral infection which was first recognised in Lassa, Nigeria in 1969 and is endemic in many parts of West Africa. Infection is usually acquired from contamination of food by the saliva or urine of infected rats of the species *Mastomys natalensis*, but spread from person to person also occurs and there have been a number of outbreaks in hospital. The Lassa virus is a member of the arenavirus genus.

The *incubation period* may be up to three weeks, but is usually 7–10 days.

Clinical Features. There is insidious onset of fever, malaise, headache and muscular aching followed in severe cases by prostration disproportionate to the pyrexia. Examination may reveal lymphadenopathy and a faint maculo-papular rash. High continuous fever may develop, with haemorrhages, serious effusions and shock and about 50 per cent of these seriously ill patients die. However, the frequent discovery of antibodies in people with no history of illness suggests that many mild cases escape recognition.

Diagnosis is established either by isolation of the virus in tissue cell culture, which takes at least 5 days, or by the demonstration of a rising antibody titre. In the U.K. specimens from patients from West Africa in whom the possibility of Lassa fever is suspected should be sent only to certain laboratories designated for the purpose.

Treatment. The administration of plasma containing Lassa fever antibodies is the only specific measure which may have a beneficial effect; in the U.K. it may be obtained from the Hospital for Tropical Diseases, London, N.W.1.

Control of Infection. Lassa fever is a notifiable disease under the Public Health (Infectious Diseases) (Amendment) Regulations 1976. A suspected patient must be admitted by special ambulance to one of the hospitals designated for the purpose; the room he occupied before admission to hospital must be disinfected; and all close contacts must be kept under surveillance.

FURTHER READING

Manson-Bahr, Sir Philip H. (Editor), *Manson's Tropical Diseases*, 17th edition, Cassell, London, 1972.
Woodruff, A. W., *Medicine in the Tropics,* Churchill Livingstone, Edinburgh and London, 1974.

CHAPTER EIGHTEEN

WORMS

1. NEMATODES (Round Worms)

THREADWORMS (*Enterobius vermicularis*)

Threadworms are extremely common, particularly in childhood. They are about ½–1 cm. long and look as their name implies, like threads of cotton. There are both male and female forms which inhabit the large bowel and rectum, being most numerous in the caecum. They may reach the anus where they cause considerable irritation.

Pairing of the worms occurs in the intestine and the eggs are passed out in the stools. These eggs may contaminate the fingers of the patient particularly if anal irritation is a feature. The eggs are then swallowed either in contaminated food or directly from sucking the fingers. The eggs then hatch and a new generation of worms develops in the intestine.

Clinical Features. Many patients may be unaware of threadworm infestation until the worms are noticed in the stools. The most common symptom is anal irritation and this may keep the child awake at night with the result that he is fretful next day.

The relationship between threadworms and acute appendicitis is still debated, but it seems probable that threadworms very rarely cause appendicular inflammation. The *diagnosis* is confirmed by finding the worm in the stools or the ova by means of perianal swabs.

Treatment. *Viprynium embenate* given either in tablet form or as a suspension as a single dose of 5·0 mg. base/kg. body weight and repeated in one week is satisfactory. It is low in side effects but colours the stools red.

Alternatively 'Pripsen', a preparation containing *piperazine* and standardised senna, is equally good. The dose for patients of six years and over is 10 g. of Pripsen granules (containing 4·0 g. of piperazine phosphate) as a single dose. Piperazine paralyses the worm which is then cleared out by the action of the senna.

Other treatment consists of general cleanliness with careful washing of the hands before meals. Anal itching may be reduced by an anti-histamine or hydrocortisone cream.

If attacks of infestation are recurrent it usually means that other members of the family are infected and it is then best to treat the whole family.

ASCARIS LUMBRICOIDES

Infection by *Ascaris lumbricoides* is acquired by swallowing the fertilised egg. In the upper small intestine the egg develops into the larval form which penetrates the intestinal wall and enters the venous system and is then swept back to the heart and passes into the lungs where it may cause a pneumonitis. The larva is then coughed up in the sputum and swallowed and in the intestine develops into the adult worm. The adult ascaris is about 6–10 in. long and is white or yellow, resembling the common earth-worm. There are males and females.

Clinical Features. Frequently there are no symptoms and the diagnosis is made by finding a worm in the stools. Occasionally the worms in the intestine give rise to intestinal colic or biliary obstruction. If the infection is heavy, the larval form may give rise to a pneumonitis or to an urticaria, which is associated with eosinophilia in the blood.

Treatment. *Piperazine* as the phosphate is satisfactory. The dose for a young child is 3·0 g. and for an older child or adult is 4·0 g. of piperazine. Only a single dose is required. The drug acts by paralysing the muscle of the worm which is then passed alive per rectum. Alternatively *bephenium hydroxynaphthoate* (Alcopar) in a single dose of 5·0 g. for adults or 2·5 g. for children is also satisfactory.

HOOK-WORMS (*Ankylostoma duodenale* and *Necator americanus*)

Hook-worm infestation is extremely common, but is confined to tropical and subtropical countries. The adult worms are about 1·0 cm. long and inhabit the duodenum and jejunum. The eggs are passed out in the faeces; if they fall on moist warm soil they develop into the larval form which penetrates the intact skin of the next human victim. The larvae then pass back to the heart and then to the lungs. They penetrate the alveoli, and passing up the trachea re-enter the intestinal tract where they develop into mature worms.

Clinical Features. The adult worms are responsible for considerable ill-health by causing chronic bleeding from the duodenum. The patient suffers from anaemia, diarrhoea, and finally cachexia and even death may occur. The larval form may lead to areas of pneumonia with an associated eosinophilia in the blood. The point of penetration of the larvae through the skin is often inflamed and is known as the 'ground itch'. It must, however, be realised that very many people harbour hook worms and suffer little if any ill health.

Treatment. *Bephenium hydroxynaphthoate* is the drug of choice. For *A. duodenale* 5·0 g. is given as a single dose. For *N. americanus* 5·0 g. is given three successive days. Side effects include nausea and diarrhoea but are minimal. If anaemia is severe it should be treated with iron.

TRICHINOSIS

The adult form of this minute round worm (*Trichinella spiralis*) lives in the intestine of the pig; embryo worms find their way into the animal's bloodstream and develop in the muscles into small cysts about ½ mm. long.

If inadequately cooked pork from such a pig is eaten, an adult worm develops in the human intestine, and in time its embryos are disseminated in the bloodstream throughout the body.

Clinical Features. Small localised outbreaks occur from the eating of pork from an infected animal; pork sausage-meat, either fried too hastily or actually eaten raw, has a bad reputation in this connection. There is often nausea and vomiting lasting a day or two immediately after the ingestion of infected meat. About a week later (when the embryos are passing into the muscles and other tissues) there is fever, muscular pains, and tenderness, and frequently oedema of the eyelids and 'splinter haemorrhages' under the nails. The urine contains protein. The cysts can be found in the muscle on biopsy. The blood always shows a great excess of eosinophil cells. This stage usually subsides slowly over several weeks, and the larvae in the muscles finally become calcified. Occasionally death occurs.

Treatment is purely symptomatic. In the stage of invasion the symptoms can best be controlled by prednisolone.

2. CESTODES (Tapeworms)

In order to complete their life cycle these parasites have to inhabit the bodies of two separate and unwilling 'hosts'. The adult tapeworm lives in the intestine of the main host, its ova passing out in the faeces. If the ova are ingested by a suitable 'intermediate host', the larval forms of the worm hatch out, gain access to the bloodstream and are distributed through the muscles of the body. If the intermediate is eaten by a main host, the cysts in the muscles develop into adult tape worms in the intestine of the latter.

Man acts as a main host for three worms. *Taenia saginata*, the common beef tapeworm, *Taenia solium*, the less common pork tapeworm, and *Diphyllobothrium latum*, the fish tapeworm. *T. saginata* and *T. solium* are the only tapeworms likely to be found in this country and infection is acquired by eating respectively imperfectly cooked beef or pork containing the larval forms. These tapeworms are white, flat, ribbon-like structures, about 1 cm. wide and many yards long, subdivided into a large number of segments, some of which break off from time to time and appear in the faeces. The head, which is no more than a pinhead in size, is firmly attached to the duodenum or upper part of the jejunum.

Clinical Features. There may be some abdominal discomfort or diarrhoea, or occasionally abnormal hunger. Frequently, however, the patient has no symptoms until he notices segments of worm in his stools. A white cell count sometimes shows an eosinophilia. Diagnosis is established by the identification of segments or ova of the tapeworm in the faeces.

Treatment. Most tapeworm infestations in Britain are due to *T. saginata*. This is best treated with *niclosamide*, which kills the worm. No preliminary starvation is necessary. Four tablets (0·5 g. each) are chewed and swallowed and the following day the dose is repeated. The treatment is nearly always successful.

With *T. solium,* niclosamide may cause disintegration of the worm with subsequent cysticercosis. The patient should, therefore, be put on a fluid diet for two days and be given a saline purge the night before treatment. He is then given *extract of male fern.* The dose is 8 ml. for an adult. It has an unpleasant taste and may be diluted in a suitably flavoured draught or given by duodenal tube. Capsules are not satisfactory as the head may be high up in the intestine and the anthelmintic may not be liberated at that level. One hour later a saline purge is given and the stools searched for the head of the worm. If it is not passed, the worm will grow again.

CYSTICERCOSIS

Cysticercosis is due to infestation of man by the cystic larval form of a cestode, usually *Taenia solium.* Infection occurs either by eating food contaminated with the eggs of *T. solium* or sometimes patients who have an adult tapeworm in the lower intestine regurgitate food and thus allow the eggs to reach the upper intestine where they develop into the larval form. These larvae then penetrate the intestinal wall and are carried in the blood stream all over the body. Common sites for cysts to develop are the subcutaneous tissues, muscles, brain, eye, lungs, and heart. In this country the disease is seen mainly in those who have spent many years in India; it is rare.

Clinical Features. Cysticercosis may produce no symptoms, as the live cysts produce little in the way of a tissue reaction. When the cysts die, however, there may be considerable inflammatory reaction. Cysts in the brain are particularly troublesome and may cause epileptic fits. The dead cysts may become calcified and will then be visible radiologically.

Treatment. There is no treatment for cysticercosis except surgical removal of the cysts and control of the epilepsy by anticonvulsants. It is important that a patient who has an infestation of the bowel with *T. solium* should be treated efficiently; mepacrine should be avoided as this is particularly liable to produce vomiting, thus leading to the escape of larval forms from the upper intestine which penetrate the intestine and lead to systemic cystericosis.

HYDATID DISEASE

Hydatid disease is due to infestation by the cystic stage of *Taenia echinococcus.* The worm is only about half a centimetre in length. It lives in the intestine of the dog. The ova are swallowed by the intermediate host, usually sheep, cattle, horses, or rarely man. The larvae then penetrate the intestinal wall and settle down in various organs and develop into the cystic form. Hydatid disease is rare in this country and is found more commonly in Australia, Iceland, South America, and the Middle East.

Clinical Features. Hydatid cysts are found most commonly in the liver and lungs. In the liver, hydatid cysts may reach a considerable size without causing symptoms. Sometimes the patient complains of a dragging pain in the abdomen. Pressure on the bile ducts may produce jaundice.

An hydatid cyst in the lungs may produce no symptoms. As it enlarges cough and sometimes haemoptysis occur. If it ruptures into a bronchus, the contents are coughed up and secondary infection develops in the cyst. Long-standing cysts may become calcified.

In hydatid disease the blood may show an eosinophilia, but this is by no means consistent. Casoni's test, which consists of the intradermal injection of fluid from an hydatid cyst, is positive in about 80 per cent of patients with the disease. False positions are, however, common.

Treatment. The treatment of hydatid cysts is either by removal of the whole cyst or by marsupialisation of the cyst which is then allowed to heal by granulation. Aspiration of the cyst is dangerous as it may lead to dissemination of daughter cysts.

GIARDIASIS

Infestation of the intestine with *Giardia lamblia* is quite common. Infection may be acquired in the Mediterranean area and in other parts of the world but it may also occur in those who have never left Britain. The presence of organisms in the bowel does not necessarily result in symptoms.

Clinical Features. Symptoms usually develop a few weeks after infection. Diarrhoea with bulky stools, abdominal distension and discomfort are common. Bleeding does not occur. These symptoms may last for several weeks or longer and may be followed by a chronic state in which steatorrhoea is associated with other manifestations of malabsorption. Diagnosis is confirmed by finding the cysts or trophozoites in the stools but this is not easy and a course of treatment may have to be given on the basis of clinical suspicion.

Treatment. Metronidazole 2·0 g. daily for three days is usually curative.

FURTHER READING

Blacklock, D. B. and Southwell, T., *Guide to Human Parasitology*, 9th edition, Lewis, London, 1973.

CHAPTER NINETEEN

DISEASES OF THE SKIN

ECZEMA AND DERMATITIS

The words 'eczema' and 'dermatitis' have been a source of confusion for many years. It is now generally accepted that they are synonymous and clinically and histologically refer to the same condition. However, because of long usage the two words are sometimes retained and eczema is used if the cause is endogenous, as in atopic eczema, and dermatitis is used if the cause is exogenous, such as in a contact dermatitis due to nickel.

Atopic eczema generally begins after the age of three months and before the age of two years. It is frequently associated with asthma and hay fever. The eczematous lesions may develop first on the face in very young children but subsequently the antecubital and popliteal fossae are the sites most commonly affected.

Some substances provoke a dermatitic reaction when applied to the skin of normal people, others only when applied to the skin of a sensitised individual. The former is often referred to as a primary irritant dermatitis and the latter as a contact dermatitis followed by the name of the causative agent.

Contact dermatitis is extremely common and the substances which may provoke this reaction can be classified into the following groups:

1. *Chemicals.* Almost any therapeutic agent applied to the skin may induce a dermatitic response, particularly if it is applied repeatedly over a period of time. Drugs such as neomycin, penicillin and streptomycin are common causes and doctors, nurses and students should be very careful when giving injections with the last two substances not to allow any of the solution to come into contact with their hands. Nickel (on rings, necklaces and brassiere clips), lipstick, nail varnish and hair dyes are common causes of a contact dermatitis and so are furs and some articles of clothing. Soaps, bleaching agents and detergents usually cause a primary irritant dermatitis rather than a true contact dermatitis.

2. *Substances of Plant Origin.* In this country the plants which may give rise to a contact dermatitis are primulas and chrysanthemums.

3. *Micro-organisms.* Skin infections such as impetigo and ringworm (tinea) may be complicated by an eczematous reaction. The diagnosis of contact dermatitis is usually suggested by taking a careful history and by the site and distribution of the lesions. It may be confirmed by a *patch test* when appropriate dilutions of the suspected substance are applied to an area of normal skin, usually on the back, covered with a micropore dress-

ing and left for 48 hrs., when it is removed. The tested area should be reviewed another 48 hrs. later. A positive result is seen with the development of a dermatitic response in the area of skin covered by the testing substance.

Treatment. The most important point is the removal of the cause if this is known. Contact with the offending agent must be prevented. If there are several possible causes, for example if the patient is a hairdresser or dentist, patch tests must be done to determine the exact cause. For local therapy treatment with a 1 per cent hydrocortisone ointment is the safest remedy. However 2½ per cent hydrocortisone, betamethasone valerate or triamcinolone acetonide are often more effective and may be needed, but these agents can induce striae formation, atrophy of the skin and telangiectasia if they are used for too long and particularly if they are applied under polythene occlusion. The stronger steroid ointments should never be used in children. If the dermatitic lesions are secondarily infected then the steroid may be combined with an antibiotic such as tetracycline. Neomycin should not be used on the skin because of the danger of sensitisation. Some other antibiotics should be avoided in topical applications because they may need to be used systemically.

DRUG ERUPTIONS

In theory nearly every drug can produce any type of skin reaction, but in practice a particular drug often produces a particular response, such as purpura. Problems must arise when a patient is on several drugs and it is often not possible to say which is the cause of his reaction. All drug therapy may have to be stopped and reintroduced one by one, when the eruption has faded. Drug eruptions are very common and may mimic the rashes of many other diseases, such as measles and scarlet fever. The *barbiturates, sulphonamides, streptomycin, gold,* and *aspirin* commonly do so and *para-amino-salicylic acid (P.A.S.), isoniazid* and *phenylbutazone* may also cause skin rashes.

Iodides are usually taken in the form of potassium iodide in a cough mixture and if taken for a long time can cause remarkable, large fungating lesions. The heavy metals such as *gold* and *arsenic* may cause a severe generalised exfoliative dermatitis which can be fatal if untreated. Twenty-five per cent of the patients on gold therapy will develop a skin eruption in time. In a sensitised individual an injection of *penicillin* may cause an urticarial rash, angioneurotic oedema or even death within a few minutes from anaphylactic shock. The last complication may occur in people who are atopic, that is they have asthma, eczema and hay fever. If a patient says he has had a rash from penicillin on no account should any more be given.

Treatment. In mild cases withdrawal of the drug is all that is needed. For relief of irritation an anti-histamine tablet should be given, such as promethazine hydrochloride 25 mg. or mepyramine maleate 100 mg. two or three times a day. All anti-histamines cause drowsiness and motor-car drivers and others should be warned of this side-effect. Chlorpheniramine maleate 4 mg. three times daily is an alternative which is said to cause less drowsiness. Promethazine 50 mg. or chlorpheniramine 10 mg. may be given intramuscularly if the need is urgent. Very severe cases should be treated with cortisone or an analogue such as prednisolone 30–40 mg. daily. The dosage is gradually tailed off over a period of two or three weeks. Dermatitis due to heavy metals such as gold can be treated with dimercaprol (B.A.L.) intramuscularly 3 mg. per kg. of body weight every 6 hrs. for 3 days.

For anaphylactic shock following injection of a drug give an immediate injection of adrenaline 1:1,000, 0·5 ml. subcutaneously, after which it may be necessary for an intravenous infusion of saline containing nor-adrenaline or aminophylline to be set up. It is a very good rule never to give any drug by injection without having a solution of adrenaline ready for use if needed.

INFECTIONS OF THE SKIN

Infection with coagulase positive staphylococci is responsible for furunculosis (boils), sycosis barbae (folliculitis of the beard area), carbuncles, axillary hidradenitis, pemphigus neonatorum, and impetigo contagiosa (which may also be due to streptococcal infection). Only the last of these will be described here.

Impetigo Contagiosa

This is a very common condition and is due to a bacterial infection of the superficial layers of the skin. If the condition does not respond to treatment, an underlying cause such as scabies or pediculosis should be suspected. As the name implies it is spread by direct contact or by the use of contaminated towels or clothes.

Clinical Features. The first lesion is a pink macule up to half an inch in diameter, but within a few hours this becomes converted into a superficial vesicle, then a pustule which soon ruptures with the formation of a typical bright yellow crust. Bullous lesions may occur in children. The face is a common site. There is rarely any fever or constitutional disturbance.

Treatment. Patients with severe infection should be given flucloxacillin 250 mg. 6 hourly by mouth. The essential local treatment is to remove the crusts with 1 per cent cetrimide (Savlon). Topical antibiotic preparations should be avoided because of the risk of sensitisation. In many cases it is essential to give a systemic antibiotic. It is important to search for and treat any associated lesion, such as scabies or pediculosis capitis. The latter is particularly likely to be found in girls with long hair. The patient must of course be kept away from other children and must have his own towel and pillow-case, which should subsequently be sterilised by boiling.

RINGWORM

This is a group of common fungus infections of the skin which affect mainly the scalp, the groin and the feet.

Tinea Capitis (Ringworm of the Scalp)

The infection is seen mainly in children under ten, particularly boys, and never persists beyond adolescence. The scalp shows a number of rounded or oval patches which are covered with fine greyish-white scales and from which most of the hairs have fallen out. The ringworm fungus fluoresces a bright green colour under Wood's light, and this examination is therefore helpful in diagnosis. The fungus can also be identified microscopically in stumps of hair removed from one of the patches.

Treatment. Griseofulvin 125 mg. four times daily for a month or 6 weeks is now the treatment of choice. Very occasionally, it may cause headache and urticaria and should be used with caution in patients sensitive to penicillin.

Tinea Cruris (Ringworm of the Groins)

This infection occurs mainly in young adults, particularly men, and may be acquired by direct contact, from infected clothing or spread from between the toes. It causes a red, slightly raised patch extending from the crutch for two or three inches down the inner aspect of each thigh. There is sometimes itching in the affected area. The infection is seen mainly in hot weather and is more common therefore in the tropics.

Treatment. Half strength Whitfield's ointment is usually very effective, but relapses in subsequent spells of hot weather are common. Griseofulvin may also prove effective.

Tinea Pedis (Athlete's Foot)

This infection occurs with two characteristic distribution patterns, but both may occur together, the first showing vesicles and subsequent desquamation on the sole of the foot, and the second causing fissuring and maceration of the skin in the clefts between the toes. Like tinea cruris, with which it may be associated, this infection is often seen in young adults and is acquired from the floors of swimming baths and changing-rooms.

Treatment. Whitfield's ointment, Castellani's paint, and undecylenic acid ointment are three among a number of effective remedies. Relapse is common, however, and to try to prevent it careful attention to the hygiene of the feet is important. They should be washed daily, carefully dried and powdered and the socks should be changed every day.

PARASITIC DISEASES

Scabies

The animal causing scabies is a mite (*Sarcoptes scabei hominis*). It has four pairs of legs and the female, which causes the trouble, is about

0·3 mm. long being therefore just visible to the naked eye. The male is smaller. The female makes a burrow up to a centimetre in length in the epidermis and lays about 30–40 eggs in it. Each egg hatches out in 4–8 days into a larval form which leaves the burrow and eventually matures into the adult form.

Infection is usually acquired by sleeping with an infected person. It may therefore be a venereal infection, or children may acquire it from their parents or from each other. Less often infected blankets, bedding, or clothes may transmit the infection.

Clinical Features. The burrow is the characteristic lesion of scabies and appears as a fine, often zig-zag, hair-like line in the epidermis, greyish or whitish in colour and 0·5–1 cm. in length. At the far end a tiny pinhead vesicle may be seen. These burrows occur mainly in the webs and sides of the fingers, the ulnar sides of the hands, the anterior axillary folds, the lower abdomen and penis and the lower part of the buttocks. They cause intense itching, particularly when the patient is warm in bed. As a result of scratching secondary infection is common and there may be an extensive papular and pustular eruption.

Diagnosis is usually easy from the history of intense itching and the discovery of typical burrows and may be confirmed by identifying the female acarus or its eggs in a microscopical preparation of scrapings from a burrow.

Treatment. This starts with a hot bath, the patient being instructed to scrub with a nail brush and soap all areas where there are burrows. After drying himself the patient is painted from head to foot with a 25 per cent emulsion of benzyl benzoate (applicatio benzylis benzoatis, B.P.C.), sparing only the head and neck, which are never affected by scabies in adults. Next morning the lotion is applied again and allowed to dry before the patient dresses. This regime is repeated for two more days. On the third night another hot bath is taken to wash off the remains of the benzyl benzoate and a complete change of clothing and bed linen is made. Gloves and other articles which are difficult to disinfect should be laid aside for three weeks, at the end of which time all acari they contain will have died. Residual itching after benzyl benzoate treatment is quite common. It is important to treat this with calamine lotion or crotamiton lotion because further applications of benzyl benzoate will make it worse by causing a dermatitis. It need hardly be said that all contacts with the patient, particularly those within his family circle, should be treated at the same time to avoid reinfection.

PEDICULOSIS

Lice are blood sucking parasites which mainly infest hairy parts of the body. The female produces several hundred eggs, each of which is attached to a hair and is commonly known as a nit. A larva is hatched out from the egg in 6–9 days and develops into a mature louse in one to two weeks.

Pediculosis Capitis (Infestation with Head Lice)

The louse concerned is the *Pediculus humanus capitis*, which is about 3 mm. long and 1 mm. broad. It infests the scalp, the nits being attached mainly to hairs at the back and sides of the head. Since the louse deposits the eggs on hairs close to the scalp and since they have hatched out by the time the hair has grown an inch or so, the search for nits should be concentrated on hair close to the head. The diagnosis depends usually on the discovery of nits, since the lice themselves are few in number and difficult to find. Nits are greyish-white, shiny, oval, opalescent structures firmly attached to the hairs.

Infection may be acquired by direct transmission from person to person or by wearing infected headgear; and since the lice flourish particularly in long hair which is seldom washed, it is now often seen in young men as well as in women living under poor hygienic conditions. However, school children are particularly liable to be infested. Patients recently infected usually complain of irritation of the scalp, but those who have had head lice for a long time often seem to suffer no inconvenience at all. When there has been much scratching septic lesions of the scalp are a common complication.

Treatment. Gamma benzene hexachloride application is effective but may have to be repeated after a week. The hair should be shampooed twelve hours after the application and combed while wet with a fine-toothed comb. It is much easier to treat short hair.

Pediculosis Corporis (Infestation with Body Lice)

Pediculus humanus corporis is similar to the head louse but slightly bigger. It normally lives in the clothes and deposits its eggs in the seams and folds of woollen undergarments.

Clinical Features. Infestation causes a variable amount of itching; scratch marks are seen mainly around the shoulders, buttocks, and the fronts of the thighs and there may be a widespread eruption from secondary bacterial infection in these situations. Tramps and vagrants after lifelong infestation may develop a generalised pigmentation of the skin like that seen in Addison's disease (*vagabond's pigmentation*). The diagnosis is established by finding the louse or its ova in the seams of the patient's underclothes.

Treatment. Gamma benzene hexachloride should be applied as a 0·6 per cent dusting powder and scrubbed on to infected hairy areas as a 2 per cent lotion in a detergent base. Underclothes must be washed and ironed and bedding and other clothing autoclaved. It is sufficient for the patient to take a hot bath before putting on clean clothes.

In some countries, in addition to their direct effects, infestation with head and body lice is important in the spread of typhus (p. 570) and relapsing fever (p. 567).

'Pediculosis' Pubis (Infestation with 'Crab' Lice)

This louse is not in fact of the species pediculus, its scientific name being *Phthirus pubis*. Its life history is similar to that of the pediculi, but it is smaller (about 2 mm. by 1·5 mm.) and does not spread typhus or any other disease.

Clinical Features. It infests the pubic region, but in very hairy men the whole of the trunk, the thighs, and the upper arms may be involved. On close inspection the adult lice can be seen, lying flat on the skin and holding on to a hair at each side; the nits are very similar to those of pediculus humanus and are closely attached to the body hairs. Infection is acquired mainly by sexual intercourse and occurs usually therefore in young adults.

Treatment is as for pediculosis corporis. Crotamiton lotion or even benzyl benzoate are alternative applications.

URTICARIA

In susceptible subjects local urticaria may follow trauma, stings, or insect bites. Generalised urticaria may be due to sensitivity to certain foods, particularly shellfish and strawberries, or to drugs, notably penicillin, or to parenteral serum or blood. In other patients the condition is associated with worm infestation; but in more than half of the cases seen with chronic urticaria the cause is never found.

Clinical Features. The typical lesion is an extremely itchy wheal surrounded by a zone of erythema. The wheals may be of any size and shape may cover the greater part of the body. There may be associated swelling (*angioneurotic oedema*) in the subcutaneous tissue and mucous membranes, particularly in the mouth and throat. Papular urticaria without much wheal formation is common in children.

Treatment. Quick relief can usually be obtained by giving 0·5 ml. 1:1,000 adrenaline hydrochloride subcutaneously. An intramuscular anti-histamine, such as promethazine hydrochloride 50 mg. may also be given. If there is laryngeal obstruction which is not quickly relieved by these measures emergency tracheotomy must be performed. Anti-histamines are given by mouth for more sustained effect; promethazine hydrochloride 25 mg. or mepyramine maleate 100 mg. are the most powerful of these but often cause troublesome drowsiness. Chlorpheniramine maleate 4 mg. has a slightly weaker anti-histamine effect but causes less sedation. The tablets are given two or three times daily. Ephedrine 30 mg. three times daily is worth trying if the symptoms persist. Cortisone suppresses the lesions, but its administration is rarely justified in this condition. The best local application is calamine lotion or 1 per cent hydrocortisone ointment.

ACNE VULGARIS

Acne is often associated with seborrhoea (that is excessive sebaceous secretion). The essential lesion is the comedo, which is a sebaceous follicle the opening of which has been blocked with sebum mixed with epithelial debris, and these comedones frequently become pustular from infection of the retained sebaceous material. They are found on the face, chest, shoulders, and back. Their formation appears to be favoured by androgens and they appear therefore in the years following puberty and more often in boys than in girls. Adolescent acne tends to disappear spontaneously in early adult life, though when it is very severe it may persist and healing of the lesions may leave permanent scarring.

Treatment. The treatment of acne falls under two headings: those applications which de-grease the skin and those which treat the secondary infection. Natural sunlight (or ultra violet light therapy) combines the two actions and is the best single treatment for acne. A hair style which keeps the hair from falling over the face is important. Daily washing with soap and water is a help in mild cases, and the patient should shampoo his scalp at least three times a week. Oral tetracycline 250 mg. twice daily for two months or longer may be of great benefit for patients with grossly infected lesions. All patients, particularly women, must be discouraged from picking and squeezing the lesions, and they should realise there is no magic cure, but patient, persistent therapy can achieve remarkable results.

PSORIASIS

The cause of this common chronic skin disorder is unknown, although heredity (polygenic inheritance) undoubtedly plays some part in its aetiology. In some patients the onset appears to be precipitated by an acute infection, by pregnancy, or by trauma.

Clinical Features. The typical lesion is a red spot or patch of varying size covered with a thick layer of scales, which can be scraped off with the finger nail or curette, and which exhibits a characteristic silvery sheen. Further gentle scraping of the exposed red shiny surface causes bleeding, but there is no exudation of serum. The lesions are most often seen on the knees and elbows, but practically the whole surface of the body may be involved. The scalp is a common site and there may be hyperkeratotic patches on the palms and soles. Affection of the nails causes them to be thickened, pitted and striated. The condition may persist for life, with occasional remissions and acute exacerbations.

Arthropathic Psoriasis

Arthropathic psoriasis is often seen in middle aged or elderly patients. There is a characteristic destructive polyarthritis of the hands and feet, associated with the skin lesions as described above, similar to that seen in rheumatoid arthritis (p. 355).

Treatment. The appearance of the lesions on exposed parts and the profuse scaling may cause great social embarrassment and it is important to stress to the patient and his relatives that the disorder is neither contagious nor infectious. He should also be encouraged to live an active normal life with as much sunshine as possible, though a period of bed rest may be very beneficial during acute exacerbations. At such times a 1 per cent hydrocortisone, Ung. emulsifications baths or even yellow vaseline (Paraff. molle flav.) should be used, but in the chronic stage preparations such as 0·1 per cent dithranol in Lassar's paste should be applied twice daily. If this causes inflammation of the skin, 3 per cent crude coal tar in a zinc or starch paste may be more suitable. Application of the newer absorbable corticosteroids under polythene occlusion at night may clear the lesions but it should be used with caution because of the danger of secondary infection. It is wise to treat only one area at a time, to use the ointment sparingly and to watch for the development of striae or atrophy of the skin. Topical steroids are helpful in the treatment of psoriasis, but the lesions are more liable to relapse than if they are treated with dithranol.

PITYRIASIS ROSEA

This is probably a virus infection and occasionally groups of three or four cases are seen in hostels and similar institutions. It produces one of the most characteristic rashes in dermatology. The first lesion (or *herald patch*) is an oval erythematous area about an inch across with a collarette of inward facing scale. It is often situated on the front of the chest. A few days later other similar but smaller oval patches appear, mainly on the trunk with long axes in line with the ribs, though there may be a few on the upper arms and thighs. There may be slight itching but this is not a striking feature and the general health is unimpaired and complete spontaneous recovery is the rule within about 6–8 weeks. No treatment is necessary, but if irritation is troublesome 1 per cent hydrocortisone ointment may be used.

LICHEN PLANUS

The cause of lichen planus is unknown. The eruption is seen only in adults and although it usually clears up spontaneously in from three to nine months, relapses are common and in some patients the lesions may persist for years. A lichenoid eruption, indistinguishable from lichen planus, may be caused by some drugs.

Clinical Features. The typical lesion is a small flat topped violaceous papule, often little bigger than a pin's head. The papules may be limited to certain situations, such as the anterior aspect of the wrists and forearms, the genitalia, or the legs, or they may be very profuse and widespread over most of the body, though the face and other exposed parts are rarely affected. Linear disposition of the lesions along scratch marks (Koëbner phenomenon) is common. In some of the patients bluish-white streaks or patches may be seen on the buccal mucosa. There is usually some irritation of the skin and sometimes this is severe.

Treatment. Confinement to bed and sedation may be necessary in very severe acute cases, but usually all that is necessary is an application such as calamine lotion to allay irritation. An anti-histamine tablet such as promethazine hydrochloride 25 mg. may help in this respect. If itching continues, 1 per cent hydrocortisone ointment may be tried. If the mouth, scalp, or genitalia are affected about a month's course of oral steroids may be given, but is seldom necessary.

ERYTHEMA MULTIFORME

This eruption consists of raised erythematous areas of irregular outline and varying size and shape; sometimes in addition there are vesicular, bullous, or nodular lesions. There may be associated ulcerative lesions on the buccal mucosa. Sometimes it appears as a cutaneous reaction to a focus of infection in the skin or elsewhere; sometimes it is a manifestation of acute rheumatism; sometimes it is a drug reaction; but usually the cause is never discovered. It may be preceded by Herpes simplex, which is often the precipitating factor.

Apart from slight fever there is little constitutional upset and spontaneous healing occurs within a couple of weeks, though recurrent attacks are common.

STEVENS-JOHNSON SYNDROME

This is the severest variety of erythema multiforme presenting acutely with fever, followed by the appearance of ulcers in the mouth and sometimes on the conjunctivae. Within a few days an erythematous and bullous eruption spreads over the body, occurring particularly on the genitalia. The patient may be gravely ill for a week or two, but rapidly recovers when the temperature settles. Ophthalmic scarring however, may lead to blindness. Prednisolone should be given, particularly if there is a rising pulse rate or falling blood pressure.

LUPUS ERYTHEMATOSUS (see p. 348)

ROSACEA

This is a chronic hyperaemia of the face, particularly the cheeks and central part of the forehead, leading to permanent dilatation of capillaries and the formation of telangiectases. The patients are often middle-aged women, many of whom also have vague digestive symptoms for which no definite cause can be found. The cosmetic disability is aggravated by the flushing associated with the menopause and with the taking of alcohol or hot spicy food, that is, anything which tends to make the face flush. There may be associated papules and pustules and sometimes hyperplasia of the sebaceous glands. Oral tetracycline 250 mg. twice daily for 2 months and application of 2 per cent sulphur in aqueous cream may be of benefit.

PEMPHIGUS

The cause of this very serious disease is unknown. Fortunately rare, it occurs equally in men and women and seldom appears before late middle age. Before cortisone therapy it was nearly always fatal within 2 years.

Clinical Features. The essential lesion is a bulla which appears on normal skin with no surrounding erythema. Crops of these bullae appear on the skin and mucous membranes and soon rupture and become infected. Constitutional disturbance is severe.

Treatment. Cortisone or an equivalent must be given in high dosage, for example prednisolone 60 mg. daily. The dose is slowly reduced when fresh blisters cease to appear, but at least 15 mg. daily should be continued until the patient has been free of symptoms for three months when the drug may be further reduced in dosage and then stopped. With this treatment a fatal outcome is not so common.

DERMATITIS HERPETIFORMIS

This disease of unknown cause has a clinical similarity to pemphigus, since the lesions are predominantly vesicular or bullous and it tends to run a chronic or relapsing course. There are however, important differences: first, the vesicles and bullae are set on an erythematous base and are often accompanied by urticarial and erythematous lesions. Second, the blisters tend to appear in clusters, particularly on the buttocks and posterior aspect of the thorax. Third, there are seldom lesions in the mouth. Fourth, constitutional upset is slight and, fifth, irritation of the skin is usually severe.

About 60 per cent of these patients have a coeliac syndrome which responds to a gluten-free diet.

Treatment. Dapsone (diamino-diphenyl sulphone) is the drug of choice and so often successful that it is sometimes used as a diagnostic test in this condition. The dose is 100–300 mg. a day by mouth. Prednisolone and sulphapyridine are now less often used.

EXFOLIATIVE DERMATITIS

Exfoliative dermatitis is a syndrome in which there is a progressive desquamation involving the whole skin. It is characterised by the shedding of large amounts of the superficial layers of the skin, and is complicated by excessive heat loss and almost always by secondary infection. There may be a generalised lymphadenopathy. If of long standing the constant skin loss causes negative nitrogen balance and hypoproteinaemia, which may result in oedema. Special skin structures (sweat and sebaceous glands and hair follicles) may be destroyed, sometimes permanently. If healing occurs these structures may not regenerate, so that the patient is left hairless and unable to sweat. This may be a considerable hazard in hot climates, and result in heat stroke.

Many causes of exfoliative dermatitis are recognised, and the commoner are numerated below.

(1) *Medicamentosa.* Arsenic, gold, streptomycin, penicillin.

(2) *External applications.* Penicillin, sulphonamides, dithranol, streptomycin.

(3) *Generalised atopic eczema.*

(4) *Generalised psoriasis.* Often after therapy which is too strong has been applied.

(5) *Generalised erythroderma* may complicate Hodgkin's disease, leukaemias and lymphosarcomas.

(6) Two rare conditions, *Mycosis fungoides* and *Pityriasis rubra pilaris.*

(7) *Idiopathic group*, which is by far the largest group.

Treatment. Secondary infection should be treated appropriately, and the patient's body kept clean and warm. All other drugs should be withdrawn. If heavy metal poisoning is suspected a course of B.A.L. should be given (p. 609). Some cases respond well to local and systemic application of steroids, but with the exception of the iatrogenic group treatment often has to be continued for months or even years.

ERYTHEMA NODOSUM

Clinical Features. In this condition there are painful red, tender nodules usually affecting the front of the lower legs, and occasionally the thighs and forearms. These subside spontaneously in three to six weeks, with some scaling of the skin and colour changes like a bruise. The nodules do not leave permanent skin changes. Occasionally the patient is pyrexial. Women are affected more commonly than men, with a peak incidence in the third decade of life.

The commonest cause is a streptococcal infection of the throat, but it is also often due to sarcoidosis or a drug such as a sulphonamide. Pulmonary tuberculosis is no longer a common cause, but it must be excluded. Less common causes are ulcerative colitis, Crohn's disease, deep fungus infections such as coccidioidomycosis and Hodgkin's disease. In Africa and Asia leprosy is a common cause.

Erythema nodosum is an important condition to recognise, because most patients need further investigations. The treatment is for the underlying condition.

FURTHER READING

Sneddon, I. B. and Church, R. E., *Practical Dermatology*, 3rd edition, Edward Arnold, London, 1976.

Hall-Smith, P. and Cairns, R. J., *Dermatology. Current Concept and Practice*, 2nd edition, Staples Press, London, 1973.

Borrie, P. (revised), *Roxburgh's Common Skin Diseases*, 14th edition, H. K. Lewis, London, 1975.

CHAPTER TWENTY

VENEREAL DISEASES

The word venereal is derived from Venus, the goddess of love, and is applied to those diseases which are communicated by sexual intercourse. The important members of this group are syphilis, gonorrhoea and other causes of urethritis and vaginitis; rarer disorders include chancroid and lymphogranuloma venereum.

GONORRHOEA

The *Neisseria gonorrhoea* is a delicate organism which does not survive for long outside the body, and gonorrhoea is almost invariably acquired by coitus with an infected person. Recovery confers no immunity and it is therefore possible for the same individual to have repeated attacks of the disease. Young girls may acquire the disease from infected bed-linen and towels, but outbreaks of vulvo-vaginitis in children are in fact more often due to other organisms.

The *Neisseria gonorrhoea* is identified in smears of purulent exudates as a gram-negative kidney-shaped diplococcus which must be seen within the cytoplasm of polymorph leucocytes before the diagnosis can be made. It is rather difficult to grow in culture unless special media and increased carbon-dioxide tension are employed.

Clinical Features

(1) **In Men.** Within about three to ten days of exposure to infection the first symptom is usually slight *scalding* on micturition, soon followed by a *purulent urethral discharge* and there may be tender swollen lymph nodes in the groin. If treatment is not given the infection tends to spread to the posterior urethra, as indicated by cloudiness in the second glass of voided urine. Infection of the *prostate* may follow and may cause acute retention of urine, while involvement of the *seminal vesicles* causes severe local pain and fever. Stricture in the posterior urethra is a late sequela. *Acute epididymitis*, indicated by severe pain, swelling, and tenderness which often spread to involve the testicle on the same side is a serious complication since it may be followed by sterility. With modern treatment spread beyond the anterior urethra is very rare.

(2) **In Women.** After a similar incubation period the disease usually presents with *painful, frequent micturition,* and *vaginal discharge,* though there may be no symptoms if the infection is confined to the cervix. Two-thirds of women infected do not seek medical advice, either through

fear or lack of presenting symptoms. Involvement of *Skene's* or *Bartholin's glands* may lead to large painful abscesses, though in fact Bartholin's abscess is much more often of streptococcal origin. If untreated the infection may spread to the uterus and Fallopian tubes, leading to the formation of a *pyosalpinx*; this presents with severe lower abdominal pain and fever and a tender adnexal mass can be felt on one or both sides on pelvic examination. It may be possible to demonstrate gonococci in cervical smears. Involvement of the tubes usually leads to permanent sterility.

Complications. Metastatic lesions due to transient bacteraemia are now very rare, but a purulent arthritis is occasionally seen. Gonorrhoeal rheumatism, however, is usually not due to bacteria in situ and may be in fact an associated Reiter's syndrome (p. 360). It may take the form of a flitting polyarthritis coming on a month or so after infection, or a single joint may be involved, particularly the knee, wrist or ankle. Associated tenosynovitis is common and iritis may occur.

Treatment. A single injection of procaine penicillin B.P., 1·2–2·4 g. (1,200,000–2,400,000 units), is usually adequate treatment for uncomplicated gonorrhoea. Women should receive the higher dose as they tend to respond less well. There are now strains of gonococci relatively resistant to penicillin; but most of the patients whose symptoms persist or relapse within a few days respond to procaine penicillin, fortified, B.P., 5 ml. (containing procaine penicillin 1·5 g. and benzylpenicillin 0·5 g.). A single injection of spectinomycin 2·0 g. for a man or 4·0 g. for a woman given I.M. is useful in patients who are sensitive to penicillin. Good results have been obtained with oral demethylchlortetracyline in a single dose of 600–900 mg., or erythromycin 500 mg. six-hourly for five days. It is important to remember that the treatment of gonorrhoea may suppress the appearance of a syphilitic lesion acquired at the same time and serological tests for the latter disease must always be made three and six months after the gonorrhoea has been treated.

SYPHILIS

As a result of improved treatment and the consequent reduced infectivity of patients with the disease, syphilis is much less common. It remains very important, however, because of the serious lesions which may appear in almost any organ of the body many years after the primary infection.

The causative organism, *Treponema pallidum*, is a thin, actively motile spirochaete from 6–14 μm. in length, which can be recognised by its characteristic movements in preparations of the serous discharge from the early infectious lesions examined by the microscopic technique known as darkground illumination (D.G.I.). It cannot withstand drying and is transmitted only by direct contact.

Congenital syphilis is contracted by the foetus through the placenta in the later months of pregnancy; acquired syphilis is nearly always the result of sexual intercourse with an infected person, though occasionally extragenital infection may be acquired, for example by doctors or nurses, by handling syphilitic lesions. Congenital syphilis is fortunately extremely rare nowadays. It is a preventible disease, since if a woman with syphilis is given adequate treatment sufficiently early in pregnancy the child escapes infection. Routine serum tests should therefore be made on all women on their first attendance at ante-natal clinics.

Clinical Features. Congenital syphilis may cause intra-uterine death and result in *miscarriage* or *stillbirth*, or the child may be born apparently healthy only to develop various stigmata of the disease during childhood. Early manifestations are failure to gain weight in the first month or two of life and an infection in the nose ('*snuffles*') which interferes with the development of the nasal bones and leads eventually to the depressed bridge of the nose which is one of the most characteristic signs of the disease. A scaly yellow or copper-coloured *rash* is also common. Among the many lesions which may appear later in childhood are notches in the incisor teeth of the second dentition, which also tend to be widely spaced and to taper from the gum margin to the cutting edge (*Hutchinson's teeth*); scars known as *rhagades* radiating from the margins of the lips; and opacity of the cornea due to *interstitial keratitis* (I.K.). Aortic lesions are very rare in congenital syphilis, but juvenile forms of *tabes* and *general paresis* are occasionally seen.

Acquired syphilis passes through three stages, known as *primary* syphilis, *secondary* syphilis, and *tertiary* syphilis. The secondary stage occurs within a few months of primary infection, but many years may elapse before a tertiary lesion appears.

Primary syphilis is characterised by the appearance of a hard chancre (pronounced 'shanker') about a month after exposure to infection. In men the chancre usually occurs on the penis; in women it appears most often on the labia or cervix and in the latter situation readily escapes notice. Much more rarely the primary sore may be on the lip, tongue, tonsil, or nipple. The chancre is a hard, painless ulcer about 1 cm. in diameter, has a thin, serous discharge and is accompanied by painless enlargement of the regional lymph nodes. *Diagnosis* depends on identifying the *Treponema pallidum* in the exudate with the use of the dark-ground microscope.

Secondary syphilis may cause some constitutional disturbance with *sore throat*, low *fever* and generalised *lymph-node enlargement*, but usually its manifestations are confined to the skin and the mucous membrane of the mouth. Various types of skin *rash* are seen, all having in common a symmetrical distribution over the body, absence of irritation, and a colour usually likened to raw ham. In the mouth painless, slimy, greyish patches known as '*snail-track ulcers*' are the typical lesions. Warty lesions known as *condylomata* may appear in the peri-anal and vulval regions. The cutaneous and mucosal lesions of the secondary stage are highly infective and the serum tests for antibody are invariably positive.

Tertiary Stage. A localised swelling known as a gumma may appear anywhere in the body many years after the primary infection; these lesions differ from those of primary and secondary syphilis in containing no spirochaetes and being therefore non-infective. In certain situations such as the liver, the lung, or the stomach, a gumma may be mistaken for a carcinoma; the distinction can be made by giving potassium iodide 1–2 g. which causes rapid disappearance of a gumma but has no effect on a carcinoma. The centre of a gumma often breaks down and leads to the formation of an ulcer with sharply punched-out margins.

Syphilitic *aortitis* is discussed on p. 152, and *neurosyphilis* on p. 298.

Treatment of Syphilis. Procaine penicillin injection B.P., 600 mg. (600,000 units), should be given daily for ten days. Alternatively itinerant or unco-operative patients may be given a single intramuscular injection of benzathine penicillin 2·4 g. (2·4 mega units) as this will maintain the necessary blood level (at least 0·03 units per ml.) for about two weeks. Patients sensitive to penicillin may be given tetracycline by mouth 750 mg. six-hourly for 10 to 15 days, though the long-term efficacy of this treatment has not yet been fully assessed. Patients with early infectious syphilis are kept under supervision for 2 years. Patients with late syphilis require two or more courses of treatment lasting 2–3 weeks each and may need prolonged follow-up. At each visit in addition to clinical examination serum tests for syphilis using specific syphilitic antigen are performed, e.g. T.P.I. (Treponema Pallidum Immobilisation) or R.P.C.F.T. (Reiter Protein Complement Fixation Test). If there are clinical indications the C.S.F. is examined also.

An acute exacerbation of the lesions may occur within a day or so of starting treatment (the *Herxheimer reaction*) but this is never harmful in early syphilis and is over in a few hours. The Herxheimer reaction may have more serious effects in patients with syphilitic aortitis or gummata in special situations such as the larynx; penicillin therapy should be started under steroid cover in such patients.

NON-SPECIFIC URETHRITIS

Following the striking decline in the numbers of patients with gonorrhoea and syphilis, non-specific urethritis has become one of the most common conditions seen in V.D. departments. It may be due to known organisms such as virus (TRIC), mycoplasma organisms, mixed bacteria, *Trichomonas vaginalis, Candida albicans,* or at times to non-infective causes. It is seen mainly in young men.

After a variable incubation period which can probably be as long as two to three months, the patient develops scalding, frequency, and a purulent urethral discharge which contains no *Neisseria gonorrhoea.* In addition to urethral discharge some patients have conjunctivitis and acute arthritis affecting one or more of the large joints of the limbs, and the condition is then known as *Reiter's syndrome* (p. 360). The urethral discharge usually subsides fairly quickly, but the arthritis when present may persist for many months. A frequent local complication is subacute prostatitis.

Tetracycline 250 mg. six-hourly for five days should be given, but the response is often unsatisfactory.

SOFT SORE (Chancroid)

Chancroid is very rare in Britain, though it is occasionally seen in seaports. The causative organism is *Haemophilus ducreyi* (Ducrey's bacillus), a gram negative bacillus about 1–2 μm. in length.

Clinical Features. After an incubation period of two to fourteen days one or more small red papules appear on the genitalia or surrounding skin and within a few days develop into necrotic ulcers with undermined edges surrounded by an area of erythema and oedema. The inguinal lymph nodes enlarge and sometimes suppurate. The important distinction from syphilis is made by the shorter incubation period, the absence of induration in the lesions, the failure to demonstrate spirochaetes on dark-ground illumination and identification of Ducrey's bacillus in stained smears and on culture.

Treatment. A course of sulphadimidine or other sulphonamide is effective.

LYMPHOGRANULOMA INGUINALE

This is also very rare in Britain. It is a virus infection with an incubation period of up to three weeks.

Clinical Features. The initial lesion may be a small vesicle or ulcer on the genitalia, but more often the first evidence of the disease is enlargement of the inguinal lymph nodes. The swelling may become quite massive and eventually suppuration may occur with the discharge of yellow pus through multiple sinuses in the skin. There is often severe constitutional reaction with high fever. In women proctitis and subsequent rectal stricture may occur; sequelae in men include scarring and elephantiasis of the genitalia.

Diagnosis A positive intradermal *Frei test* indicates that the patient now has or has had the disease.

Treatment. Some success may be achieved with either the sulphonamides or the tetracyclines, or the two drugs may be combined. Sulphonamides such as sulphadimidine should be given in doses of 3–4 g. daily for three to six weeks; tetracycline dosage is 500 mg. six-hourly for five days followed by 250 mg. six-hourly for three to six weeks or longer. Fluctuant buboes should be aspirated rather than incised.

FURTHER READING

Catterall, R. D., *A Short Textbook of Venereology*, Hodder and Stoughton Educational, 2nd edition, 1974.

King, A. and Nicol, C., *Venereal Diseases*, 3rd Edition, Baillière Tindall, London, 1975.

CHAPTER TWENTY-ONE

ABNORMAL REACTIONS TO DRUGS

INTRODUCTION

Drug reactions are becoming increasingly important as the range of substances used for diagnostic and therapeutic purposes is increased. The classification of these reactions is difficult for their underlying mechanism is often not fully understood.

(1) **Overdosage.** This term is self-explanatory. It must be realised, however, that patients vary in the amount of drug required to produce symptoms and signs of overdosage. Patients who develop evidence of overdosage with small doses are said to show *intolerance* to the drug.

(2) **Side Effects.** These effects although not therapeutically useful are inherent in the action of the drug. The constipation which complicates the use of ganglion blocking agents is a good example.

(3) **Secondary Effects.** These effects are not due to any action of the drug, but are a consequence of that action.

(4) **Idiosyncrasy.** This means that the subject reacts to the drug in some abnormal way.

(5) **Hypersensitivity Reactions.** These reactions imply that the patient is sensitive to the drug, usually from previous contact, and that the reaction is mediated by an antigen-antibody reaction.

(6) **Drug Interactions.**

In practice it is often very difficult to decide into which group a drug reaction falls, particularly to distinguish between idiosyncracy and hypersensitivity reactions.

The following is a description of a number of clinical syndromes which may occur as a result of taking drugs. The majority of these syndromes are hypersensitivity reactions.

ACUTE HYPERSENSITIVITY REACTION

This reaction occurs within a few minutes of administration of the drug. The main features are chest pain, dyspnoea, cyanosis, and a rapid fall in blood pressure. There is often, but not always, a history of previous exposure to the drug. This type of reaction is more common in those with a history of atopic disorders. It seems probable that these subjects are particularly liable to produce antibodies of the IgE class (see p. 339). These antibodies become attached to the surface of mast cells and when they combine with the appropriate antigen pharmacologically active substances such as histamine, bradykinin and 5-hydroxytryptamine are released from the cell.

Treatment begins with prophylaxis. It is important to ask the patient if he is sensitive to the drug about to be administered. If a reaction occurs adrenaline 0·5 ml. of 1:1,000 solution, must be given subcutaneously together with an anti-histamine (chlorpheniramine maleate 10·0 mg. I.V.).

DELAYED HYPERSENSITIVITY REACTION

The onset of symptoms with this type of reaction usually occurs from seven to fourteen days after the start of taking the drug. There is often a history of previous drug exposure. The common symptoms are *fever, skin rashes, joint pains*, and *lymphadenopathy*. The skin rashes although usually urticarial may occasionally be purpuric and sometimes even an exfoliative dermatitis occurs.

Among the drugs which produce these symptoms are the barbiturates, the sulphonamides, streptomycin, thiouracil, and particularly penicillin. Exfoliative dermatitis may follow the heavy metals, particularly gold or arsenic, as well as penicillin and the sulphonamides.

Treatment consists of stopping the drug. Usually this is sufficient. The disappearance of symptoms may be aided by an anti-histamine (promethazine hydrochloride 25 mg. twice daily or chlorpheniramine maleate 4 mg. three times daily). Prednisolone is occasionally required in severe cases. If the rash is troublesome the local application of calamine lotion reduces the itching.

BLOOD DYSCRASIAS

Blood dyscrasias are among the most important drug reactions. It would seem that many of them are hypersensitivity reactions and are due to combination of antigen, antibody and complement on the cell. Others are due to a direct effect on the blood cells or their precursors.

Agranulocytosis

This may occur with a number of drugs including amidopyrine, the sulphonamides, thiouracil, carbimazole, tridione, isoniazid, phenylbutazone, chloramphenicol, gold, and arsenic. In addition large doses of most cytotoxic drugs such as nitrogen mustard will produce agranulocytosis. With most drugs the agranulocytosis is reversible, provided the drug is not continued for too long, but with chloramphenicol recovery may not occur.

Clinical Features. There may be no symptoms and the depression in the granulocytes may be found by a routine blood count. Such patients are susceptible to infection and may present with general malaise, fever, and some infective process, usually a severe throat infection.

Treatment

(1) *Prophylaxis.* The patient should always be asked if he is susceptible to the drug before it is given. Certain drugs such as amidopyrine and chloramphenicol should be avoided if possible. It is doubtful if routine blood counts on patients taking drugs which may cause agranulocytosis are much help as the fall in granulocytes may be sudden. The patient must, however, be told to report to the doctor if he becomes ill and in particular if he develops a sore throat; a blood count must then be performed.

(2) *Curative.* The drug must be stopped immediately. If the white count does not improve within a few days, prednisolone 30 mg. daily should be given. Infections should be treated as they arise with the appropriate antibiotic. The majority of patients will recover on this treatment. When granulopenia is due to heavy metals it should be treated with dimercaprol (p. 609).

Thrombocytopenia

Thrombocytopenia may occur as a result of drug administration. It has been described with sedormid, tridione, chloramphenicol, thiazide, gold, sulphonamides, and quinine. It may occur with excessive dosage of cytoxic drugs. Clinical features include purpura and bleeding from various sites.

Treatment. The drug should be stopped immediately. Prednisolone 30 mg. daily is the most effective treatment. It is doubtful whether blood transfusion is helpful and it should be reserved for those patients who require transfusion because of excessive blood loss. Fresh blood should be used, because transfused platelets are effective for only a few hours. Platelet transfusions will however raise the plasma platelet count for a few days.

Aplastic Anaemia

Aplastic anaemia is not common following the taking of drugs. It may occur with benzol and its derivatives, with chloramphenicol and with a number of other drugs including gold and the sulphonamides. It may be associated with depression of other elements of the blood.

Treatment. The drug should be stopped. Repeated transfusion may be required. Prednisolone is not usually very helpful, but it is worth a trial in patients who are not recovering. If poisoning is due to heavy metals, dimercaprol should be used. Provided the drug is stopped quickly, recovery usually occurs. The exception is chloramphenicol, which rarely causes bone-marrow dyscrasias and usually only after repeated courses; if they occur, however, they are usually irreversible and ultimately prove fatal.

Haemolytic Anaemia

Drugs can occasionally cause haemolysis. It seems that a number of mechanisms may be responsible. Quinine has long been known to precipitate the acute haemolysis occurring in association with malaria and called *blackwater fever*. It is most likely that this is some kind of hypersensitivity reaction.

Potassium chlorate in large doses will produce haemolysis by a direct action on the cell; occasionally this occurs with quite a small dose of the drug and it can then be classed as an example of intolerance.

Finally in about 10% of American negroes there appears to be a deficiency in glucose 6 phosphate dehydrogenase which is normally responsible for the integrity of the red cells. This results in acute haemolysis when such subjects take primaquine sulphonamides, nitrofurantoins and other drugs and is an example of true idiosyncrasy to a drug.

Methaemoglobinaemia and Sulphaemoglobinaemia

These changes in the haemoglobin may occur with certain drugs, including phenacetin, potassium chlorate, and the sulphonamides. The patient appears cyanosed, but is not distressed or dyspnoeic. The diagnosis is confirmed by finding the absorption spectra of methaemoglobin or sulphaemoglobin in the blood. The only treatment usually required is to stop the offending drug. Methaemoglobinaemia can be temporarily reversed by giving methylene blue as a 1 per cent solution intravenously, the dose for an adult being 5 ml.

Megaloblastic Anaemia

Certain drugs including pyrimethamine and the anticonvulsants primidone and phenytoin may produce a megaloblastic anaemia which can be reversed by folic acid 10 mg. daily.

LIVER DAMAGE (see p. 89)

DRUG REACTIONS AND COLLAGEN DISEASES

Although some authors include a wide variety of syndromes under the term collagen diseases, this term should be confined to rheumatic fever, rheumatoid arthritis, disseminated lupus erythematosus, polyarteritis nodosa, dermatomyositis, and giant-cell arteritis. There has been considerable discussion whether drug reactions can cause these conditions. There is no doubt that a clinical picture similar to that of disseminated lupus erythematosus can be produced by *hydralazine* and by *procaineamide*, but it differs from the true disease in that recovery occurs when the drug is stopped. In addition, transient arteritis can occur in association with hypersensitivity reaction to a number of drugs, including *penicillin* and the *sulphonamides*. Whether such reactions play any part in the pathogenesis of true polyarteritis nodosa is more doubtful and it is unlikely that drug reactions are causally related to any of the other collagen diseases.

Other types of connective tissue disease can be drug induced. *Methysergide* causes a retroperitoneal fibrosis which may affect the mediastinum. It is a rare cause of ureteric obstruction. *Practolol* produces various disorders including skin rashes, sclerosis of the cornea and peritoneal fibrosis. The cause of these changes is not known.

SERUM REACTIONS

Serum reactions can be divided into:

      (a) Immediate reactions.
      (b) Delayed reactions (serum sickness).

They are hypersensitivity reactions and are more common in those who have had serum before and in those with a history of allergic diseases such as asthma, hay fever, urticaria, or infantile eczema.

Immediate Serum Reactions

Clinical Features. Immediate serum reactions appear within a few minutes of injection and vary greatly in their severity. There may be merely swelling, with perhaps some local urticaria in the region of the injection. There may be a generalised rash without any other upset. In severe cases the patient complains of feeling unwell, with tightness in the chest and faintness, followed by collapse with cyanosis, a falling blood pressure and occasionally death.

Treatment. Mild reactions respond to the application of calamine lotion to the rash and an anti-histamine by mouth for a few days (chlorpheniramine maleate 4 mg. t.d.s. or promethazine 25 mg. b.d.). In severe cases subcutaneous adrenaline 0·5 ml. of 1:1,000 solution should be given immediately and may have to be repeated. This should be followed by an anti-histamine given by slow intravenous injection (chlorpheniramine maleate 10 mg. or promethazine hydrochloride 25 mg.). Rarely, hydrocortisone hemisuccinate 100 mg. intravenously will be required.

Delayed Serum Reaction (Serum Sickness)

This is due to a circulating antigen/antibody complement complex which causes transient damage to certain tissues.

Clinical Features. About a week to ten days after the patient has received serum he develops a rash, usually urticarial, pain and stiffness with some swelling in the joints, and usually a fever. Sometimes there is enlargement of the lymph nodes and a transient albuminuria. Rarely, a shock-like state develops with low blood pressure. This condition usually clears up in a few days.

Treatment. Local application of calamine lotion helps to relieve the itching. An anti-histamine such as chlorpheniramine maleate 4 mg. t.d.s. shortens the duration of the illness. In severe or resistant cases, prednisolone 20 mg. for a day or two and then tailed off will usually relieve the symptoms.

AVOIDANCE OF SERUM REACTIONS

When serum is given to a patient the following rules should be observed.

(1) The patient should be asked whether he has had serum before or whether he suffers from allergic diseases such as asthma, hay fever, eczema, or urticaria.

(2) If the answer to these questions is negative, 0·1 ml. of serum is injected subcutaneously. If there is no local or general reaction within half an hour, the full dose of serum is given intramuscularly.

(3) If the patient has a history of allergic disease or has had serum before, 0·1 ml. of serum diluted 1:10 is given subcutaneously; if there is no reaction within half an hour 0·1 ml. of serum is given subcutaneously; if after a further half an hour there is still no reaction, the full dose of serum is given intramuscularly.

(4) If the patient has a history of serum reactions or has a reaction to the test dose, he should be admitted to hospital. He is then given an anti-histamine followed by the serum in gradually increasing doses. It is usual to start with 0·1 ml. of a 1:100 dilution of serum and if this causes no reaction in half an hour the dose is doubled and so on until enough serum has been given. It is a very tedious process.

(5) Whenever serum is given it is essential that a syringe of fresh 1:1,000 adrenaline solution be at hand and also an anti-histamine suitable for I.V. injection (chlorpheniramine maleate 10 mg.). Whenever patients are given serum they must be observed for half an hour after the injection and must be warned of the possibility of a delayed serum reaction.

(6) Intravenous injections of serum should be avoided if possible. Where they are necessary, the same precautions should be adopted. Intravenous serum should not be given to those who have previously had serum or who have allergic disorders and in addition a test dose of 0·1 ml. of serum should also be given intramuscularly. As a general rule intravenous serum should be given only to patients in hospital.

(7) Following the administration of serum the patient should be actively immunised against the appropriate diseases. This should be delayed until at least one month after he has received the serum, as the circulating antibody from the serum may prevent the antigen from provoking active immunity.

GENETICALLY DETERMINED DRUG REACTIONS

Reactions to drugs may be due to specific hereditary enzymatic deficiency. About 10 per cent of American Negroes develop haemolytic anaemia when exposed to primaquine and other related drugs. It is now clear that these individuals lack the enzyme glucose-6-phosphate dehydrogenase and this deficiency is sex-linked. Precipitation of acute porphyria in genetically predisposed individuals by ingestion of barbiturates is well known. A dangerously prolonged response to the muscle relaxant succinyl-choline may be due to a deficiency of the hereditary serum enzyme pseudo-cholinesterase. The height of the blood level of isoniazid which follows an oral dose depends on whether it is 'rapidly' or 'slowly' inactivated (acetyla-ted). The gene for 'slow' inactivator is recessive and patients who are 'slow' inactivators, although they have a more rapid bacteriological response to isoniazid, are more likely to exhibit drug reactions than 'rapid' inactiva-tors.

DRUG INTERACTION

The increasing use of drugs, particularly the prescribing of more than one drug at a time, has made drug interaction an important problem. Interaction may occur at several stages in the passage of drugs through the body:

(1) **In the gastro-intestinal tract** drugs may combine or their physical state may be altered so that absorption is modified. For example, iron combines with tetracycline decreasing its absorption and leading to lower blood levels of the antibiotic.

(2) **Competition for Transport Sites on the Plasma Proteins.** Many drugs are transported to their sites of action partially or almost totally bound to plasma proteins. When bound in this way they cannot produce their pharmacological effects and are not available to be metabolised or ex-creted. The activity of the drug depends on the unbound fraction.

When two drugs compete for a limited number of protein-binding sites there is a decrease in the bound fraction of each and an increase in the amount of free drug, with a corresponding enhancement of the pharmaco-logical effect. The anticoagulant Warfarin, for example, is normally about 98 per cent bound to plasma protein. If phenylbutazone is given con-currently competition for sites occurs and the bound fraction of Warfarin may drop to 96 per cent; the amount of active Warfarin is therefore doubled and signs of overdosage may result. Other drugs which are protein bound and may compete for sites are tolbutamide, chlorpro-pamides, sulphonamides and indomethacin.

(3) **Modification at Sites of Action.** The pharmacological action of a drug can be modified in several ways by the concurrent administration of another drug. For example:

(1) Hypokalaemia produced by *diuretics* enhances the action of *digitalis* on the heart.

(2) *Tricyclic antidepressants* reverse the effect of *adrenergic blocking hypotensive* agents, possibly by increasing the amount of noradrenaline at the adrenergic nerve endings. They also enhance the effect of *sympathomimetic amines*, which for example may be added to a local anaesthetic.

(3) The action of central nervous depressants such as barbiturates and alcohol is additive.

(4) *Monoamine Oxidase Inhibitors* (*MAO Inhibitors*). These interact in two ways:

(a) Certain drugs, particularly sympathomimetic drugs such as phenylpropanolamine or tyramine, release the excess noradrenaline which accumulates in nerve endings of the subject taking MAO inhibitors, resulting in a hypertensive crisis. Tyramine is found in certain foods.

(b) The effect of some central depressants, particularly pethidine, is enhanced.

(4) **Enzyme Induction.** Many drugs are metabolised by enzymes, usually in the liver. Certain drugs increase the activity of these enzymes so that drug breakdown is enhanced. For example, if a patient on an oral anticoagulant is given phenobarbitone the barbiturate increases the enzyme activity and the anticoagulant is metabolised more rapidly. An increased dose is therefore necessary to produce a satisfactory anticoagulant effect. Conversely, if the phenobarbitone is stopped enzyme activity decreases and signs of anticoagulant overdosage may appear.

(5) **Enzyme Inhibition.** Sulphonamides decrease the rate of breakdown of tolbutamide. Allopurinol decreases the rate of breakdown of 6-mercaptopurine.

(6) **Renal Excretion.** Competition for pathways in the kidney by two drugs given together may reduce the rate of excretion of both. Use is made of this phenomenon when probenecid is given with penicillin to reduce its excretion and so achieve a higher level of penicillin in the blood.

CHAPTER TWENTY-TWO

POISONING

Poisoning is responsible for about 10 per cent of all acute admissions to hospital in the U.K. It may be due to:

(a) *Self Poisoning*. This may be a serious suicide attempt, or more often an attempt to draw the attention of relatives, friends or doctors to some intolerable situation in the patient's life.

(b) *Accidental*.

(c) *Rarely homicidal*.

Preliminary Assessment. When a diagnosis of poisoning is made it is important to determine:

(a) The nature of the poison or poisons. More than one poison has often been taken.

(b) Any other complicating factors such as injuries, etc.

(c) The severity of the poisoning.

The assessment of the severity of the poisoning will be based on three criteria.

(1) *Level of Consciousness*. This is usually divided into:

Grade I   Drowsy but responds to mild stimulation.
Grade II   Unconscious but responds to mild stimulation.
Grade III   Unconscious but responds to severe stimulation.
Grade IV   Unconscious and unresponsive.

(2) *Circulation*. Many drugs cause acute circulatory failure (p. 107). This can be assessed by the blood pressure and by the peripheral blood flow (temperature of extremities, etc.). An apparently normal blood pressure may however be associated with inadequate peripheral perfusion.

(3) *Respiration*. Central depression of respiration is caused by many drugs. A crude assessment may be obtained from the respiration rate and presence or absence of cyanosis. Blood gases should be measured if there is any doubt.

Treatment

Non-specific Measures. Certain measures are common in the management of most types of poisoning. They consist of:

(a) *Maintenance of Adequate Ventilation*. This includes keeping a clear airway in the unconscious patient and the use of a ventilator in severe poisoning.

(b) *Emptying the Stomach.* In all patients who are conscious except those who have taken corrosive poisons, vomiting should be precipitated by making the patient drink a pint of warm water and then stimulating the pharynx with the fingers. This must be followed, except with corrosive poisons, by gastric lavage. A 30 English gauge Jacques tube is passed and 250 ml. of warm water is run into the stomach and then syphoned out. This should be repeated at least six times. If the nature of the poison is known, a suitable antidote may be left in the stomach (see below).

It is very important to avoid inhalation of gastric contents by the patient and during gastric lavage he should lie in the prone position with the head and shoulders lower than the rest of the body.

In the unconscious patient the risk of inhalation is increased. In these patients the help of an anaesthetist is advisable for gastric lavage which should be preceded by the passing of a cuffed endotracheal tube.

After four hours most poisons have left the stomach and so very little will be recovered by gastric lavage. Salicylates however cause pyloric spasm and gastric lavage is useful for up to 24 hours.

Finally, all vomit and the first return from gastric lavage should be kept and carefully labelled for further analysis.

(c) *Forced Alkaline Diuresis.* Excretion of certain poisons (particularly phenobarbitone and salicylates) can be accelerated by producing an alkaline diuresis. A central venous pressure line is useful to guard against overloading the circulation and the bases of the lungs should be examined regularly for signs of pulmonary oedema. In the first hour 500 ml. of $1 \cdot 2$ per cent sodium bicarbonate (or $\frac{1}{6}$ M sodium lactate)$+20$ mg. of frusemide, followed by $1 \cdot 0$ litre of 5 per cent dextrose$+20$ mg. of frusemide are given intravenously. At the end of the hour the urinary flow should be greater than $3 \cdot 0$ ml./min. Subsequent rate of infusion will depend on central venous pressure and urinary volume. Every third bottle (500 ml.) of infusion fluid should contain 150 mEq. of sodium and every bottle of infusion fluid $10 \cdot 0$ mEq. of potassium. Diuresis can be maintained either by adding mannitol (not more than 20 g./hour) to the infusion fluid or by further injections of frusemide intravenously. The urinary pH must be kept above $7 \cdot 5$.

If a diuresis is not produced by the end of the first hour there is probably impairment of renal function and dialysis will be required.

BARBITURATE POISONING

Barbiturate poisoning is the commonest type of poisoning in Great Britain and stands second to carbon monoxide as a cause of death. Chronic addiction to barbiturates also occurs.

Acute Poisoning

Barbiturates are usually taken in a deliberate suicidal attempt; occasionally by accident. Barbiturate and alcohol poisoning may be combined;

these two drugs certainly have an additive effect, and it is believed by some that their actions are synergistic.

The speed of action and duration of effect depend on the type of barbiturate used.

Clinical Features. The symptoms of mild barbiturate overdosage are mental confusion with slurred speech, nystagmus, and unsteady gait. These are followed by deep sleep from which the patient can be roused though perhaps with difficulty. The corneal and pharyngeal reflexes remain and respiration is not markedly depressed. A bullous rash occurs in about 10 per cent of patients with barbiturate overdosage.

In severe barbiturate overdosage there is deep coma, the patient cannot be roused and reflexes have disappeared. Finally death occurs from respiratory depression complicated by circulatory failure. The diagnosis can be confirmed by finding the drug in the urine, blood, or gastric contents.

The blood level of barbiturate is a poor guide as to prognosis as patients vary in their sensitivity to the drug.

Treatment. If the patient is conscious, no treatment will usually be required unless a large dose has just been taken, when it should be removed by gastric lavage.

In the unconscious patient management is:

(1) Ensure a clear airway, if the cough reflex is absent, an endotracheal tube should be introduced.
(2) Ensure adequate ventilation; in a cyanosed patient with respiratory depression some form of mechanical ventilation will be required.
(3) Gastric contents should be aspirated and the stomach washed out only if the drug has been taken within the previous four hours.
(4) Maintain hydration by giving 2·0 litres of intravenous fluid in 24 hours (N/5 dextrose saline).
(5) Treat intercurrent chest infections as they arise.

In severe intoxication however (absent reflexes—depressed respiration), an attempt should be made to increase the rate of barbiturate elimination. Renal excretion of phenobarbitone can be increased by producing a high flow rate of alkaline urine. This is not however effective with the short acting barbiturates which are largely broken down in the liver. For method see p. 605).

The death rate from hospital admission with barbiturate poisoning is about 2–5 per cent.

Chronic Barbiturate Addiction

Chronic barbiturate addiction is by no means uncommon. Patients may indulge in bursts of intoxication or may take the drug regularly. Most addicts suffer from some form of psychological abnormality. If the drug is suddenly stopped a well-marked withdrawal syndrome occurs with weakness, nausea and vomiting, anxiety, and often convulsions.

ETHYL ALCOHOL

Most subjects with acute alcoholic intoxication will sleep it off. In severe cases the stomach should be washed out if the alcohol has been taken recently, and treatment continued as in barbiturate poisoning. Forced alkaline diuresis is not used. Various substances, including vitamins B and C and fructose, have been claimed to sober up a patient, but there is little evidence that they are of practical use in the treatment of acute alcoholic poisoning.

The combination of alcohol and barbiturates is additive and can be very dangerous.

MORPHINE POISONING

Acute morphine poisoning may result from overdosage during the therapeutic use of the drug or from a suicidal attempt. The lethal dose is variable, but has been given as between 60–240 mg., but it must be realised that repeated dosage quickly produces tolerance of the drug.

Clinical Features. The patient is comatose and cannot be wakened. The respiration rate is very slow. The skin is cyanosed and is cold and clammy. The pupils are pin-point in size. With severe poisoning the blood pressure may fall. Death results from respiratory depression.

Treatment. (1) If the drug has been taken by mouth, wash out the stomach with 1 : 2,000 potassium permanganate solution.

(2) *Nalorphine* is a specific antidote for morphine. The dose is 10 mg. intravenously repeated as required every 15 minutes until a total of 40 mg. has been given. The effects of nalorphine usually last for about two hours and if relapse occurs at this time the drug should be repeated. The aim of the treatment with nalorphine is to restore the respiratory rate to normal. Wakening the patient is not necessary. Alternatively *naloxone* 0·4 mg. I.V. can be given and repeated at three minute intervals if a satisfactory response is not obtained. It has the advantage of being effective against pethidine and other synthetic opiates. These drugs will produce acute withdrawal symptoms in morphine addicts.

(3) If there is severe respiratory depression with cyanosis, oxygen should be given and artificial respiration may be required.

(4) Occasionally respiratory stimulants such as nikethamide 4 ml. of a 25 per cent solution intravenously, or aminophylline 0·5 g. intravenously are useful in patients only partially relieved by nalorphine.

Glutethimide

Glutethimide is occasionally used as a suicide agent. It produces deep unconsciousness with dilated pupils, in severe poisoning periods of apnoea may occur and these are associated with the development of papilloedema. The fatal dose is in the region of 10 g.

Treatment. Dialysis is not useful and treatment is largely supportive. If papilloedema develops 500 ml. of 20 per cent mannitol should be given intravenously over twenty minutes followed by 500 ml. of 5 per cent dextrose over the ensuring four hours.

Phenothiazines

The dose response curve of the phenothiazines is fairly flat so there is a wide safety margin. Overdosage produces unconsciousness associated with extrapyramidal signs and with torticollis. Cardiac arrythmias, hypotension and hypothermia occur.

Treatment. If the extrapyramidal signs are severe they respond to benztropine 2·0 mg. I.V. otherwise treatment is supportive.

Benzodiazepines

This group of drugs has a very wide safety margin so that they rarely produce anything more than unconsciousness and no specific treatment is required.

Methaqualone

This drug is a relatively mild hypnotic but is combined with diphenhydramine in the preparation *Mandrax* which is both powerful and quick acting. Overdosage produces a rather characteristic clinical state with coma combined with increased muscle tone and reflexes.

TRICYCLIC ANTIDEPRESSIVES

This group includes imiprimine, nortriptyline and amitriptyline.

These drugs have become common agents in attempted suicide. The clinical picture is one of excitement followed by coma and sometimes convulsions. The pupils are dilated, the reflexes increased and the plantars extensor. In severe overdosage special features are hypotension, tachycardia and the occurrence of cardiac arrythmias. Frequently they may be combined with a phenothiazine or with a benzodiazepine compound such as chlordiazepoxide which produces a complicated clinical picture.

Treatment. There is no specific antidote and symptoms must be treated as they arise. Fits can be controlled by diazepam. The cardiac arrythmias should be treated along the usual lines (see p. 117). Hypotension is difficult to treat and both vaso-constriction and cautious infusion with plasma volume expanders such as dextran have been used. Forced diuresis and dialysis are *not* effective.

ARSENICAL POISONING

Inorganic arsenic, usually in the form of the oxide, acquired notoriety as a homicidal poison and is still sometimes taken with suicidal intent.

Poisoning may also occur as a result of exposure to arsenical dusts which are produced in various industrial processes. It produces its toxic action by inhibiting the intracellular sulphydril enzymes which are essential to metabolism.

Acute Poisoning

Clinical Features. The main symptoms of acute poisoning by arsenic are burning in the throat, vomiting, abdominal pain, and diarrhoea. In severe cases circulatory collapse and death may follow.

Treatment. (1) The stomach should be emptied and then washed out with freshly prepared ferric hydroxide, which is made by adding 45 g. of ferric chloride to 15 g. of sodium carbonate (washing soda) in half a tumbler of water.

(2) *Dimercaprol* (B.A.L.) 300 mg. in oily solution is given I.M. six-hourly for two days and then decreased over the next few days. The action of dimercaprol is to offer SH groups with which the arsenic combines; it is thus unable to combine with the SH groups in intracellular enzymes.

Chronic Poisoning

The symptoms and signs of chronic arsenical poisoning are variable, but include:

(1) Pigmentation of the skin which has a typical mottled ('raindrop') appearance.
(2) Polyneuritis.
(3) Hyperkeratosis of the palms of hands and soles of the feet.
(4) Chronic pharyngitis and perforation of the nasal septum.
(5) Chronic diarrhoea.

Treatment. The patient should be removed from exposure to arsenic and given dimercaprol as for acute poisoning.

POISONING BY FERROUS COMPOUNDS

This form of poisoning has become common; it is usually due to children eating sugar-coated ferrous sulphate tablets in mistake for sweets.

Clinical features, Initially there is vomiting and diarrhoea often associated with haematemesis and melaena. After a few hours the patient becomes confused and this may be followed by coma, convulsion and shock. Acute liver necrosis can occur.

Treatment. (1) Vomiting should be induced.

(2) The stomach should then be washed out with a solution containing 2·0 g. of desferrioxamine per litre and 5·0 g. in 50 ml. should be left in the stomach in adults. Desferrioxamine is an iron chelating agent.

(3) 2·0 g. of desferrioxamine are given intramuscularly twice daily.

In severe cases desferrioxamine can be given intravenously in 5 per cent glucose solution at a rate of 15 mg./kg. per hour to a maximum of 80 mg./kg. per 24 hours.

(4) The patient must be kept in bed and under observation for at least 48 hours after apparent recovery.

ANTICHOLINESTERASE POISONING

A number of these substances are used in medicine and also as insecticides. They also have a potential use in war, and are known as 'nerve gases'. They inhibit the enzyme cholinesterase either temporarily or for long periods, so that there is widespread overactivity of the parasympathetic nervous system and also neuromuscular block in voluntary muscle. Symptoms may include colicky abdominal pain, excess salivation, respiratory paralysis and the pupils are constricted.

Treatment. Atropine should be given in doses of 2·0 mg. intravenously or intramuscularly, and repeated as required. This will not however relieve neuromuscular block. Cholinesterase can be reactivated by pralidoxime 1·0 g. in 5 ml. of water I.V. or I.M., and repeated at four-hourly intervals as required. In severe cases some form of assisted ventilation may be necessary.

PARAQUAT

Paraquat is normally used as a weed killer and is very toxic. More than 30 ml. of the concentrated drug is dangerous. With massive overdosage, death may occur from acute renal failure, with smaller doses it is usually due to lung damage and may be delayed for one to two weeks. There is no known antidote.

SALICYLATE POISONING

Poisoning by salicylates is common; it may be suicidal, or in children it may be accidental. The fatal dose in adults is in the region of 25 g. Doses of 2–4 g. have proved toxic in children. In addition, some subjects, particularly asthmatics, develop a hypersensitivity reaction with salicylates and death has occurred after as little of 0·3 g. of aspirin.

Clinical Features. In mild cases the main symptoms are nausea, vomiting, tinnitus and increased respirations. After larger doses there is mental confusion, the patient is flushed and sweating with a full pulse and overbreathing is very striking. In the early stages hyperventilation lowers the pCO_2 of the plasma and leads to a respiratory alkalosis; with increasing absorption of salicylate there is a metabolic acidosis with a fall in plasma bicarbonate. In children acidosis is common, whereas in adults a raised blood pH is more usual. In addition vomiting and sweating lead to dehydration and oliguria.

The urine gives a positive reaction to ferric chloride and may contain protein.

Treatment. (1) In salicylate poisoning it is always worthwhile to wash out the stomach with water. If the patient is in coma a cuffed intratracheal tube should be passed beforehand to avoid possible aspiration of vomited material into the lungs.

(2) In mild cases 5 per cent sodium bicarbonate solution should be given orally in doses of 2 g. four-hourly for 24 hours. Sodium bicarbonate, by making the urine alkaline, increases the rate of excretion of salicylate by the kidneys.

(3) In severe cases (plasma salicylate level of more than 30 mg./100 ml. in children and 50 mg./100 ml. in adults) treatment is aimed at correcting dehydration and producing a diuresis of alkaline urine and thus rapidly clearing salicylate from the body. Owing to the complex acid/base disorder which occurs in salicylate poisoning, it is important to estimate plasma pH, bicarbonate and pCO_2. For method of forced diuresis see p. 605.

(4) 25 mg. of phytomenadione should be injected intravenously to prevent bleeding.

By this method a majority of adult patients with salicylate poisoning can be resuscitated. In a few patients with high plasmas salicylate levels (over 100 ml./100 ml.) and with renal or circulatory failure, haemadialysis will be required. Children are more sensitive to the toxic effects of salicylate.

PARACETAMOL

Overdosage by paracetamol is dangerous and a single dose of over 10 g. can produce serious liver damage. With the normal therapeutic dose of paracetamol a toxic metabolite is produced which however is mopped up by glutathione in the liver. With overdose the glutathione mechanism is saturated and the metabolite combines with the liver cell macromolecules causing cell death. Liver damage is probable if the blood level of paracetamol exceeds 300 mcg./ml. at four hours or 50 mcg./ml. at twelve hours after ingestion.

Clinical Features. Nausea and vomiting may occur after ingestion of the drug but symptoms and signs of liver failure may be delayed for some days.

Treatment. The stomach should be washed out. There is some evidence that methionine orally or cysteamine intravenously will decrease the liver damage if given within ten hours of taking the drug. These drugs alter the metabolism of paracetamol and reduce the production of toxic metabolites.

CARBON MONOXIDE POISONING

Excluding road accidents, carbon monoxide is the commonest cause of accidental death in Great Britain; it is also used by the suicide. Poisoning may result from the escape of carbon monoxide from gas lights or gas fires, from car exhausts, from combustion stoves in a poorly ventilated room or from coal-mine explosions.

Carbon monoxide is odourless and lighter than air. It has a far greater affinity for haemoglobin than oxygen and forms a compound, carboxy-haemoglobin, which is bright-red colour. The carboxyhaemoglobin cannot carry oxygen and tissue anoxia results.

Clinical Features. Symptoms are minimal if less than 30 per cent of haemoglobin is combined with carbon monoxide and consist of nausea, lassitude, and headache. With higher concentrations the onset of symptoms is rapid. There is a transient increase in pulse rate and respiration followed by weakness, dimness of vision and finally coma, respiratory depression, and death.

The patient with carbon monoxide poisoning is often pale and cyanosed. The typical cherry red colour due to carboxyhaemoglobin is usually only seen at post mortem. The presence of this compound in the blood may be confirmed by its characteristic absorption spectrum.

Treatment. The patient must be removed from the poisoned atmosphere. Artificial respiration should be started immediately. If possible, pure oxygen should be given by the best available method. Cerebral oedema may develop in severe cases. The diagnosis is suggested by papilloedema and it should be treated by 500 ml. of 20 per cent mannitol by infusion. Several days in bed are required after apparent recovery. Occasionally patients show evidence of permanent brain or cardiac damage after recovery.

CYANIDE POISONING

Hydrocyanic acid and potassium or sodium cyanide are very powerful poisons. They act by inhibiting a number of enzymes, the most important of which is cytochrome oxidase. They are used as pesticides and in metallurgy.

Clinical Features. The inhalation of hydrocyanic acid (which is a gas) results in death within a few minutes. After ingestion of cyanide salts, death may occur in anything from a few minutes up to several hours, depending on the dose. Generally speaking the absorption of about 1 mg. of cyanide is fatal.

Treatment. The aim of treatment in cyanide poisoning is to give substances which will combine with cyanide and prevent interference with enzyme systems. The following steps should be taken as rapidly as possible.

(1) Crush ampoules of amyl nitrite and allow the patient to inhale the vapour; this will form some methaemoglobin which combines with cyanide. This should be followed by sodium nitrite 0·3 g. in 10 ml. of water given I.V. over three minutes, to form more methaemoglobin.

(2) Sodium thiosulphate 50 ml. of 50 per cent solution should be given I.V. over ten minutes; this also combines with cyanide.

(3) The stomach should be washed out with 5 per cent sodium thiosulphate.

(4) Oxygen and artificial respiration may be required.

If available 20 ml. of a 1·5 per cent solution of cobalt edetate given intravenously over one minute is a specific remedy. It can be repeated if the response is adequate.

INSECT STINGS

Stings by bees, wasps, and other insects are very common. Usually except for some local pain and swelling which subsides in a few days, these stings cause little trouble. Rarely, a generalised reaction occurs which is occasionally fatal. This is seen particularly in those with a history of allergy.

Treatment consists in the local application of an anti-histamine cream. In the case of the bee, the sting is left behind and may be scraped out. If a severe general reaction occurs 0·5 ml. of 1:1,000 adrenalin is given subcutaneously and an anti-histamine is given intramuscularly (promethazine hydrochloride 50 mg. is satisfactory). In very severe cases hydrocortisone hemisuccinate 100 mg. should be given intravenously. Subjects who have had a severe reaction may be desensitised.

LEAD POISONING

Lead poisoning may occur in a number of industries including lead smelting and lead burning, the manufacture of white and red lead and the making of accumulators. Children may also develop lead poisoning from sucking lead-containing paint. Poisoning is infinitely more probable when lead is absorbed through the lungs as dust or fumes rather than when taken by mouth. If lead is absorbed slowly it is stored in the bones. The development of the symptoms of lead poisoning depends not so much on the total amount of lead in the body, but on its rate of absorption or mobilisation from the bones.

Clinical Features

Lead Colic. Intestinal colic and constipation are the most common symptoms of lead poisoning. The pain is usually peri-umbilical and there are no abnormal signs in the abdomen.

Lead Neuropathy. In lead poisoning weakness develops in certain groups of muscles, usually the extensor muscles of the wrist and rarely of the foot. Sensory changes do not occur. The site of the lesion in lead 'neuropathy' is not certain, but is probably in the muscles.

Lead Encephalopathy. This manifestation of lead poisoning is rare. The patient complains of severe headaches and may suddenly develop epileptic fits.

Anaemia. A normocytic hypochromic anaemia occurs in lead poisoning, usually with punctate basophilia.

Gums. Patients with lead poisoning may show a bluish stippled line on the gum margin. It is only found in association with gingivitis and is due to the deposition of lead sulphide in the gums. The lead line may be found in patients without other manifestations of lead poisoning.

Other symptoms consist of weakness, loss of weight, joint pains, and a metallic taste in the mouth.

Generally speaking, a blood level of 80–100 microgrammes of lead per 100 ml. of blood or 200 microgrammes of lead per litre of urine are associated with symptoms of lead poisoning.

Treatment. Lead colic can be relieved by intravenous injections of 10 ml. of a 10 per cent solution of calcium gluconate. Lead can be cleared from the body by using a chelating agent. Certain of these substances form compounds with lead which are soluble and which are excreted by the kidneys. The agent of choice is sodium calcium edetate. The lead in the body displaces the calcium from this chelating agent and the resulting compound is excreted. The adult dose is 1 g. twice daily, given by slow intravenous infusion in saline, at intervals of twelve hours. Such treatment may be carried out for five days and then repeated if necessary. A high calcium diet should be given after treatment.

Prophylaxis. Prophylactic measures include:

(1) Avoidance of exposure to lead dust or fumes by ventilation, hygiene, and by wearing masks.

(2) Avoidance of absorption from the intestine by personal cleanliness, including washing of the hands, etc., before meals.

(3) Regular medical examination of those exposed to lead.

(4) A high calcium diet helps to prevent lead poisoning.

FOOD POISONING

Food poisoning may be due to bacteria or viruses, or their products, in the food, to poisonous substances or to allergy to something ingested.

BACTERIAL FOOD POISONING

(1) Staphylococcal

Some strains of staphylococci produce an entero-toxin which is fairly stable to heat and will resist boiling. The chief symptoms which start abruptly in from one to six hours, are nausea, vomiting, intestinal colic, and diarrhoea. The attack is short-lived and is all over within a few hours. It is not usually serious, but rarely there may be collapse with dehydration and deaths have occurred, particularly in young children and the aged.

Treatment. In most cases rest in bed with frequent sips of fluid and mist. kaolin and morphine (B.P.C.) 15 ml. four-hourly will control the symptoms. Rarely if there is collapse with severe dehydration and sodium chloride deficiency, intravenous fluids will be required.

(2) Salmonella

Certain of the salmonella group of organisms produce specific diseases such as typhoid and paratyphoid fevers. Others of the group, particularly *S. typhi-murium, S. Newport, S. St. Paul, S. Thompson,* and *S. Dublin,* produce an acute gastroenteritis which presents as a food poisoning.

Clinical Features. The onset is usually within forty-eight hours of eating infected food. The main symptoms are general malaise, headache, and fever combined with vomiting, intestinal colic, and diarrhoea. Occasionally there may be high fever with rigors, suggesting a septicaemia and the spleen may be palpable. The disease usually lasts several days.

The diagnosis is confirmed by culture of the pathogenic organism from the stools. This is important in indicating the most appropriate treatment and in helping to trace the source of infection.

Treatment. General measures include rest in bed and sips of fluid by mouth. If the diarrhoea has been severe, the oral fluids should consist of N/3 saline flavoured with fruit juice. Occasionally when vomiting is severe and prolonged, fluids and electrolytes must be given intravenously and this requires a daily estimation of the blood electrolytes and a full record of fluid balance. The diarrhoea and colic can be controlled by mist. kaolin and morphine 15 ml. four-hourly.

There is little evidence that antibiotic treatment modifies the course of Salmonella gastroenteritis.

3) Virus

There is no doubt that certain outbreaks of gastroenteritis are due to a virus; they are usually mild and respond to symptomatic treatment.

MUSHROOM POISONING

Mushroom poisoning is usually due to *Amanita phalloides*. This mushroom has a yellow or olive yellow cap with white gills and there is a volva (cup) at the base of the stem.

Clinical Features. There is often a delay of several hours before the onset of symptoms. This is followed by severe abdominal colic with bloody diarrhoea and vomiting. Death may occur from shock or collapse. If the patient survives this stage, acute liver necrosis may develop and prove fatal.

Treatment. The stomach should be washed out. Atropine 1 mg. should be given intravenously and repeated as required. Fluid and electrolyte replacement will be necessary and this will have to be given intravenously. Antiphallinic serum should be given if available. It has been suggested that mashed rabbit stomach and brain should be given as these animals are resistant to mushroom poisoning. Otherwise, treatment is symptomatic.

ALLERGY TO FOOD

Some patients are hypersensitive to certain articles of food and may suffer from urticarial rashes, vomiting, diarrhoea, and even attacks of asthma. It is best for them to avoid such foods although desensitisation can be attempted.

Treatment. An attack due to allergy to food is treated as a sensitisation reaction (p. 597). If diarrhoea is a prominent symptom it can be relieved by a mixture containing morphine, such as mist. kaolin and morphine (N.F.) 15 ml. four-hourly.

FURTHER READING

Matthew, H. and Lawson, A. H. H., *Treatment of Common Acute Poisoning*, 3rd edition, Livingstone, 1974.

CHAPTER TWENTY-THREE

DISEASES DUE TO PHYSICAL AGENTS

DECOMPRESSION SICKNESS

Decompression sickness occurs when people who have been working at a high atmospheric pressure, such as workers in a caisson or diving bell, are suddenly decompressed. It may also occur in a subject who rises quickly to a height above 25,000 ft. In both circumstances, nitrogen rapidly comes out of solution both in the blood and in the tissues and forms bubbles. Oxygen and carbon dioxide also come out of solution, but rapidly diffuse away. These bubbles occur particularly in the nervous system and in adipose tissue, as nitrogen is soluble in fat.

Clinical Features. Within a few hours of decompression the patient complains of severe pain in the muscles and joints. This may be followed by evidence of involvement of the central nervous system, including vertigo, weakness of the limbs, and sphincter disturbances. Various skin rashes may develop.

Treatment. *Preventive.* Where possible workers should not be exposed to pressures greater than 18 lb. to the sq. in., for below this pressure sickness does not occur. If they work under higher pressures they should be slowly decompressed. *Curative.* If decompression sickness develops the subject should be recompressed again and then very slowly decompressed.

MOTION SICKNESS

Motion sickness may occur as a result of sea, land, or air travel. Although the exact mechanism is not known it would seem that repetitive stimulation of the vestibular apparatus plays a large part; it is not possible to produce sickness in animals who have had their vestibular apparatus removed, nor are deaf mutes seasick. Susceptibility to motion sickness varies, but is particularly common in migrainous subjects.

Clinical Features. The victim of motion sickness complains of feeling unwell with nausea, headache, and sometimes faintness. Finally symptoms are such as to require a rapid withdrawal from company and terminate in severe vomiting. The duration of the attack is variable and may last only a few hours, although susceptible subjects may be prostrate for several days.

Treatment. People susceptible to motion sickness should avoid undue movement. When at sea they should remain near the centre of the ship and if possible lie down with the eyes closed. In an aeroplane the head should be rested back on the head rest. Some food should be taken and if this is not possible, barley sugar should be sucked.

Certain drugs diminish the liability to sea-sickness. They are the hyoscine group and the anti-histamines. The most satisfactory drug is not decided, but there is a little evidence that hyoscine is better for short journeys and the anti-histamines for longer ones. The doses are:

Hyoscine, 0·5 mg.–1 mg. according to weight, taken 20 minutes before starting, is suitable for journeys lasting up to four hours. Side effects include dry mouth and paralysis of accommodation.

Cyclizine, 50 mg. three times daily or meclozine 50 mg. daily, are suitable for longer journeys.

Dimenhydrinate (Dramamine) 25 mg. three times daily is also suitable, but rather liable to produce drowsiness.

These drugs can be used for children in reduced dosage.

DISORDERS DUE TO HEAT

A number of syndromes may appear in those exposed to heat. They are more liable to occur in subjects who have had no opportunity to become acclimatised, in the very young, the elderly and in association with heavy exertion.

Heat Stroke (Heat Hyperpyrexia)

Heat stroke is due to a failure of the heat-controlling mechanism. It may occur merely as a result of exposure to heat or may complicate some pyrexial illness such as malaria. The symptoms are mental confusion, headaches, and inco-ordination proceeding to delirium, convulsions, and death. The body temperature is raised and may be 41° C. or higher. The skin is hot and dry, the sweating mechanism having failed.

Treatment. Heat stroke is a medical emergency and the body must be cooled as rapidly as possible until the rectal temperature is 39° C. This may be achieved by keeping the body surface moist by sponging or by sprays of water and encouraging evaporation by means of fans. The possibility of some complicating infection such as malaria must be remembered and appropriate treatment given.

Heat Exhaustion

Heat exhaustion may occur for a number of reasons and has to be subdivided on this basis:

(a) Salt Deficiency Heat Exhaustion

This is due to salt loss with inadequate replacement.

Clinical Features. The symptoms are those of salt deficiency, i.e. weakness, cramps, vomiting, and collapse with a low blood pressure. The plasma sodium and chloride levels are reduced and the urine may be low in chlorides.

Treatment is aimed at replacing the salt loss and this may be done by mouth, or by intravenous infusion if vomiting is troublesome.

(b) Anhidrotic Heat Exhaustion

Clinical Features. This form of heat exhaustion is usually associated with prickly heat. The symptoms are weakness and irritability and if exertion is attempted the patient may collapse. Examination shows that sweating is confined to localised areas, usually the face and axillae and sometimes the hands and feet. The condition may proceed to heat stroke.

Treatment is to remove the subject to a cooler environment.

In addition, heat exhaustion on effort may occur without clear evidence of either salt deficiency or anhidrosis.

Prickly Heat

Prickly heat is due to excessive sweating. It is a fine papular rash which sometimes becomes vesicular and usually gives a sensation of prickling (thus the name). It may become infected.

Treatment is removal to a cooler and less humid atmosphere.

Sunburn

Sunburn is due to the ultra-violet fraction of sunlight. It may be merely an erythema but if severe the erythema will be accompanied by some local oedema and sometimes headache and pyrexia.

Treatment. Sunburn may be prevented by graduated exposure to direct sunlight and by applying creams which exclude part of the ultra-violet end of the spectrum. If sunburn has occurred further exposure to sunlight should be avoided and some soothing lotion such as oily calamine applied.

DISORDERS DUE TO COLD

They may be either local or general. Local effects in temperate climates are commonly chilblains or Raynaud's phenomenon (p. 186). If cold is extreme, then the tissues of the extremities may freeze, and frostbite result. General effects result from the progressive cooling of the whole body, the syndrome of hypothermia.

Hypothermia

Immersion in cold water causes rapid heat loss and hypothermia, and in water near to freezing point death occurs within an hour. Hypothermia in air in this country usually affects the elderly.

Old people may lose heat from their bodies faster than it can be generated, despite apparently adequate insulation with bedding or clothes, and so pass gradually into hypothermia. This occurs only when the external temperature is very cold.

Aggravating features are malnutrition, loss of mobility from arthritis or paralysis, urinary incontinence, dementia, and myxoedema.

Clinically, the patients become confused, then drowsy, and fall asleep, often in exposed positions. Unless rescued they pass into coma and ultimately die. On examination, their bodies are cold, and the rectal temperature low (usually 30° C.). Respiration is slow and shallow, the

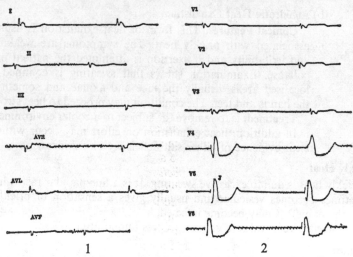

E.C.G. in hypothermia, showing J waves from male, aged 80, rectal temperature 24·5°C., pulse rate 16/min

pulse very slow, and the blood pressure low. The E.C.G. is characteristic (above). Treatment is by warming the body with relays of hot blankets, correcting electrolyte abnormalities which may be present, and administering intravenous hydrocortisone (100 mg. I.V.) 4 hourly and an antibiotic. Prognosis depends upon how cold the body is on discovery, how old and how frail the patient is, and on co-incident disease. In general it is not good.

ALTITUDE SICKNESS

Altitude sickness is due to hypoxia occurring as a result of the decrease in the partial pressure of oxygen in the atmosphere at high altitudes. It may arise as a result of flying or mountain climbing. Up to 8,000 ft. no symptoms occur, but over 10,000 ft. symptoms may begin to appear. The susceptibility of people varies considerably, being less in the young and healthy and more marked in the elderly and those with respiratory or cardiac disease.

Some acclimatisation can occur to high altitudes. This is brought about by increased respiration, by increase in the pulmonary vascular diffusing surface and by polycythaemia.

Clinical Features

The earliest symptoms are some blunting of mental acuity with motor inco-ordination and slurred speech. These may be followed by headache and weakness. If the degree of hypoxia is increased there will be loss of consciousness and convulsions and finally death.

FURTHER READING

Hunter. D., *Diseases of Occupations*, 6th edition, Hodder and Stoughton Educational, 1978.

CHAPTER TWENTY-FOUR

THE STEROIDS

There are now a number of substances which in structure and actions are similar to cortisone and which are collectively known as the steroids. They all have the following actions to a greater or lesser extent.

(1) *Carbohydrate and protein metabolism.* The steroids cause breakdown of protein and the release of glucose, with increased resistance to the action of insulin. Occasionally patients receiving steroid hormones develop *diabetes mellitus.* Prolonged treatment with high doses of steroids causes withdrawal of bone matrix (osteoporosis, p. 373). This is associated with loss of calcium from the skeleton and a negative calcium balance. Rarely necrosis of the head of the femur develops with disorganisation of the joint and pain on movement.

(2) *Electrolyte balance.* This group of drugs leads to retention of sodium and water and loss of potassium through the kidneys. Oedema of the ankles and eventually hypertension may develop.

Potassium deficiency can be avoided in patients taking large doses of steroids over a long period by giving potassium as a slow release compound by mouth.

(3) *Effect on the inflammatory reaction.* The steroids suppress both the local and general response to infection. This may lead to a rapid spread of the infection without the usual symptoms and signs.

(4) *Effect on allergic reaction.* These drugs suppress both the allergic reaction and the formation of antibodies.

(5) *Peptic ulceration.* Corticosteroids may cause peptic ulcers or exacerbations of those already present. The reason for this is not known.

(6) *The eye.* Steroids may precipitate glaucoma in those prone to this condition. Prolonged use may also cause cataracts. Local steroids must be used with great care in infectious conditions of the eye as unless the infection is controlled it will spread with disastrous results.

(7) *Other effects.* Prolonged treatment with these drugs leads to an appearance similar to that found in Cushing's disease. In addition, mental disturbances may occur, particularly in people who have previously been unstable mentally; such a history is therefore an important contra-indication to treatment with corticosteroids.

(8) *Steroid therapy* which has persisted for six months or longer leads to atrophy of the adrenal cortex. This is a potentially dangerous situation, since the adrenals can no longer react to stress by boosting the secretion of cortical hormones and a state of collapse similar to an Addisonian crisis may be induced by any acute infection, injury, or emotional shock. Such

Addisonian shock may occur not only in patients still receiving long-term steroid therapy, but for up to two years after it has been discontinued. These patients must be warned that if they contract any acute illness or injury steroid therapy must be resumed immediately, or if they are still being treated the dose must be increased to two or three times its maintenance level until the acute episode is over.

Short courses of injections of ACTH every few months are sometimes given to patients on long-term corticosteroid therapy to stimulate and so prevent atrophy of the adrenal cortex. Unfortunately this may suppress ACTH release and has not been shown to be effective in practice.

Therapeutic Use

These drugs are used in the treatment of a number of diseases. They can be given locally or systemically. The more important diseases which can be treated are:

(1) *Collagen diseases.*	Rheumatoid arthritis.	
	Rheumatic fever.	
	Systemic lupus erythematosus.	
	Polyarteritis nodosa.	
	Giant-cell arteritis (temporal arteritis).	
(2) *Allergic diseases.*	Asthma.	
	Hay fever.	
	Angioneurotic oedema.	
	Eczema (applied locally).	
	Serum sickness.	
(3) *Blood diseases.*	Acute and chronic haemolytic anaemia.	
	Idiopathic thrombocytopenic purpura.	
	Acute leukaemia.	
	Drug-induced bone-marrow depression.	
(4) *Miscellaneous group.*	Nephrotic syndrome.	
	Ulcerative colitis.	
	Sarcoidosis.	
(5) *Eye disease.*	Applied locally in various inflammatory diseases of the eye.	
(6) *Replacement therapy.*	Addison's disease or after adrenalectomy.	

The following preparations are available and are given with equivalent doses:

(1) Cortisone 100 mg.   (4) Prednisone 20 mg.
(2) Hydrocortisone 80 mg.   (5) Triamcinolone 16 mg.
(3) Prednisolone 20 mg.   (6) Methyl prednisolone 16 mg.
(7) Dexamethasone 3·0 mg.

It is difficult to decide which is the best steroid to use. Except for replacement therapy, the steroid with the maximum therapeutic effect and the least salt-retaining properties would be the most satisfactory. It would appear that on these grounds dexamethasone is the best, but clinical experience is not very large with this drug. It is recommended, therefore, that prednisolone, with which there is a considerable amount of experience, should be used, but it is possible that it will be replaced by a better steroid in the future.

For replacement therapy, cortisone is usually the best, as a certain amount of salt retention is required in these circumstances.

Dosage

The correct dose of a steroid is the minimum amount of drug required to produce the desired effect, and it varies considerably. In general, if the dose does not exceed 10 mg. of prednisolone daily, side effects are much less common than with higher doses. For replacement therapy the dose usually is 50 mg. of cortisone; for other purposes it is usually necessary to start with 200–300 mg. of cortisone, though for maintenance of the effect as little as 25–50 mg. may be enough. Patients taking cortisone should be seen regularly and the following points noted:

(1) *General appearance*—any evidence of Cushing-like appearance.

(2) *Any dyspepsia suggestive of peptic ulcer.* If ulcer symptoms develop the steroid is usually stopped. If steroid therapy is vital it will have to be continued together with a full ulcer regime.

(3) *Blood pressure.*

(4) *Urine* must be tested for sugar.

(5) *Blood electrolytes* must be estimated in patients undergoing prolonged therapy with these drugs, particularly if there is evidence of renal damage. A close watch should be kept for undue potassium loss or sodium retention.

(6) *Any evidence of infection* (note that the symptoms may be masked). See under (8) on p. 621.

(7) Enquire about backache, which might suggest the development of osteoporosis.

(8) Patients on long term steroids should be given a card which records the details of their treatment.

ANTIBIOTICS

Drug	Dose	Sensitive Organisms	Side Effects	Comments
Sulphonamides	*Orally*			High fluid intake required with rapidly absorbed sulphonamides except sulphamethizole. Sulphadiazine penetrates meninges very well.
Rapidly absorbed				
Sulphadimidine	3 g. stat			
Sulphadiazine	1 g. 4 or 6 hourly			
Sulphafurazole				
Sulphamethizole	0·1 g. 4 or 6 hourly		Precipitation in the urinary tract. Nausea and vomiting. Rashes. Drug fever Agranulocytosis	
Poorly absorbed		Strep. pneumoniae		Poorly absorbed group used for intestinal infection and sterilising gut.
Succinylsulphathiazole	4 g. stat. 3 g.	Strep. pyogenes		
Phthalylsulphathiazole	6 or 8 hourly	Meningococcus		
		Gonococcus		
Long acting		Shigellae		High degree of protein binding leads to slow excretion and prolonged action.
Sulphamethoxypyridazine	1 g. stat. 0·5 g. daily	E. coli		
Sulphamethoxydiazine				
Co-trimoxazole (Septrin–Bactrim) *Each tablet contains 80 mg. Trimethoprim and 400 mg. Sulphamethoxazole.*	tabs. 1–2 twice daily orally	Most pyogenic cocci and many Gram-negative organisms.		Most useful in bronchitis and urinary infections.
Nitrofurantoin	50–100 mg. t.d.s.	E. coli B. Proteus.	Nausea (give after food) Neuritis Hyperpyrexia	Concentrated by the kidney and only used for renal infection.

Drug	Dose	Administration	Sensitive Organisms	Side Effects	Comments
Penicillin Benzylpenicillin	300 mg. (500,000 units) per injection 20,000 units	Intramuscularly Intrathecally	Strep. pyogenes Strep. pneumoniae Staph. aureus	Sensitisation reactions. Skin rashes and rarely collapse.	Benzylpenicillin rapidly absorbed from injection site and excreted, must be given 6 hourly.
Procaine penicillin	600 mg. (600,000 units) per injection	Intramuscularly	Strep. viridans		Procaine penicillin more slowly mobilised 12 hourly injection satisfactory.
Benzathine penicillin	600,000 units	Intramuscularly	Meningococcus		Benzathine penicillin slowly excreted. One injection adequate for sensitive organism.
Oral penicillins Phenoxymethylpenicillin Phenethicillin	250 mg. q.i.d. 250 mg. q.i.d.	Oral	Gonococcus B. anthracis Treponema pallidum Actinomyces bovis		Very little to choose between them. Effective in all but severe infections provided organism is sensitive.
Ampicillin Amoxycillin	250 mg. q.i.d. 250 mg. t.d.s. or q.i.d.	Oral Oral	Similar to above with addition of Salmonellae Shigellae E. coli & H. influenzae		Useful in urinary and gut infection, and in chronic bronchitis.
Cloxacillin	500 mg. q.i.d. 250 mg. 4 hourly	Oral Intramuscular	Effective against resistant staphs.		Reserved for severe staph. infections.
Flucloxacillin	250 mg. q.i.d.	Oral			

Penicillin is the most generally useful antibiotic. A satisfactory treatment for infection by a sensitive organism is benzylpenicillin 300 mg. followed by either procaine penicillin 600 mg, 12 hours or phenoxymethylpenicillin 250 mg. q.i.d. In mild infections oral penicillin alone is adequate. In overwhelming infection or that by partially resistant organism larger doses must be given by injection. Penicillin does not cross the meningeal barrier in adequate concentrations and must be given intrathecally in meningitis. Hypersensitivity reactions are not uncommon and the patient must always be asked if he is sensitive to penicillin before treatment.

Drug	Dose	Administration	Sensitive Organisms	Side Effects	Comments
Tetracycline Chlortetracycline Oxytetracycline	250 mg. q.i.d.	oral	Broad Spectrum	1. Diarrhoea. 2. Gut superinfection with staphs. 3. Candida mouth infection. 4. Discoloration of growing teeth.	Particularly useful in recurrent bronchitis, urinary infections, lymphogranuloma brucellosis, typhus.
Doxycycline	1000 mg. daily	oral			Similar to above but longer action.

In spite of their wide antibacterial spectrum tetracycline must not be used indiscriminately because of side effects. Particular care is required in pregnancy and infancy, when they should be avoided if possible.

Chloramphenicol	500 mg. q.i.d. 3·0 g. daily	oral IV drip	Broad Spectrum including Salm. typhii H. influenzae and rickettsiae	Marrow aplasia rare but usually fatal.	H. influenzae meningitis Typhoid

Owing to side effects, chloramphenicol should only be used as indicated or in a severe infection resistant to other antibiotics.

Erythromycin	250 mg. q.i.d.	oral	Str. pneumoniae „ pyogenes „ viridans Staphs. C. diphtheriae N. gonorrhoea H. influenzae and H. pertussis Mycoplasma		Resistant staphs., H. influenzae infection—Diphtheria. Useful in patient sensitive to penicillin.

Drug	Dose	Administration	Sensitive Organisms	Side Effects	Comments
Cephalorin	500 mg. q.i.d.	I.M.	Broad spectrum including penicillin resistant staphs, E. coli and proteus.	Possibly skin rashes	
Cephalexin	0·5–1·0 g. three times daily	oral	Broad spectrum		
Rifampicin	450–600 mg. daily	oral	Many gram + and some gram + organisms and M. tuberculosis.	Colours urine and sputum red. Disturbs hepatic function tests	Useful in tuberculosis.
Streptomycin	0·5 g. b.d. 2·0–3·0 g. daily	I.M. oral	Myco. tuberculosis, E. coli, H. influenzae, Shigellae; orally for gut infections	8th nerve damage: particularly in elderly and in renal failure.	Tuberculosis—Short courses in other infections by sensitive organisms.
Gentamicin	1·0–1·5 mg./kg. 8 hourly	IM or IV	Gram – organisms staphylococol	8th nerve damage	Severe urinary infections and gram – septicaemias. Reduce dose with impaired renal function
Colistin	50,000 units/kg./ 24 hours	I.M. Locally	P. pyocyaneus	Rashes	Pyocyaneus infections.
Sodium fusidate	500 mg. three times daily	oral	Staphylococci		Used largely for resistant staphylococci.
Lincomycin Clindamycin	500 mg. 150 mg.	oral oral	Similar to Benzylpencillin	Diarrhoea, rarely pseudo-membranous colitis	Useful in subjects sensitive to pencillin and also osteomyalitis due to high concentration in bone

CONVERSION SCALES FOR S.I. UNITS WITH NORMAL RANGE

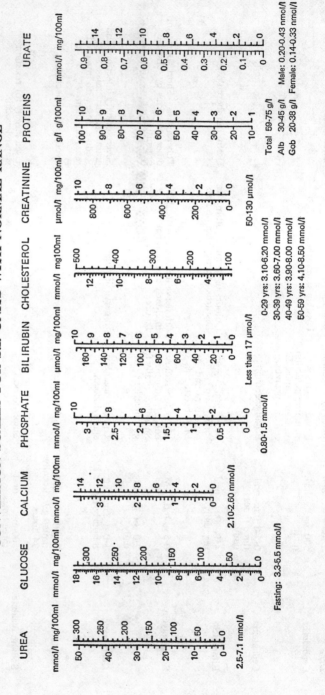

INDEX

INDEX